Clinical Arthritis

Clinical Arthritis

Edited by Mary Kellar

hayle medical
New York

Hayle Medical,
750 Third Avenue, 9th Floor,
New York, NY 10017, USA

Visit us on the World Wide Web at:
www.haylemedical.com

ISBN: 978-1-63241-483-0

The publisher's policy is to use permanent paper from mills that operate a sustainable forestry policy. Furthermore, the publisher ensures that the text paper and cover boards used have met acceptable environmental accreditation standards.

Printed in China.

Cataloging-in-Publication Data

Clinical arthritis / edited by Mary Kellar.
p. cm.
Includes bibliographical references and index.
ISBN 978-1-63241-483-0
1. Arthritis. 2. Joints--Diseases. I. Kellar, Mary.
RC933 .C55 2018
616.722--dc23

Table of Contents

Preface IX

Chapter 1 ***PADI4* and HLA-DRB1 are Genetic Risks for Radiographic Progression in RA Patients, Independent of ACPA Status: Results from the IORRA Cohort Study** 1
Taku Suzuki, Katsunori Ikari, Koichiro Yano, Eisuke Inoue, Yoshiaki Toyama, Atsuo Taniguchi, Hisashi Yamanaka, Shigeki Momohara

Chapter 2 **Synergistic Effects of Ethanol and Isopentenyl Pyrophosphate on Expansion of γδ T Cells in Synovial Fluid from Patients with Arthritis** 9
Agneta J. Laurent, Niels Bindslev, Björn Johansson, Louise Berg

Chapter 3 **Mannose Binding Lectin and Susceptibility to Rheumatoid Arthritis in Brazilian Patients and their Relatives** 22
Isabela Goeldner, Thelma L. Skare, Shirley R. Utiyama, Renato M. Nisihara, Hoang van Tong, Iara J. T. Messias-Reason, Thirumalaisamy P. Velavan

Chapter 4 **Glycyrol Suppresses Collagen-Induced Arthritis by Regulating Autoimmune and Inflammatory Response** 34
Yanxia Fu, Hailing Zhou, Shuangyan Wang, Qun Wei

Chapter 5 **Analyzing Genome-Wide Association Studies with an FDR Controlling Modification of the Bayesian Information Criterio** 43
Erich Dolejsi, Bernhard Bodenstorfer, Florian Frommlet

Chapter 6 **Identification of Autoantibodies against Transthyretin for the creening and Diagnosis of Rheumatoid Arthritis** 56
Saurabh Sharma, Sreejoyee Ghosh, Lalit Kumar Singh, Ashish Sarkar, Rajesh Malhotra, Onkar Prasad Garg, Yogendra Singh, Radhey Shyam Sharma, Darshan Singh Bhakuni, Taposh Kumar Das, Sagarika Biswas

Chapter 7 **Cellular Adhesion Gene *SELP* is Associated with Rheumatoid Arthritis and Displays Differential Allelic Expression** 68
Jana Burkhardt, Mechthild Blume, Elisabeth Petit-Teixeira, Vitor Hugo Teixeira, Anke Steiner, Elfi Quente, Grit Wolfram, Markus Scholz, Céline Pierlot, Paola Migliorini, Stefano Bombardieri, Alejandro Balsa, René Westhovens, Pilar Barrera, Timothy R. D. J. Radstake, Helena Alves, Thomas Bardin, Bernard Prum, Frank Emmrich, François Cornelis, Peter Ahnert, Holger Kirsten

Chapter 8 **B Cell Receptor Signaling-Based Index as a Biomarker for the Loss of Peripheral Immune Tolerance in Autoreactive B Cells in Rheumatoid Arthritis** 78
Taras Lyubchenko, Gary O. Zerbe

Chapter 9 **The Impact of DMARD and Anti-TNF Therapy on Functional Characterization of Short-Term T-Cell Activation in Patients with Rheumatoid Arthritis** 85
Balázs Szalay, Áron Cseh, Gergő Mészáros, László Kovács, Attila Balog, Barna Vásárhelyi

Chapter 10 **Bead Arrays for Antibody and Complement Profiling Reveal Joint Contribution of Antibody Isotypes to C3 Deposition** 92
Burcu Ayoglu, Eszter Szarka, Krisztina Huber, Anita Orosz, Fruzsina Babos, Anna Magyar, Ferenc Hudecz, Bernadette Rojkovich, Tamás Gáti, György Nagy, Jochen M. Schwenk, Gabriella Sármay, József Prechl, Peter Nilsson, Krisztián Papp

Chapter 11 **Clinical and Serological Features of Patients Referred through a Rheumatology Triage System because of Positive Antinuclear Antibodies** 105
Christie Fitch-Rogalsky, Whitney Steber, Michael Mahler, Terri Lupton, Liam Martin, Susan G. Barr, Dianne P. Mosher, James Wick, Marvin J. Fritzler

Chapter 12 **Accelerating Translational Research by Clinically Driven Development of an Informatics Platform** 113
Imad Abugessaisa, Saedis Saevarsdottir, Giorgos Tsipras, Staffan Lindblad, Charlotta Sandin, Pernilla Nikamo, Mona Ståhle, Vivianne Malmström, Lars Klareskog, Jesper Tegnér

Chapter 13 **Evolution of Direct Costs in the First Years of Rheumatoid Arthritis: Impact of Early versus Late Biologic Initiation - An Economic Analysis based on the ESPOIR Cohort** 131
Karine Chevreul, Georges Haour, Sandy Lucier, Stephanie Harvard, Marie-Laure Laroche, Xavier Mariette, Alain Saraux, Isabelle Durand-Zaleski, Francis Guillemin, Bruno Fautrel

Chapter 14 **Usual Interstitial Pneumonia Preceding Collagen Vascular Disease: A Retrospective Case Control Study of Patients Initially Diagnosed with Idiopathic Pulmonary Fibrosis** 140
Masato Kono, Yutaro Nakamura, Noriyuki Enomoto, Dai Hashimoto, Tomoyuki Fujisawa, Naoki Inui, Masato Maekawa, Takafumi Suda, Thomas V. Colby, Kingo Chida

Chapter 15 **Decreased Circulating Visfatin is Associated with Improved Disease Activity in Early Rheumatoid Arthritis: Data from the PERAC Cohort** 150
Ondřej Sglunda, Heřman Mann, Hana Hulejová , Markéta Kuklová, Ondřej Pecha, Lenka Pleštilová, Mária Filková, Karel Pavelka, Jiří Vencovský, Ladislav Šenolt

Chapter 16 **Plasma Levels of IL-37 and Correlation with TNF-α, IL-17A, and Disease Activity during DMARD Treatment of Rheumatoid Arthritis** 155
Ping-Wei Zhao, Wei-Guang Jiang, Li Wang, Zhen-Yu Jiang, Yu-Xing Shan, Yan-Fang Jiang

Chapter 17 **An Osteoprotegerin Gene Polymorphism is Associated with an Increased Risk of Hip Fracture in Japanese Patients with Rheumatoid Arthritis: Results from the IORRA Observational Cohort Study** 162
Shinji Yoshida, Katsunori Ikari, Takefumi Furuya, Yoshiaki Toyama, Atsuo Taniguchi, Hisashi Yamanaka, Shigeki Momohara

Chapter 18 **From Synovial Tissue to Peripheral Blood: Myeloid Related Protein 8/14 is a Sensitive Biomarker for Effective Treatment in Early Drug Development in Patients with Rheumatoid Arthritis**..........167
Ivy Y. Choi, Danielle M. Gerlag, Dirk Holzinger, Johannes Roth, Paul P. Tak

Chapter 19 **Inhibition of HMGB1-Induced Angiogenesis by Cilostazol via SIRT1 Activation in Synovial Fibroblasts from Rheumatoid Arthritis**..........172
Hye Young Kim, So Youn Park, Sung Won Lee, Hye Rin Lee, Won Suk Lee, Byung Yong Rhim, Ki Whan Hong, Chi Dae Kim

Chapter 20 **iNitro-Tyr: Prediction of Nitrotyrosine Sites in Proteins with General Pseudo Amino Acid Composition**..........183
Yan Xu, Xin Wen, Li-Shu Wen, Ling-Yun Wu, Nai-Yang Deng, Kuo-Chen Chou

Chapter 21 **Comparative Persistence of the TNF Antagonists in Rheumatoid Arthritis - A Population-Based Cohort Study**..........193
Anat Fisher, Ken Bassett, James M. Wright, M. Alan Brookhart, Hugh Freeman, Colin R. Dormuth

Chapter 22 **Identification of Urinary Peptide Biomarkers Associated with Rheumatoid Arthritis**..........201
Angelique Stalmach, Hanna Johnsson, Iain B. McInnes, Holger Husi, Julie Klein, Mohammed Dakna, William Mullen, Harald Mischak, Duncan Porter

Chapter 23 **Effect of Combination Therapy on Joint Destruction in Rheumatoid Arthritis: A Network Meta-Analysis of Randomized Controlled Trials**..........210
Niels Graudal, Thorbjørn Hubeck-Graudal, Simon Tarp, Robin Christensen, Gesche Jürgens

Permissions

List of Contributors

Index

Preface

This book has been a concerted effort by a group of academicians, researchers and scientists, who have contributed their research works for the realization of the book. This book has materialized in the wake of emerging advancements and innovations in this field. Therefore, the need of the hour was to compile all the required researches and disseminate the knowledge to a broad spectrum of people comprising of students, researchers and specialists of the field.

Arthritis is a disorder that affects joints. The symptoms mostly include swelling, redness and pain in the affected area. The two commonly occurring arthritis are osteoarthritis and rheumatoid arthritis. The treatment for arthritis includes pain medications and physiotherapy. This book presents researches and studies performed by experts across the globe. It is a vital tool for all those who are researching or studying the subject matter as it gives incredible insights into the diagnosis and treatment of arthritis.

At the end of the preface, I would like to thank the authors for their brilliant chapters and the publisher for guiding us all-through the making of the book till its final stage. Also, I would like to thank my family for providing the support and encouragement throughout my academic career and research projects.

Editor

PADI4 and HLA-DRB1 Are Genetic Risks for Radiographic Progression in RA Patients, Independent of ACPA Status: Results from the IORRA Cohort Study

Taku Suzuki[1,2,9], Katsunori Ikari[1*,9], Koichiro Yano[1,9], Eisuke Inoue[1], Yoshiaki Toyama[2], Atsuo Taniguchi[1], Hisashi Yamanaka[1], Shigeki Momohara[1]

1 Institute of Rheumatology, Tokyo Women's Medical University, Shinjuku, Tokyo, Japan, **2** Department of Orthopaedic Surgery, Keio University School of Medicine, Shinjuku, Tokyo, Japan

Abstract

Introduction: Rheumatoid arthritis (RA) is a systemic, chronic inflammatory disease influenced by both genetic and environmental factors, leading to joint destruction and functional impairment. Recently, a large-scaled GWAS meta-analysis using more than 37,000 Japanese samples were conducted and 13 RA susceptibility loci were identified. However, it is not clear whether these loci have significant impact on joint destruction or not. This is the first study focused on the 13 loci to investigate independent genetic risk factors for radiographic progression in the first five years from onset of RA.

Methods: Sharp/van der Heijde score of hands at 5-year disease duration, which represents joint damage, were measured retrospectively and used as an outcome variable in 865 Japanese RA patients. Genetic factors regarded as putative risk factors were RA-susceptible polymorphisms identified by the Japanese GWAS meta-analysis, including HLA-DRB1 (shared epitope, SE), rs2240340 (*PADI4*), rs2230926 (*TNFAIP3*), rs3093024 (*CCR6*), rs11900673 (*B3GNT2*), rs2867461 (*ANXA3*), rs657075 (*CSF2*), rs12529514 (*CD83*), rs2233434 (*NFKBIE*), rs10821944 (*ARID5B*), rs3781913 (*PDE2A-ARAP1*), rs2841277 (*PLD4*) and rs2847297 (*PTPN2*). These putative genetic risk factors were assessed by a stepwise multiple regression analysis adjusted for possible non-genetic risk factors: autoantibody positivity (anti-citrullinated peptide antibody [ACPA] and rheumatoid factor), history of smoking, gender and age at disease onset.

Results: The number of SE alleles ($P = 0.002$) and risk alleles of peptidyl arginine deiminase type IV gene (*PADI4*, $P = 0.04$) had significant impact on progressive joint destruction, as well as following non-genetic factors: ACPA positive ($P = 0.0006$), female sex ($P = 0.006$) and younger age of onset ($P = 0.02$).

Conclusions: In the present study, we found that *PADI4* risk allele and HLA-DRB1 shared epitope are independent genetic risks for radiographic progression in Japanese rheumatoid arthritis patients. The results of this study give important knowledge of the risks on progressive joint damage in RA patients.

Editor: Sunil K. Ahuja, South Texas Veterans Health Care System and University Health Science Center San Antonio, United States of America

Funding: This work was supported by grants provided by the Japanese Ministry of Education, Culture, Sports, Science and Technology Grant-in-Aid for Scientific Research (KI), the Japanese Ministry of Health, Labour and Welfare (SM, HY) and the Japan Science and Technology Agency (HY). The IORRA cohort was supported by non-restricted research grants from commercial companies (Asahikasei Kuraray Medical Co., Ltd., Abbott Japan Co., Ltd., Asahikasei Pharma Corporation, Astellas Pharma Inc., AstraZeneca K. K., Bristol-Myers Squibb, Chugai Pharmaceutical Co., Ltd., Daiichi Fine Chemical Co., Ltd., Daiichi Sankyo Co., Ltd., Dainippon Sumitomo Pharma Co., Ltd., Dentsu, Sudler & Hennessey Inc., Eisai Co., Ltd., GlaxoSmithKline K. K., Hisamitsu Pharmaceutical Co.,Inc., Janssen Pharmaceutical K. K., Japan Tobacco Inc., Kaken Pharmaceutical Co., Ltd., Kissei Pharmaceutical Co., Ltd., Kowa Pharmaceutical Co., Ltd., Mitsubishi Chemical Medience Corporation, Mitsubishi Tanabe Pharma Corporation, Mochida Pharmaceutical Co., Ltd., MSD K. K., Mundipharma K.K., Nippon Chemiphar Co., Ltd., Nippon Shinyaku Co., Ltd., Novartis Pharma K. K., Otsuka Pharmaceutical Co., Ltd., Pfizer Japan Inc., Sanofi-Aventis K. K., Santen Pharmaceutical Co., Ltd., Sanwa Kagaku Kenkyusho Co., Ltd., Sekisui Medical Co., Ltd., Taishotoyama Pharmaceutical Co., Ltd., Takeda Pharmaceutical Company Limited, Teijin Pharma Limited, Torii Pharmaceutical Co., Ltd., UCB Japan Co., Ltd., ZERIA Pharmaceutical Co., Ltd.). However, these funders had no role in study design, data collection and analysis, decision to publish, or preparation of the manuscript. This does not alter the authors' adherence to all the PLOS ONE policies on sharing data and materials.

Competing Interests: This work was supported by grants provided by the Japanese Ministry of Education, Culture, Sports, Science and Technology Grant-in-Aid for Scientific Research (KI), the Japanese Ministry of Health, Labour and Welfare (SM, HY) and the Japan Science and Technology Agency (HY). The IORRA cohort was supported by non-restricted research grants from commercial companies (Asahikasei Kuraray Medical Co., Ltd. Abbott Japan Co., Ltd. Asahikasei Pharma Corporation Astellas Pharma Inc. AstraZeneca K.K. Bristol-Myers Squibb Chugai Pharmaceutical Co., Ltd. Daiichi Fine Chemical Co., Ltd. Daiichi Sankyo Co., Ltd. Dainippon Sumitomo Pharma Co., Ltd. Dentsu, Sudler & Hennessey Inc. Eisai Co., Ltd. GlaxoSmithKline K.K. Hisamitsu Pharmaceutical Co.,Inc. Janssen Pharmaceutical K.K. Japan Tobacco Inc. Kaken Pharmaceutical Co., Ltd. Kissei Pharmaceutical Co., Ltd. Kowa Pharmaceutical Co., Ltd. Mitsubishi Chemical Medience Corporation Mitsubishi Tanabe Pharma Corporation Mochida Pharmaceutical Co., Ltd. MSD K.K., Mundipharma K.K. Nippon Chemiphar Co., Ltd. Nippon Shinyaku Co., Ltd. Novartis Pharma K.K. Otsuka Pharmaceutical Co., Ltd. Pfizer Japan Inc. Sanofi-Aventis K.K. Santen Pharmaceutical Co., Ltd. Sanwa Kagaku Kenkyusho Co., Ltd. Sekisui Medical Co., Ltd. Taishotoyama Pharmaceutical Co., Ltd. Takeda Pharmaceutical Company Limited Teijin Pharma Limited Torii Pharmaceutical Co., Ltd. UCB Japan Co., Ltd. ZERIA Pharmaceutical Co., Ltd). However, these funders had no role in study design, data collection and analysis, decision to publish, or preparation of the manuscript. This does not alter the authors' adherence to all the PLOS ONE policies on sharing data and materials.

* E-mail: kikari@ior.twmu.ac.jp

9 These authors contributed equally to this work.

Introduction

Rheumatoid arthritis (RA) is a common autoimmune disease characterized by the chronic synovitis and the localized destruction of cartilage and bone resulting in deteriorated physical function and reduced quality of life. It has been recognized that early therapeutic intervention can prevent progress of joint damage and provide long-term benefits to the patients of RA. The therapeutic recommendations for the management of RA indicate patients may use non-biologic and/or biologic disease-modifying anti-rheumatic drugs (DMARDs) in consideration of the presence of poor prognostic factors.[1–3].

To date, prognostic markers of joint damage have been studied extensively and reported; anti-cyclic citrullinated peptides antibody (ACPA) positive,[4–7] rheumatoid factor (RF) positive, [6,7] the history of smoking, [8,9] the high level of disease activity measured using composite measures,[10–12] gender [4,13] and the age of disease onset.[13–15].

Since RA is a complex disease influenced by both genetic and environmental factors, susceptibility genes to the disease have been widely investigated and identified, especially in the era of genome-wide association studies (GWAS) and GWAS meta-analyses.[16–18] Recently, a large-scaled GWAS meta-analysis was conducted using samples from more than 9,000 Japanese RA patients and 38,000 controls. As a result, nine novel RA susceptibility loci were identified; *B3GNT2*, *ANXA3*, *CSF2*, *CD83*, *NFKBIE*, *ARID5B*, *PDE2A-ARAP1*, *PLD4* and *PTPN2*. [16] The study also showed that some previously reported RA susceptibility genes satisfied the genome-wide significance threshold ($P<5.0 \times 10^{-8}$); HLA-DRB1, *PADI4*, *TNFAIP3* and *CCR6*. [16] Of these 13 RA-susceptible loci, HLA-DRB1 shared epitope (SE) have been reported to have impact on disease severity.[19–21] However, the question remains whether if the other RA-susceptible genes have significant impact on joint destruction.

The purpose of this study is to explore genetic risk factors associated with radiographic progression in RA patients.

Methods

Patients and Evaluation of Radiographic Joint Damage

Tokyo Women's Medical University Genome Ethics Committee approved the present study and each individual signed an informed consent form after receiving a verbal explanation of the study. All the patients satisfied the American College of Rheumatology 1987 revised criteria for RA. [22] DNA samples from RA patients were obtained from the IORRA (Institute of Rheumatology Rheumatoid Arthritis cohort study) DNA collection. [16] IORRA is a project of observational RA cohort with an enrollment of over 5,000 Japanese RA patients, and DNA samples were collected from 2,068 patients. [23,24] All these DNA samples were included in the Japanese GWAS meta-analysis. [16].

Radiographic data at 5-year disease duration were collected retrospectively from the medical records of the patients. Of the patients who donated DNA samples, Sharp/van der Heijde score (SHS) of the hands representing radiographic joint damage (a higher score indicating more damage) was available in 865 patients who have not received biologic agents. [25] Proper anteroposterior radiographs of the hands were scored by a single experienced reader as described elsewhere. [26] Since it has been well known that the rate of radiologic progression develops rapidly in early disease course of RA, joint damage scores of the same disease duration, 5 years, were used. Interobserver and intraobserver agreements (0.85 and 0.95, respectively) indicated good reliability.

The reasons of the exclusion for the patients who treated with biologic agents were as follows: the apparent reported dissociation between clinical and radiologic outcomes in patients with RA who are treated with biologic agents, which could be a confounding factor for the study; [27] the year of RA onset for most patients in this study was before 2000 (70.2%), while the first biologic agent was not launched in the Japanese market until 2003, and the number of the patients who have ever used biologic agents in the first 5-year of disease duration was not sufficient for the sub-analysis targeted on biologic agents.

Assessment Measures, Non-genetic Factors

From the IORRA database and medical records of the patients, demographic, clinical, biological and therapeutic data during the first 5-year after onset of RA were collected, including ACPA status (ACPA titers were measured with second [MESACUP CCP test, Medical and biological laboratories] or third generation [QUANTA Lite CCP3 IgG ELISA, Inova Diagnostics] kit), [28] RF status (determined by a latex agglutination turbidimetric immunoassay method), history of smoking, gender and the age at onset. The age at onset was defined as the age at the onset of first symptoms, according to the patient's self-report, and it did not mean the age that satisfied the 1987 ACR criteria.

ACPA, RF, history of smoking and gender were categorized into two dichotomous variables: ACPA (positive [$>=$4.5 IU/ml] = 1, negative = 0), RF (positive [$>=$15.0 IU/ml] = 1, negative = 0; maximum value in the first 5 years was used), history of smoking (ever smoked = 1, never = 0) and gender (female = 1, male = 0). Data of age at onset was used as continuous variables.

Assessment Measures, Genetic Factors

HLA-DRB1 SE and twelve single nucleotide polymorphisms that have been reported as RA susceptibility polymorphisms using a large-scaled GWAS meta-analysis of Japanese were chosen for the study. [16] There were rs2240340 (*PADI4*, peptidyl arginine deiminase type IV), rs2230926 (*TNFAIP3*, tumor necrosis factor, alpha-induced protein 3), rs3093024 (*CCR6*, C-C chemokine receptor type 6), rs11900673 (*B3GNT2*, UDP-GlcNAc:betaGal beta-1,3-N-acetylglucosaminyltransferase 2), rs2867461 (*ANXA3*, annexin A3), rs657075 (*CSF2*, colony stimulating factor 2), rs12529514 (*CD83*, CD83 molecule), rs2233434 (*NFKBIE*, nuclear factor of kappa light polypeptide gene enhancer in B-cells inhibitor, epsilon), rs10821944 (*ARID5B*, AT rich interactive domain 5B [MRF1-like]), rs3781913 (*PDE2A-ARAP1*, *PDE2A*; phosphodiesterase 2A, cGMP-stimulated, *ARAP1*; ArfGAP with RhoGAP domain, ankyrin repeat and PH domain 1), rs2841277 (*PLD4*, phospholipase D family, member 4) and rs2847297 (*PTPN2*, protein tyrosine phosphatase, non-receptor type 2). The risk alleles were defined as the allele that increases the risk of RA based on a prior report. [16].

Genotyping

Duplicate samples and negative controls were included to ensure accuracy of genotyping. High-resolution polymerase chain reaction (PCR) based DNA typing of HLA-DRB1 locus was performed using the sequence-based typing method with the AlleleSEQR DRB1 typing kit (Abbott Japan), according to the manufacturer's instructions. Assignment of HLA-DRB1 alleles was performed using Assign software. HLA-DRB1 SE were defined as alleles encoding amino acid sequences of QKRAA/QRRAA/RRRAA in positions 70–74 of HLA-DRB1. Genotyping of non-HLA RA susceptibility single-nucleotide polymorphisms (SNPs) were performed using the TaqMan fluorogenic 5′ nuclease assay according to the manufacturer's instructions (Applied Biosystems,

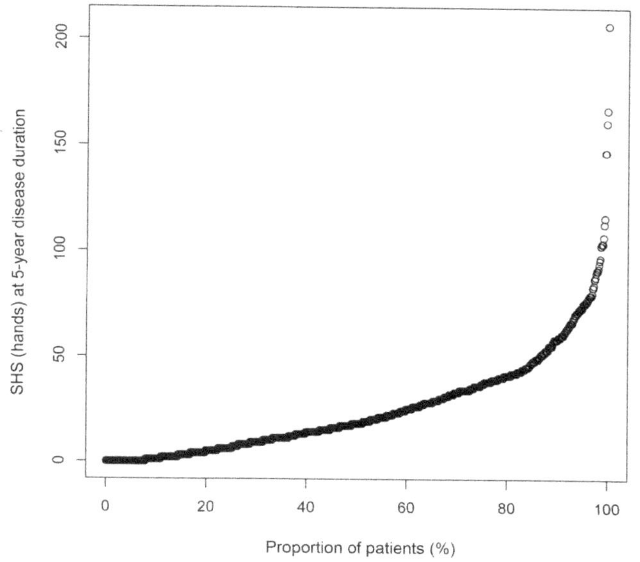

Figure 1. Probability plot of Sharp/van der Heijde score of the hands at the 5-year disease duration. Each point on the plot represents the Sharp/van der Heijde score (SHS) of the hands at the 5-year disease duration, which representing approximate value of the radiographic progression in the first 5 years after onset of RA, in an individual patient. A zero value represents a patient without any radiographic progression, and the right-side tail represents patients with the most progression.

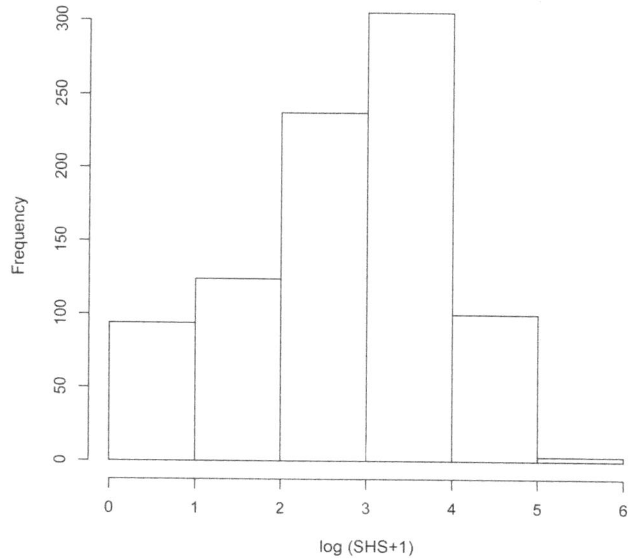

Figure 2. Histogram of distribution of the log-transformed SHS (hands).

Tokyo, Japan) as described elsewhere. [16] All PCRs were performed using GeneAmp PCR System 9700 (Applied Biosystems), DNA sequencing for HLA typing on 3130×l Genetic Analyzer (Applied Biosystems) and endpoint fluorescent readings for TaqMan assays on ABI PRISM 7900 HT Sequence Detection System (Applied Biosystems).

Statistical Analysis

First, the putative risk factors including non-genetic factors on joint damage were assessed using univariate linear regression analyses (univariate-based feature selection process). Any variable showing a significance level (alpha = 0.05) was selected as a candidate for a stepwise multiple regression analysis (backward elimination) to evaluate the putative risk factor as an independent risk of radiographic damage in RA patients. Number of reported risk alleles on disease susceptibility (0, 1 and 2) was used for the RA susceptible polymorphisms to test the additive effect of the alleles. [16] The dependent variable was the radiographic progression in the first 5 years after onset of RA, calculated as SHS of hands at the 5-year disease duration. Since some RA patients may show more rapid radiographic progression than others[29–31], the SHS (hands) were log-transformed to obtain a normal distribution for all statistical analyses. [32,33].

All valuables were standardized using "scale" command in R software to calculate standardized regression coefficients (ß) in the stepwise multiple regression analysis. Statistical analyses were performed using the R software package (http://www.r-project.org/).

Results

Demographic, Clinical and Biological Characteristics of the Patients

Demographic, clinical, biological and therapeutic characteristics of the patients are shown in Table 1. Median age of the patients at

Table 1. Demographic and clinical characteristics of patients at 5 years from onset.

Age at 5-year disease duration, years	54 (46–62)
Sex, female	738 (85.3)
Year of disease onset	
<1990	141 (16.3)
1990<1995	195 (22.5)
1995<2000	271 (31.3)
2000<	258 (29.8)
SHS (hands)	18 (6–37)
ACPA, positive*	739 (87.8)
RF, positive†	781 (90.3)
History of smoking, ever	301 (35.2)
Medication in the first 5-year from the onset	
DMARDs use, ever	735 (92.3)
Methotrexate use, ever	399 (50.1)
Biologic agents use, ever	0 (0)
Corticosteroid use, ever	375 (47.4)

Data are presented as median (interquartile range) or n (%).
*Cut-off = 4.5 IU/ml.
†Maximum value in the first 5-year period of the disease was used, cut-off = 15.0 IU/ml.
SHS, Sharp/van der Heijde score; ACPA, anti-citrullinated peptide antibody; RF, rheumatoid factor; DMARDs, disease-modifying anti-rheumatic drugs.

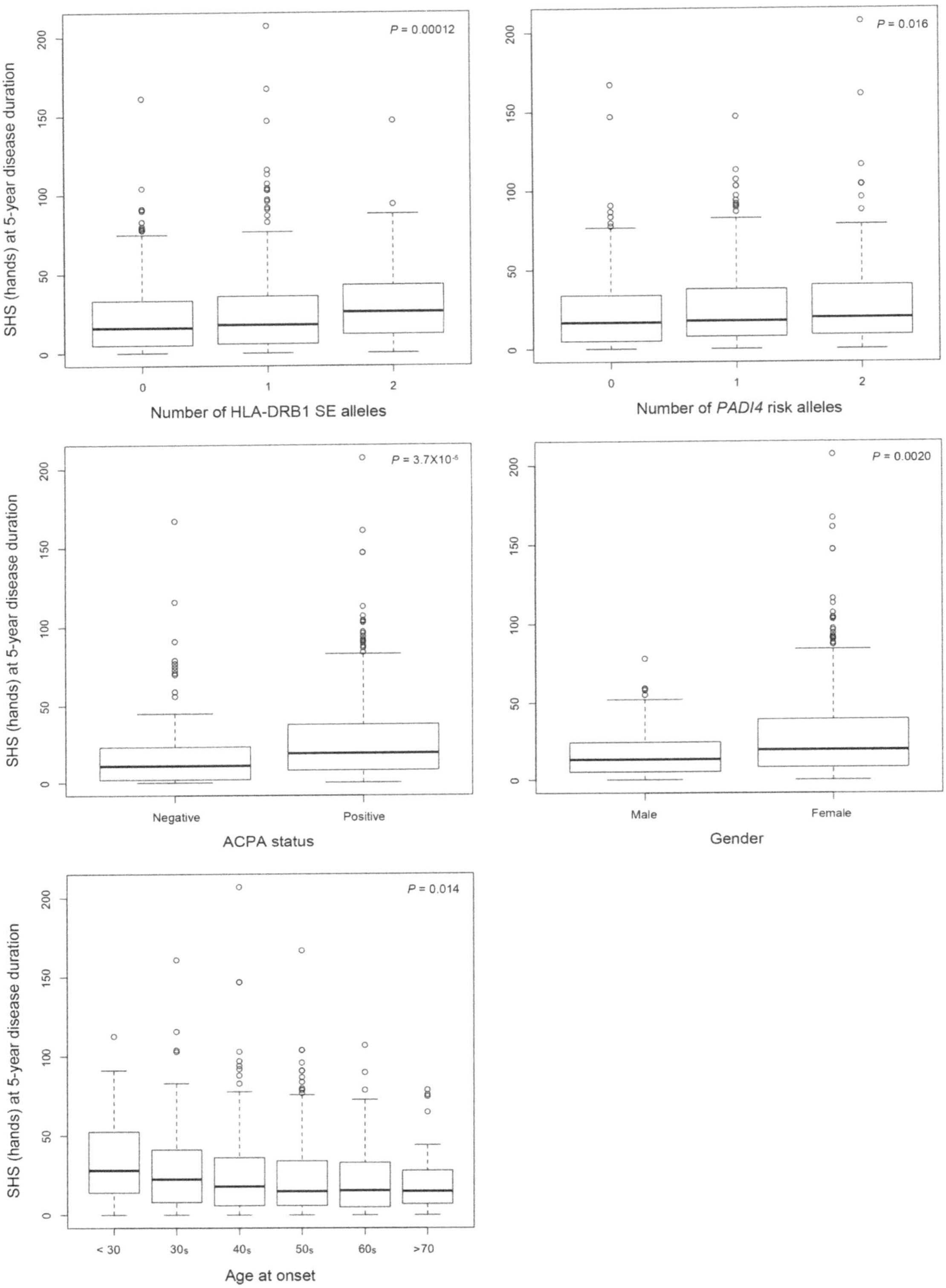

Figure 3. Boxplots representing the distribution of Sharp/van der Heijde score (SHS) of the hands in each category of independent risk factors for joint destruction. Risk factors; the number of HLA-DRB1 shared epitope, the number of PADI4 risk alleles, ACPA status (negative [<4.5 IU/ml] and positive), gender (female and male) and age at onset (categorized as "age under 30", "30 s", "40 s", "50 s", "60 s" and "age over 70"). Each box represents the interquartile range of values, with the bold line showing the median value. The vertical lines show maximum and minimum value that fall within 1.5 box lengths, the open circles show extreme values >1.5 box plot lengths. The P values were given by the univariate linear regression analyses (a log-transformed SHS was used as the dependent variable). PADI4, peptidyl arginine deiminase type IV ACPA, anti-citrullinated peptide antibody.

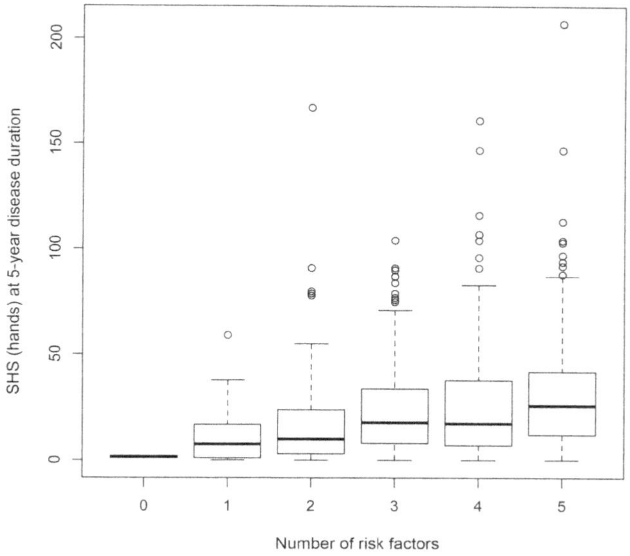

Figure 4. Boxplots representing the distribution of Sharp/van der Heijde score (SHS) of the hands according to the number of the risk factors. Risk factors; SE allele carrier, PADI4 risk allele carrier, ACPA positive, female and age at onset under 50. Each box represents the interquartile range of values, with the bold line showing the median value. The vertical lines show maximum and minimum value that fall within 1.5 box lengths, the open circles show extreme values >1.5 box plot lengths. PADI4, peptidyl arginine deiminase type IV ACPA, anti-citrullinated peptide antibody.

5-year disease duration was 54 years, 85.3% of the patients were female, 87.8% were ACPA positive and 90.3% were RF positive. Median SHS (hands) at 5-year disease duration was 18 (inter-quartile range 6–37) and yearly progression rate (SHS/disease duration) was 3.6 (Figure 1 and 2). The distribution of SHS (hands) was similar to those in recent clinical studies in which some patients had extreme progressive joint destruction compared to others.[29–31] Half of the patients had prior use of MTX (50.1%) for their treatment of RA in the first 5 years of the disease. The patients who had used biologic agents in the first 5-year disease duration were excluded from the study. Since ACPA measurements started only in the early 2000 s in Japan, data of ACPA in the first 5-years from the onset could not be collected in most patients in this study, and they were substituted by recent data.

SNPs and HLA-DRB1 Genotyping

The overall genotyping success rate was 98.1% and the genotype concordance rate was 100% as assessed by duplicate samples. After the application of quality control criteria for genotyping (remove samples that consistently fail for ≥20% [3/13] SNPs, SNP call rate >95% overall after removing samples that consistently fail), 857 of 865 samples and all polymorphisms passed for the analyses. The following HLA-DRB1 alleles were classified as belonging to SE: DRB1*0101, DRB1*0401, DRB1*0404, DRB1*0405, DRB1*0410, DRB1*1001, DRB1*1402 and DRB1*1406. Frequency of SE carrier was 70.4% (n = 605) and 130 patients were homozygous for SE (15.1%).

Risk Factors for Radiographic Joint Damage

The univariate analysis identified 6 covariates initially as potential candidates; ACPA positive, RF positive, female sex, younger age at onset, HLA-DRB1 SE and *PADI4* risk allele (Table 2). The stepwise multiple regression analysis revealed all tested candidates except RF as independent risks for radiographic joint destruction (Table 3 and Figure 3). Patients with higher number of risk factors had more joint damage (Figure 4). Patients with extremely high joint damage score (SHS [hands] at 5-year disease duration more than 100, n = 13) were all females and had either SE or *PADI4* risk allele.

In the power calculation with a sample size of 830 (the number of samples used in the stepwise multivariate analysis), a 22% change of SHS of the hands with and without a risk by power 0.69 and an 11% change by power 0.23 could be detected.

Discussion

To date, a lot of studies focused on disease severity of RA have been conducted using various endpoints: radiographic progression, disease activity, functional impairment, presence of extra-articular features, complication or death.[34–36] Since a major symptom of RA is the chronic synovitis of multiple joints, which leads to highly damaged joints, restriction of activities of daily living and deterioration of quality of life, SHS that represent radiographic damage in joints has been thought to be a reliable index to assess the disease severity.

One of the difficulties in a study using joint damage score to evaluate RA severity is that the radiographic change is highly influenced by the disease duration. The patients with longer disease duration tend to have more accumulated damage; furthermore, rates of progression in joint damage are nonlinear, it is significantly faster in the early stage than the late phase of the disease. [37] Though the problem can be solved by using the radiographic joint damage score of the same disease duration, such data must be collected from a large number of patients. One of the strong points of this study was that we could obtain hundreds of SHS data from the same disease duration of 5 years, from a large RA cohort project, IORRA. As a result, we were able to perform powerful statistical analyses on joint destruction.

RA is caused by a combination of genetic and environmental factors, and to date, plenty of RA-susceptible polymorphisms have been identified, especially in the era of GWAS. However, genetic factors associated with joint destruction in RA patients have not been extensively studied. Although we had tested the association between joint destruction and some susceptible polymorphisms, no significant association was found thus far. [26,38,39] One of the reasons for the negative association may be due to the small sample size. By utilizing a larger size of DNA samples, we could find that HLA-DRB1 SE and *PADI4* risk allele were genetic risk factors for joint destruction in RA patients.

Hence, the genetic background of disease severity of RA is not yet fully known, although one thing may be for sure; there is little doubt that HLA-DRB1 SE, the strongest genetic factor to RA susceptibility, has impact on the disease severity, as was confirmed in this study.[19–21,40] HLA-DRB1 SE may play a central role for genetic component of RA, and the association between HLA-DRB1 SE and RA susceptibility or severity has been repeatedly reported across the different ethnic populations.

However, RA susceptible genes outside the HLA region have not been fully replicable across racial or ethnic groups. A representative example is *PADI4*, which was first reported in 2003 as RA susceptible gene in a Japanese population. [41] Since then, several reports using Caucasian samples showed negative association between RA susceptibility and *PADI4* polymorphisms, while the association was repeatedly confirmed in Asian populations.[42–47] Currently, based on amassing of research evidence,

Table 2. Univariate linear regression analysis on putative risk factors for radiographic progression: non-genetic and genetic factors.

Putative risk/gene(s)	Polymorphism	alleles *	MAF	risk allele	n	ß	*P* value
ACPA (positive)					834	0.14	3.7×10^{-5}†
RF (positive)					857	0.12	0.00043†
Smoking status (ever)					848	−0.056	0.10
Gender (female)					857	0.11	0.0020†
Age of onset					857	−0.084	0.014†
HLA-DRB1	SE	+/−	0.428	SE	853	0.13	0.00012†
PADI4	rs2240340	G/A	0.442	A	856	0.082	0.016†
TNFAIP3	rs2230926	T/C	0.089	C	847	−0.027	0.43
CCR6	rs3093024	C/T	0.487	T	852	−0.011	0.74
B3GNT2	rs11900673	C/T	0.320	T	852	0.015	0.66
ANXA3	rs2867461	A/G	0.454	G	822	−0.020	0.56
CSF2	rs657075	G/A	0.391	A	832	0.019	0.59
CD83	rs12529514	T/C	0.163	C	843	−0.030	0.39
NFKBIE	rs2233434	T/C	0.239	C	828	0.028	0.42
ARID5B	rs10821944	T/G	0.398	G	842	−0.032	0.35
PDE2A-ARAP1	rs3781913	A/C	0.278	A	848	0.062	0.073
PLD4	rs2841277	T/C	0.287	T	853	−0.013	0.70
PTPN2	rs2847297	A/G	0.360	G	854	−0.032	0.36

*Alleles shown as major allele/minor allele.
†$P<0.05$.
ACPA, anti-citrullinated peptide antibody; RF, rheumatoid factor. MAF; Minor allele frequency in the tested population, SE, shared epitope; *PADI4*, peptidyl arginine deiminase type IV; *TNFAIP3*, tumor necrosis factor, alpha-induced protein 3; *CCR6*, C-C chemokine receptor type 6; *B3GNT2*, UDP-GlcNAc:betaGal beta-1,3-N-acetylglucosaminyltransferase 2; *ANXA3*, annexin A3; *CSF2*, colony stimulating factor 2; *CD83*, CD83 molecule; *NFKBIE*, nuclear factor of kappa light polypeptide gene enhancer in B-cells inhibitor, epsilon; *ARID5B*, AT rich interactive domain 5B [MRF1-like]; *PDE2A*, phosphodiesterase 2A, cGMP-stimulated; *ARAP1*, ArfGAP with RhoGAP domain, ankyrin repeat and PH domain 1; *PLD4*, phospholipase D family, member 4; *PTPN2*, protein tyrosine phosphatase, non-receptor type 2.

PADI4 is considered as RA susceptibility gene even in Caucasian populations though its impact on disease susceptibility is lower than in Asian populations. [16].

It is interesting that *PADI4* risk allele had impact on joint damage independent of ACPA status, which is the most significant finding of this study. *PADI4* gene encodes one of PADI enzymes that catalyse the post-translational modification reaction generating citrulline residues from arginine, [41] and the serum titer of antibodies against citrullinated peptides, ACPA, which is an established prognostic marker for joint destruction in RA patients, is significantly correlated to *PADI4* risk alleles.[48–50] Thus, to date, the relationship between *PADI4* gene and disease severity of RA have been reported mainly in the context of association of *PADI4* haplotypes (or alleles) with serum titer (or positivity) of ACPA.[41,48–50] Recently, Bang et al. [51] indicated that *PADI4* gene contributed to the development of RA, regardless of ACPA status. Combined with our results, the *PADI4* gene is likely to play an additional role in the development and disease progression of RA along with its role in ACPA formation. Subsequent studies should elucidate the unidentified role of *PADI4* in the pathogenesis of RA.

Table 3. Stepwise multiple regression analysis on risk factors for radiographic progression (n = 830).

Risk factors	ß	95% CI for ß	*P* value
ACPA (positive)	0.12	0.05–0.17	0.00056
Gender (female)	0.09	0.03–0.16	0.0059
Age of onset	−0.07	−0.14– −0.01	0.024
HLA-DRB1 SE	0.11	0.04–0.17	0.0021
PADI4 risk allele	0.07	0.004–0.14	0.037

Multiple R squared value = 0.055.
95% CI, 95% confidence interval; ACPA, anti-citrullinated peptide antibody; SE, shared epitope; *PADI4*, peptidyl arginine deiminase type IV.

Numerous clinical studies have indicated that severe, tight control with aggressive treatment in RA patients with remission as a target would help to lower the risk of progression of joint damage, which is especially critical in patients with uncontrollable risk factors. Although prediction of progressive joint damage in RA patients is still far from perfect, the use of identified risk factors (HLA-DRB1-SE positive, *PADI4* risk allele positive, ACPA positive, younger age of onset and female sex) should make it easier for rheumatologists to make their treatment decisions in the future.

Our cohort study has strong points, but also still has some limitations. Since the study was a retrospective cohort study, we were able to collect radiographic data from only 865 of 2,068 patients with DNA sample. Loss of patients could affect the results, although the baseline characteristics of the patients with radiographic data were similar to the whole DNA cohort of IORRA. As a result of the limited sample size, the study was underpowered to detect minor effect on joint destruction. Though we used the data of SHS (hands) at the same disease duration, because radiographs at baseline (onset of the disease) were not available in most patients, they are only approximate values of delta-SHS in the first 5 years of the disease.

Conclusions

In conclusion, we have identified HLA-DRB1 SE and *PADI4* risk alleles as independent risk factors for progressive joint destruction in the first five years from onset of RA, as well as several non-genetic factors; ACPA positive, younger age of onset and female sex. Results of this study may help patients with these risk factors receive early aggressive intervention to change their natural disease course of RA.

Acknowledgments

We thank all DNA donors for making this study possible. We appreciate the members of Institute of Rheumatology, Tokyo Women's Medical University for their effort on the IORRA cohort. We are also grateful to the members of the Genetics and Allied research in Rheumatic diseases Networking (GARNET) consortium for their helpful advices in conducting the study. We also thank Ms Kaori Arai for her technical assistance, and Dr. Noriko Iikuni for her assistance in preparing the manuscript.

Author Contributions

Conceived and designed the experiments: KI. Performed the experiments: TS KI EI. Analyzed the data: TS KI KY EI. Contributed reagents/materials/analysis tools: KI KY YT AT HY SM. Wrote the paper: TS KI.

References

1. Smolen JS, Aletaha D, Bijlsma JW, Breedveld FC, Boumpas D, et al. (2010) Treating rheumatoid arthritis to target: recommendations of an international task force. Ann Rheum Dis 69: 631–637.
2. Smolen JS, Landewe R, Breedveld FC, Dougados M, Emery P, et al. (2010) EULAR recommendations for the management of rheumatoid arthritis with synthetic and biological disease-modifying antirheumatic drugs. Ann Rheum Dis 69: 964–975.
3. Singh JA, Furst DE, Bharat A, Curtis JR, Kavanaugh AF, et al. (2012) 2012 update of the 2008 american college of rheumatology recommendations for the use of disease-modifying antirheumatic drugs and biologic agents in the treatment of rheumatoid arthritis. Arthritis Care Res (Hoboken) 64: 625–639.
4. Syversen SW, Gaarder PI, Goll GL, Odegard S, Haavardsholm EA, et al. (2008) High anti-cyclic citrullinated peptide levels and an algorithm of four variables predict radiographic progression in patients with rheumatoid arthritis: results from a 10-year longitudinal study. Ann Rheum Dis 67: 212–217.
5. Forslind K, Ahlmen M, Eberhardt K, Hafstrom I, Svensson B (2004) Prediction of radiological outcome in early rheumatoid arthritis in clinical practice: role of antibodies to citrullinated peptides (anti-CCP). Ann Rheum Dis 63: 1090–1095.
6. Berglin E, Johansson T, Sundin U, Jidell E, Wadell G, et al. (2006) Radiological outcome in rheumatoid arthritis is predicted by presence of by IgA-RF at disease onset. Ann Rheum Dis 65: 453–458.
7. Lindqvist E, Eberhardt K, Bendtzen K, Heinegard D, Saxne T (2005) Prognostic laboratory markers of joint damage in rheumatoid arthritis. Ann Rheum Dis 64: 196–201.
8. Manfredsdottir VF, Vikingsdottir T, Jonsson T, Geirsson AJ, Kjartansson O, et al. (2006) The effects of tobacco smoking and rheumatoid factor seropositivity on disease activity and joint damage in early rheumatoid arthritis. Rheumatology (Oxford) 45: 734–740.
9. Wolfe F (2000) The effect of smoking on clinical, laboratory, and radiographic status in rheumatoid arthritis. J Rheumatol 27: 630–637.
10. van der Heijde DM, van Riel PL, van Leeuwen MA, van 't Hof MA, van Rijswijk MH, et al. (1992) Prognostic factors for radiographic damage and physical disability in early rheumatoid arthritis. A prospective follow-up study of 147 patients. Br J Rheumatol 31: 519–525.
11. Welsing PM, Landewe RB, van Riel PL, Boers M, van Gestel AM, et al. (2004) The relationship between disease activity and radiologic progression in patients with rheumatoid arthritis: a longitudinal analysis. Arthritis Rheum 50: 2082–2093.
12. Aletaha D, Funovits J, Breedveld FC, Sharp J, Segurado O, et al. (2009) Rheumatoid arthritis joint progression in sustained remission is determined by disease activity levels preceding the period of radiographic assessment. Arthritis Rheum 60: 1242–1249.
13. Kuiper S, van Gestel AM, Swinkels HL, de Boo TM, da Silva JA, et al. (2001) Influence of sex, age, and menopausal state on the course of early rheumatoid arthritis. J Rheumatol 28: 1809–1816.
14. van der Heijde DM, van Riel PL, van Leeuwen MA, van 't Hof MA, van Rijswijk MH, et al. (1991) Older versus younger onset rheumatoid arthritis: results at onset and after 2 years of a prospective followup study of early rheumatoid arthritis. J Rheumatol 18: 1285–1289.
15. Pease CT, Bhakta BB, Devlin J, Emery P (1999) Does the age of onset of rheumatoid arthritis influence phenotype?: a prospective study of outcome and prognostic factors. Rheumatology (Oxford) 38: 228–234.
16. Okada Y, Terao C, Ikari K, Kochi Y, Ohmura K, et al. (2012) Meta-analysis identifies nine new loci associated with rheumatoid arthritis in the Japanese population. Nat Genet 44: 511–516.
17. Zhernakova A, Stahl EA, Trynka G, Raychaudhuri S, Festen EA, et al. (2011) Meta-analysis of genome-wide association studies in celiac disease and rheumatoid arthritis identifies fourteen non-HLA shared loci. PLoS Genet 7: e1002004.
18. Stahl EA, Raychaudhuri S, Remmers EF, Xie G, Eyre S, et al. (2010) Genome-wide association study meta-analysis identifies seven new rheumatoid arthritis risk loci. Nat Genet 42: 508–514.
19. Marotte H, Farge P, Gaudin P, Alexandre C, Mougin B, et al. (2006) The association between periodontal disease and joint destruction in rheumatoid arthritis extends the link between the HLA-DR shared epitope and severity of bone destruction. Ann Rheum Dis 65: 905–909.
20. Wagner U, Kaltenhauser S, Pierer M, Seidel W, Troltzsch M, et al. (2003) Prospective analysis of the impact of HLA-DR and -DQ on joint destruction in recent-onset rheumatoid arthritis. Rheumatology (Oxford) 42: 553–562.
21. Gorman JD, Lum RF, Chen JJ, Suarez-Almazor ME, Thomson G, et al. (2004) Impact of shared epitope genotype and ethnicity on erosive disease: a meta-analysis of 3,240 rheumatoid arthritis patients. Arthritis Rheum 50: 400–412.
22. Arnett FC, Edworthy SM, Bloch DA, McShane DJ, Fries JF, et al. (1988) The American Rheumatism Association 1987 revised criteria for the classification of rheumatoid arthritis. Arthritis Rheum 31: 315–324.
23. Yamanaka H, Inoue E, Singh G, Tanaka E, Nakajima A, et al. (2007) Improvement of disease activity of rheumatoid arthritis patients from 2000 to 2006 in a large observational cohort study IORRA in Japan. Mod Rheumatol 17: 283–289.
24. Yamanaka H, Tohma S (2006) Potential impact of observational cohort studies in Japan on rheumatoid arthritis research and practice. Mod Rheumatol 16: 75–76.
25. van der Heijde DM (2000) How to read radiographs according to the Sharp/van der Heijde method. J Rheumatol 27: 261–263.
26. Nishimoto K, Kochi Y, Ikari K, Yamamoto K, Suzuki A, et al. (2010) Association study of TRAF1-C5 polymorphisms with susceptibility to rheumatoid arthritis and systemic lupus erythematosus in Japanese. Ann Rheum Dis 69: 368–373.
27. Keystone EC (2009) Clinical implications of understanding radiographic findings in relation to clinical outcomes in rheumatoid arthritis. J Rheumatol Suppl 82: 11–16.
28. Shidara K, Inoue E, Tanaka E, Hoshi D, Seto Y, et al. (2011) Comparison of the second and third generation anti-cyclic citrullinated peptide antibody assays in the diagnosis of Japanese patients with rheumatoid arthritis. Rheumatol Int 31: 617–622.
29. Ideguchi H, Ohno S, Hattori H, Senuma A, Ishigatsubo Y (2006) Bone erosions in rheumatoid arthritis can be repaired through reduction in disease activity with conventional disease-modifying antirheumatic drugs. Arthritis Res Ther 8: R76.
30. Landewe R, van der Heijde D (2005) Radiographic progression in rheumatoid arthritis. Clin Exp Rheumatol 23: S63–68.
31. de Vries-Bouwstra JK, Goekoop-Ruiterman YP, Verpoort KN, Schreuder GM, Ewals JA, et al. (2008) Progression of joint damage in early rheumatoid arthritis: association with HLA-DRB1, rheumatoid factor, and anti-citrullinated protein antibodies in relation to different treatment strategies. Arthritis Rheum 58: 1293–1298.
32. Keene ON (1995) The log transformation is special. Stat Med 14: 811–819.
33. McDonald JH (2009) Handbook of Biological Statistics. Baltimore: Sparky House Publishing. 160–164 p.
34. Tanaka E, Mannalithara A, Inoue E, Hara M, Tomatsu T, et al. (2008) Efficient management of rheumatoid arthritis significantly reduces long-term functional disability. Ann Rheum Dis 67: 1153–1158.
35. Nakajima A, Inoue E, Tanaka E, Singh G, Sato E, et al. (2010) Mortality and cause of death in Japanese patients with rheumatoid arthritis based on a large observational cohort, IORRA. Scand J Rheumatol 39: 360–367.
36. Nakajima A, Inoue E, Shidara K, Hoshi D, Sato E, et al. (2011) Standard treatment in daily clinical practice for early rheumatoid arthritis improved disease activity from 2001 to 2006. Mod Rheumatol 21: 594–597.
37. van der Heijde DM (1995) Joint erosions and patients with early rheumatoid arthritis. Br J Rheumatol 34 Suppl 2: 74–78.
38. Tsukahara S, Shinozaki M, Ikari K, Mochizuki T, Inoue E, et al. (2008) Effect of matrix metalloproteinase-3 functional SNP on serum matrix metalloproteinase-3 level and outcome measures in Japanese RA patients. Rheumatology (Oxford) 47: 41–44.
39. Kobayashi S, Ikari K, Kaneko H, Kochi Y, Yamamoto K, et al. (2008) Association of STAT4 with susceptibility to rheumatoid arthritis and systemic

lupus erythematosus in the Japanese population. Arthritis Rheum 58: 1940–1946.
40. Rojas-Villarraga A, Diaz FJ, Calvo-Paramo E, Salazar JC, Iglesias-Gamarra A, et al. (2009) Familial disease, the HLA-DRB1 shared epitope and anti-CCP antibodies influence time at appearance of substantial joint damage in rheumatoid arthritis. J Autoimmun 32: 64–69.
41. Suzuki A, Yamada R, Chang X, Tokuhiro S, Sawada T, et al. (2003) Functional haplotypes of PADI4, encoding citrullinating enzyme peptidylarginine deiminase 4, are associated with rheumatoid arthritis. Nat Genet 34: 395–402.
42. Kang CP, Lee HS, Ju H, Cho H, Kang C, et al. (2006) A functional haplotype of the PADI4 gene associated with increased rheumatoid arthritis susceptibility in Koreans. Arthritis Rheum 54: 90–96.
43. Iwamoto T, Ikari K, Nakamura T, Kuwahara M, Toyama Y, et al. (2006) Association between PADI4 and rheumatoid arthritis: a meta-analysis. Rheumatology (Oxford) 45: 804–807.
44. Barton A, Bowes J, Eyre S, Spreckley K, Hinks A, et al. (2004) A functional haplotype of the PADI4 gene associated with rheumatoid arthritis in a Japanese population is not associated in a United Kingdom population. Arthritis Rheum 50: 1117–1121.
45. Burr ML, Naseem H, Hinks A, Eyre S, Gibbons LJ, et al. (2010) PADI4 genotype is not associated with rheumatoid arthritis in a large UK Caucasian population. Ann Rheum Dis 69: 666–670.
46. Martinez A, Valdivia A, Pascual-Salcedo D, Lamas JR, Fernandez-Arquero M, et al. (2005) PADI4 polymorphisms are not associated with rheumatoid arthritis in the Spanish population. Rheumatology (Oxford) 44: 1263–1266.
47. Too CL, Murad S, Dhaliwal JS, Larsson PT, Jiang X, et al. (2012) Polymorphisms in peptidylarginine deiminase (PADI) associate with rheumatoid arthritis in diverse Asian populations: evidence from MyEIRA study and meta-analysis. Arthritis Res Ther 14: R250.
48. Hoppe B, Haupl T, Egerer K, Gruber R, Kiesewetter H, et al. (2009) Influence of peptidylarginine deiminase type 4 genotype and shared epitope on clinical characteristics and autoantibody profile of rheumatoid arthritis. Ann Rheum Dis 68: 898–903.
49. Harris ML, Darrah E, Lam GK, Bartlett SJ, Giles JT, et al. (2008) Association of autoimmunity to peptidyl arginine deiminase type 4 with genotype and disease severity in rheumatoid arthritis. Arthritis Rheum 58: 1958–1967.
50. Cha S, Choi CB, Han TU, Kang CP, Kang C, et al. (2007) Association of anti-cyclic citrullinated peptide antibody levels with PADI4 haplotypes in early rheumatoid arthritis and with shared epitope alleles in very late rheumatoid arthritis. Arthritis Rheum 56: 1454–1463.
51. Bang SY, Han TU, Choi CB, Sung YK, Bae SC, et al. (2010) Peptidyl arginine deiminase type IV (PADI4) haplotypes interact with shared epitope regardless of anti-cyclic citrullinated peptide antibody or erosive joint status in rheumatoid arthritis: a case control study. Arthritis Res Ther 12: R115.

2

Synergistic Effects of Ethanol and Isopentenyl Pyrophosphate on Expansion of γδ T Cells in Synovial Fluid from Patients with Arthritis

Agneta J. Laurent[1,3]*, Niels Bindslev[2], Björn Johansson[3], Louise Berg[1]

1 Rheumatology Unit, Department of Medicine, Karolinska Institutet, Stockholm, Sweden, **2** Department of Biomedical Sciences, Faculty of Health and Medical Sciences, University of Copenhagen, Copenhagen, Denmark, **3** Neurogenetics Unit, Department of Molecular Medicine and Surgery, Karolinska Institutet, Stockholm, Sweden

Abstract

Low to moderate ethanol consumption has been associated with protective effects in autoimmune diseases such as rheumatoid arthritis, RA. An expansion of γδ T cells induced by isopentenyl pyrophosphate, IPP, likewise seems to have a protective role in arthritis. The aim of this project was to test the hypothesis that low doses of ethanol can enhance IPP-induced expansion of synovial fluid γδ T cells from patients with arthritis and may thereby potentially account for the beneficial effects of ethanol on symptoms of the arthritic process. Thus, mononuclear cells from synovial fluid (SF) from 15 patients with arthritis and from peripheral blood (PB) from 15 healthy donors were stimulated with low concentrations of ethanol and IPP for 7 days *in vitro*. IPP in combination with ethanol 0.015%, 2.5 mM, equivalent to the decrease per hour in blood ethanol concentration due to metabolism, gave a significantly higher fractional expansion of SF γδ T cells compared with IPP alone after 7 days (ratio 10.1+/−4.0, $p<0.0008$, $n=12$) in patients with arthritis. Similar results were obtained for PB γδ T cells from healthy controls (ratio 2.0+/−0.4, $p<0.011$, $n=15$). The augmented expansion of γδ T cells in SF is explained by a higher proliferation ($p=0.0034$, $n=11$) and an increased survival ($p<0.005$, $n=11$) in SF cultures stimulated with IPP plus ethanol compared to IPP alone. The synergistic effects of IPP and ethanol indicate a possible allosteric effect of ethanol. Similar effects could be seen when stimulating PB with ethanol in presence of risedronate, which has the ability to increase endogenous levels of IPP. We conclude that expansion of γδ T cells by combinatorial drug effects, possibly in fixed-dose combination, FDC, of ethanol in the presence of IPP might give a protective role in diseases such as arthritis.

Editor: Hiranmoy Das, Ohio State University Medical Center, United States of America

Funding: This study was financed by Börje Dahlin's Foundation and Polysackaridforskning i Uppsala AB. This does not alter the authors' adherence to all the PLOS ONE policies on sharing data and materials. The funders had no role in study design, data collection and analysis, decision to publish, or preparation of the manuscript.

Competing Interests: This study was financed by Polysackaridforskning i Uppsala AB. This does not alter the authors' adherence to all the PLOS ONE policies on sharing data and materials.

* Email: agneta.laurent@comhem.se

Introduction

Rheumatoid arthritis, RA, is a systemic, inflammatory, autoimmune disorder [1] affecting about 0.5–1% of the adult population worldwide [2]. It is characterized by inflammation in joints causing both bone and cartilage destruction [1]. The destruction of bone and cartilage is dependent on different mechanisms in which autoantibodies, osteoclasts, activated T cells and fibroblast-like synoviocytes are involved [1]. Fibroblast-like synoviocytes (FLS) residing in the inner synovial lining of two cell layers, which together form the healthy synovial membrane, produce synovial fluid to the inner cavity of the joint [2]. RA pathogenesis is characterized by inflammatory cell infiltration, supported by proliferation of FLS and angiogenesis. Synovial hyperplasia eventually develops a so called pannus tissue, which invades and destroys the cartilage and the underlying bone [2].

Low to moderate alcohol consumption has been shown to have protective effects in several chronic inflammatory diseases such as rheumatoid arthritis and cardiovascular diseases [3]. Epidemiological studies have analyzed the risk factor of alcohol consumption in developing rheumatoid arthritis and showed a preventive effect of alcohol in rheumatoid arthritis [4–13]. In a mouse model of arthritis, ethanol has been shown to lower the chemotactic activity of leukocytes and down-regulate NF-κB activity [14]. The molecular mechanisms behind the protective effects of low to moderate alcohol consumption in humans remain to be elucidated.

T cells bearing the γδ T cell receptor normally constitute 2–5% of peripheral blood T cells [15], are evolutionary conserved, and have specific tissue distribution and functions [16]. There are two major γδ T cell subsets, Vδ1 and Vδ2, of which the Vδ2 T cells are the most common. Vδ2 T cells are predominantly found in peripheral blood, and Vδ1 T cells are most abundant in gut mucosa [16]. In contrast to αβ T cells the activation of γδ T cells is not dependent on antigen presentation by major histocompatibility complex (MHC) class I or II molecules. Instead, Vδ1 T cells respond to stress-induced cell-surface major histocompatibility class-I related proteins MICA and MICB [16], while Vδ2 T cells proliferate in response to prenyl pyrophosphates such as isopentenyl pyrophosphate (IPP), an intermediate in the mevalonate pathway, with an EC_{50} of 1 μM [15]. Further, Vδ2 T cells are stimulated by (*E*)-4-hydroxy-3-methyl-but-2-enyl pyrophosphate (HMBPP), produced by bacteria and parasitic protozoa, with an even higher potency of $EC_{50} = 32$ pM [15]. In an indirect mechanism, Vδ2 T cells are also stimulated by bisphosphonates and alkylamines, in part by increasing intracellular levels of IPP [15,17].

It has been suggested that rheumatoid arthritis is associated with alterations in the different subsets of γδ T cells [18]. In RA, γδ T cells constitute a smaller fraction of total T cells in blood and synovial fluid (SF) compared to controls. In addition, the ratio of Vδ2/Vδ1 T cells in blood and synovial fluid is lower in RA patients compared to controls [19]. Moreover a greater proportion of IPP responsive γδ T cells have been found in patients who recovered from disease [20].

Fibroblast-like synoviocytes (FLS) in the synovium of patients with RA show abnormal behavior including increased proliferation and production of proinflammatory mediators and enzymes [21]. Thus, it has recently been shown that IPP stimulated SF γδ T cells can induce apoptosis of FLS *in vitro* [22], which could argue for a protective role of γδ T cells in the inflamed joint. Furthermore, an increased ratio of SF γδ T cells in proportion to FLS increased apoptosis of FLS [23].

Evidently, ethanol potentiates proliferation of mitogen-activated T lymphocytes in blood from humans [24]. However, studying effects of ethanol on proliferation of T lymphocytes from *synovial fluid* seems more relevant for future alcohol related treatment of arthritic symptoms. We therefore asked whether ethanol may have an enhancing effect on IPP stimulated synovial fluid γδ T cells. We also asked if there is an additive or synergistic mechanism behind possible ethanol-enhancing effects on expansion with IPP. Our results show that a low dose of ethanol can indeed enhance the expansion of IPP stimulated SF γδ T cells *in vitro*, and that this ethanol enhancing effect is synergistic at certain IPP-ethanol concentration combinations.

Materials and Methods

Patients

Of eighteen patients included in this study, seventeen were attending the Rheumatology Unit at Karolinska University Hospital in Solna and one at the University Hospital in Uppsala. Clinical characteristics and medication of patients are shown in table 1. 15 healthy volunteers, 9 women and 6 men, median age 46 (27–79) years were included. The study was approved by The Regional Ethical Review Board in Stockholm (Regionala Etikprövningsnämnden i Stockholm), number 2010/351-31/2. At the time of sampling, patients were informed of the study and of the possibility of donating samples to research. Oral consent was obtained and documented by the physician in the patients' electronic records, as is the normal procedure in Sweden. The oral consent was in accordance with Swedish law and practice and approved by The Regional Ethical Review Board in Stockholm.

Isolation of synovial fluid mononuclear cells or peripheral blood mononuclear cells

Freshly collected heparinized synovial fluid mononuclear cells (SFMCs) from patients and peripheral blood mononuclear cells (PBMCs) from both patients and controls were isolated by Ficoll-Paque density gradient centrifugation (GE Healthcare, Little Chalfont, United Kingdom) by standard procedures.

Flow cytometry

Cells were stained with fluorochrome conjugated monoclonal antibodies: PerCP or APC (from Biolegend, San Diego, California, USA) or Brilliant Violet 421 (from BD Biosciences, Franklin Lakes, New Jersey, USA), antihuman CD3, clone UCHT1, together with PE conjugated anti-human TCR γδ, clone B1 (from Biolegend) or APC anti-human TCR γδ, clone B1 (BD Biosciences) and APC conjugated anti-human CD27, clone L128, and PE-cy7 conjugated anti-human CD45RA, clone L48

Table 1. Characteristics of the 18 patients participating in the study.

Patient	Diagnosis	Sex	Age	Treatment
1	Psoriatic arthritis	F	53	Prednisone
2	Psoriatic arthritis	F	38	Local steroid injection
3	Psoriatic arthritis	F	40	Prednisone
4	Seropositive RA	F	72	Methotrexate, tocilizumab
5	Polyarthrit unspec	M	24	Methotrexate
6	Oligoarthritis	M	49	Naproxen, local steroid injection
7	Psoriatic arthritis	F	66	Untreated
8	Juvenile arthritis	F	32	Golimumab
9	Pelvospondylitis	M	22	Diclofenac
10	Spondylitis	M	62	Adalimumab, methotrexate, prednisone
11	Spondyloarthritis	M	38	Methotrexate, prednisone, golimumab, ketoprofen
12	Psoriatic arthritis	F	69	Methotrexate, infliximab
13	Oligoarthritis	F	67	Methotrexate, ketoprofen
14	Seropositive RA	F	51	Prednisone, methotrexate
15	Juvenile arthritis	M	47	Methotrexate, prednisone, golimumab
16	Systemic lupus arthritis+juvenile arthritis	F	35	Prednisone, methotrexate
17	Sjögren's syndrome+polyarthritis	F	56	Abatacept, calcium carbonate/cholecalciferol
18	Seronegative, polyarthritis	F	26	Celecoxib, omeprazole

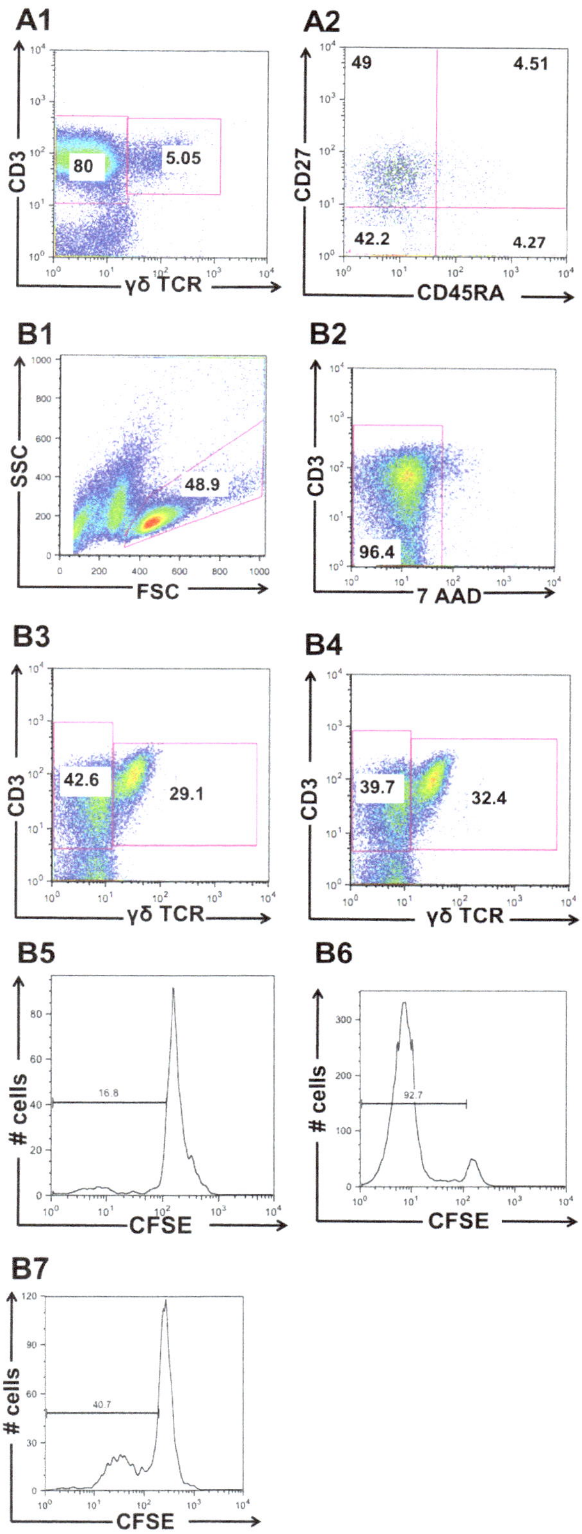

Figure 1. Phenotypic characterization and proliferative response of SFMCs. (**A**) SFMCs at start stained with antibodies to γδ TCR (A1) and γδ TCR gated cells stained with CD45RA and CD27 (A2). Representative FACS dot plots of two stainings. (**B**) Representative FACS dot plots of CFSE-labeled SFMCs in a single patient (pat no 10) after 7 days in culture. Gating of lymphocytes, FSC = Forward Scatter, SSC = Side scatter (B1). Gating of live 7-AAD$^-$ lymphocytes (B2). Gating of γδ T cells stimulated with 0.25 μM IPP+IL2 (B3) and 0.25 μM IPP+0.015% ethanol+IL2 (B4). γδ T cells with different CFSE intensity bar show CFSE^{low} with no stimulation (B5) and with stimulation of 0.25 μM IPP+0.015% ethanol+IL2 after 7 days (B6) and after 4 days (B7).

(both from BD Biosciences) for 30 min at 4°C. The cells were then stained with 7-aminoactinomycin D (7-AAD, BD Biosciences Pharmingen) for 10 min at 4°C for visualization of viable 7-AAD negative cells (7-AAD$^-$) and analyzed on a BD FACS Sort using the CellQuest software (BD Biosciences) or Beckman Coulter Gallios. Further analysis was performed using the software FlowJo 9.4.10 (Tree Star Inc, Ashland, Oregon, USA). APC conjugated anti-human IFN-γ clone B27 (Biolegend) was used for intracellular staining.

In vitro proliferation assay, stimulation with IPP and ethanol

To assess the proliferative response, SFMCs were stained with carboxyfluorescein succinimidyl ester, (CFSE, Invitrogen, Carlsbad, California, USA). Cells were incubated at 37°C for 15 minutes and washed twice in PBS (Sigma, St Louise, Missouri, USA)+0.5% fetal calf serum (Sigma). The proliferative response was calculated based on the fraction of γδ or αβ T cells with low CFSE intensity.

Cells (1×10^6 cells/ml) were cultured for 4 and 7 days in 24 well plates (Sarstedt, Nümbrecht, Germany) in 1 ml RPMI-1640 medium (Sigma) supplemented with 5% heat-inactivated human serum (Sigma), 2 mM L-glutamine (Sigma), 100 U/ml penicillin (Sigma), 100 μg/ml streptomycin (Sigma) and 20 U/ml recombinant human interleukin 2 (Pepro Tech, Rocky Hill, New Jersey, USA) at 37°C in 5% CO_2. The cells were stimulated at start of culturing with IPP (Sigma), range 0.00025–250 μM or risedronate from the University of Eastern Finland, range of 0.00001–1000 μM and ethanol in a range from 0.00015–15 vol/vol %. The number of viable cells, as assessed by Trypan blue (Sigma) staining, was counted under microscope after 4 and 7 days incubation. The percentage of γδ and αβ T cells was measured with flow cytometry at start and after 4 and 7 days of culture, and the absolute numbers of viable and proliferating CFSE^{low} γδ T cells were calculated. To obtain dose-response curves for survival, proliferation and expansion, cells were cultured in 96 well plates, 1×10^6 cells/200 μL RPMI, and supplemented as indicated above.

Intracellular staining

To measure intracellular cytokine accumulation, SFMCs were re-stimulated after 7 days culture for 6 hours with either 0.25 μM IPP, 0.015% ethanol, 0.25 μM IPP+0.015% ethanol or 20 ng/mL phorbol 12-myristate 13-acetate (PMA, Sigma)+0.1 μM ionomycin (Sigma), and the last 4.5 hours of the 6 hours with Golgi Stop (BD Biosciences) diluted 1:1500. This was followed by standard procedures for fixation and permeabilization using BD Cytofix/Cytoperm (BD Biosciences) and staining.

Data analysis - definitions and statistical analysis

The total number of γδ T cells was calculated as: % γδ T cells x total number of viable cells per well at the end of culturing. The expansion, or fold-increase, was calculated as the total number of γδ T cells at the end of culturing over the total number of γδ T cells at start. Proliferation and survival were calculated first as absolute number of CFSE^{low} and CFSE^{high} cells per well respectively at the end of culturing. Both fractional expansion,

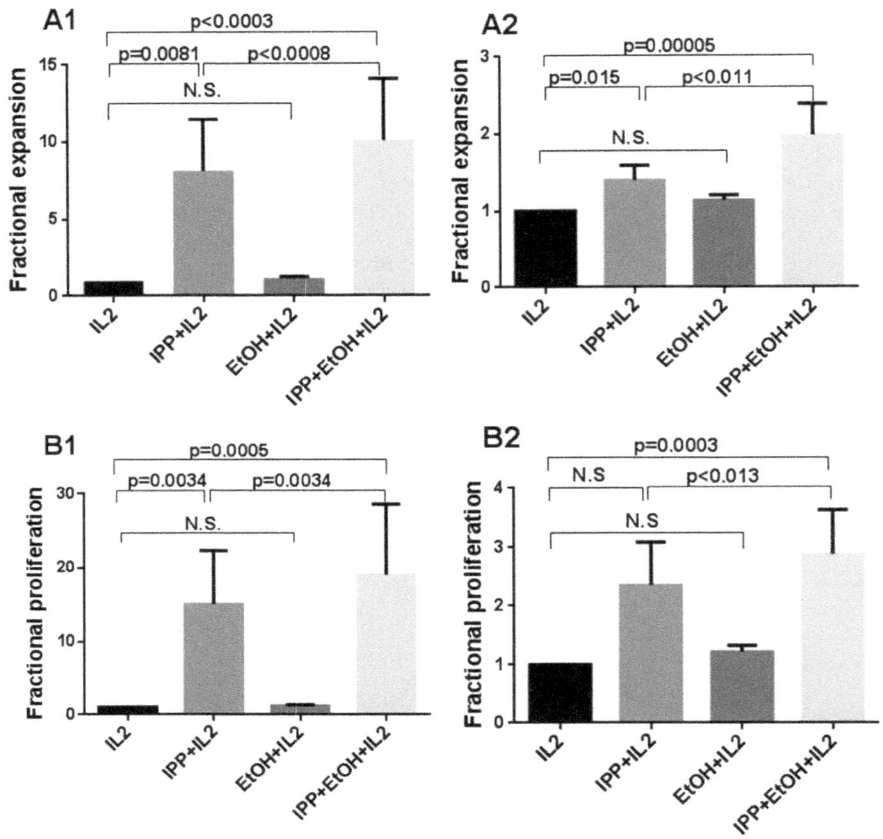

Figure 2. Expansion and proliferation of γδ T cells stimulated with IPP and ethanol for 7 days. SFMCs from patients and PBMCs from healthy controls were stimulated with 0.25 μM IPP, 0.015% ethanol or 0.25 μM IPP+0.015% ethanol, all in presence of IL2. Fractional A) expansion, showing fold-increase of total number of A1) SF γδ T cells from patients, n = 12 and A2) PB γδ T cells, n = 15 from healthy controls B) proliferation, showing total number of B1) CFSE^{low} SF γδ T cells from patients, n = 11 and B2) CFSE^{low} PB γδ T cells from healthy controls, n = 15, all normalized to IL2 = 1. The different growth conditions were compared using Wilcoxon signed rank test one-sided. Bars show means +/− SEM.

- proliferation and - survival are given by values normalized to unity.

Wilcoxon signed rank-test was used to analyze significance between groups. Values reported are means +/− SEM. Prism 6 (Graph Pad Software, Inc, La Jolla, USA) was used for statistical analysis.

For doubling times, the rate constant k was adjusted to fit the equation $N\ cells_t = N\ cells_{t=0} \times e^{kt}$ to data, in which cell doubling time (T) is equal to $\ln 2/k$.

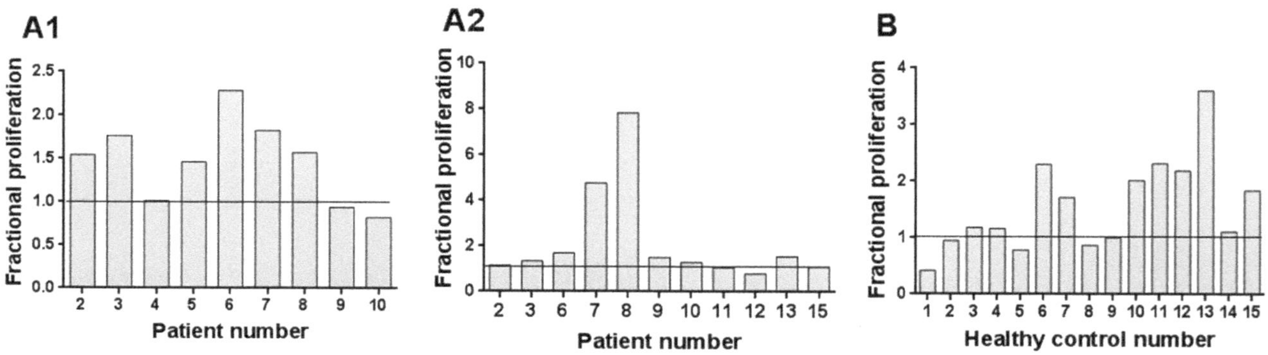

Figure 3. Relative proliferation of γδ T cells from different patients and healthy controls by adding 0.015% ethanol. Proliferation, showing total number of A) CFSE^{low} SF γδ T cells from patients incubated for A1) 4 days and A2) 7 days and B) CFSE^{low} PB γδ T cells from healthy controls incubated for 7 days, all normalized to 0.25 μM IPP = 1.

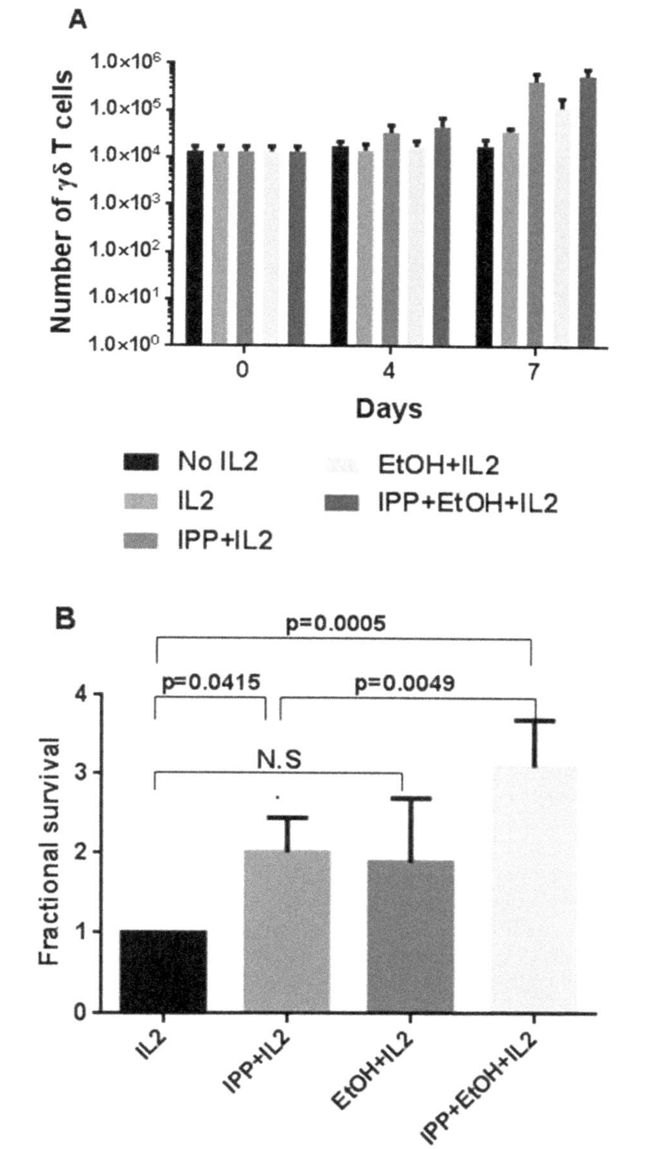

Figure 4. Growth data of total number of γδ T cells and survival of CFSE^{high} γδ T cells. A) SFMCs were untreated or treated with IL2 alone or together with 0.25 μM IPP, with 0.015% ethanol or with 0.25 μM IPP plus 0.015% ethanol for 7 days. Bars show means +/−SEM from five individual experiments. B) Relative response of adding 0.015% ethanol on the survival of CFSE^{high} γδ T cells stimulated for 7 days. SFMCs were stimulated with IL2 alone or in combination with 0.25 μM IPP, with 0.015% ethanol, or with 0.25 μM IPP+0.015% ethanol for 7 days. The number of surviving cells was calculated as viable γδ T cells CFSE^{high}. Values are normalized to IL2 = 1. Wilcoxon signed rank test, one-sided, n = 11. Bars show means +/− SEM.

Concentrations of IPP and ethanol were varied independently and in combination, and possible synergistic effects are presented in 3D surface response plots using Sigmaplot version 12.3.

Bell-shaped dose-response curves for IPP were analyzed by a simplified version of the homotropic two-state model, HOTSM, without spontaneous activity (parameter $L = 0$) [25].

Results

Low doses of ethanol enhance the proliferation and expansion of IPP stimulated γδ T cells

The study was carried out to determine if low doses of ethanol could potentiate the effects of low doses of IPP in expansion of γδ T cells from inflamed joints. Thus, CFSE-stained SFMCs from patients with different arthritic diagnoses were stimulated *in vitro* with IPP and IPP in combination with ethanol, each in presence of IL2, for 4 and 7 days. The proportion of viable CFSE^{low} proliferating γδ T cells was measured by flow cytometry, Fig. 1, B5-B7. A concentration of ethanol at 0.015% was chosen as it represents the approximate blood concentration after one glass of wine or a shot of aquavit and is equivalent to the normal decrease in blood concentration per hour when ingested ethanol is metabolized [26].

IPP, 0.25 μM, in combination with 0.015% ethanol gave a significantly higher fractional expansion, mean ratio 10.1+/−4.0 ($p<0.0008$, $n = 12$) and proliferation, mean ratio 19.1+/−9.5 ($p = 0.0034$, $n = 11$), compared with IPP alone after 7 days of SFMC culture, Fig. 2 A1 and B1. The effect of ethanol could be seen already after 4 days for expansion ($p = 0.04$) and for proliferation ($p = 0.02$) compared with IPP alone ($n = 9$), data not shown. In spite of a great variation in response to IPP between patients, Fig. 3 A1-A2, significant effects of ethanol were obtained in the rather small group of patients studied, Figs. 2 A1, B1 and 4. Considerably more patients would be needed to check for response differences between diagnostic subgroups. In addition, PBMC γδ T cells from healthy controls showed a higher fractional expansion, mean ratio 2.0+/−0.4 ($p<0.011$, $n = 15$) and proliferation, mean ratio 3.0+/−0.7 ($p<0.013$, $n = 15$) compared with IPP after 7 days, Fig. 2 A2 and B2. Similarly to the patient data, the effect of ethanol could be seen already after 4 days (data not shown), and a great variation was found in the response between subjects, Fig. 3 B.

Effect of low doses of ethanol on cell-doubling time and survival of IPP stimulated γδ T cells

T cell proliferation may be analyzed by different factors such as initial cell death and cell doubling time [27]. To analyze the effects of low doses of ethanol on IPP stimulation of γδ T cells, we first investigated the cell population doubling time, equal to the first doubling time, using experimental growth curves as described in Materials and Methods. Doubling times are based on data for growth in figure 4 A. Adding 0.015% ethanol significantly reduces the cell doubling time from 52 to 34 hours, ($p = 0.03$, $n = 5$). Another factor we analyzed was the survival of cells. We found that by adding 0.015% ethanol, the number of surviving non-proliferating (7AAD$^-$ CFSE^{high}) γδ T cells after 7 days in culture was significantly higher compared to cells stimulated with IPP alone, normalized mean ratio 3.1+/−0.6 ($p<0.005$, $n = 11$), Fig. 4 B. Both the reduced doubling time and the augmented survival due to ethanol are part of the observed increase in IPP expansion induced by ethanol.

Effect of ethanol on expansion of αβ T cells and on IFN-γ producing capacity

We questioned if only γδ T cells were expanded and found that also αβ T cells from both patients and healthy controls were expanding when adding IPP and ethanol in combination. IPP alone had no effects on the expansion of αβ T cells above the effect of IL2, Fig. 5.

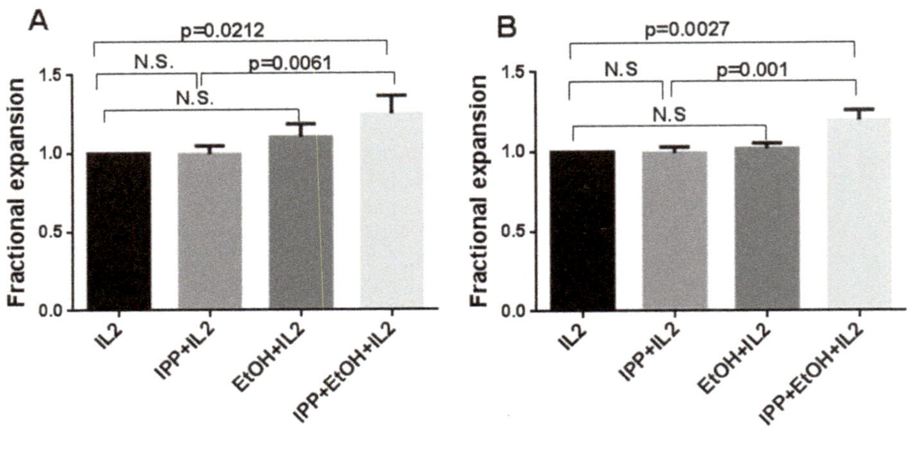

Figure 5. Effects of ethanol and IPP on expansion of αβ T cells. SFMCs from patients and PBMCs from healthy controls were stimulated with IL2 alone or in combination with 0.25 μM IPP or 0.25 μM IPP+0.015% ethanol for 7 days. Relative response of adding 0.015% ethanol on the expansion of A) SF αβ T cells from patients, n = 12 and B) PB αβ T cells from healthy controls, n = 15. Values are normalized to IL2 = 1. Bars show means +/− SEM.

We next asked what the effects of adding 0.015% ethanol had on the IFN-γ producing capacity. The percentage of IFN-γ producing SF T cells was not affected by 0.25 μM IPP or 0.015% ethanol compared with IL2 added alone, and the per cell production of IFN-γ was not elevated as measured by median fluorescence intensity, MFI, of IFN-γ producing SF T cells, Fig 6.

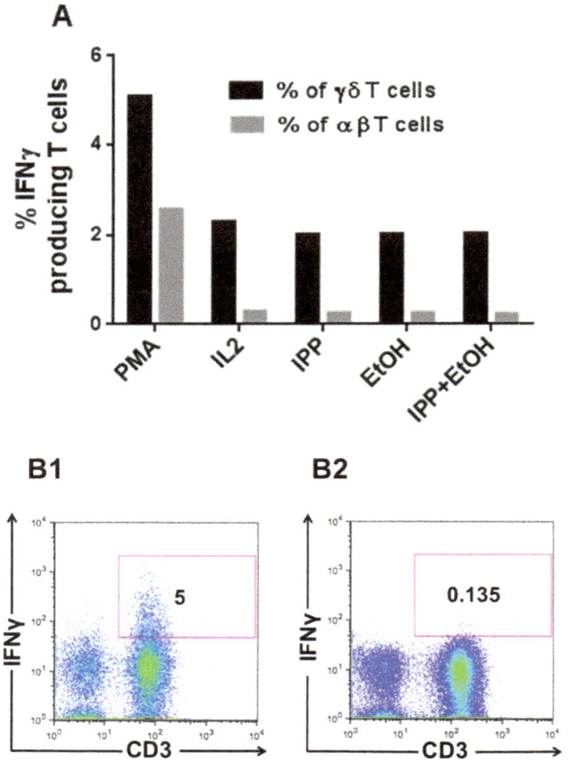

Figure 6. Effects of ethanol and IPP on cytokine production. SFMCs from patients were stimulated with IL2 alone or in combination with 0.25 μM IPP or 0.25 μM IPP+0.015% ethanol for 7 days. A) Effect on the number of IFN-γ producing SF T cells by adding 0.015% ethanol. Bars shows means, n = 5. Representative FACS dot plots of % IFN-γ producing T cells stimulated with PMA (B1) and 0.25 μM IPP+0.015% ethanol (B2).

Auto-inhibition by IPP

Increasing IPP concentrations in absence of ethanol resulted in a bell-shaped dose-response curve for proliferation, Fig. 7. Such an auto-inhibition dose-response curve may indicate a receptive unit with two binding sites or two separate receptors for IPP of which an inhibitory site or receptor has the lowest association constant. The IPP auto-inhibitory relationship in figure 7 was analyzed with a homotropic two-state model, HOTSM [25]. Since the spontaneous activity in absence of IPP is almost zero and because data are limited, we used a simplified form of HOTSM with spontaneous activity equal to zero ($L = 0$). Equilibrium association constants for binding at a high affinity stimulatory site/receptor, A_s, and at a low affinity inhibitory site/receptor, A_m, were estimated by fitting of the HOTSM to data, yielding $A_s = 5.37+/-0.96$ and $A_m = 0.91+/-3.32$ (μM^{-1}) combined with a binding cooperativity coefficient $c = 0.105+/-1.48$ and a maximum fractional proliferation factor at 18.47+/−0.80. These data for auto-inhibition by IPP is compared and discussed with similar observations in the literature, see Discussion.

Synergistic and inhibitory effect of ethanol on proliferation of IPP stimulated γδ T cells

To further investigate the effects of ethanol on the proliferation of γδ T cells with IPP, we studied the auto-inhibition of IPP stimulated proliferation in the presence of ethanol. As shown in figure 7 there is a left-ward shift of the activated leg of IPP stimulated γδ T cells with low doses of ethanol. Since cotreatment with ethanol and IL2 did not stimulate γδ T cell expansion or proliferation more than IL2 alone as shown in Fig. 2, the ethanol enhancement of IPP stimulation resembles a synergistic rather than an additive effect of ethanol on IPP stimulation of γδ T cells. To document these potency effects of ethanol, we analyzed the shifts in dose-response curves of IPP-induced proliferation by ethanol with Michaelis-Menten kinetics. The potency effect, as an apparent decrease in the high-affinity EC_{50} values, is shown as an example in figure 7, where the leftward shift by adding 0.015% ethanol decreases the EC_{50} value fivefold from 0.19 μM+/−

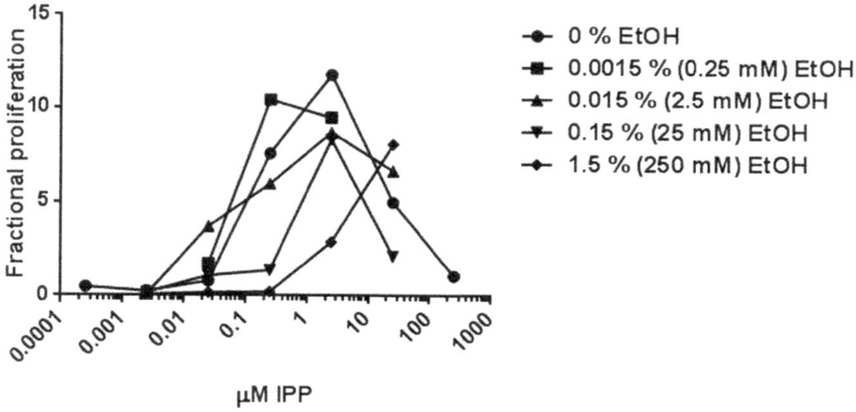

Figure 7. Effect of IPP in combination with ethanol on proliferation of γδ T cells. SFMC from patients with arthritis were stimulated for 7 days by varying concentrations of the agonist IPP and at different concentrations of the modulator ethanol together with IL2. The proliferations were determined for each combination. The data represents one single patient (no 12) and is one example of three performed experiments with similar results. Values are normalized to the absolute number of γδ T cells per culture well at start of experiment sat to unity.

0.036 µM to 0.04 µM+/−0.019 µM, the same as a fivefold increase in affinity for IPP, or its potency. In case ethanol has activity in its own right and also lifts the max IPP effect, this is an allo-ago-synergy or additive effect. Alternatively, if ethanol does not stimulate in its own right but still lifts the max IPP effect, it is an allo-synergy or classical synergy effect [28]. However, there is a decrease in the max IPP effect, seen in figure 7 as a decrease in the maximum number of proliferating γδ T cells in proportion to γδ T cells at start from 12.83+/−0.61 to 8.15+/−0.75, indicating a lower efficacy with ethanol. Thus ethanol, cause both enhancement with a lower EC_{50} value (leftward-shift of the left leg) and efficacy inhibition (lower max IPP effect) [28].

Response surface plots for concentration range of synergy

To better demonstrate possible synergistic effects of ethanol at various combinations of drug concentrations, we performed experiments to create response surface plots. We first prepared dose-response curves to illustrate the effect of either IPP or ethanol alone on proliferation, survival and expansion. Concentrations of either IPP (agonist) or ethanol (modulator) were then varied, while keeping the other at a constant concentration. These results are shown as examples of expansion, proliferation and survival of SF γδ T cells in figure 8. These plots are more for illustrative purposes than for calculating parameters.

An example of expansion is shown in figure 8A, where the maximal effect (plateau) is lifted by ethanol at concentrations between 10^3 and 10^4 µM in combination with IPP concentrations of around 10^{-3} and 10^{-4} µM, demonstrating a clear synergistic effect of ethanol on IPP-expansion. An example of the effects of ethanol on proliferation can be seen in figure 8B, where a maximal peak effect by IPP around 10^{-1} µM IPP is lowered (in general) with ethanol concentrations above 10^3 µM. Finally an example of survival is shown in figure 8C. IPP at low concentration in combination with ethanol can enhance the expansion, but as can be seen from the survival response surface plot, IPP and ethanol effects on survival have a rather complex interaction with several peaks indicating an intricate synergy. Presently we have no suggestion for possible mechanisms behind the observed synergy peaks on survival shown in figure 8C.

Effect of ethanol on expansion and proliferation of risedronate stimulated γδ T cells

It has been suggested that bisphosphonates stimulate γδ T cells indirectly by inhibiting farnesyl diphosphate synthase leading to the accumulation of endogenously produced IPP [17]. We therefore asked whether ethanol could enhance the expansion and proliferation of γδ T cells stimulated with bisphosphonate induced IPP. We found that ethanol has similar enhancing effect under these circumstances, Fig. 9. PBMC γδ T cells from healthy controls stimulated with 0.025 µM risedronate in combination with 0.015% ethanol showed a higher fractional expansion ($p < 0.016$, $n = 6$, Fig. 9 A1) and proliferation ($p < 0.016$, $n = 7$) compared with risedronate and IL2 alone. Ethanol and IL2 did not have any effects above IL2 alone. The effect of ethanol on risedronate stimulated γδ T cells could be seen already after 4 days (data not shown), and a great variation was found in the response between subjects, Fig. 9 A2. The enhancing effect of ethanol was further demonstrated in figure 9 B1–B2. The risedronate concentration 0.025 µM was chosen based on dose-response experiments, Fig. 9B and earlier studies [17,29].

Discussion

Our investigation shows that low to moderate doses of ethanol in presence of low concentrations of IPP can enhance the *in vitro* expansion of synovial fluid γδ T cells from patients with inflammatory arthritis. Several studies have documented the effect of ethanol on lymphocytes in blood from humans [24,30]. It has been shown that ethanol can augment mitogen-induced T cell proliferation with phytomhemagglutinin (PHA) and concanavalin A (ConA) [24]. PHA and ConA have also been shown to be γδ T cell stimulatory reagents [31,32] and PHA has been shown to give proliferative effect on T cells in synovial fluid [33]. It is therefore possible that ethanol may enhance or synergize other γδ T cell stimulatory reagents, beside IPP. To our knowledge, however, this is the first time results are obtained on ethanol stimulated proliferation of *synovial fluid* γδ T cells *in vitro* in humans at a blood alcohol concentration range equivalent to what is obtained with one or two glasses of wine. This knowledge may eventually lead to better diagnostics and treatment of arthritic diseases.

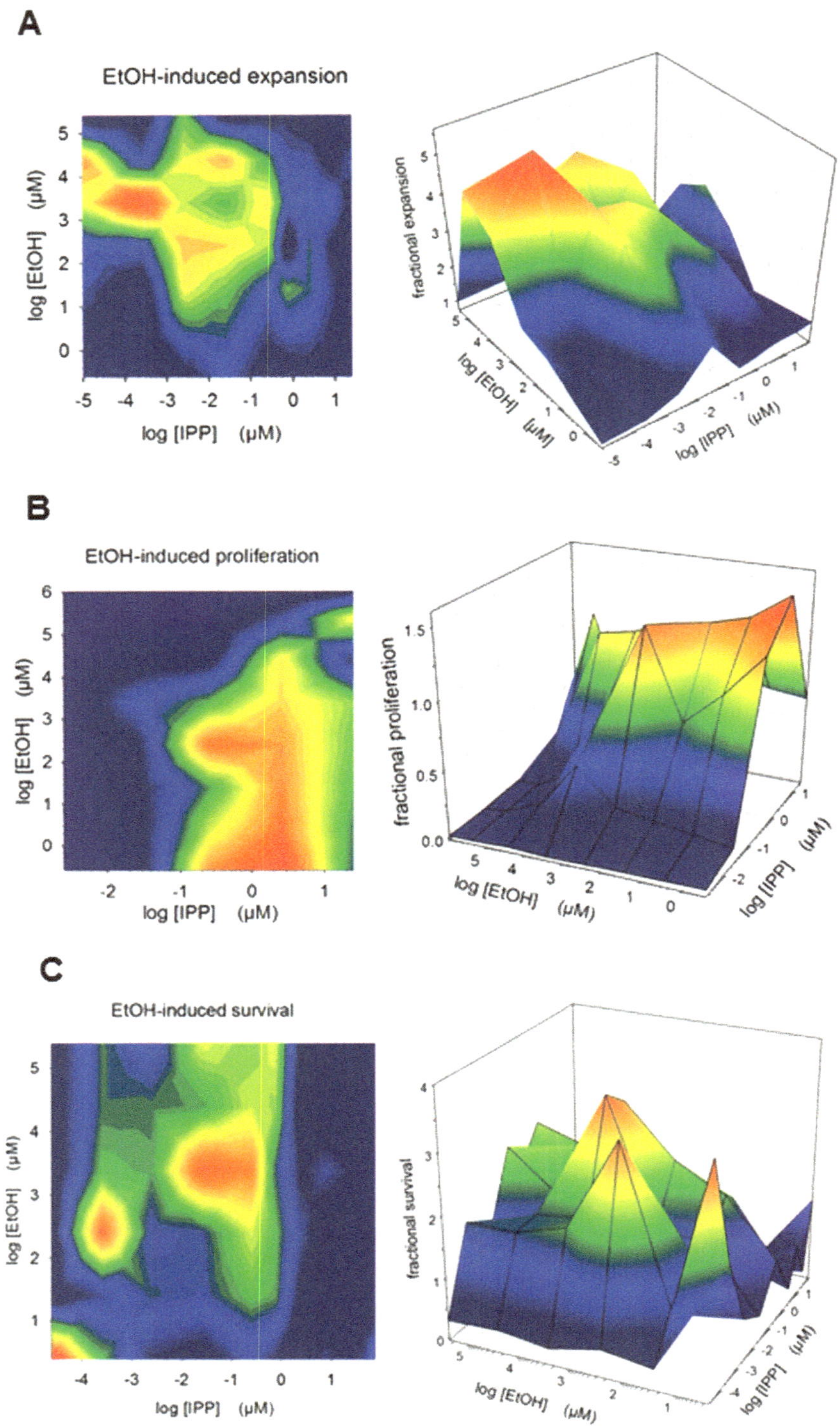

Figure 8. Effects of IPP in combination with ethanol on expansion, proliferation and survival of γδ T cells. SFMC from patients with arthritis were stimulated for 7 days with various concentrations of IPP and ethanol all in combination with IL2. The plots are representative of four independent experiments showing the fractional response normalized to 0.25 µM IPP = 1 for each combination, where the plots show A) expansion, data from patient no 15, B) proliferation, data from patient no 12 and C) survival, data from patient no 15.

Effects of IPP on expansion of SF γδ T cells

In this study SF γδ T cells showed proliferation capacity at 0.25 µM IPP, a response which is normally found for memory cells [34]. Indeed, γδ T cells from SF of patients with inflammatory arthritis are generally of a memory subtype [35]. There are essentially no cells in uninflamed healthy joint fluid [36], so control data from healthy patients are therefore not possible to present. However, our preliminary data indeed indicate that the ethanol

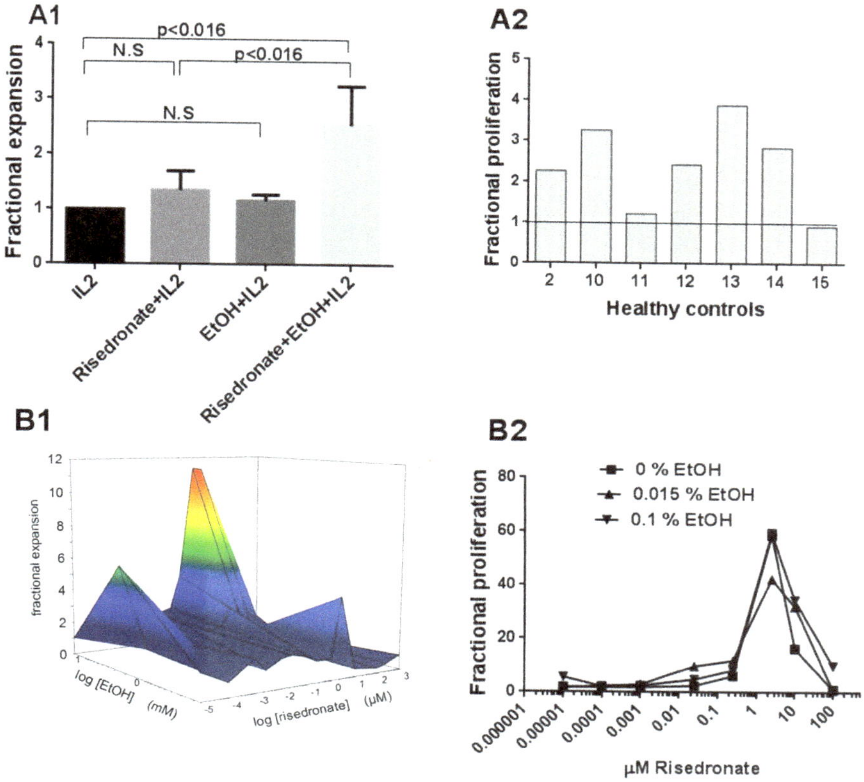

Figure 9. Expansion and proliferation of γδ T cells stimulated with risedronate and ethanol for 7 days. A) PBMCs from healthy controls were stimulated with 0.025 μM risedronate, 0.015% ethanol or 0.025 μM risedronate+0.015% ethanol, all in presence of IL2. A1) Fractional expansion, showing fold-increase of total number of PB γδ T cells, n = 6 from healthy controls. A2) Fractional proliferation, showing total number of CFSE^{low} PB γδ T cells from healthy controls, n = 7, all normalized to 0.025 μM risedronate = 1. The different growth conditions were compared using Wilcoxon signed rank test one-sided. Bars show means +/− SEM. B) PBMC from healthy controls were stimulated for 7 days with various concentrations of risedronate and ethanol all in combination with IL2. The plots are representative of three independent experiments showing the fractional response normalized to IL2 = 1 for each combination, where the plots show B1) expansion, data from healthy control no 2 and B2) proliferation, data from healthy control no 13.

enhancing effect is general, as we see similar effects on PBMC both from patients with arthritis (data not shown) as well as from healthy donors. Our results also show similar enhancing effects of ethanol on risedronate stimulated PBMCs from healthy donors. To our knowledge, there are currently no data available in the literature on the levels of IPP in plasma or in the inflamed joint *in vivo*, but farnesyl pyrophosphate has been measured in blood from healthy humans at a concentration of 0.017 μM [37], which is slightly below the concentration of IPP used in our study, 0.25 μM. SF αβ T cells from arthritic patients have shown a general hyporesponsiveness [38]. Meanwhile, other studies show proliferative response of SF γδ T cells in patients with arthritis stimulated with IPP [20,23], synthetic alkyl phosphates [39] or with eubacteria using the MEP pathway [1-deoxy-D-xylulose 5-phosphate (DXP) pathway] such as *Mycobacterium tuberculosis* [33] and *Yersinia enterocolitica* [40,41]. Further studies are needed to determine the IPP levels *in vivo* in the synovial fluid and the synovial lining in patients with arthritis.

A possible homotropic allostery of IPP proliferation

Studying a range of IPP concentrations, we observed a bell-shaped dose-response of SF γδ T cell proliferation with a maximum at around 1 μM IPP, Fig. 7. We question if concentrations above 1 μM of IPP are toxic for SF γδ T cells or have a regulatory function, thereby balancing their proliferation. In case IPP at higher concentrations down-regulate proliferation it may be due to an inhibitory modulation through binding to a low affinity site. Bell-shaped dose-response curves are often observed in effectors as receptors, transporters and enzymes when an agonist itself binds to a modulator site and thereby affects its own function. Our observation of a bell-shaped proliferation induced by IPP is consistent with other studies, e.g., the study by Dieli et al [34] demonstrating bell-shaped IPP-induced proliferation of Vδ2 T cells in blood from healthy individuals. In another study, Tanaka and coworkers showed bell-shaped proliferation of SF γδ T cells with alkyl phosphates [39]. The lowered proliferation at higher IPP concentrations could be due to IPP binding to an inhibitory allosteric receptor site with low affinity, or due to a stimulatory allosteric site that activates cell death, possibly by death signals including Fas/FasL and others [42]. In Dieli's study [34] naïve γδ T cells show a bell-shaped dose-response as well, although it has been shown that naïve T cells do not express FasL [43]. Accordingly, we assume that there can be alternative explanations for the bell-shaped dose-response besides activation by Fas/FasL.

Therefore, due to the lack of a clear explanation for the bi-phasic effect, we suggest that the observed bell-shaped IPP dose-response relation covers regulatory auto-inhibition, homotropic allostery, and may be analyzed by a homotropic two-state model, HOTSM. HOTSM is an auto-regulatory reaction scheme with spontaneous activity, Fig. 10 [25]. Table 2 lists fitted values for

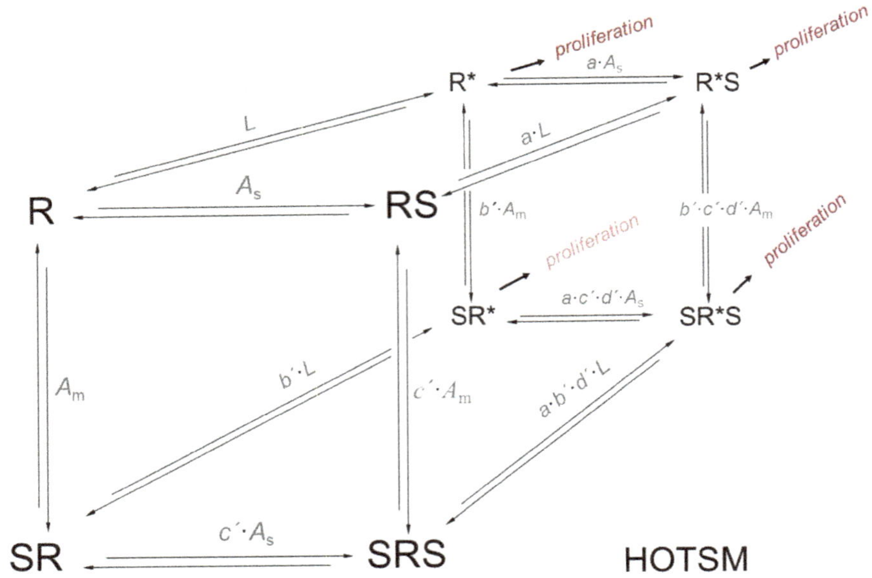

Figure 10. Homotrophic two-state model, HOTSM. An agonist or substrate, S, can bind to two sterically separate sites in a receptor R. An unbound receptor in such a system can be in two conformations, an inactive form, R, and active form, R*. The displayed HOTSM is a thermodynamically complete reaction scheme for such a system. Bell-shaped dose-response relations, as for the IPP effect on $\gamma\delta$ T cell proliferation, may be analyzed according to this HOTSM scheme. S = agonist. R and R* are receptor in inactive and active conformations respectively. L = the isomerization constant between unbound R* and R, L = R*/R. A_s = the equilibrium association constant for S at the orthosteric site of R. A_m = is equilibrium association constant for S at the allosteric site of R. a = efficacy constant for RS ⇄ R*S when S is already bound to the orthosteric site. b = efficacy constant for SR ⇄ SR* when S is already bound to the allosteric site. c = co-operativity coefficient for binding of S at either site to an already liganded R. d = co-operativity coefficient for efficacy induced by one ligand on binding when another ligand is already bound to R*s or an efficacy coefficient when two ligands are already bound

HOTSM parameters A_s, A_m and c for the IPP bell-shaped response in our study. These values fall within the range of values for the same parameters extracted with the HOTSM from the study by Dieli et al [34]. We note that the values of A_s, A_m and c for IPP from the bell-shaped profile in this study are within less than a factor of 10 of those for the memory CD45RA$^-$CD27$^+$ cells studied by Dieli et al. Much higher concentrations of IPP as well induced a bell-shaped proliferation of naïve Vδ2 T cells [34], probably due to lower affinity constants compared to memory cells. Thus, the same parameter values for naïve cells in their study are off by factors of more than 500, Table 2.

A possible mechanism for synergistic effects of ethanol and IPP

Ethanol may act not only through the disordering of lipids in cell membranes [44], but also more specifically on enzymes and ion channels [45]. Ethanol has low binding affinity to proteins, thus normally concentrations 15 to 150 mM are required for detectable binding, although alcohol binding to alcohol-dehydrogenase is in a low millimolar concentration range [45].

With low doses of IPP present, we show an increased proliferation of SF $\gamma\delta$ T cells by adding a moderate dose of 0.015% (2.5 mM) ethanol, Fig. 2B1 and 3A. This concentration of alcohol lies within the blood alcohol concentration range reached when alcohol is consumed socially, while it is more than three

Table 2. Best fit values for parameters of the homotropic two-state model, HOTSM, based on IPP-proliferation of $\gamma\delta$ T cells.

Parameter	Dieli 1 (memory)	Present study	Dieli 2 (naïve)
A_s (μM^{-1})	52.2	5.37	0.0104
A_m (μM^{-1})	0.321	0.912	0.000309
c (factor)	0.373	0.105	0.350
Proliferation	52.8 (cpm·10^{-3})	18.5 (fractional)	29.4 (cpm·10^{-3})

Values for equilibrium association constants A_s and A_m and the cooperative binding constant c were extracted by fitting the HOTSM relation [25] to bell-shaped dose-response curves of IPP activation-inhibition of $\gamma\delta$ T cell proliferation from this study and data in the literature [34], Fig. 4A. As our experiments indicated almost no response in the absence of ligands IPP and EtOH, parameter L was kept at zero symbolizing no spontaneous activity. Values for our proliferative response of T cells - most likely as memory CD45RA$^-$CD27$^+$ cells - to IPP in a concentration range from 3×10^{-3} to 3×10^{2} µM are within a factor of 10 to the data set for memory cells in Dieli et al's 2003 study, columns 2 and 1.

orders above the normal 15 μM of ethanol in blood [46]. Further, we show that SF γδ T cells expand more, Fig. 4A, that non-proliferating SF γδ T cells survive better, Fig. 4B, and that SF αβ T cells increase in numbers when a low dose of ethanol is added together with IPP, Fig. 5A.

Figure 7 shows the effects of combining ethanol with the IPP-induced bell-shaped response on proliferation of SF γδ T cells. In the presence of moderate doses of ethanol, the width of the IPP bell-shaped response is broadened both left and right. At the bell's left leg with low doses of IPP present there is an enhanced proliferation at moderate doses of ethanol on the expansion of SF γδ T cells. This indicates an ethanol-induced increase in affinity for IPP. At the bell's right leg with high doses of IPP, there is a shift to the right in the presence of moderate doses of ethanol. This points to a decrease in the IPP affinity at an inhibitory site for IPP, elicited as a mixed inhibition by ethanol. In the HOTSM for IPP, these effects of alcohol may be interpreted as an increase in parameter A_s ($1/EC_{50}$) and a decrease in parameter A_m ($1/IC_{50}$) for IPP when adding ethanol. Further, the peak of the IPP-induced bell-shaped response is lowered by moderated doses of ethanol, Fig. 7. This may be interpreted either as an effect on the cooperative binding coefficient c for IPP induced by ethanol at both IPP binding sites or as an ethanol-induced proportional down-regulation of both types of IPP receptors due to the symmetry of reduction. Thus, if our model for the combined effects of IPP and ethanol is valid, ethanol binding at a single site elicits synergistic conformational changes in both a stimulatory and an inhibitory site for IPP-regulated proliferation.

Meanwhile, we cannot exclude that the shift to the left by ethanol of the bell-shaped curve in figure 7 is due to a bitopic ligand formed by IPP and ethanol or their metabolites such as acetaldehyde. Our results show that ethanol has an enhancing effect on IPP stimulated γδ T cell expansion, also when endogenous IPP is generated by pharmacological means, using risedronate. Earlier studies have shown that IPP generated from bisphosphonates may react with metabolites forming new compounds [47]. Future studies may clarify if this may be an explanation for our results. Alternatively, the observed left-ward shift may indicate binding sites at low concentrations of both compounds, where a putative binding site for ethanol is either upstream or downstream of the binding sites for IPP proliferation.

When increasing the concentration of ethanol above 25 mM, the IPP bell-shaped response in figure 7 is lowered from its maximum. We would have expected an increase in proliferation of IPP stimulated γδ T cells at these concentrations since earlier studies have shown an enhancing effect on mitogen-activated T cells at a concentration of 150 mM ethanol [24]. Our findings at the higher ligand concentrations indicate mixed competition between IPP and ethanol [28]. Other studies have shown that ethanol by stimulating cyclic adenosine monophosphate (cAMP) can activate protein kinase A (PKA) which would block γδ T cell proliferation via the mitogen-activated protein kinase (MAPK) pathway. Meanwhile, ethanol up to 200 mM may have an effect on cAMP without activating PKA [24,48]. It is possible that the effects of ethanol on cAMP in the presence of IPP can give signals via MAPK by a different route such as via exchange proteins activated by cAMP (EPAC), or protein kinase C (PKC) and escape the blockade from PKA [49,50], thereby also overcoming the inhibitory effects of prostaglandin E2 (PGE_2) on γδ T cell proliferation and cytotoxicity described in other studies [51,52].

Effects of low concentrations of ethanol and IPP on proliferation of different T cell populations

Ethanol may have different effects on different T cell populations. Other studies have shown that ethanol at 150 mM *in vitro* can augment mitogen-induced T cell proliferation in human blood stimulated with mitogens, ConA or PHA [24], but a lower concentration of 25 mM of ethanol could at the same time inhibit proliferation of activated antigen-specific T cells [24]. Because γδ T cells are not MHC dependent, an enhancing effect of ethanol on expansion of γδ T cells together with IPP could be expected. In this study we also found an increased proliferation of αβ T cells when low to moderate levels of ethanol together with low concentration of IPP was added. Transient increases in αβ T cells have also been found in studies of macaques when stimulated with HMBPP [53]. It is conceivable that if γδ T cells secrete IL2, an increased number of IL2 secreting SF γδ T cells could also stimulate an expansion of SF αβ T cells.

Effects of ethanol on cytokine production

Central memory T_{CM} cells ($CD45RA^-CD27^+$) can be further differentiated into different effector subgroups such as effector memory T_{EMh} cells ($CD45RA^-CD27^-$) which are perforin^{low} IFN-γ^{high}, resembling the Th1 cells, or the more cytotoxic T_{EMRA} cells ($CD45RA^+CD27^-$) which are IFN-γ^{low} and perforin^{high} [54]. In one study, IPP stimulation of SF cells from juvenile arthritis gave an increased proportion of IFN-γ cells [23]. Another study has shown that stimulation with IPP only of memory PB γδ T $CD45RA^-CD27^+$ cells in arthritis expands T_{EM} $CD45RA^-CD27^-$ after 7–14 days in culture [35]. In contrast, in our study we found that SF γδ and αβ T cells did not respond with increased IFN-γ secretion when stimulated with the lower concentrations of IPP with or without ethanol. Our preliminary results show instead that adding ethanol gives the more cytotoxic perforin producing T_{EMRA} cells (preliminary results, data not shown). Effector cytokines such as perforin produced at the peak expansion coinciding with the increase in αβ T has been found also in the study with macaques stimulated with HMBPP [53].

The benefit of alcohol to treat rheumatoid arthritis has been known for a long time. Aquavit as a remedy for alleviation of arthritic pain was described already in a booklet from 1843 [55]. "Drink a spoonful each morning for several weeks and scrub it with help of a brush to the painful parts each morning and evening". What the inventor of the aquavit treatment, William Lee, did not know, was that his prescription may have an effect on the activation of γδ T cells. Indeed the prescribed amount of ethanol is likely to be within the range of a stimulating concentration on Vδ2 T cells. Thus, our findings provide a possible mechanistic explanation for the historical observation of William Lee.

In conclusion, we have demonstrated that an ethanol concentration equivalent to one glass of wine can enhance expansion of IPP stimulated γδ T cells. If these expanded γδ T cells can target FLS this could be one explanation of the protective role of ethanol in arthritis and possibly in other diseases as well.

Acknowledgments

The authors gratefully acknowledge Assistant Professor Alexander Espinosa and Professor Henrik Dohlman for stimulating consultations and valuable comments on the manuscript; PhD Catarina Björklund, Lab Manager Peri Noori, MD Hristo Zlatev and Professor Seppo Auriola for helpful advice and contributions, Professor Jouko Vepsäläinen for the generous gift of risedronate and the volunteers for their kind participation in the study.

Author Contributions

Conceived and designed the experiments: AL NB LB. Performed the experiments: AL. Analyzed the data: AL NB BJ LB. Contributed reagents/materials/analysis tools: NB LB. Wrote the paper: AL NB BJ LB.

References

1. Klareskog L, Catrina AI, Paget S (2009) Rheumatoid arthritis. Lancet 373: 659–672.
2. Noss EH, Brenner MB (2008) The role and therapeutic implications of fibroblast-like synoviocytes in inflammation and cartilage erosion in rheumatoid arthritis. Immunol Rev 223: 252–270.
3. Ronksley PE, Brien SE, Turner BJ, Mukamal KJ, Ghali WA (2011) Association of alcohol consumption with selected cardiovascular disease outcomes: a systematic review and meta-analysis. BMJ 342: d671.
4. Hazes JM, Dijkmans BA, Vandenbroucke JP, de Vries RR, Cats A (1990) Lifestyle and the risk of rheumatoid arthritis: cigarette smoking and alcohol consumption. Ann Rheum Dis 49: 980–982.
5. Aho K, Heliovaara M (1993) Alcohol, androgens and arthritis. Ann Rheum Dis 52: 897.
6. Voigt LF, Koepsell TD, Nelson JL, Dugowson CE, Daling JR (1994) Smoking, obesity, alcohol consumption, and the risk of rheumatoid arthritis. Epidemiology 5: 525–532.
7. Myllykangas-Luosujarvi R, Aho K, Kautiainen H, Hakala M (2000) Reduced incidence of alcohol related deaths in subjects with rheumatoid arthritis. Ann Rheum Dis 59: 75–76.
8. Cerhan JR, Saag KG, Criswell LA, Merlino LA, Mikuls TR (2002) Blood transfusion, alcohol use, and anthropometric risk factors for rheumatoid arthritis in older women. J Rheumatol 29: 246–254.
9. Pedersen M, Jacobsen S, Klarlund M, Pedersen BV, Wiik A, et al. (2006) Environmental risk factors differ between rheumatoid arthritis with and without auto-antibodies against cyclic citrullinated peptides. Arthritis Res Ther 8: R133.
10. Kallberg H, Jacobsen S, Bengtsson C, Pedersen M, Padyukov L, et al. (2009) Alcohol consumption is associated with decreased risk of rheumatoid arthritis: results from two Scandinavian case-control studies. Ann Rheum Dis 68: 222–227.
11. Maxwell JR, Gowers IR, Moore DJ, Wilson AG (2010) Alcohol consumption is inversely associated with risk and severity of rheumatoid arthritis. Rheumatology (Oxford) 49: 2140–2146.
12. Di Giuseppe D, Alfredsson L, Bottai M, Askling J, Wolk A (2012) Long term alcohol intake and risk of rheumatoid arthritis in women: a population based cohort study. BMJ 345: e4230.
13. Scott IC, Tan R, Stahl D, Steer S, Lewis CM, et al. (2013) The protective effect of alcohol on developing rheumatoid arthritis: a systematic review and meta-analysis. Rheumatology (Oxford) 52: 856–867.
14. Jonsson IM, Verdrengh M, Brisslert M, Lindblad S, Bokarewa M, et al. (2007) Ethanol prevents development of destructive arthritis. Proc Natl Acad Sci U S A 104: 258–263.
15. Morita CT, Jin C, Sarikonda G, Wang H (2007) Nonpeptide antigens, presentation mechanisms, and immunological memory of human Vgamma2V-delta2 T cells: discriminating friend from foe through the recognition of prenyl pyrophosphate antigens. Immunol Rev 215: 59–76.
16. Hayday AC (2000) [gamma][delta] cells: a right time and a right place for a conserved third way of protection. Annu Rev Immunol 18: 975–1026.
17. Wang H, Sarikonda G, Puan KJ, Tanaka Y, Feng J, et al. (2011) Indirect stimulation of human Vgamma2Vdelta2 T cells through alterations in isoprenoid metabolism. J Immunol 187: 5099–5113.
18. Bank I, Cohen L, Mouallem M, Farfel Z, Grossman E, et al. (2002) gammadelta T cell subsets in patients with arthritis and chronic neutropenia. Ann Rheum Dis 61: 438–443.
19. Lunardi C, Marguerie C, Walport MJ, So AK (1992) T gamma delta cells and their subsets in blood and synovial fluid from patients with rheumatoid arthritis. Br J Rheumatol 31: 527–530.
20. Berkun Y, Bendersky A, Gerstein M, Goldstein I, Padeh S, et al. (2011) GammadeltaT cells in juvenile idiopathic arthritis: higher percentages of synovial Vdelta1+ and Vgamma9+ T cell subsets are associated with milder disease. J Rheumatol 38: 1123–1129.
21. Bottini N, Firestein GS (2013) Duality of fibroblast-like synoviocytes in RA: passive responders and imprinted aggressors. Nat Rev Rheumatol 9: 24–33.
22. Bendersky A, Markovits N, Bank I (2010) Vgamma9+ gammadelta T cells in systemic sclerosis patients are numerically and functionally preserved and induce fibroblast apoptosis. Immunobiology 215: 380–394.
23. Bendersky A, Marcu-Malina V, Berkun Y, Gerstein M, Nagar M, et al. (2012) Cellular interactions of synovial fluid gammadelta T cells in juvenile idiopathic arthritis. J Immunol 188: 4349–4359.
24. Szabo G, Verma B, Catalano D (1993) Selective inhibition of antigen-specific T lymphocyte proliferation by acute ethanol exposure: the role of impaired monocyte antigen presentation capacity and mediator production. J Leukoc Biol 54: 534–544.
25. Bindslev N (2004) A homotropic two-state model and auto-antagonism. BMC Pharmacol 4: 11.
26. Siegel JA, Saukko PJ, Knupfer GC (2000) Encyclopedia of forensic sciences. San Diego: Academic Press.
27. Deenick EK, Gett AV, Hodgkin PD (2003) Stochastic model of T cell proliferation: a calculus revealing IL-2 regulation of precursor frequencies, cell cycle time, and survival. J Immunol 170: 4963–4972.
28. Bindslev N (2013) Allosteric transition: a comparison of two models. BMC Pharmacol Toxicol 14: 4.
29. Das H, Wang L, Kamath A, Bukowski JF (2001) Vgamma2Vdelta2 T-cell receptor-mediated recognition of aminobisphosphonates. Blood 98: 1616–1618.
30. Atkinson JP, Sullivan TJ, Kelly JP, Parker CW (1977) Stimulation by alcohols of cyclic AMP metabolism in human leukocytes. Possible role of cyclic AMP in the anti-inflammatory effects of ethanol. J Clin Invest 60: 284–294.
31. Bukowski JF, Morita CT, Brenner MB (1994) Recognition and destruction of virus-infected cells by human gamma delta CTL. J Immunol 153: 5133–5140.
32. Siegers GM, Felizardo TC, Mathieson AM, Kosaka Y, Wang XH, et al. (2011) Anti-leukemia activity of in vitro-expanded human gamma delta T cells in a xenogeneic Ph+ leukemia model. PLoS One 6: e16700.
33. Holoshitz J, Koning F, Coligan JE, De Bruyn J, Strober S (1989) Isolation of CD4- CD8- mycobacteria-reactive T lymphocyte clones from rheumatoid arthritis synovial fluid. Nature 339: 226–229.
34. Dieli F, Poccia F, Lipp M, Sireci G, Caccamo N, et al. (2003) Differentiation of effector/memory Vdelta2 T cells and migratory routes in lymph nodes or inflammatory sites. J Exp Med 198: 391–397.
35. Hu C, Qian L, Miao Y, Huang Q, Miao P, et al. (2012) Antigen-presenting effects of effector memory Vgamma9Vdelta2 T cells in rheumatoid arthritis. Cell Mol Immunol 9: 245–254.
36. van de Putte LB, Meijer CJ, Lafeber GJ, Kleinjan R, Cats A (1975) Lymphocytes in rheumatoid and nonrheumatoid synovial fluids. Nonspecificity of high T-cell and low B-cell percentages. Ann Rheum Dis 35: 451–455.
37. Saisho Y, Morimoto A, Umeda T (1997) Determination of farnesyl pyrophosphate in dog and human plasma by high-performance liquid chromatography with fluorescence detection. Anal Biochem 252: 89–95.
38. Emery P, Panayi GS, Nouri AM (1984) Interleukin-2 reverses deficient cell-mediated immune responses in rheumatoid arthritis. Clin Exp Immunol 57: 123–129.
39. Tanaka Y, Sano S, Nieves E, De Libero G, Rosa D, et al. (1994) Nonpeptide ligands for human gamma delta T cells. Proc Natl Acad Sci U S A 91: 8175–8179.
40. Young JL, Goodall JC, Beacock-Sharp H, Gaston JS (1997) Human gamma delta T-cell recognition of Yersinia enterocolitica. Immunology 91: 503–510.
41. Hermann E, Lohse AW, Mayet WJ, van der Zee R, Van Eden W, et al. (1992) Stimulation of synovial fluid mononuclear cells with the human 65-kD heat shock protein or with live enterobacteria leads to preferential expansion of TCR-gamma delta+ lymphocytes. Clin Exp Immunol 89: 427–433.
42. Kabelitz D, Janssen O (1997) Antigen-induced death of T-lymphocytes. Front Biosci 2: d61–77.
43. Hamann D, Baars PA, Rep MH, Hooibrink B, Kerkhof-Garde SR, et al. (1997) Phenotypic and functional separation of memory and effector human CD8+ T cells. J Exp Med 186: 1407–1418.
44. Szabo G, Dolganiuc A, Dai Q, Pruett SB (2007) TLR4, ethanol, and lipid rafts: a new mechanism of ethanol action with implications for other receptor-mediated effects. J Immunol 178: 1243–1249.
45. Harris RA, Trudell JR, Mihic SJ (2008) Ethanol's molecular targets. Sci Signal 1: re7.
46. Geigy Scientific Tables, 8th Rev edition, pp 165–177. Edited by C Lentner, West Cadwell, N.J.: Medical education Div., Ciba-Geigy Corp., Basel, Switzerland c 1981–11992.
47. Monkkonen H, Auriola S, Lehenkari P, Kellinsalmi M, Hassinen IE, et al. (2006) A new endogenous ATP analog (ApppI) inhibits the mitochondrial adenine nucleotide translocase (ANT) and is responsible for the apoptosis induced by nitrogen-containing bisphosphonates. Br J Pharmacol 147: 437–445.
48. Yoshimura M, Tabakoff B (1999) Ethanol's actions on cAMP-mediated signaling in cells transfected with type VII adenylyl cyclase. Alcohol Clin Exp Res 23: 1457–1461.
49. Gerits N, Kostenko S, Shiryaev A, Johannessen M, Moens U (2008) Relations between the mitogen-activated protein kinase and the cAMP-dependent protein kinase pathways: comradeship and hostility. Cell Signal 20: 1592–1607.
50. Nedellec S, Bonneville M, Scotet E (2010) Human Vgamma9Vdelta2 T cells: from signals to functions. Semin Immunol 22: 199–206.
51. Martinet L, Fleury-Cappellesso S, Gadelorge M, Dietrich G, Bourin P, et al. (2009) A regulatory cross-talk between Vgamma9Vdelta2 T lymphocytes and mesenchymal stem cells. Eur J Immunol 39: 752–762.
52. Martinet L, Jean C, Dietrich G, Fournie JJ, Poupot R (2010) PGE2 inhibits natural killer and gamma delta T cell cytotoxicity triggered by NKR and TCR

through a cAMP-mediated PKA type I-dependent signaling. Biochem Pharmacol 80: 838–845.
53. Ali Z, Shao L, Halliday L, Reichenberg A, Hintz M, et al. (2007) Prolonged (E)-4-hydroxy-3-methyl-but-2-enyl pyrophosphate-driven antimicrobial and cytotoxic responses of pulmonary and systemic Vgamma2Vdelta2 T cells in macaques. J Immunol 179: 8287–8296.
54. Angelini DF, Borsellino G, Poupot M, Diamantini A, Poupot R, et al. (2004) FcgammaRIII discriminates between 2 subsets of Vgamma9Vdelta2 effector cells with different responses and activation pathways. Blood 104: 1801–1807.
55. Lee W (1843) Bränwin och salt, ett läkemedel emot gikt, rheumatism, asthma, lungsot och andra åkommor, uppfunnet af William Lee, Esq. med Tillägg innehållande sednare upplysningar, utdragna af ett i England nyligen utkommet läkarvetenskapligt verk öfver denna kurmethod. Translated from English. Christiania. PT Mallings förlag.

3

Mannose Binding Lectin and Susceptibility to Rheumatoid Arthritis in Brazilian Patients and Their Relatives

Isabela Goeldner[1,2], Thelma L. Skare[3], Shirley R. Utiyama[1], Renato M. Nisihara[1], Hoang van Tong[2], Iara J. T. Messias-Reason[¶1*], Thirumalaisamy P. Velavan[¶2,4*]

1 Department of Medical Pathology, Federal University of Paraná, Curitiba, Brazil, **2** Institute of Tropical Medicine, University of Tübingen, Tübingen, Germany, **3** Rheumatology Unit, Evangelical Hospital, Curitiba, Brazil, **4** Fondation Congolaise pour la Recherche Medicale, Brazzaville, Republic of Congo

Abstract

Introduction: Rheumatoid arthritis (RA) is a commonly occurring systemic inflammatory auto immune disease and is believed to be associated with genetic factors. The innate immune complement protein Mannose binding lectin (MBL) and their *MBL2* genetic variants are associated with different infectious and autoimmune diseases.

Methods: In a Brazilian cohort, we aim to associate the functional role of circulating MBL serum levels and *MBL2* variants in clinically classified patients (n = 196) with rheumatoid arthritis including their relatives (n = 200) and ethnicity matched healthy controls (n = 200). MBL serum levels were measured by ELISA and functional *MBL2* variants were genotyped by direct sequencing.

Results: The exon1+54 *MBL2**B* variant was significantly associated with an increased risk and the reconstructed haplotype *MBL2**LYPB* was associated with RA susceptibility. Circulating serum MBL levels were observed significantly lower in RA patients compared to their relatives and controls. No significant contribution of MBL levels were observed with respect to functional class, age at disease onset, disease duration and/or other clinical parameters such as nodules, secondary Sjögren syndrome, anti-CCP and rheumatoid factor. Differential distribution of serum MBL levels with functional *MBL2* variants was observed in respective RA patients and their relatives.

Conclusions: Our results suggest MBL levels as a possible marker for RA susceptibility in a Brazilian population.

Editor: Cordula M. Stover, University of Leicester, United Kingdom

Funding: This work was partially supported by grants from the Araucária Foundation (No. 412/2009, protocol 5103), as well as by fellowship from the Coordination for the Improvement of Higher Level Personnel (CAPES). The authors acknowledge the partial support by the Open Access Publishing Fund of Tuebingen University. The funders had no role in study design, data collection and analysis, decision to publish, or preparation of the manuscript.

Competing Interests: The authors have declared that no competing interests exist.

* E-mail: velavan@medizin.uni-tuebingen.de (TPV); iarareason@hc.ufpr.br (IJTMR)

¶These authors share the last authorship.

Introduction

Rheumatoid arthritis (RA) is one of the most common inflammatory rheumatic diseases and is closely related to significant increase in healthcare costs and social burden [1]. The early diagnosis and appropriate management of the disease have been established as an effective strategy to minimize the risk of complications and co-morbidities. Nevertheless, tools for RA early diagnosis are still scarce [2]. Genetic factors contribute to at least 60% of the risk of developing this disease [3–5] and relatives have an increased risk to develop RA and other autoimmune diseases [6–8]. Although extensive research into the pathogenesis of RA, many aspects of the disease are still unclear and the main cause of RA remains unknown.

Complement system is a key component of the innate immunity. The lectin pathway is one of the three pathways of the complement system and can be triggered by pattern-recognition receptors, mainly mannose-biding lectin (MBL), ficolins and collectin 11 [9]. These innate recognitions elements such as MBL and ficolins were associated with susceptibility to various clinical infectious diseases [10–14]. These proteins bind to pathogen- or damage-associated molecular patterns and together with MBL-associated serine proteases, activates a cascade of events resulting in membrane attack complex. Although the complement system plays a vital role in pathogen recognition and elimination, there is substantial evidence on its contribution towards immune homeostasis [15]. It recognizes self and nonself antigens and is believed to modulate immunological tolerance towards self antigens avoiding auto immune reactions. Complement system has been related to the development and clinical presentation of many autoimmune diseases [16–18].

The etiology of RA is believed to be influenced by genetic and immunological factors. During RA, our own immune system attacks and causes inflammation. The inflammatory process modulates the glycosylation profile of IgG antibodies [19]. Studies have shown that MBL interacts with the IgG G0 glycoform through the exposed GlcNac and thus activating the complement system [20]. Studies have suggested that decreased galactosylation of IgG with high expression MBL2 genotypes are involved in the pathophysiology of RA [21]. Lectin pathway has been involved in the pathology of many rheumatological disorders [22]. In RA, immune complexes are recognized by MBL, leading to complement activation and intense inflammatory response. In this context, higher MBL levels exacerbate complement activation in rheumatic joints, accelerating articular destruction and worsening prognosis [23]. Moreover, high MBL levels have been already related to cardiovascular commitment and premature death in these patients [24]. Interestingly, MBL serum levels were suggested to be elevated in RA patients compared to their first degree relatives, thus revealing their potential significance as a susceptibility marker [25]. On the other hand, low MBL levels have been related to earlier RA development and poor prognosis [26–29].

The human MBL encoded on *MBL2* gene is located on chromosome 10. Three single nucleotide polymorphisms (SNPs) in the exon1 of the human *MBL2* gene at codons 52 (*p.Arg52Cys, MBL2*D*), 54 (*p.Dly54Asp, MBL2*B*), and 57 (*p.Gly57Glu, MBL2*C*), interfere with the formation of higher *MBL* oligomers. These genetic variants modulate the functional activity of the MBL protein and their circulating levels in addition to reduced binding that affects the complement activation [30–34]. In addition, two strongly linked SNPs in the proximal promoter (−551 L/H and −221 X/Y), as well as a SNP in the 5′UTR (+4 P/Q); together are linked to three independent non-synonymous SNPs (i.e. *MBL2*B, C* and *D*) and had been shown to partially account for alterations in complement activation and decreased circulating levels of MBL [35]. In particular, a base substitution at −221 (G to C; promoter allele *X*) is associated with lower MBL serum concentration [36]. Studies have documented that these SNPs contribute to the circulating levels against the seven common secretor haplotypes (namely *HYPA, HYPD, LXPA, LYPA, LYPB, LYQA* and *LYQC*) [36]. The *HYPA, LYQA* and *LYPA* are associated with high expression of MBL protein whereas *LXPA, HYPD, LYPB* and *LYQC* are associated with low expression of the MBL [37]. The variant alleles have been designated as *O* haplotype, whereas the common *MBL2* allele is designated as *A* [30]. A total of 24 allelic haplotypes were predefined for *MBL2* [38]. Functional MBL deficiency occurs mostly in *MBL2*B/B* or *MBL2*B/C* carriers whereas the *MBL2*D* variant has less influence on MBL structure [32]. The functional *MBL2* alleles and their respective haplotypes have been distributed as different geographical patterns in world populations [39]. Different population specific alleles have shown to contribute to different clinical significance on infectious and auto immune diseases [34]. In the present study, we analyzed the functional role of *MBL2* genetic variants (two strongly linked SNPs in the proximal promoter, one in the 5′UTR and three in exon1) and circulating serum MBL levels and investigate their possible role as a marker for susceptibility and prognosis for RA in a Brazilian cohort.

Materials and Methods

Patients

One-hundred and ninety-six (n = 196) adult RA patients were consecutively included from August 2007 till April 2009. All were diagnosed RA according to the American College of Rheumatology (ACR) criteria [40]. Clinical and demographic data were obtained from medical records and interviews using a standard questionnaire (Table 1). Steinbrocker functional classification was applied to determine the extent of physical disability in RA patients. According to this index of disease activity, patients are classified on a four-level scale, ranging from class I (complete functional capacity to carry out all usual duties) to class IV (largely or wholly incapacitated). In the present study, classes III and IV were grouped due to the low number of patients in each representative class. The anti-cyclic citrullinated peptide (anti-CCP) is auto antibody which is used as surrogate markers for diagnosis and prognosis in RA. The Anti-CCP and rheumatoid factor were determined according to standard procedures described elsewhere [6]. Two hundred relatives (n = 200) were also enrolled on this study based on their mutual consent and donated blood samples after their signed consent. Demographic data and articular symptoms suggestive of RA (swollen or tender joints) were investigated using a questionnaire and clinical examination (Table 1). Two hundred healthy matched unrelated individuals (n = 200) from the same geographical area were used as a control group.

Ethnicity was defined according to physical characteristics and informed ethnic background and divided in European; African or Amerindian ancestry. Considering the same ascendency definition, Euro-Brazilians from Southern Brazil have genotype distribution of *MBL2* haplotypes homogeneous with the *MBL2* genotype distribution of most European populations, whereas Afro-Brazilians are similar to eastern Africans [41]. Three ml of venous blood was collected with anticoagulant EDTA. The samples were centrifuged at 800 g for 15 minutes, sera and buffy coat was stored as aliquots at −80°C until used. DNA was extracted from peripheral blood mononuclear cells through DNAzol genomic DNA isolation reagent (Molecular Research Center, Inc., Cincinnati, EUA) according to the manufacturer's instruction.

Ethical Statement

Informed written consent was obtained from all study participants or from the parents, whose child was less than 18 years of age. This study was approved by the Ethics Research Committee of the Sociedade Evangélica Beneficiente, Curitiba, Brazil.

MBL2 Genotyping

MBL2 polymorphisms at promoter [−550G/C (H/L), −221G/C (Y/X) and 5′UTR +4C/T (P/Q)] and in exon 1 at codons [52C/T (*MBL2*D*), 54G/A (*MBL2*B*) and 57G/A (*MBL2*C*)] were amplified by PCR and subsequently sequenced utilizing appropriate primers. A 696 bp fragment in the promoter region was amplified using the primer pairs MBL-PromF (5′-GGCCAACGTAGTAAGAAATTTCCAGAGA-3′) and MBL-PromR (5′-GAGGGAGTGATGGAAACAGGGACA-3′). In brief: 2 µl of genomic DNA was amplified in a 20 µl volume of reaction mixture containing 2.5 µl of 10xPCR reaction buffer (20 mM Tris-HCl pH 8.4, 50 mM KCl and 1.5 mM $MgCl_2$), 0.2 µl dNTPs 10 mM, 0.5 µl $MgCl_2$ 25 mM, 0.25 mM of each primer and 1 U Taq polymerase (QIAGEN). Thermal cycling conditions were 95°C for 4 min; 35 cycles of 95°C for 30 s, 65°C for 30 s, 72°C for 1 min, with a final extension of 72°C for 2 min. Similarly, a 343 bp fragment in the exon 1 was amplified using primer pairs MBL-Ex1F (5′-GTGGCAGCGTCTTACTCA-GAAAC-3′) and MBL-Ex1R (5′-TGGGCTGGCAAGACAAC-TATTAG-3′). Similar cycling conditions as for the promoter fragment amplification were used, except for the annealing temperature which was 61°C for the exon 1 amplification. The amplified PCR fragments were stained with SybrGreen I (Applied Biosystems, Foster City, California, USA) and were visualized on a

Table 1. Clinical and demographic features of the RA patients, relatives and healthy controls.

Characteristics	Cases n = 196(%)	Relatives n = 200(%)	Controls n = 200(%)	P value
Age (years)	53 [18–84]	36 [7–91]	46 [24–89]	<0.0001
Gender (Male/Female)	24/132	78/122	40/160	<0.0001
Ethnicity (Afro/Euro/Indian)				NS
Afro-Brazilian	113 (72.5)	154 (77.0)	156 (78.0)	
Euro-Brazilian	42 (26.9)	46 (23.0)	41 (20.5)	
Amerindian	1 (0.6)	0 (0)	3 (1.5)	
Age at disease onset	44 [16–83]	ND	ND	NA
Disease duration	6 [0–60]	ND	ND	NA
Anti-CCP (IU/ml)	110 [6–253]	ND	ND	NA
Number of positive (≥20)	152 (77.5)			
Number of negative (<20)	48 (24.5)			
Rheumatoid factor (IU/mL)	139 [0–7680]	16 [0–1280]	ND	NA
Functional class (Steinbrock)		ND	ND	NA
Class I	90 (45.9)			
Class II	79 (40.3)			
Class III+IV	27 (13.8)			
Nodules (Yes)[a]	15 (7.6)	ND	ND	NA
Sjögren's syndrome (Yes)[a]	45 (29.2)	ND	ND	NA
Recurrent infections[b]	25 (33.8)	ND	ND	NA
Articular symptom (swollen or tender joints)	ND	47 (23.5)	ND	NA

Anti-CCP: anti-cyclic citrullinated peptide antibody, ([a]): Total of samples with available data are 154; ([b]): Total samples with available data are 74.
NS: Not significant; NA: not available; ND: not determined. Values expressed in medians and interquartiles range.

1.5% agarose gel. The PCR products were purified by using the illustra GFX PCR and Gel Band Purification kit following manufacturer's instructions (GE Healthcare, Little Chalfont, UK).

The entire promoter fragment including the 5′ UTR (+4 P/Q) was sequenced with the MBL-PromR and with an internal reverse primer (5′-TCTGCCACCTGAATCCCATCTTTGTATC-3′). A single sequencing reaction was made for the exon 1 fragment with the MBL-Ex1F primer. Purified PCR products were then sequenced with the BigDye Terminator v1.1 Cycle Sequencing Kit (Applied Biosystems, Foster City, CA, USA). Sequencing reactions were analyzed on an automated sequencer (ABI Prism 3130XL Genetic Analyzer, Applied Biosystems). The resulting DNA sequences were aligned using using Codon code Aligner 4.0 software and were reconfirmed visually from their respective electropherograms.

MBL Levels

MBL serum levels were measured in patients, relatives and healthy control by ELISA as described earlier [42] using monoclonal anti-human MBL antibody HYB131-01 (BioPorto Diagnostics A/S, Copenhagen, Denmark). Individuals with a MBL concentration ≤100 ng/ml were considered MBL low producers or deficient whereas individuals between 100–1000 ng/ml as medium producers and >1000 ng/ml considered as high secretors. The assay cut-off value was 100 ng/ml.

Statistical Analysis

Direct counting was used to estimate genotype, allele and haplotype frequencies. Tests of independence between RA patients and the comparison group, as well as possible associations between *MBL2* genotypes, alleles or haplotypes and clinical/demographical characteristics were analyzed using logistical regression implicated in Intercooled Stata v 9.2. The odds ratios (OR) and respective *P* values were adjusted for age, gender and ethnicity to exclude the influence of different cofactors to RA susceptibility. The comparison of MBL levels between different groups and the correlations of clinical and demographical characteristics were executed using the SPSS v.19 software by nonparametric Kruskal-Wallis or Mann-Whitney tests and Pearson's correlation tests, respectively. Deviations from Hardy-Weinberg equilibrium and from the hypothesis of homogeneity between haplotype distributions were tested using the Arlequin software package version 3.1. In all comparisons *P* values less than 0.05 were considered significant.

Results

Baseline Characteristics of the Study Cohort

The baseline clinical and demographic characteristics of the RA patients, their relatives and healthy controls are summarized in Table 1. Significant differences were observed in distributions of age, sex and ethnicity in all the three studied groups. The median age at disease onset was 44 (min: 16–max: 83 years) and the median disease duration was 6 years (min: 0–max: 60 years). A significantly weak correlation between anti-CCP levels and the age of patients was observed, of which the elderly patients had higher anti-CCP levels (Pearson's $r = 0.22$, $P = 0.006$). We also observed a significant difference in anti-CCP levels as segregated to different age groups. Additionally, correlation between anti-CCP levels and age at disease onset (Pearson's $r = 0.17$, $P = 0.024$) remained significant. Patients between 30 to 60 years of disease onset had higher anti-CCP levels compared to those with age higher than 60

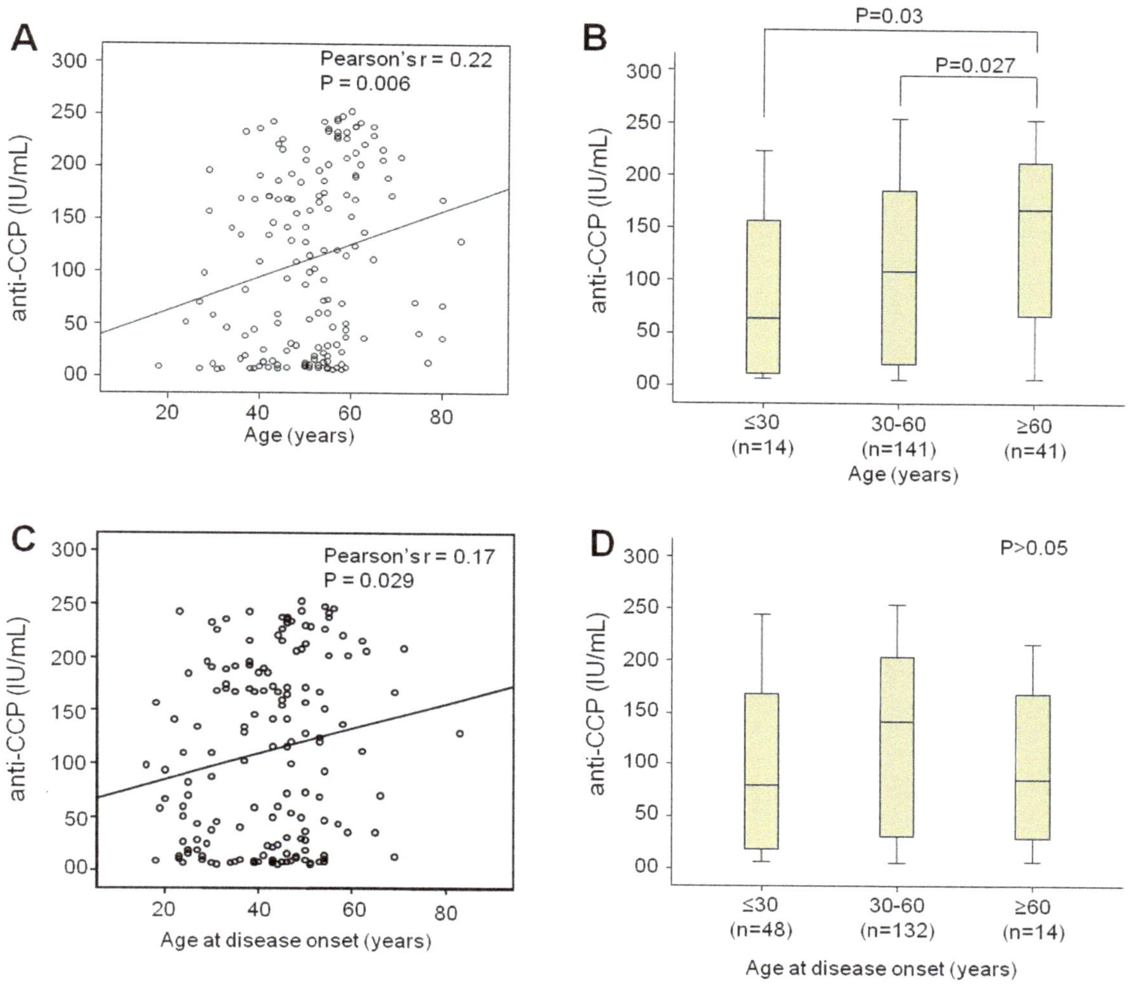

Figure 1. Correlations between anti-CCP and patient's age and age at disease onset. Anti-CCP correlated with the age of patients (A) and age at disease onset (C). Anti-CCP studied according to patient's age (B) and age at disease onset (D).

years (Figure 1). High levels of rheumatoid factor were observed significantly higher in RA patients compared to their relatives. Furthermore, RA patients were also classified based on Steinbrocker, with or without nodules as well as with or without Sjögren's syndrome (Table 1).

Functional *MBL2* Variants and RA

The genotype and allele frequencies for the analyzed functional *MBL2* SNPs in patients, relatives and controls were in Hardy-Weinberg equilibrium (P>0.05) except for one variant at codon 54 (rs1800450G/A *MBL2*B*) in the relatives (P<0.05). The distribution of observed *MBL2* genotype and their respective allele frequencies across different studied variants in different study groups are listed in Table 2. Linkage disequilibrium (LD) pattern of studied *MBL2* variants revealed that variants in the promoter region were in strong LD in RA patients and controls (data not shown).

The minor allele *−221X* in the promoter region was observed significantly higher in the control individuals compared to relatives (OR = 0.6, 95%CI = 0.4–0.99, P = 0.047) whereas the minor allele *MBL2*B* (codon 54 *rs1800450A*) in exon 1 was observed more frequently in RA patients compared to controls (OR = 1.28, 95%CI = 1.04–1.6, P = 0.018) suggesting an increased susceptibility to RA. In addition, the variant allele *O* of exon 1 was observed to contribute significantly to RA susceptibility in the dominant genetic model (OR = 1.29, 95%CI = 1.03–1.6, P = 0.026) and marginally associated in allelic model (OR = 1.2, 95%CI = 1.0–1.4, P = 0.058). No significant differences were observed for other studied variants in comparisons between the RA patients and controls and/or between relatives and controls. Furthermore, there were no significant differences in genotype and allele frequencies of other studied variants in all comparisons irrespective of patient functional classes (data not shown).

We observed nine secretor haplotypes in our study. The distribution of the reconstructed *MBL2* secretor haplotypes in the studied cohort is presented in Table 3. The *MBL2* haplotypes were further divided into those associated with high expression (*LYPA+LYQA+HYPA*) and low expression (*LYQC+LXPA+HYPD+LYPB*) of MBL. The *LYPB* haplotype was observed more frequent in RA patients than in controls (OR = 1.28, 95%CI = 1.04–1.6, P = 0.018) suggesting a possible risk factor whereas *LXPA* was observed more frequently in controls compared to relatives (OR = 0.6, 95%CI = 0.4–0.99, P = 0.047). The haplotypes associated with low MBL expression were

Table 2. Distribution of MBL2 genotypes and alleles in RA patients, relatives and healthy controls.

SNP position	Genotype	Patients	Relatives	Controls	Patients vs. Controls		Relatives vs. Controls		Patients vs. Relatives	
		n = 156(%)	n = 120(%)	n = 200 (%)	OR (95% CI)	*P* value#	OR (95% CI)	*P* value#	OR (95% CI)	*P* value#
(−221G/C)										
GG	*YY*	109 (69.9)	91 (75.8)	130 (65)						
GC	*YX*	38 (24.3)	28 (23.3)	58 (29)						
CC	*XX*	9 (8.8)	1 (0.8)	12 (6)						
G	*Y*	256 (82.1)	210 (87.5)	318 (79.5)						
C	*X*	56 (17.9)	30 (12.5)	82 (20.5)		NS	**0.6 (0.4–0.99)**	**0.047**		NS
Dominant						NS		NS		NS
Recessive						NS		NS		NS
Exon1 (codon54)										
GG	*AA*	96 (61.5)	79 (65.8)	148 (74)						
GA	*AB*	55 (35.3)	41 (34.2)	45 (22.5)						
AA	*BB*	5 (3.2)	0	7 (3.5)						
G	*A*	247 (79.2)	199 (82.9)	341 (85.3)						
A	*B*	65 (20.8)	41 (17.1)	59 (14.7)	**1.28 (1.04–1.6)**	**0.018**		NS		NS
Dominant						NS		NS		NS
Recessive						NS		NS		NS
Exon1 (codon52+54+57)										
	AA	75 (48.1)	62 (51.7)	119 (59.5)						
	AO	73 (46.8)	58 (48.3)	73 (36.5)						
	OO	8 (5.1)	0	8 (4)						
	A	223 (71.4)	182 (75.8)	311 (77.8)						
	O	89 (28.6)	58 (24.2)	89 (22.2)	1.2 (1–1.4)	0.058		NS		NS
Dominant					**1.29 (1.03–1.6)**	**0.026**		NS		NS
Recessive						NS		NS		NS

NS: not significant; NA: not applicable;
#P values were calculated by logistic regression adjusted for age, gender and ethnicity.
Dominant genetic model: Major genotype vs. Heterozygote+Minor genotype; Recessive genetic model: Minor genotype vs. Major+heterozygote genotype.

Table 3. Distribution of observed MBL2 haplotype in RA patients, relatives and healthy controls.

MBL2 **Haplotype**	**Patients**	**Relatives**	**Controls**	**Patients vs. Controls**		**Relatives vs. Controls**		**Patients vs. Relatives**	
	n = 312(%)	**n = 240(%)**	**n = 400(%)**	**OR (95% CI)**	***P* value#**	**OR (95% CI)**	***P* value#**	**OR (95% CI)**	***P* value#**
HYPA	80 (25.6)	70 (29.2)	113 (28.3)		NS		NS		NS
LYPB	65 (20.8)	41 (17.1)	59 (14.8)	**1.28 (1.04–1.6)**	**0.018**		NS		NS
LXPA	56 (17.9)	30 (12.5)	82 (20.5)		NS	**0.6 (0.4–0.99)**	**0.047**		NS
LYQA	53 (17)	44 (18.3)	79 (19.8)		NS		NS		NS
LYPA	26 (8.3)	30 (12.5)	33 (8.3)		NS		NS		NS
HYPD	22 (7.1)	15 (6.3)	22 (5.5)		NS		NS		NS
LYQC	10 (3.2)	10 (4.2)	9 (2.3)		NS		NS		NS
LYPD	0	0	2 (0.5)		NA		NA		NA
HYPC	0	0	1 (0.3)		NA		NA		NA
High expression of MBL									
LYPA+LYQA+HYPA	159 (51)	144 (60)	225 (56.3)		reference		reference		reference
Low expression of MBL									
LYQC+LXPA+HYPD+LYPB	153 (49)	96 (40)	172 (43)		NS		NS		NS

NS: not significant; NA: not applicable.
#P values were calculated by logistic regression adjusted for age, gender and ethnicity.

observed more frequently in RA patients compared to relatives (OR = 1.44, 95%CI = 1.01–2.1, P = 0.038), however no significant distribution was observed after adjusted for age, gender and ethnicity (Table 3).

MBL Levels and Rheumatoid Arthritis

MBL serum levels in RA patients, relatives and controls are presented in Figure 2. RA patients had significantly lower MBL levels compared to relatives and controls ($P = 0.006$ and $P = 0.004$, respectively). No significant differences in distribution were observed between relatives and controls (Figure 2A). MBL levels were higher in the patients with age at disease onset lower than 30 years, and decreased MBL levels in the patients with age at disease onset of more than 30 years (Figure 2C). No significant distributions of MBL levels segregated according to functional classes or disease duration (Figure 2B and 2D) was observed. MBL levels were segregated according to clinical parameters. No significant differences were observed between patients positive and negative for nodules, Sjögren's syndrome, anti-CCP and rheumatoid factor (Figure 3). Nevertheless, we observed that patients with recurrent infections had lower MBL levels than those without it ($P = 0.02$).

MBL2 Variants and MBL Serum Levels in RA Patients

The serum MBL levels were observed to segregate according to different *MBL2* genotypes in the investigated cohort. Our results indicate that the presence of minor alleles *−550H* and *−4Q* contributed significantly to higher MBL serum levels whereas minor alleles *MBL2*D*, *MBL2*B* and *MBL2*C* at codons 52, 54 and 57, respectively contributed significantly to lower MBL levels (Figure 4). The homozygous variant genotype *−221XX* presented lower MBL serum levels compared to homozygous wild type genotype *−221YY* and heterozygote genotype *−221XY*. We also observed a similar trend for the effects of *MBL2* variants on MBL levels with relatives (Figure 4).

A base substitution at −221 (G to C; promoter allele *X*) is associated with lower MBL serum concentrations [34]. The *MBL2* diplotypes were reconstructed from promoter variant −221X/Y and variants in exon1 (Codon 52+54+57, A/O) and divided into high (*YA/YA*), intermediate (*YA/YO*, *XA/XA* and *XA/YA*) and low MBL producers (*YO/YO*, *XA/YO*). MBL levels were significantly distributed across high, intermediate and low MBL producers in both RA patients and their relatives (Figure 5A). In addition, the MBL serum levels were significantly distributed across haplotypes in both RA patients and relatives. Patients with *HYPA*, *LYQA* and

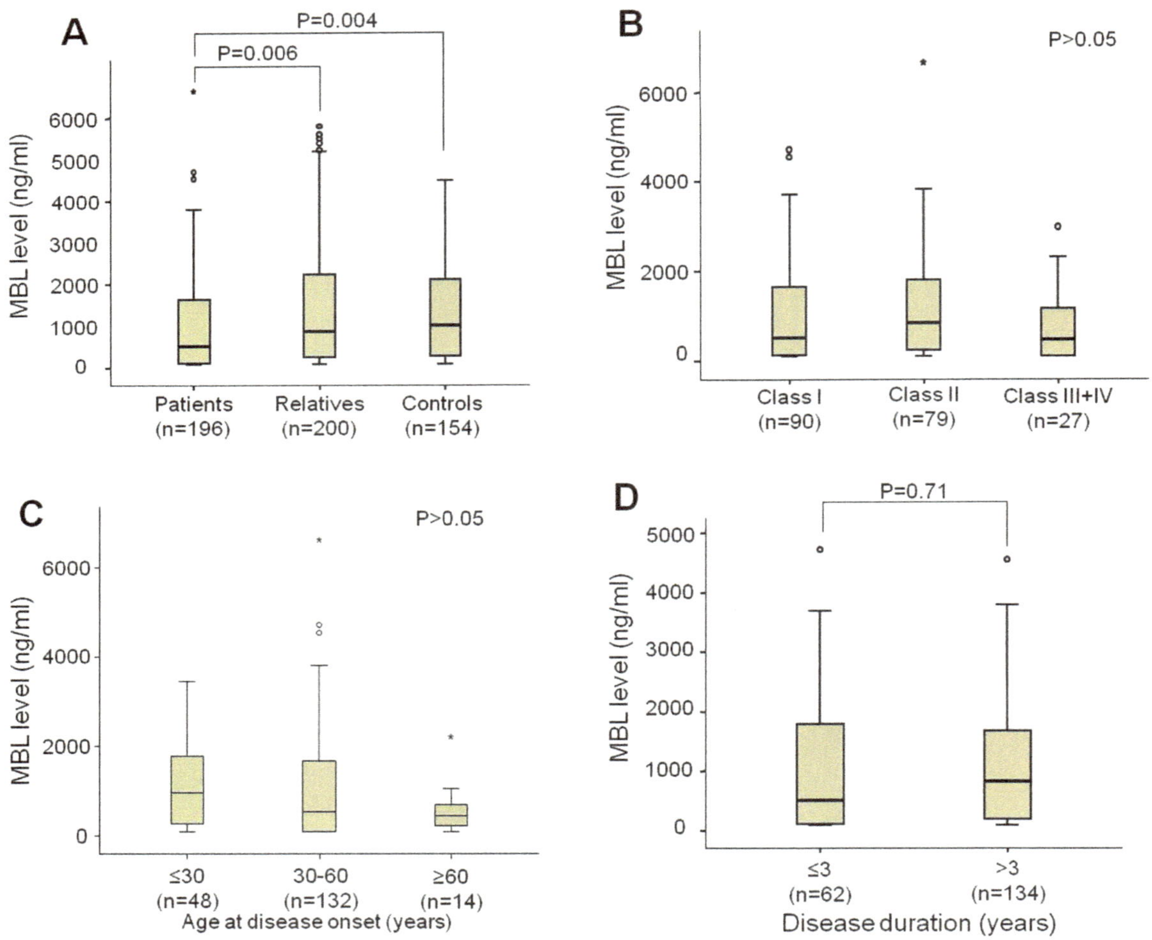

Figure 2. Distribution of MBL levels in studied Brazilian cohort. Distribution of MBL levels in patients, relatives and controls (A), according to different functional classes (B), according to age at disease onset (C) and according to disease duration (D). Open circles indicate possible outliers in each group and the *represents significant distribution amongst the investigated groups.

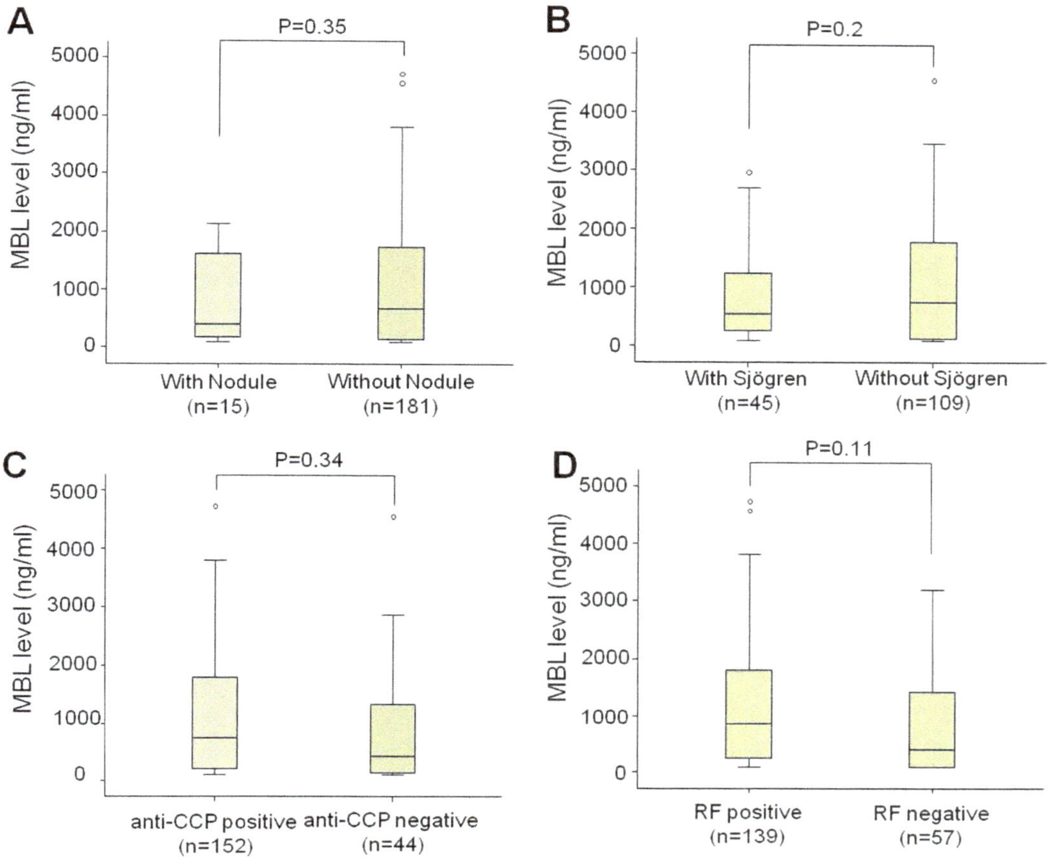

Figure 3. Distribution of MBL levels in RA patients segregated by clinical parameters. Distribution of MBL levels according to presence of nodules (A), Secondary Sjögren's syndrome (B), positivity for anti-CCP (C) and positivity for Rheumatoid factor (D).

LYPA haplotypes had higher MBL levels compared to other observed haplotypes (Figure 5B and 5C).

Discussion

Rheumatoid arthritis is an autoimmune disease that involves a complex interplay between environmental and genetic factors. Many immune regulatory factors underlie the initial stage and development of this disease [4,5,43]. The activation of innate immune system has been associated with both RA susceptibility and pathophysiology as well as to others autoimmune and infectious diseases [4].

In the present study, we observed that functional *MBL2* variants and MBL levels are significantly associated with RA and equally towards clinical progression in the studied Brazilian cohort. We demonstrated that the allele(s) *MBL2*B*, the variant allele *O* in the exon 1, the *MBL2*LYPB* haplotype and lower MBL serum levels as factors for RA development. The association of genetic factors including gene polymorphisms with RA susceptibility has been widely described including *HLA-DRB1* locus, rs2476601 variant in the protein tyrosine phosphatase gene (*PTPN22*), in IL2 receptor genes (rs2104286 in *IL2RA* and rs743777 and *IL2RB*) and in TNF pathway genes such as tumour necrosis factor (*TNF*), alpha-induced protein 2 (*TNFAIP2*) [4,43–46]. Of interest, the innate immune system represented by complement components has been demonstrated to be involved in the development of RA [47–49]. Measurements of C5a levels suggested the that complement is activated in rheumatoid joints and it could induce the acute inflammatory process [50]. In RA, the interaction between autoantibodies joint structures, can activate the complement system, triggering inflammatory and adaptive immune response [49]. Mannose-biding lectin (MBL), ficolins and collectin 11 are three major pattern-recognition receptors which initiate the complement system through lectin pathway.

The *MBL2* polymorphisms and MBL serum levels were involved in different infectious diseases such as malaria and schistosomiasis [34,51,52] and in autoimmune diseases such as systemic lupus erythematosus and ankylosing spondylitis [20,53–55]. Particularly, the *MBL2* polymorphisms and MBL serum levels have been shown to play an important role in RA susceptibility and its pathophysiology in different populations including Brazil [20,24,41,56]. A previous study, conducted in Brazilian population, showed that genotype *OO* was observed more frequently in the RA patients with rheumatoid nodules [41]. In our study, the alleles *MBL2*D*, *MBL2*B* and *MBL2*C* (allele *O*) that reduces the MBL serum levels was observed to be a risk factor for RA. The secretion profiles of haplotypes observed in our study are in accordance with other published study on RA that has demonstrated the distribution of secretor haplotypes based on MBL levels in a larger Caucasian population of Dutch descent [57]. Recently a meta-analysis investigation has shown that *MBL2*B* (codon 54) variant is not associated with RA across all published study subjects irrespective of ethnicity, however when stratified by

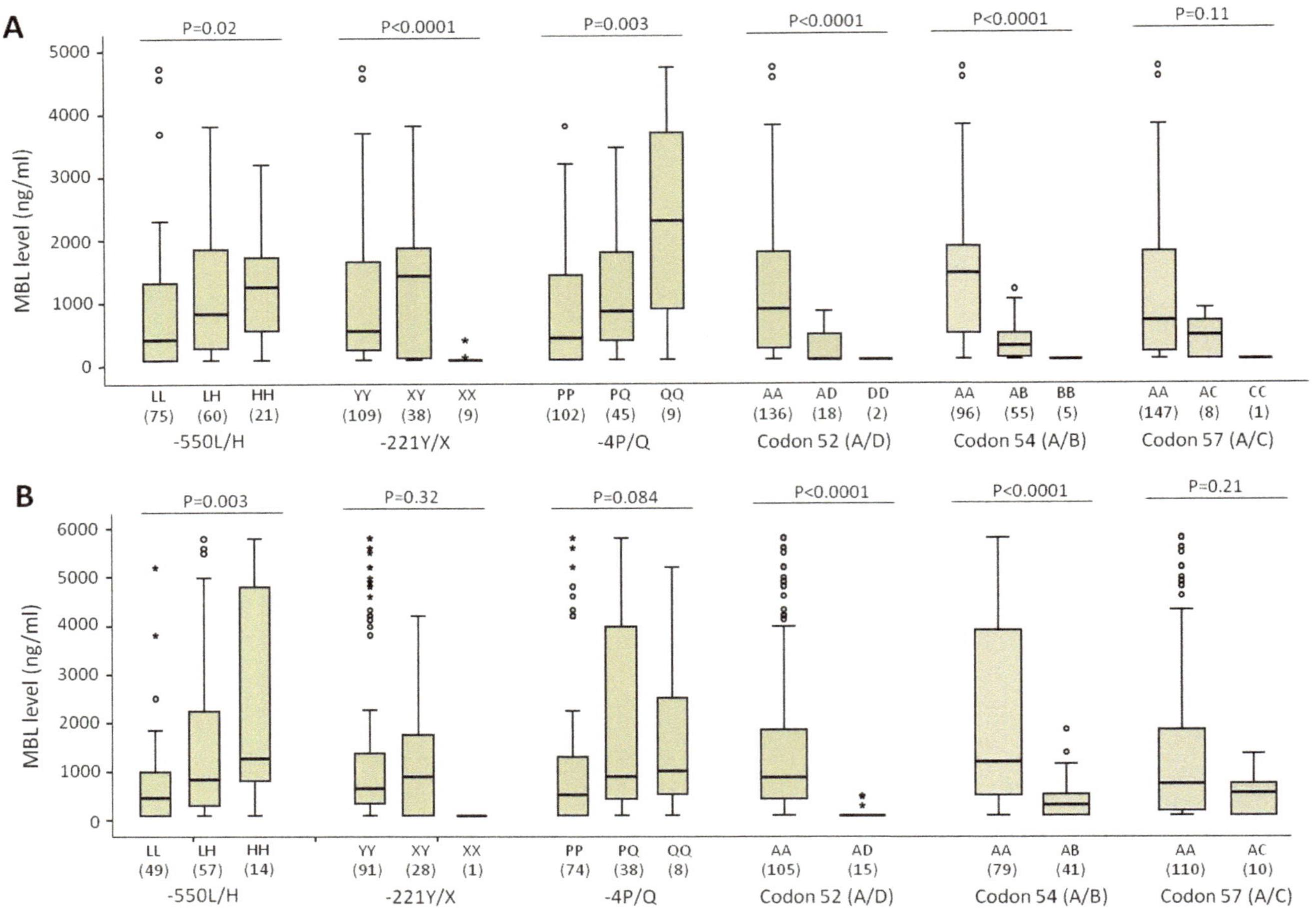

Figure 4. Distribution of MBL levels in different *MBL2* genotypes. Serum MBL levels according to different genotypes of studied *MBL2* variants in RA patients (A) and relatives (B).

ethnicity in Asian populations, a significant contribution of *MBL2*B* (codon 54) variant was observed [58].

As described in previously published studies [20,26,27,29,56], the MBL serum levels were significantly decreased in RA patients compared to controls and in addition no significant difference of MBL serum levels between RA patients and their relatives was observed. A high proportion of RA patients lacked detectable MBL in serum in a longitudinal follow up study and concluded that MBL insufficiency may be a contributing pathogenetic factor in RA [26]. Another chinese study reported that low MBL serum levels predisposes to the development of RA [27]. A yet another study concluded that MBL insufficiency as a significant risk factor for rapid progression of RA [29]. All these studies corroborate our findings that MBL serum levels were significantly decreased in RA patients compared to controls. However a study reported that RA patients had higher MBL levels than their close relatives and controls [25], which was contradictory to the observed findings in this study [25]. High MBL production was associated with an increased overall mortality in RA patients that points to a dual role of this protein in this rheumatic disease [59].

Some studies point to a septic origin of RA and is believed that microbes such as *Porphyromonas gingivalis* are involved in RA pathogenesis that are rich in sugar moieties that are recognized by MBL [60]. We hypothesized, that such pathogens could take advantage of MBL-deficiency and concomitantly induce autoimmune responses against the host. However, this hypothesis must be confirmed by further studies. Considering that RA therapy frequently involves patients immunosuppression, we suggest that MBL levels should be taken to account when choosing the therapeutic strategy.

Although the presence of low producing *MBL2* variants explains the finding of low serum MBL levels, the consumption of this protein during the inflammatory response including in the joints may offer an alternative explanation. As mentioned earlier, complement consumption within the joints has already been described for other complement components, such as C5a [50]. In this situation the reduced MBL levels could also be due to diffusion of this component into the joint cavity favored by increased synovial permeability. Sequestration of complement proteins in synovial cavity has been described to be greater in RA in comparison to other arthropathies [61,62]. Furthermore, we observed a trend of increased MBL serum levels in the patients with rheumatoid factor and anti-CCP positive in comparison to those with rheumatoid factor and anti-CCP negative. This result suggested that high MBL serum levels regulated by functional *MBL2* variants might possibly affect the pathophysiology of RA. Similar to MBL, ficolins (including ficolin-1, ficolin-2 and ficolin-3 encoded by *FCN1*, *FCN2* and *FCN3*, respectively) are also innate immune recognition proteins that activate complement system

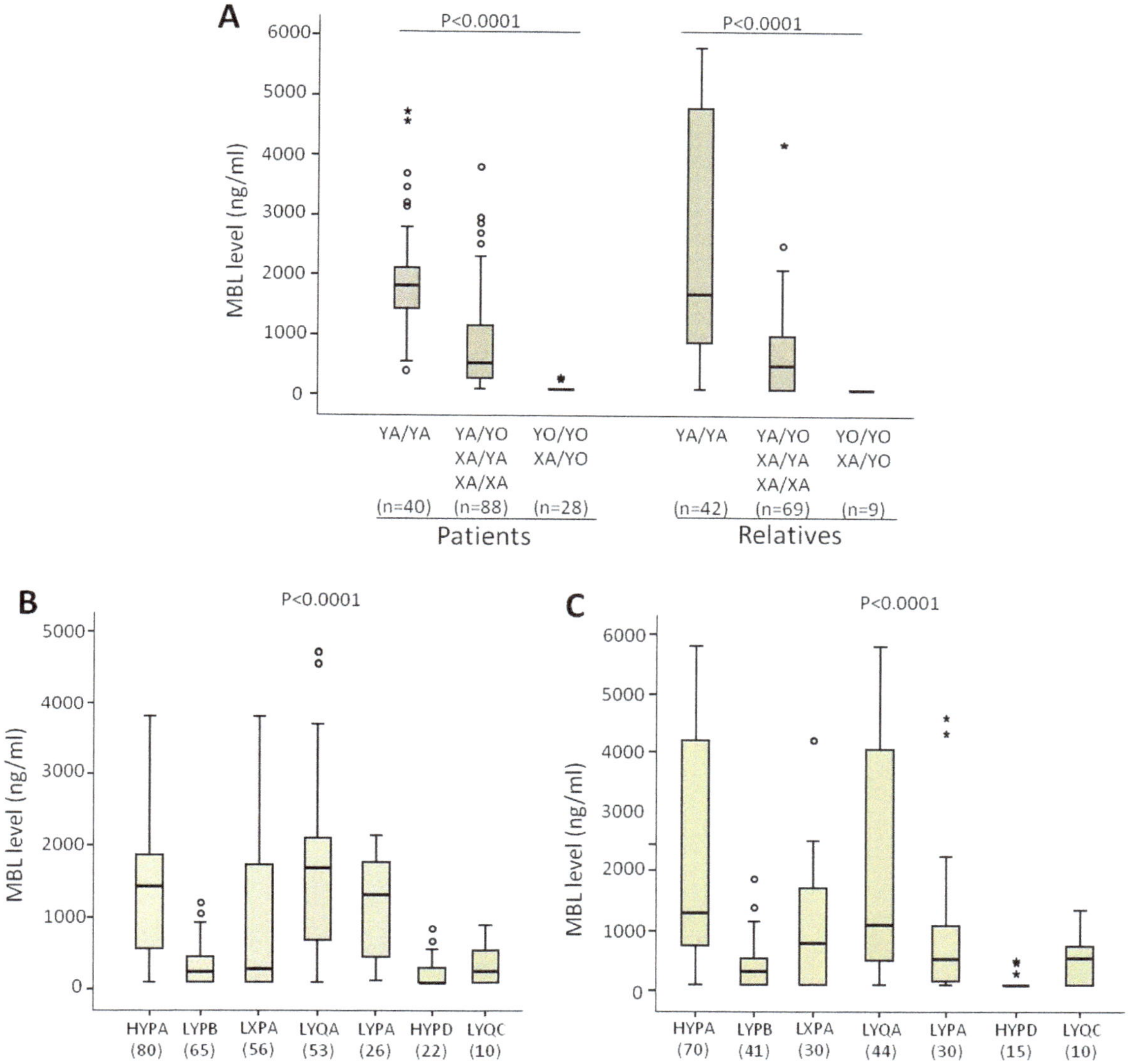

Figure 5. Distribution of MBL levels in different *MBL2* haplotypes and diplotypes. *MBL2* diplotypes were reconstructed from promoter variant −221X/Y and variants in exon1 (Codon 52+54+57, A/O) and divided into high MBL producers (*YA/YA*), intermediate (*YA/YO, XA/XA* and *XA/YA*) and low MBL producers (*YO/YO, XA/YO*). Serum MBL levels were segregated according to different *MBL2* diplotypes in patients and relatives (A), and different *MBL2* secretor haplotypes in RA patients (B) and relatives (C).

[10,12,63]. However, only polymorphisms in *FCN1* gene are significantly associated with RA development [64].

Due to the high prevalence of familial RA susceptibility, RA patient's relatives have also been analyzed. No significant differences in patients and their relatives could be detected in *MBL2* genotype and haplotype frequencies as well as in MBL levels. These results suggest that the *MBL2* functional variants may not be a key genetic factor for RA development, but probably play an inherent cofactor for pathophysiology in RA. Because RA risk is higher in female gender [4] and our study cohort was comprised by diverse ethnicities all the results of the contribution of different cofactors along with *MBL2* polymorphisms to RA susceptibility were adjusted for age, gender and ethnicity. As lower MBL serum levels affects infection's predisposition [17] this could be an important cofactor for RA susceptibility. More studies in a larger cohort in different world population with more clinical parameters of RA will be essential to validate the role of MBL and other complementary components on the pathophysiology of RA.

In conclusion, our results suggest a significant association of functional *MBL2* polymorphisms and MBL serum levels with RA susceptibility in the Brazilian population. MBL levels may be considered when choosing the therapeutic strategy for RA patients.

Acknowledgments

We would like to thank all the patients and volunteers from the Rheumatological Unit of the Evangelical Hospital of Curitiba (Brazil) for their participation and support during sample collection.

Author Contributions

Conceived and designed the experiments: IJTMR TPV. Performed the experiments: IG TLS RMN. Analyzed the data: HvT TPV. Contributed reagents/materials/analysis tools: TPV TLS SRU. Wrote the paper: IG TPV HvT.

References

1. Bansback N, Marra CA, Finckh A, Anis A (2009) The economics of treatment in early rheumatoid arthritis. Best Pract Res Clin Rheumatol 23: 83–92.
2. Aletaha D, Neogi T, Silman AJ, Funovits J, Felson DT, et al. (2010) 2010 Rheumatoid arthritis classification criteria: an American College of Rheumatology/European League Against Rheumatism collaborative initiative. Arthritis Rheum 62: 2569–2581.
3. MacGregor AJ, Snieder H, Rigby AS, Koskenvuo M, Kaprio J, et al. (2000) Characterizing the quantitative genetic contribution to rheumatoid arthritis using data from twins. Arthritis Rheum 43: 30–37.
4. McInnes IB, Schett G (2011) The pathogenesis of rheumatoid arthritis. N Engl J Med 365: 2205–2219.
5. Wordsworth P, Bell J (1991) Polygenic susceptibility in rheumatoid arthritis. Ann Rheum Dis 50: 343–346.
6. Goeldner I, Skare TL, de Messias Reason IT, Nisihara RM, Silva MB, et al. (2010) Anti-cyclic citrullinated peptide antibodies and rheumatoid factor in rheumatoid arthritis patients and relatives from Brazil. Rheumatology (Oxford) 49: 1590–1593.
7. Goeldner I, Skare TL, de Messias Reason IT, Nisihara RM, Silva MB, et al. (2011) Association of anticyclic citrullinated peptide antibodies with extra-articular manifestations, gender, and tabagism in rheumatoid arthritis patients from southern Brazil. Clin Rheumatol 30: 975–980.
8. Hemminki K, Li X, Sundquist K, Sundquist J (2009) Shared familial aggregation of susceptibility to autoimmune diseases. Arthritis Rheum 60: 2845–2847.
9. Runza VL, Schwaeble W, Mannel DN (2008) Ficolins: novel pattern recognition molecules of the innate immune response. Immunobiology 213: 297–306.
10. Carroll MV, Sim RB (2011) Complement in health and disease. Adv Drug Deliv Rev 63: 965–975.
11. Assaf A, Hoang TV, Faik I, Aebischer T, Kremsner PG, et al. (2012) Genetic evidence of functional ficolin-2 haplotype as susceptibility factor in cutaneous leishmaniasis. PLoS One 7: e34113.
12. Hoang TV, Toan NL, Song lH, Ouf EA, Bock CT, et al. (2011) Ficolin-2 levels and FCN2 haplotypes influence hepatitis B infection outcome in Vietnamese patients. PLoS One 6: e28113.
13. Luz PR, Boldt AB, Grisbach C, Kun JF, Velavan TP, et al. (2013) Association of L-ficolin levels and FCN2 genotypes with chronic Chagas disease. PLoS One 8: e60237.
14. Ouf EA, Ojurongbe O, Akindele AA, Sina-Agbaje OR, van TH, et al. (2012) Ficolin-2 levels and FCN2 genetic polymorphisms as a susceptibility factor in schistosomiasis. J Infect Dis 206: 562–570.
15. Ricklin D, Hajishengallis G, Yang K, Lambris JD (2010) Complement: a key system for immune surveillance and homeostasis. Nat Immunol 11: 785–797.
16. Degn SE, Jensenius JC, Thiel S (2011) Disease-causing mutations in genes of the complement system. Am J Hum Genet 88: 689–705.
17. Heitzeneder S, Seidel M, Forster-Waldl E, Heitger A (2012) Mannan-binding lectin deficiency - Good news, bad news, doesn't matter? Clin Immunol 143: 22–38.
18. Chen M, Daha MR, Kallenberg CG (2010) The complement system in systemic autoimmune disease. J Autoimmun 34: J276–J286.
19. Magorivska I, Jeremic I, Herman S, Munoz LE, Bilyy R, et al. (2014) 1.58 rheumatoid factor binding is influenced by the N-Glycans of their IGG targets. Ann Rheum Dis 73 Suppl 1: A25.
20. Troelsen LN, Jacobsen S, Abrahams JL, Royle L, Rudd PM, et al. (2012) IgG glycosylation changes and MBL2 polymorphisms: associations with markers of systemic inflammation and joint destruction in rheumatoid arthritis. J Rheumatol 39: 463–469.
21. Troelsen LN, Jacobsen S, Abrahams JL, Royle L, Rudd PM, et al. (2012) IgG glycosylation changes and MBL2 polymorphisms: associations with markers of systemic inflammation and joint destruction in rheumatoid arthritis. J Rheumatol 39: 463–469.
22. Boldt AB, Goeldner I, de Messias-Reason IJ (2012) Relevance of the lectin pathway of complement in rheumatic diseases. Adv Clin Chem 56: 105–153.
23. Sato R, Matsushita M, Miyata M, Sato Y, Kasukawa R, et al. (1997) Substances reactive with mannose-binding protein (MBP) in sera of patients with rheumatoid arthritis. Fukushima J Med Sci 43: 99–111.
24. Troelsen LN, Garred P, Christiansen B, Torp-Pedersen C, Christensen IJ, et al. (2010) Double role of mannose-binding lectin in relation to carotid intima-media thickness in patients with rheumatoid arthritis. Mol Immunol 47: 713–718.
25. Saevarsdottir S, Steinsson K, Grondal G, Valdimarsson H (2007) Patients with rheumatoid arthritis have higher levels of mannan-binding lectin than their first-degree relatives and unrelated controls. J Rheumatol 34: 1692–1695.
26. Graudal NA, Homann C, Madsen HO, Svejgaard A, Jurik AG, et al. (1998) Mannan binding lectin in rheumatoid arthritis. A longitudinal study. J Rheumatol 25: 629–635.
27. Ip WK, Lau YL, Chan SY, Mok CC, Chan D, et al. (2000) Mannose-binding lectin and rheumatoid arthritis in southern Chinese. Arthritis Rheum 43: 1679–1687.
28. Graudal N (2004) The natural history and prognosis of rheumatoid arthritis: association of radiographic outcome with process variables, joint motion and immune proteins. Scand J Rheumatol Suppl 118: 1–38.
29. Graudal NA, Madsen HO, Tarp U, Svejgaard A, Jurik G, et al. (2000) The association of variant mannose-binding lectin genotypes with radiographic outcome in rheumatoid arthritis. Arthritis Rheum 43: 515–521.
30. Velavan TP, Boldt AB, Tomiuk J, Seibold F, Schoepfer AM, et al. (2010) Variant alleles of the mannose binding lectin 2 gene (MBL2) confer heterozygote advantage within Crohn's families. Scand J Gastroenterol 45: 1129–1130.
31. Boldt AB, Messias-Reason IJ, Meyer D, Schrago CG, Lang F, et al. (2010) Phylogenetic nomenclature and evolution of mannose-binding lectin (MBL2) haplotypes. BMC Genet 11: 38.
32. Larsen F, Madsen HO, Sim RB, Koch C, Garred P (2004) Disease-associated mutations in human mannose-binding lectin compromise oligomerization and activity of the final protein. J Biol Chem 279: 21302–21311.
33. Madsen HO, Garred P, Thiel S, Kurtzhals JA, Lamm LU, et al. (1995) Interplay between promoter and structural gene variants control basal serum level of mannan-binding protein. J Immunol 155: 3013–3020.
34. Antony JS, Ojurongbe O, van TH, Ouf EA, Engleitner T, et al. (2013) Mannose-binding lectin and susceptibility to schistosomiasis. J Infect Dis 207: 1675–1683.
35. Madsen HO, Garred P, Thiel S, Kurtzhals JA, Lamm LU, et al. (1995) Interplay between promoter and structural gene variants control basal serum level of mannan-binding protein. J Immunol 155: 3013–3020.
36. Dommett RM, Klein N, Turner MW (2006) Mannose-binding lectin in innate immunity: past, present and future. Tissue Antigens 68: 193–209.
37. Madsen HO, Satz ML, Hogh B, Svejgaard A, Garred P (1998) Different molecular events result in low protein levels of mannan-binding lectin in populations from southeast Africa and South America. J Immunol 161: 3169–3175.
38. Bernig T, Taylor JG, Foster CB, Staats B, Yeager M, et al. (2004) Sequence analysis of the mannose-binding lectin (MBL2) gene reveals a high degree of heterozygosity with evidence of selection. Genes Immun 5: 461–476.
39. Verdu P, Barreiro LB, Patin E, Gessain A, Cassar O, et al. (2006) Evolutionary insights into the high worldwide prevalence of MBL2 deficiency alleles. Hum Mol Genet 15: 2650–2658.
40. Arnett FC, Edworthy SM, Bloch DA, McShane DJ, Fries JF, et al. (1988) The American Rheumatism Association 1987 revised criteria for the classification of rheumatoid arthritis. Arthritis Rheum 31: 315–324.
41. Martiny FL, Veit TD, Brenol CV, Brenol JC, Xavier RM, et al. (2012) Mannose-binding lectin gene polymorphisms in Brazilian patients with rheumatoid arthritis. J Rheumatol 39: 6–9.
42. Petersen SV, Thiel S, Jensen L, Steffensen R, Jensenius JC (2001) An assay for the mannan-binding lectin pathway of complement activation. J Immunol Methods 257: 107–116.
43. (2007) Genome-wide association study of 14,000 cases of seven common diseases and 3,000 shared controls. Nature 447: 661–678.
44. MacKay K, Eyre S, Myerscough A, Milicic A, Barton A, et al. (2002) Whole-genome linkage analysis of rheumatoid arthritis susceptibility loci in 252 affected sibling pairs in the United Kingdom. Arthritis Rheum 46: 632–639.
45. Begovich AB, Carlton VE, Honigberg LA, Schrodi SJ, Chokkalingam AP, et al. (2004) A missense single-nucleotide polymorphism in a gene encoding a protein tyrosine phosphatase (PTPN22. is associated with rheumatoid arthritis. Am J Hum Genet 75: 330–337.
46. Hinks A, Eyre S, Barton A, Thomson W, Worthington J (2007) Investigation of genetic variation across the protein tyrosine phosphatase gene in patients with rheumatoid arthritis in the UK. Ann Rheum Dis 66: 683–686.
47. Di MG, Perricone C, Ballanti E, Kroegler B, Greco E, et al. (2011) Complement system and rheumatoid arthritis: relationships with autoantibodies, serological, clinical features, and anti-TNF treatment. Int J Immunopathol Pharmacol 24: 357–366.
48. Ballanti E, Perricone C, Di MG, Kroegler B, Chimenti MS, et al. (2011) Role of the complement system in rheumatoid arthritis and psoriatic arthritis: relationship with anti-TNF inhibitors. Autoimmun Rev 10: 617–623.
49. Okroj M, Heinegard D, Holmdahl R, Blom AM (2007) Rheumatoid arthritis and the complement system. Ann Med 39: 517–530.
50. Jose PJ, Moss IK, Maini RN, Williams TJ (1990) Measurement of the chemotactic complement fragment C5a in rheumatoid synovial fluids by radioimmunoassay: role of C5a in the acute inflammatory phase. Ann Rheum Dis 49: 747–752.
51. Boldt AB, Messias-Reason IJ, Lell B, Issifou S, Pedroso ML, et al. (2009) Haplotype specific-sequencing reveals MBL2 association with asymptomatic Plasmodium falciparum infection. Malar J 8: 97.
52. Jha AN, Sundaravadivel P, Singh VK, Pati SS, Patra PK, et al. (2014) MBL2 variations and malaria susceptibility in Indian populations. Infect Immun 82: 52–61.
53. Glesse N, Monticielo OA, Mattevi VS, Brenol JC, Xavier RM, et al. (2011) Association of mannose-binding lectin 2 gene polymorphic variants with

susceptibility and clinical progression in systemic lupus erythematosus. Clin Exp Rheumatol 29: 983–990.

54. Im CH, Kim J, Lee YJ, Lee EY, Lee EB, et al. (2012) Mannose-binding lectin 2 gene haplotype analysis in Korean patients with ankylosing spondylitis. Rheumatol Int 32: 2251–2255.
55. Sandrin-Garcia P, Brandao LA, Coelho AV, Guimaraes RL, Pancoto JA, et al. (2011) Mannose binding lectin gene (MBL2) functional polymorphisms are associated with systemic lupus erythematosus in southern Brazilians. Hum Immunol 72: 516–521.
56. Saevarsdottir S, Ding B, Steinsson K, Grondal G, Valdimarsson H, et al. (2011) Mannan Binding Lectin (MBL) genotypes coding for high MBL serum levels are associated with rheumatoid factor negative rheumatoid arthritis in never smokers. Arthritis Res Ther 13: R65.
57. van de Geijn FE, Hazes JM, Geleijns K, Emonts M, Jacobs BC, et al. (2008) Mannose-binding lectin polymorphisms are not associated with rheumatoid arthritis–confirmation in two large cohorts. Rheumatology (Oxford) 47: 1168–1171.
58. Xie Q, Wang SC, Bian G, Zhan FL, Xie JK, et al. (2012) Association of MIF-173G/C and MBL2 codon 54 gene polymorphisms with rheumatoid arthritis: a meta-analysis. Hum Immunol 73: 966–971.
59. Troelsen LN, Garred P, Jacobsen S (2010) Mortality and predictors of mortality in rheumatoid arthritis–a role for mannose-binding lectin? J Rheumatol 37: 536–543.
60. Maffei G, Brouwer N, Dolman KM, van d, V, Roos D, et al. (2005) Plasma levels of mannan-binding lectin in relation to periodontitis and smoking. J Periodontol 76: 1881–1889.
61. Ammitzboll CG, Thiel S, Ellingsen T, Deleuran B, Jorgensen A, et al. (2012) Levels of lectin pathway proteins in plasma and synovial fluid of rheumatoid arthritis and osteoarthritis. Rheumatol Int 32: 1457–1463.
62. Swaak AJ, Van RA, Planten O, Han H, Hattink O, et al. (1987) An analysis of the levels of complement components in the synovial fluid in rheumatic diseases. Clin Rheumatol 6: 350–357.
63. Ojurongbe O, Ouf EA, van TH, Toan NL, Song lH, et al. (2012) Reliable and rapid characterization of functional FCN2 gene variants reveals diverse geographical patterns. BMC Med Genet 13: 37.
64. Vander CB, Nuytinck L, Boullart L, Elewaut D, Waegeman W, et al. (2007) Polymorphisms in the ficolin 1 gene (FCN1) are associated with susceptibility to the development of rheumatoid arthritis. Rheumatology (Oxford) 46: 1792–1795.

4

Glycyrol Suppresses Collagen-Induced Arthritis by Regulating Autoimmune and Inflammatory Responses

Yanxia Fu, Hailing Zhou, Shuangyan Wang, Qun Wei*

Department of Biochemistry and Molecular Biology, Beijing Normal University, Gene Engineering and Biotechnology Beijing Key Laboratory, Beijing, P. R. of China

Abstract

Glycyrol is a natural compound extracted from *Glycyrrhiza uralensis*, first reported by us to be a new immunosuppressant. Here, we demonstrate its beneficial effect in collagen-induced arthritis (CIA) in mice, a model for rheumatoid arthritis (RA) in man, and we document the underlying mechanisms. Peroral administration of glycyrol significantly reduced clinical scores, alleviated cartilage and bone erosion and reduced levels of serum inflammatory cytokines. Glycyrol also decreased delayed-type hypersensitivity, improved carbon clearance and reduced acetic acid-induced capillary permeability. Furthermore, glycyrol decreased NF-κB and NFAT transcriptional activities and inhibited IL-2 expression. The therapeutic effect of glycyrol was associated with down-regulation of both autoimmune and inflammatory reactions. In addition, we demonstrated that glycyrol has minimal acute toxicity in mice. Therefore, we propose that glycyrol may hold promise for future treatment of RA.

Editor: Pierre Bobé, INSERM-Université Paris-Sud, France

Funding: The work was supported by the National Natural Science Foundation of China, the National Important Novel Medicine Research Project, the Fundamental Research Funds for the Central Universities and the special fund of the co-construction project from the Beijing Education Committee. The funders had no role in study design, data collection and analysis, decision to publish, or preparation of the manuscript.

Competing Interests: The authors have declared that no competing interests exist.

* Email: weiq@bnu.edu.cn

Introduction

Rheumatoid arthritis (RA) is an autoimmune disease characterized by synovial hyperplasia and inflammatory cell recruitment eventually leading to destruction of cartilage and bone [1,2]. It afflicts approximately 1% of the worldwide population [3]. Despite intensive research, the exact etiology of RA remains obscure, and a satisfactory cure remains elusive [4]. Nonsteroidal anti-inflammatory drugs are widely used, but carry the risk of gastrointestinal toxicity [5]. Cytokine antagonists likewise decrease inflammation and joint destruction but interfere with immune defense. Additionally, these inhibitors must be injected parenterally, thereby increasing the risk of infections [6,7]. Immunosuppressive agents, such as cyclosporin A (CsA) and tacrolimus (FK506), which have been used widely in organ transplantation and autoimmune diseases, are also useful [8,9]. However, their use is plagued by severe side effects, notably nephrotoxicity and hepatotoxicity [10,11,12]. Therefore, a need is felt to develop perorally administered drugs with minimal toxicity to reduce inflammation responses and inhibit autoimmune responses. Due to the side effects of anti-arthritis drugs, an increasing proportion of patients with arthritis are resorting to complementary and alternative medicine (CAM) for their health needs. The most popular CAM treatments for inflammatory and immune disorders are found among natural plant products [13].

Our group has focused on the immunosuppressant screening of natural products with calcineurin (CN) as the target enzyme. In our previous work, we screened glycyrol from *Glycyrrhiza uralensis*, and showed that it is an immunosuppressive agent; as its intraperitoneal injection could prolong graft survival in allogeneic skin transplantation [14]. It has been reported that CN plays crucial roles in the autoimmune and inflammatory responses and that the activity of CN correlates well with the severity of arthritis in an animal model of RA. Therefore, we used collagen-induced arthritis (CIA) in mice to study the potential beneficial effect of glycyrol on the pathogenesis of arthritis. Tests for delayed type hypersensitivity (DTH) and carbon clearance were used evaluate the influenceon the immunoregulation of mice, and the acetic acid-induced capillary permeability test was used to detect the influence of glycyrol on inflammatory reactions. We show that treatment with glycyrol has great benefits at both the clinical and the pathological levels and that the therapeutic effect is associated with the down-regulation of both inflammatory and autoimmune reactions.

Materials and Methods

2.1 Ethics statement

All animal experimental procedures were approved by the Animal Ethics Committee of Beijing Normal University and were conducted in strict accordance with institutional guidelines. All efforts were made to minimize the number of animals used and to reduce their suffering.

2.2 Materials

Glycyrol ($C_{21}H_{18}O_6$, MW:366.4, purity>95%) was synthesized by Shuangyan Wang according to the published procedure [15]. For peroral administration to mice, the compound was dissolved in peanut oil containing 1% DMSO and infused into the oesophagus through a canula. Bovine type II collagen and complete Freund's adjuvant were purchased from Chondrex (USA). Specific-pathogen free male DBA/1J mice were acquired from the National Resource Center for Mutant Mice Model Animal Research Center of Nanjing University (Nanjing, China). Specific pathogen-free male BALB/c mice (6–8 weeks of age) were purchased from the Vital River Laboratories (Beijing, China). ELISA kits were purchased from Hin Bo Sheng Biological Technology Co, Ltd. (Beijing, China). TRIzol reagent was purchased from Bio Teke corporation (Beijing, China). p-IkBα antibodies were purchased from Cell Signaling Technology (USA). CsA was purchased from Shanghai Pureone Biotechnology (Shanghai,China). Dual-Luciferase Reporter Kits were purchased from Promega (USA).

2.3 Induction of CIA

CIA was induced as previously described [16]. Briefly, male DBA/1J mice were injected intradermally at the base of the tail with 100 μl of a 1/1 (v/v) emulsion of 0.1 M acetic acid containing 100 μg of bovine type II collagen (Chondrex) and complete Freund's adjuvant containing 100 μg of heat-killed *Mycobacterium tuberculosis*. The day of the first immunization was defined as day 0. Three weeks after the primary immunization, the mice were boosted with 100 μg of collagen II in Freund's incomplete adjuvant via the same route.

2.4 Clinical assessment of arthritis

The severity of arthritis was quantified every other day by visual inspection, as described previously [17]. The clinical severity of arthritis in the paws was evaluated double-blindly using the following semi-quantitative scoring system: (0) no evidence of erythema and swelling, (1) swelling and erythema of the digit, (2) mild erythema of the limb, (3) gross erythema and swelling of the digit, and (4) ankylosis of the limb or gross swelling deformity and inability to use the limb. The clinical score for each mouse was the sum of the four paw scores, which results in a maximum score of 16. On the final day of the experiments, all mice were anesthetized with pentobarbital, and their blood was collected by cardiac puncture. In addition, their hind paws and knee joints were harvested for histological examination.

2.5 Histopathologic Analysis

Removed hind paws were fixed in 4% phosphate-buffered paraformaldehyde solution, decalcified in 30% formic acid and citric acid, and then embedded in paraffin. The tissues were longitudinally cut into 5-μm serial sections and stained with hematoxylin and eosin (H&E). The histopathological changes in the joints were examined under light microscopy and scored with a value ranging from 0 to 3, where 0 = normal, 1 = mild synovitis or slight cartilage erosion, 2 = moderate synovitis and cartilage erosion, and 3 = erosion of the cartilage or bone destruction [18].

2.6 DNFB-induced DTH assay

DTH assays were conducted as previously described [19]. The fur was removed (2 cm*2 cm) to expose the abdomen. The mice were initially sensitized by uniformly painting 50 μL of 1% 2,4-dinitrofluorobenzene (DNFB) dissolved in acetone and peanut oil (1:1) on their shaved abdomens on days 1 and 2. The mice in the negative control group were painted with 50 μL of solvent without DNFB. Three days after the second sensitization (day 5), all mice were treated with 10 μL of 1% DNFB on both sides of their right ear, and the left ears were treated with solvent alone. The mice were killed by cervical dislocation 24 h after treatment, and the spleen and thymus were immediately removed and weighed. The spleen and thymus indexes were expressed as spleen weight (mg) per 10 g of body weight and the thymus weight (mg) per 10 g of body weight, respectively. The ear swelling was expressed as the difference between the weights of the left and right ear patches obtained from 8-mm punches 24 h after the third sensitization.

2.7 Carbon particle clearance test

A carbon clearance experiment [20] was used to test the effect of glycyrol on the phagocytic activity of macrophages. Indian ink was centrifuged for 10 min at 3000 rpm; the supernatant was diluted 1:4 with sterile physiological saline and then injected into the tail vein of BALB/c mice (0.1 ml per 10 g body weight) 30 min after the last peroral administration. 2 min (T1) and 10 min (T2) after the injection of the ink, 20 μL of blood obtained from the retro-orbital venous plexus was added into 2 mL of 0.1% solution of Na_2CO_3 to lyse the red cells. The absorbances at 675 nm of the blood collected at 2(C1) and 10 min (C2) were measured, and the absorbance of the blood from the normal control group was set to zero. The mice were sacrificed by cervical dislocation, and the liver and the spleen weights were measured. The clearance index (K) and the phagocytic index (α) were calculated using the following equations: $k = (\lg C1 - \lg C2)/(T2-T1)$ and $\alpha = \left(1/3\sqrt{k} \times \text{body weight}\right)/(\text{liver weight} + \text{spleen weight})$, respectively.

2.8 Acute toxicity test

The mice were subjected to an acute toxicity test using the fixed-dose procedure, which is a sequential testing scheme that was proposed by the British Toxicology Society in1984 as an alternative for the assessment of acute peroral toxicity via estimation of the Lethal Dose 50 (LD_{50}). The procedure is incorporated into the European Community Directive guidelines as the acute peroral toxicity test [21]. Briefly, an initial dose of 5, 50, 500, or 2000 mg per kg of body weight can be selected to evaluate the toxicity of the substance being investigated. Either 5 or 2000 mg per kg can serve as the starting dose. The procedure is terminated when either toxicity or death is observed.

2.9 Acetic acid-induced capillary permeability test

0.5% Evan's blue solution in saline (0.1 mL per 10 g of body weight) was injected into the tail vein 30 min after the last peroral administration. After 20 min, 0.6% acetic acid in saline (0.1 mL per 10 g of body weight) was injected into the peritoneal cavity to increase the capillary permeability. 20 minutes after the acetic acid injection, the mice were sacrificed by cervical dislocation, and saline (5 mL per mouse) was injected into the abdominal cavity. After a gentle knead of the abdominal region, the peritoneal fluid was collected and centrifuged at 3000 rpm for 10 min. The supernatants were collected and color was measured photometrically as absorbance at 590 nm wavelength [22].

2.10 Western blot analysis of IκB-α in Jurkat cells

The phosphorylation of IκB-α was induced by incubating $1*10^6$ Jurkat cells with 100 ng/ml phorbol 12-myristate 13-acetate (PMA) plus 1 μM Ionomycin (Ion) or a combination of glycyrol and PMA plus Ion. After 24 h, the cells were harvested by centrifugation and washed twice with phosphate-buffered saline. The cells were lysed on ice for 20 min,the cell-free supernatant was collected for Western blot analysis. The protein quantification was performed using abicinchoninic acid protein quantitation kit. The samples were separated using discontinuous SDS-PAGE. The separated proteins were transferred to polyvinylidene fluoride membranes and then soaked in 5% non-fat dried milk in Tris-buffered saline for 1 h. The membrane was incubated with the primary antibody at room temperature for 1 h, incubated with a

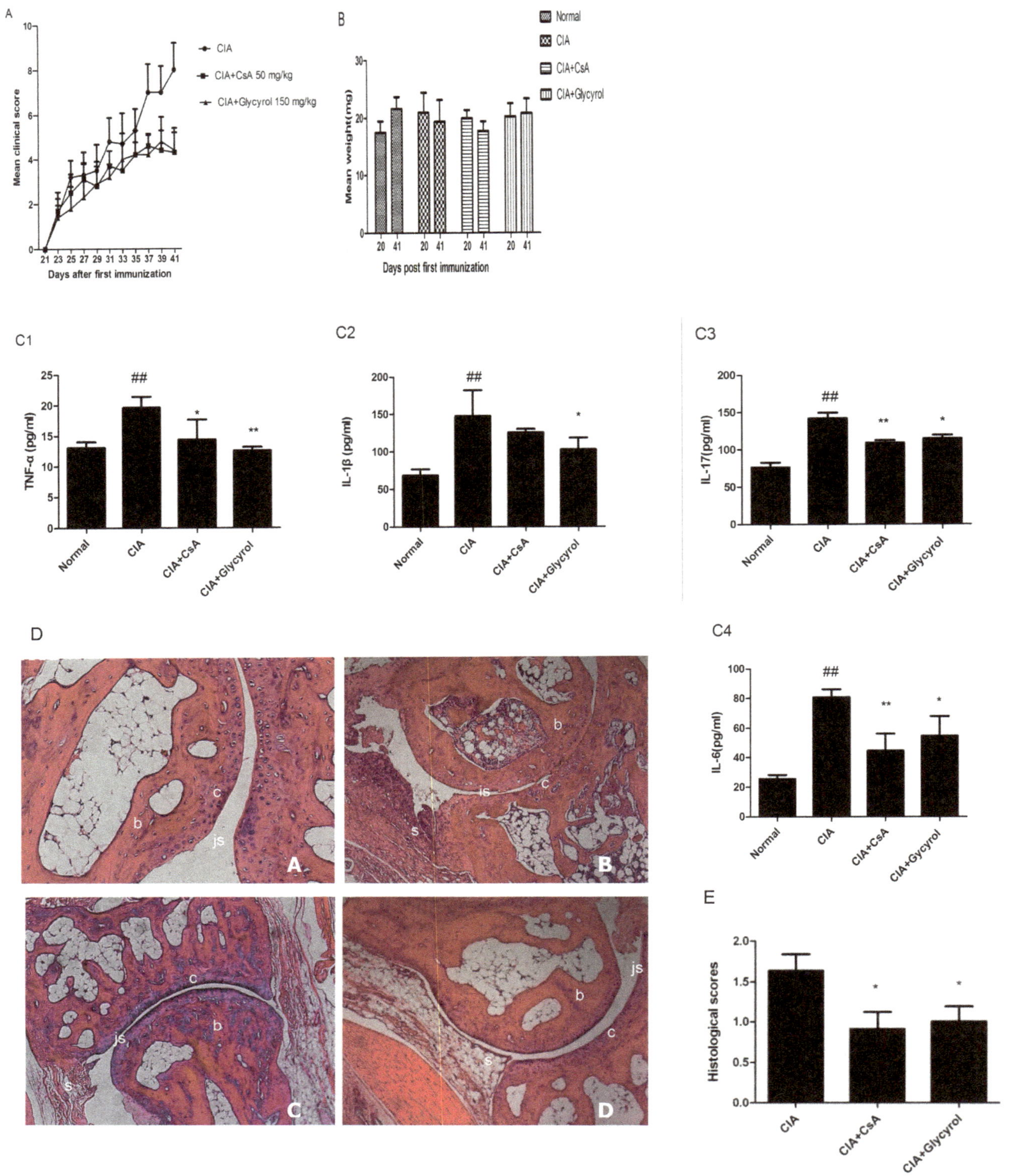

Figure 1. Glycyrol attenuates collagen-induced arthritis. CIA was induced by intradermal injection collagen II in Freund's adjuvant as described in Materials and Methods. A – C. Glycyrol and CsA were administered perorally every day from days 21 to 42. A: Time-dependent mean clinical scores (±SD) of four paws; B: Body weight changes (mean±SD); C1: TNF-α levels in serum on day 42; C2: IL-1β levels in serum on day 42; C3: IL-17 levels in serum on day 42; C4: IL-6 in serum on day 42. Data points are means ± SD of 7 mice. Differences between groups were tested by Student's t-test. # $P<0.05$ for comparison with Normal group, *$P<0.05$ for comparison with CIA group. D. Histopathologic features of representative ankle joints of male DBA/1J mice obtained on day 42 and stained with H&E (100x original magnification). "A" represents non-immunized mice showing normal articular cartilage, absence of infiltrate in the synovium and open joint space, "B" indicates CIA mice showing marked infiltration of inflammatory cells, narrow joint space with synovial hyperplasia, and "C" and "D" represent CIA mice treated with CsA or glycyrol, respectively,

showing less inflammatory cell infiltration, well-preserved joint spaces, and minimal synovial hyperplasia. "b" denotes bone tissue, whereas "c", "s", and "js" indicate cartilage, synovium, and joint space, respectively. E. Quantification of histological changes. Data represent means ±SD from 7 mice. *P<0.05 for comparison with CIA group.

biotinylated secondary antibody for 1 h, and then developed with peroxidase-conjugated streptavidin for 1 h. The specific bands were visualized using an electrochemiluminescence kit. Reactions were performed in triplicate.

2.11 Dual-luciferase reporter gene assay

The NFAT and NF-κB transcriptional activity was investigated using two reporter gene assay systems. RAW 264.7 macrophage cells plated in 24-well plates were co-transfected with the p-firefly luciferase (FL)-NFAT or NF-κB plasmid and the p-renilla luciferase (RL)-SV40 endogenous control plasmid, respectively. 24 hours after transfection, the cells were incubated with PMA plus Ion in the presence or absence of glycyrol. The NFAT and NF-κB transcriptional activity was measured using Dual-Luciferase Reporter Kit according to the manufacturer's protocol. Reactions were performed in triplicate.

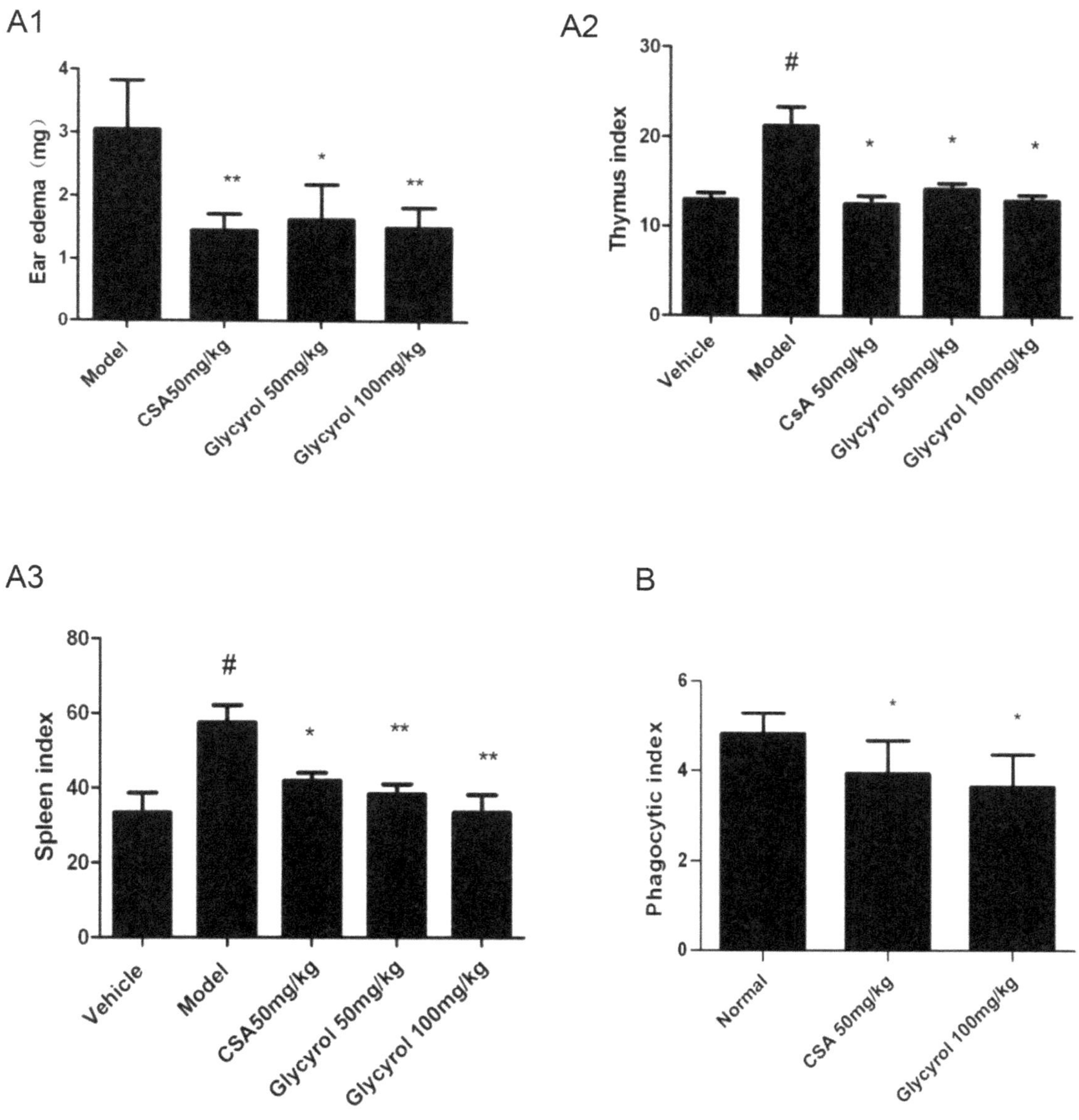

Figure 2. Effect of the peroral administration of glycyrol on immunoregulation *in vivo*. DNFB-induced DTH reaction (panel A) and carbon particle clearance test (panel B) conducted on mice given glycyrol (50 or 100 mg/kg) or CsA (50 mg/kg). The mice were initially sensitized by 50 μL of 1% DNFB on abdomens 30 min after drug administration on days 1 and 2. On day 5, 30 min after drug administration, mice were treated with 10 μL of 1% DNFB on both sides of their right ear. The mice were killed by cervical dislocation 24 h after the third sensitization. A1: ear swelling; A2: thymus; A3: spleen; B: phagocytic index. Data are shown as means ±SD from 8 mice. Differences between groups were tested by Student's t-test. # P<0.05 for comparison with Vehicle group, *P<0.05 for comparison with Model group.

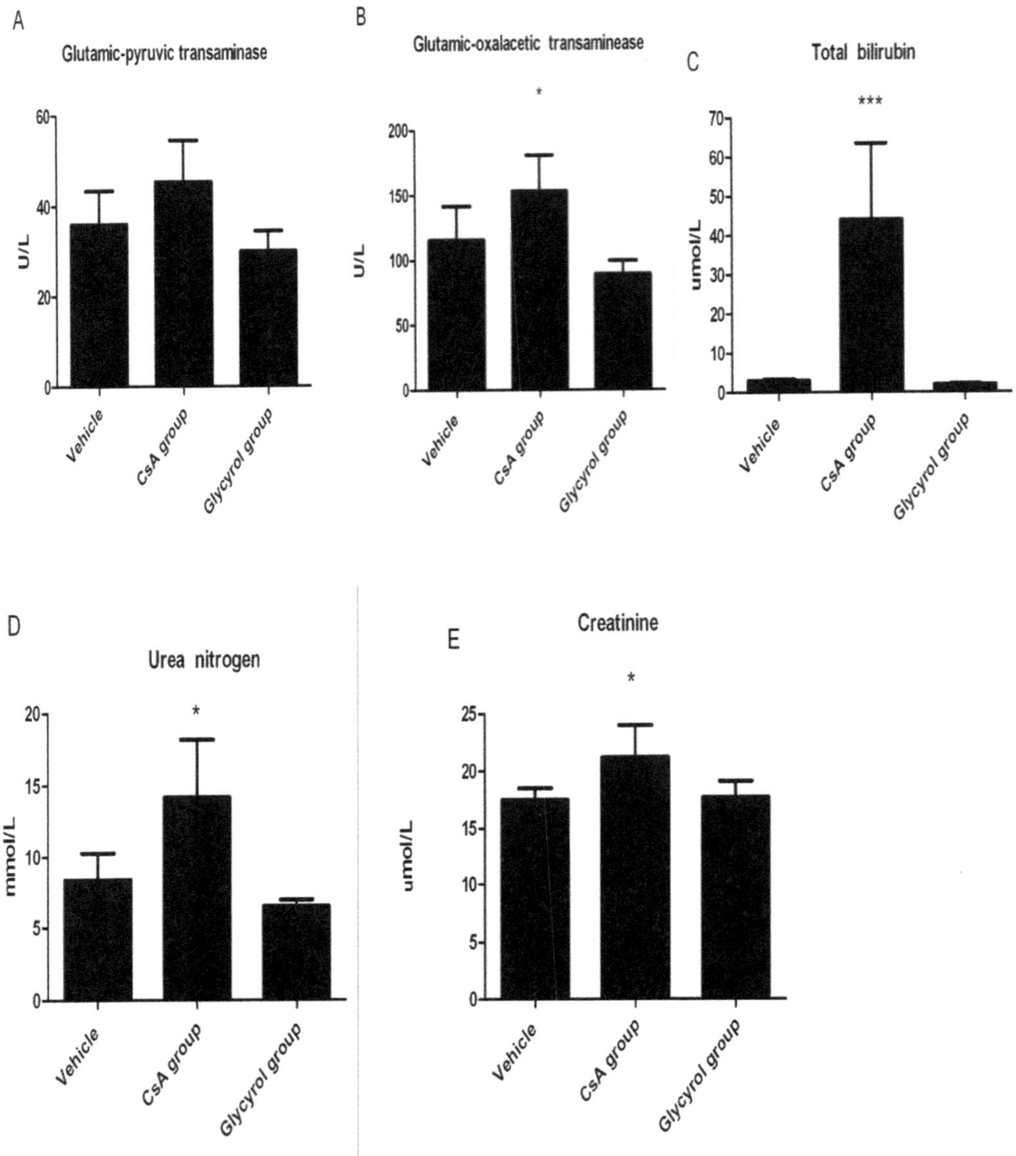

Figure 3. Acute toxicity of glycyrol in mice. Biochemistry in serum of mice treated with CsA or glycyrol. Dosage schedule: 500 mg/kg on day 0, 100 mg/kg on days 1 and 2; blood sampling on day 4. A: Glutamic-pyruvic transaminase; B: Glutamic-oxaloacetic transaminase; C: Total bilirubin; D: Urea nitrogen; E: Serum creatinine. Bars represent means ±SD from 7 mice. *P<0.05, **P<0.01 and ***P<0.001 for comparison with Vehicle group.

2.12 Real-time quantitative PCR for IL-2

The RNA was extracted from the RAW264.7 macrophages using the TRIzol reagent as described by the manufacturer. Real-time quantitative PCR was performed to detect the transcriptional level of IL-2. The primer sequences for IL-2 were 5′-CCTGAG-CAGGATGGA GAATTACA-3′ (forward) and 5′-TCCAGAA-CATGCCGCAGAG -3′ (reverse).β-actin:5′-AGA GGGAAATC-GTGCGTGAC-3′(forward), and5-'CAATAGTGATGACCTG-GCCGT-3′ (reverse). β-actin was used as an endogenous control gene. The real-time quantitative PCR was performed on an Applied Biosystems 7500 Real-Time PCR System using SYBR Green Dye. The reactions were performed in triplicate and the results are shown as the means ± SD.

2.13 Statistical analysis

Statistical comparisons were performed using one-way ANOVA and paired samples were compared by the Student's t-test using SPSS 11.0 software. The GraphPad Prism5 software was employed to calculate and draw plots. Values of P< 0.05 were considered as indicative of statistical significance.

Results

3.1 Glycyrol attenuates collagen-induced arthritis

Mice were immunized to induce CIA (see Materials and Methods). After the secondary immunization, they were randomly divided into four groups of 7: (1) normal non-immunized group, (2) CIA group, (3) CIA plus CsA group (50 mg per kg), and (4) CIA

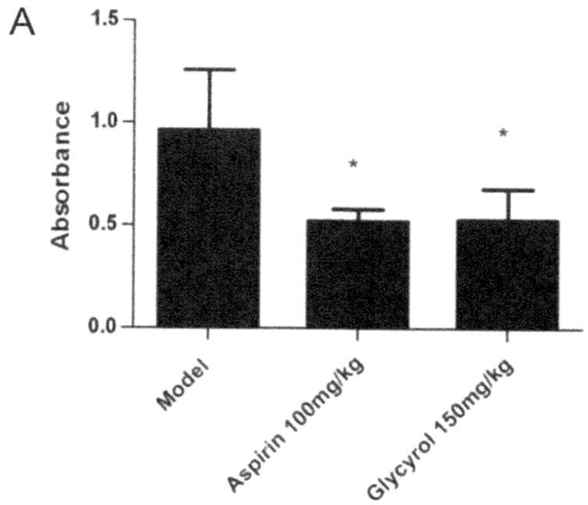

Figure 4. The action of glycyrol on acute inflammation *in vivo.* Acetic acid-induced capillary permeability test. Mice were given 150 mg/kg glycyrol perorally for 5 consecutive days before the acute inflammatory test. 0.5% Evan's blue was injected into the tail vein 30 min after the last peroral administration. Permeability scored by Evans Blue concentration in peritoneal fluid (light absorbance at 590 nm). Columns represent means ±SD from 8 mice. Differences between groups were tested by Student's t-test. *P<0.05 for comparison with Model group.

plus glycyrol group (150 mg per kg). Glycyrol and CsA were administered perorally every day from days 21 to 42. On the final day, blood samples were collected via cardiac punctures. The contents of TNF-α, IL-1β, IL-6, and IL-17 in the serum were measured using ELISA kits according to the manufacturers' instructions. The measurements were done in triplicate. The experimental results show that both the CsA and the glycyrol treatments reduced the mean arthritis scores (Figure 1A), and reduced the contents of IL-1β, TNF-α, IL-6, and IL-17(Figure 1C) in the serum. By the final day of the experiments, the weights of the normal and the glycyrol-treated mice had increased, whereas those of the mice in the CIA and CsA groups had decreased (Figure 1B). The histopathological changes in the joints were examined under light microscopy and scored with a value ranging from 0 to 3 based on the observed synovitis and cartilage/bone destruction. As the analysis of the histological changes (Figures 1D and 1E) suggests, there was obvious evidence of synovial hyperplasia, joint space narrowing, and bone and cartilage erosion in the joints of the mice in the CIA group, whereas these changes were scarcely observed in the mice in the glycyrol-treated group.

3.2 Inhibitory effect of glycyrol on immunoregulation

The DTH reaction and the carbon particle clearance test were employed to evaluate the influence of glycyrol on immunoregulation. Our previous work had demonstrated that mice injected intraperitoneally with glycyrol showed significantly decreased DTH and exhibited prolonged graft survival in allogeneic skin transplantation. To adapt to the characteristics of arthritis patients, who take drug over a long period of time, we decided to test peroral administration of glycyrol. For the DTH test, 40 male BALB/c mice were randomly divided into five groups of 8: a negative control group, a model group, a CsA group, and two glycyrol groups. The mice in the CsA group received peroral doses of 50 mg/kg CsA daily for six days, and the mice in the glycyrol groups received 50 or 100 mg/kg peroral glycyrol daily for six days. The mice were initially sensitized by DNFB on abdomens 30 min after drug administration on days 1 and 2, then on both sides of their right ear 30 min after drug administration on day 5. Figure 2A shows that the administration of glycyrol has a dose-dependent effect on DNFB-induced DTH because the ear swelling was significantly lower in the glycyrol-treated groups than in the model group. The results indicate that both glycyrol and CsA inhibit the increase in the spleen and thymus indexes induced by DNFB and that the inhibitory effect of glycyrol on the spleen index is better than that on the thymus index. Furthermore, the inhibitory effect of glycyrol on the spleen index is better than that of CsA (Figure 2A).

For the carbon clearance test, 24 male BALB/c mice were randomly divided into 3 groups of 8: a normal group, a CsA group (50 mg/kg), and a glycyrol group (100 mg/kg). The mice in CsA or glycyrol group were administered perorally every day for three days. 30 min after the last dose, indian ink diluted with sterile physiological saline was injected into the caudal vein of every mouse. Figure 2B shows that both glycyrol and CsA reduced phagocytosis by monocytes.

3.3 Acute toxicity of glycyrol in mice

In the European Community, the estimated LD_{50} is used mainly to place a substance under investigation into one of four categories. The substance is classified as 'very toxic' if the estimated LD_{50} is less than 25 mg per kg body weight, as 'toxic' if it is between 25 and 200 mg per kg body weight, and as 'harmful' if it is between 200 and 2000 mg per kg body weight. Substances with an estimated LD_{50} larger than 2000 mg per kg body weight are termed 'unclassified' [23].

Fourteen male BALB/c mice were divided into two groups of 7. Glycyrol was administered perorally at a single dose of 500 mg per kg to one group and at a dose of 2000 mg per kg to the other group. The mice were then observed over a period of two weeks to assess any changes in reactivity, gait, motor activity, respiration rate, and especially death. Mice given 2000 mg/kg body weight (n = 7) glycyrol did not show any difference in their gross general behavior; no death or obvious weight changes were observed over the 14 days that the mice were observed. Thus, the LD_{50} of glycyrol is more than 2000 mg/kg, which indicates that glycyrol can be categorized as 'unclassified.'

To further investigate the effect of glycyrol on the function of the liver and the kidney of animals, 21 male BALB/c mice were randomly divided into three groups of 7: a control group, a CsA group, and a glycyrol group. The dosage schedule was: 500 mg/kg perorally on day 0 and 100 mg/kg on days 1 and 2. The mice in the control group received an equivalent amount of the solvent. On day four, the mice were anesthetized with pentobarbital and blood was collected to determine the levels of glutamic-pyruvic transaminase, glutamic-oxaloacetic transaminase, total bilirubin, urea nitrogen, and creatinine in the serum.

Tests on the liver and kidney function showed blood biochemistry differences between the CsA-treated and the control groups. Treatment with CsA increased the blood biochemistry characteristics of the liver and the kidney, whereas minimal changes were observed in the glycyrol group (Figure 3). Thus, glycyrol had fewer adverse effects than CsA in our experimental animals.

3.4 Effects of glycyrol on acetic acid-induced capillary permeability

Acetic acid-induced capillary permeability was used to evaluate the action of glycyrol on inflammation *in vivo*. 24 male BALB/c mice were randomly divided into 3 groups of 8: control group, aspirin group, and glycyrol group. Peroral treatment with glycyrol or aspirin was administered on five consecutive days before inducing the capillary permeability test. The mice in the aspirin

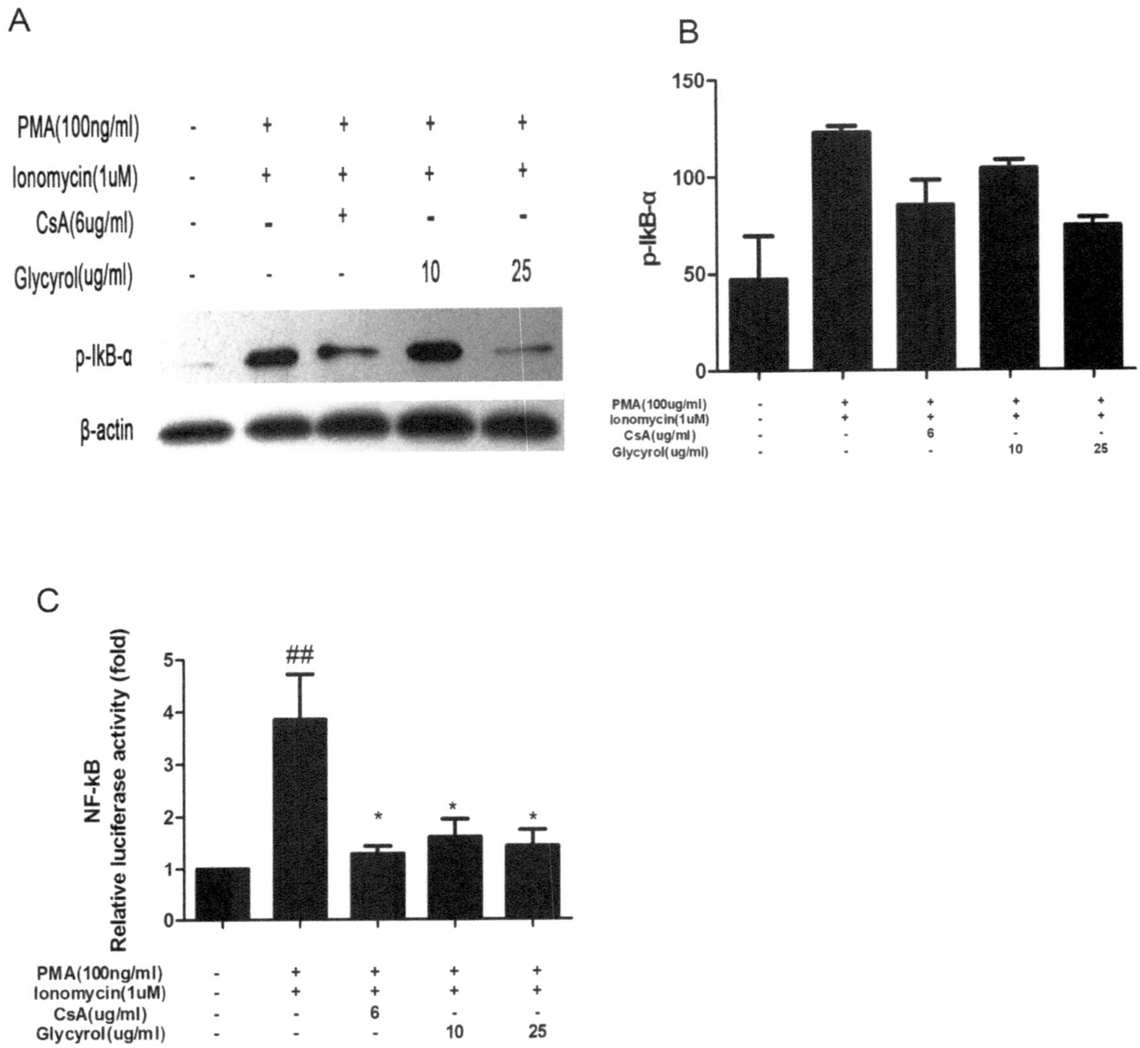

Figure 5. Glycyrol inhibits expression of p-IκB and NF-κB. A & B: Jurkat cells were stimulated with PMA plus Ion or a combination of indicated concentrations glycyrol or CsA and PMA plus Ion for 24 h to induce IκB-α expression. A: Western blot picture of p-IκB-α; B: Quantification of Western blot. C: RAW 264.7 cells were induced with PMA plus Ion or a combination of indicated concentrations glycyrol or CsA and PMA plus Ion for 24 h to induce NF-κB expression, and measured by dual-reporter gene assay system. Assays were performed in triplicate. Data represent means ±SD over three independent experiments. # $P<0.05$ for comparison with naïve group, *$P<0.05$ for comparison with PMA plus Ion-stimulated group.

group received peroral doses of 100 mg/kg aspirin daily for 5 days, and the mice in the glycyrol groups received 150 mg/kg peroral glycyrol daily for five days. Figure 4 shows that glycyrol substantially reduces the increase in capillary permeability stimulated by acetic acid.

3.5 Glycyrol inhibits the activity of NF-κB

IκB is an endogenous inhibitor of the transcription factor nuclear factor kappa B (NF-κB) which, upon phosphorylation by IκB kinase, is rapidly degraded, and this allows translocation of NF-κB to the nucleus [24]. NF-κB plays an important role in the inflammatory response. Hence, we tested the effects of glycyrol on expression of IκB-α in Jurkat cells and on NF-κB expression in RAW 264.7 cells. Cells were stimulated with PMA plus Ion or a combination of different doses glycyrol (as indicated in Figure 5) and PMA plus Ion for 24 h. Cells incubated only with plain medium or PMA plus Ion served as negative and positive controls, respectively. As shown in Figure 5, the phosphorylation of p-IκB and the transcriptional activity of NF-κB increased after stimulation with PMA plus Ion, increments that were partially prevented by simultaneous treatment with glycyrol or CsA.

3.6 Glycyrol inhibits NFAT activity and IL-2 transcription

CsA displays its immunosuppressive effect by inhibiting the NFAT/IL-2 signaling pathway. To determine whether glycyrol influences the NFAT/IL-2 signaling pathway, two reporter gene assays and real-time quantitative PCR were employed to test NFAT activity and IL-2 transcription, in RAW 264.7 macrophages, respectively. Cells were stimulated with PMA plus Ion or a combination of glycyrol or CsA and PMA plus Ion for 24 h. The data in Figure 6 suggest that glycyrol dose-dependently inhibits both NFAT and IL-2.

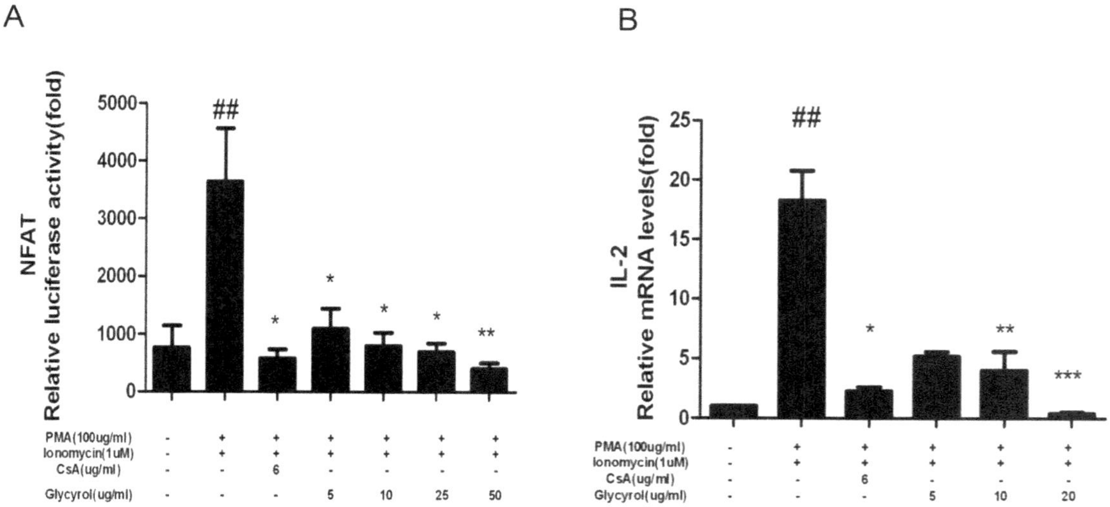

Figure 6. Glycyrol inhibits transcription of NFAT and IL-2genes. RAW 264.7 cells were stimulated with PMA plus Ion or a combination of indicated concentrations glycyrol or CsA and PMA plus Ion for 24 h to induce NFAT and IL-2 gene transcription. Panel A: NFAT transcription was measured using the dual-reporter gene assay system; Panel B: IL-2 gene transcription was detected by Real-time quantitative PCR. Assays were performed in triplicate. Data represent means ± SD over three independent experiments. Statistical significance was calculated using one-way analysis of variance (ANOVA) and Bonferroni post-test. # $P<0.05$ for comparison with naïve group, *$P<0.05$ for comparison with PMA plus Ion-stimulated group.

Discussion

We proved in this study that perorally administered glycyrol is effective in slowing down CIA as it lowered the clinical (Figure 1A) and pathological scores (Figure 1E), reduced blood levels of inflammatory cytokines (Figure 1C), and prevented joint damage (Figure 1D). We also present evidence showing that this therapeutic effect of glycyrol on arthritis is associated with a reduction in the two deleterious components of the disease, namely the autoimmune and the inflammatory responses. CN plays crucial roles in both these responses [25]. It acts mainly on T-lymphocytes and other immune cells, particularly via the CN-NFAT signaling pathway. Activated CN dephosphorylates NFAT, leading to its nuclear localization and the activation of the expression of its target genes, such as IL-2 [26,27]. Both DTH and CIA have been identified as Th1-mediated diseases [28]. Peroral administration of glycyrol significantly inhibited CIA (Figure 1) and DNFB-induced DTH (Figure 2A), demonstrating the suppressive effect of glycyrol on T-cell-dependent immune responses. In addition, peroral administration of glycyrol was found to inhibit the phagocytosis of macrophages (Figure 2B) in the carbon clearance experiment, which suggests that glycyrol can also adjust inherent immunity.

It has been reported that the pathogenesis process of rheumatoid arthritis is mainly driven by nuclear transcription factors, such as NF-κB, which is a transcription factor that plays an important role in regulating the expression of many genes involved in immune responses, including the cytokines TNF-α, IL-1β, MMP-1, and MMP-3, all of which are closely involved in the pathogenesis of RA. CsA, which inhibit RA, hampers the activity of NF-κB and NFAT [9]. Figures 5 and 6 show that, similar to CsA, glycyrol can inhibit the activation of NF-κB and NFAT *in vitro*.

Although the precise mechanism of RA is unknown, it is clear that cytokines play a key role in the inflammation processes of RA [29]. The monocyte/macrophage product TNF-α plays a central role in joint inflammation because TNF-α is at the top of a pro-inflammatory cytokine cascade [30,31]. IL-17 is a T cell-derived cytokine that leads to angiogenesis, joint inflammation, cartilage destruction, and bone erosion in RA [32,33]. In several animal models of arthritis, the inhibition of IL-17 has been found to limit inflammation and joint erosion [34]. Glycyrol treatment reduced levels of TNF-α, IL-17, IL-6, and IL-1β (Figure 1C) in the serum of CIA. Furthermore, it decreased the MMPs and NO contents in the of primary and inhibited the impression of inducible nitric oxidase synthase (iNOS) and cyclooxygenase-2 (COX-2) (data not shown). Thus, it appears that glycyrol attenuates CIA through its influence on the inflammatory response.

As a whole, the therapeutic effect of glycyrol was associated with down-regulation of both the inflammatory and the autoimmune reactions. It is well established that there are some interactions between inflammatory factors and immune cells. Because NF-κB plays a key role in both the inflammation and the autoimmune responses, there are many intersections between the autoimmune and the inflammation reactions. Thus, it is difficult to precisely state how much of the RA pathogenesis is autoimmune and how much is due to inflammatory reactions. However, the effective dose in DTH and in the carbon clearance test was100 mg per kg of body weight, whereas the effective dose in the acetic acid-induced capillary permeability test was150 mg per kg of body weight ($P<0.05$). Thus, glycyrol maybe more powerful as an immunosuppressant than as an anti-inflammatory agent.

In this study, the acute toxicity of glycyrol was tested in mice over a period of 14 days. No mice died or exhibited behavioral changes during this period, even in the high-dose group (2000 mg per kg), which indicates that the median lethal dose (LD_{50}) of glycyrol is greater than 2000 mg per kg. Our previous work on the maximum dose tolerance in mice proved that intraperitoneal administration of 400 mg/kg glycyrol three times a day also did not cause death or behavioral changes. Therefore, we can conclude that glycyrol has no or minimal toxicity. Because RA is a chronic autoimmune disease, which requires drug treatment for several months, a higher dose was employed to further test whether glycyrol impacts the liver and kidney functions. In this study, we found that the levels of total bilirubin, glutamic-pyruvic transaminase, glutamic-oxaloacetic transaminase, urea nitrogen, and creatinine (Figures 3) were increased in mice administered large peroral doses of CsA but not in mice treated with glycyrol. Overall, the results show that glycyrol has fewer adverse effects than CsA on experimental animals.

From the prescription of the medication Sandimmune (Cyclosporine), we have learned that the initial oral dosage for transplantation is 14 to 18 mg/kg in most clinical trials. The usual oral dose for autoimmune disease is 5 mg/kg, and this dose must be taken for three to six months according to the instructions. For CIA, a peroral dose of 50 mg/kg is a moderate dose for mice because this dosage is equivalent to 4 mg/kg for humans, as determined through a dose conversion using experimental pharmacological methods. In the 20-day period during which the drug was taken after the second immunization, the weight of the mice in the CsA-treated (50 mg per kg) group decreased by 11% and that of the mice in the CIA group decreased by 7%, whereas the weight of the mice in the glycyrol-treated (150 mg/kg) group increased by 2%. This result may be further proof that glycyrol is less toxic than CsA. Therefore, we have reason to expect that it will become a potential candidate drug in the future.

Author Contributions

Conceived and designed the experiments: YF QW. Performed the experiments: YF HZ. Analyzed the data: HZ YF. Contributed reagents/materials/analysis tools: SW HZ YF. Wrote the paper: YF QW.

References

1. Vinay DS, Kwon BS (2012) Targeting TNF superfamily members for therapeutic intervention in rheumatoid arthritis. Cytokine. 57:305–12
2. Pierer M, Wagner U, Rossol M, Ibrahim S (2011) Toll-like receptor 4 is involved in inflammatory and joint destructive pathways in collagen-induced arthritis in DBA1J mice. PLoS One 6:e23539
3. Gabriel SE, Michaud K (2009) Epidemiological studies in incidence, prevalence, mortality, and comorbidity of the rheumatic diseases. Arthritis Res. Ther. 11:229
4. Umar S, Asif M, Sajad M (2012) Anti-inflammatory and antioxidant activity of Trachyspermumammi seeds in collagen induced arthritis in rats. J Drug Dev Res 4:210–9
5. Wang JH, Shih KS, Liou JP, Wu YW, Chang AS, et al. (2012) Anti-arthritic effects of magnolol in human interleukin 1beta-stimulated fibroblast-like synoviocytes and in a rat arthritis model. PLoS One 7:e31368
6. McInnes IB, Schett G (2007) Cytokines in the pathogenesis of rheumatoid arthritis. Nat. Rev. Immunol. 7:429–42
7. Scott DL, Wolfe F, Huizinga TW (2010) Rheumatoid arthritis. Lancet. 376:1094–108
8. Yocum DE, Furst DE, Kaine JL, Baldassare AR, Stevenson JT, et al. (2003) Efficacy and safety of tacrolimus in patients with rheumatoid arthritis: a double-blind trial. Arthritis Rheum. 48:3328–37
9. Kitahara K, Kawai S (2007) Cyclosporine and tacrolimus for the treatment of rheumatoid arthritis. Curr. Opin. Rheumatol. 19:238–45
10. Hong JC, Kahan BD (2000) Immunosuppressive agents in organ transplantation: past, present, and future. Semin. Nephrol. 20:108–25
11. Bennett WM, Norman DJ (1986) Action and toxicity of cyclosporine. Annu. Rev. Med. 37:215–24: 215–24
12. Thomson AW, Whiting PH, Simpson JG (1984) Cyclosporine: immunology, toxicity and pharmacology in experimental animals. Agents Actions. 15:306–27
13. Venkatesha SH, Rajaiah R, Berman BM, Moudgil KD (2011) Immunomodulation of Autoimmune Arthritis by Herbal CAM. Evid. Based. Complement Alternat. Med. 2011:986797. doi: 10.1155/2011/986797. Epub;%2010 Dec 22.:986797
14. Li J, Tu Y, Tong L, Zhang W, Zheng J, et al. (2010) Immunosuppressive activity on the murine immune responses of glycyrol from Glycyrrhiza uralensis via inhibition of calcineurin activity. Pharm. Biol. 48:1177–84
15. Jin Y, Kim S, Kim Y, Kim S, Kim H (2008) The first total synthesis of glycyrol. Tetrahedron Letters 49:6835–7
16. Brand DD, Latham KA, Rosloniec EF (2007) Collagen-induced arthritis. Nat. Protoc. 2:1269–75
17. Nishikawa M, Myoui A, Tomita T, Takahi K, Nampei A, et al. (2003) Prevention of the onset and progression of collagen-induced arthritis in rats by the potent p38 mitogen-activated protein kinase inhibitor FR167653. Arthritis Rheum. 48:2670–81
18. Strid J, Tan LA, Strobel S, Londei M, Callard R (2007) Epicutaneous immunization with type II collagen inhibits both onset and progression of chronic collagen-induced arthritis. PLoS One 2:e387
19. Feng YH, Zhou WL, Wu QL, Li XY, Zhao WM, et al. (2002) Low dose of resveratrol enhanced immune response of mice. Acta Pharmacol. Sin. 23:893–7
20. Hua Y, Gao Q, Wen L, Zhao M (2012) Structural characterisation of acid-soluble polysaccharides in the fruiting body of *Dictyophora indusiata* and their immunomodulatory activities. Food Chem 132:739–43
21. Stallard N, Whitehead A (1995) Reducing animal numbers in the fixed-dose procedure. Hum. Exp. Toxicol. 14:315–23
22. Huang LJ, Gao WY, Li X, Zhao WS, Huang LQ, et al. (2010) Evaluation of the in vivo anti-inflammatory effects of extracts from Pyrus bretschneideri Rehd. J. Agric. Food Chem. 58:8983–7
23. Cen J, Shi M, Yang Y, Fu Y, Zhou H, et al. (2013) Isogarcinol is a new immunosuppressant. PLoS One 8:e66503
24. Kockx M, Jessup W, Kritharides L (2010) Cyclosporin A and atherosclerosis–cellular pathways in atherogenesis. Pharmacol. Ther. 128:106–18
25. Yoo SA, Park BH, Park GS, Koh HS, Lee MS, et al. (2006) Calcineurin is expressed and plays a critical role in inflammatory arthritis. J. Immunol. 177:2681–90
26. Rusnak F, Mertz P (2000) Calcineurin: form and function. Physiol Rev. 80:1483–521
27. Baksh S, Burakoff SJ (2000) The role of calcineurin in lymphocyte activation. Semin. Immunol. 12:405-15
28. Mauri C, Williams RO, Walmsley M, Feldmann M (1996) Relationship between Th1/Th2 cytokine patterns and the arthritogenic response in collagen-induced arthritis. Eur. J Immunol. 26:1511–8
29. Brennan FM, McInnes IB (2008) Evidence that cytokines play a role in rheumatoid arthritis. J. Clin. Invest. 118:3537–45
30. Kim HS, Kim AR, Park HJ, Park DK, Kim dK, et al. (2011) Morus bombycis Koidzumi extract suppresses collagen-induced arthritis by inhibiting the activation of nuclear factor-kappaB and activator protein-1 in mice. J. Ethnopharmacol. 136:392–8
31. Gorman CL, Cope AP (2008) Immune-mediated pathways in chronic inflammatory arthritis. Best. Pract. Res. Clin. Rheumatol. 22:221–38
32. Lubberts E, van den BL, Oppers-Walgreen B, Schwarzenberger P, Coenen-de Roo CJ, et al. (2003) IL-17 promotes bone erosion in murine collagen-induced arthritis through loss of the receptor activator of NF-kappa B ligand/osteoprotegerin balance. J Immunol. 170:2655–62
33. Pickens SR, Volin MV, Mandelin AM, Kolls JK, Pope RM, et al. (2010) IL-17 contributes to angiogenesis in rheumatoid arthritis. J. Immunol. 184:3233–41
34. van den Berg WB, Miossec P (2009) IL-17 as a future therapeutic target for rheumatoid arthritis. Nat. Rev. Rheumatol. 5:549–53

5

Analyzing Genome-Wide Association Studies with an FDR Controlling Modification of the Bayesian Information Criterion

Erich Dolejsi[1], Bernhard Bodenstorfer[2], Florian Frommlet[1]*

1 Center for Medical Statistics, Informatics, and Intelligent Systems/Section of Medical Statistics, Medical University Vienna, Vienna, Austria, **2** cogiti e.U., Karlstift, Austria

Abstract

The prevailing method of analyzing GWAS data is still to test each marker individually, although from a statistical point of view it is quite obvious that in case of complex traits such single marker tests are not ideal. Recently several model selection approaches for GWAS have been suggested, most of them based on LASSO-type procedures. Here we will discuss an alternative model selection approach which is based on a modification of the Bayesian Information Criterion (mBIC2) which was previously shown to have certain asymptotic optimality properties in terms of minimizing the misclassification error. Heuristic search strategies are introduced which attempt to find the model which minimizes mBIC2, and which are efficient enough to allow the analysis of GWAS data. Our approach is implemented in a software package called MOSGWA. Its performance in case control GWAS is compared with the two algorithms HLASSO and d-GWASelect, as well as with single marker tests, where we performed a simulation study based on real SNP data from the POPRES sample. Our results show that MOSGWA performs slightly better than HLASSO, where specifically for more complex models MOSGWA is more powerful with only a slight increase in Type I error. On the other hand according to our simulations GWASelect does not at all control the type I error when used to automatically determine the number of important SNPs. We also reanalyze the GWAS data from the Wellcome Trust Case-Control Consortium and compare the findings of the different procedures, where MOSGWA detects for complex diseases a number of interesting SNPs which are not found by other methods.

Editor: María Mar Abad-Grau, University of Granada - Q1818002F, Spain

Funding: This research has been funded by the Vienna Science and Technology Fund (http://www.wwtf.at/) through project MA09-007a. All three authors received funding. The funders had no role in study design, data collection and analysis, decision to publish, or preparation of the manuscript.

Competing Interests: The co-author Bernhard Bodenstorfer runs the company cogiti e.U., which provides information technology services such as programming, consultancy and technology management. However, this does not alter the authors' adherence to PLOS ONE policies on sharing data and materials. In particular, the program developed has been openly published on sourceforge.net under the GNU GPL version 3 open license for the scientific community to freely use, as the authors have indicated in their submitted paper.

* Email: Florian.Frommlet@meduniwien.ac.at

Introduction

Recently there has been growing interest in model selection approaches to GWAS analysis. Although it is still common practice in published GWAS to perform statistical analysis for each SNP individually, there is increasing awareness that this kind of single marker analysis has certain deficiencies in case of complex traits. Several authors have commented that marginal tests will suffer from lack of power to detect SNPs because the effect of other causal SNPs remains unaccounted for [23,29]. It has been argued that this shortcoming of single marker tests might play a significant role in the widely discussed phenomenon of "missing heritability" in GWAS [43].

A slightly more sophisticated and less known problem is that single marker tests have serious difficulties to rank important SNPs correctly [23]. This is obvious for SNPs which are not directly associated with a trait, but which have an important effect conditional on the presence of other SNPs. However, even in case of SNPs with marginal effects it turns out that due to small sample correlations some important SNPs might have rather small probability to be detected, whereas other SNPs which are not associated at all with the trait might be selected with large probability. This result puts in question the common practice to report those SNPs in GWAS which have lowest ranking marginal p-values.

Given these deficiencies of single marker tests one can expect that the use of multi marker models to analyze GWAS will become more and more important. Multiple linear regression models for quantitative traits and logistic regression models for case control studies have a long history in genetic association studies. To facilitate their use for GWAS there is a strong demand of two things: A thorough theoretical understanding of different model selection strategies in high dimensions to find the regression model which includes important SNPs, as well as the availability of software packages which make modern statistical methodology applicable to GWAS analysis.

Concerning the theory of high dimensional data analysis the last two decades have seen a large number of innovations. One milestone was the development of LASSO [39], which paved the way for a large number of other new approaches to model selection. Bühlmann and van de Geer [12] give a comprehensive presentation of the theoretical foundations of LASSO and its many extensions like adaptive LASSO, group lasso or the elastic net. In the context of GWAS several algorithms have been implemented based on LASSO or one of its extensions [26,30,42].

From a Bayesian perspective the LASSO is equivalent to model selection with a double exponential (DE) distribution as shrinkage prior. Among the first software packages which allowed to perform multi marker analysis of GWAS was HLASSO [29], which uses not only DE priors, but alternatively considers normal exponential Gaussian (NEG) priors. The NEG distribution is more pointed than DE at 0, resulting in the selection of potentially smaller models. More recently a Bayesian version of the LASSO was introduced for GWAS analysis [31].

The LASSO itself was originally developed for model selection problems of moderate size, whereas in GWAS one usually is confronted with up to a million SNPs or more. For such ultra-high dimensional problems, Fan et al. [17] suggested sure independence screening (SIS) as a convenient way of dimension reduction. In case of regression models SIS is nothing else but preselecting a certain number of markers based on marginal tests. After SIS more refined methods like LASSO or SCAD can be applied to select a model. Using tests conditional on that selected model over all remaining markers one can apply another SIS step. Iterating SIS and refined model selection gives the procedure called ISIS.

A startlingly simple but computationally intensive method to improve the performance of model selection procedures in high dimensions is stability selection [33], where random subsamples of the data are drawn repeatedly and a given model selection procedure like LASSO is performed on each of these subsamples. The final model is then obtained by considering those regressors which have appeared consistently over the repeated samples.

One of the more prominent model selection packages for GWAS is GWASelect [26], which combines ISIS with stability selection based on 50 random subsamples, where the refined model selection procedure in ISIS is LASSO. GWASelect itself uses a prespecified size of the model, but there exists a 'dynamic' version d-GWASelect which uses cross-validation to fit the LASSO parameter and which determines the number of selected SNPs using stability selection. Thus in this article GWASelect actually refers to d-GWASelect, the algorithm which allows to determine the number of interesting SNPs.

An alternative approach to model selection in high dimensions which is currently gaining popularity is based on information criteria. Among the large number of SNPs genotyped in GWAS one expects only a moderate number of SNPs to have a strong effect. In such a sparse setting classical information criteria like Akaike's AIC or Schwarz's Bayesian information criterion (BIC) [38] have been shown to select too large models [11]. Consequently, Bogdan et al. [8] introduced a modification of BIC called mBIC which is designed to control the family wise error rate (FWER) of selected markers in sparse regression [9]. A rather similar criterion called EBIC was presented by Chen and Chen [14], where consistency results for EBIC under sparsity were shown even in case when the number of markers is growing faster than the number of observations.

Here we will focus on mBIC2, a modification of BIC which has the property of controlling the false discovery rate (FDR). The false discovery rate is the expected proportion of incorrectly rejected null hypotheses, and was introduced by Benjamini and Hochberg [6] as a measure of type I error control in multiple testing which is less stringent than the family-wise error rate. Frommlet et al. [21] introduced the criterion mBIC2 to control the FDR in a model selection context. Further background information on mBIC2 is given by Frommlet et al. [23], where extensive GWAS simulations of quantitative traits based on real SNP data show that mBIC2 is considerably more powerful to detect causal SNPs than mBIC, while controlling the FDR at a fixed level.

In this article we will focus on case control studies, where the model selection task is performed using logistic regression models. Modifications of BIC for generalized linear models were studied already in the context of QTL mapping [45]. However, for GWAS the task of minimizing the criterion over all possible models is much more challenging than in QTL mapping due to the much larger number of genetic markers involved. In case of logistic regression computing maximum likelihood estimates for each model becomes much more time consuming than for quantitative traits, and therefore one needs to develop rather involved search strategies trying to find models which minimize mBIC2. The resulting algorithm is implemented in the software package MOSGWA, and we compare its performance with single marker tests and with other variable selection methods, in particular with HLASSO [29] and GWASelect [26]. The main reason for this choice is that He and Lin [26] performed already a comparison with several other methods for GWAS analysis, where HLASSO and GWASelect gave the most convincing results. We will report results from an extensive simulation study to compare the performance of the different procedures, and we will reanalyze the GWAS data from the Wellcome Trust Case-Control Consortium (WTCCC) [41].

Methods

Selection criterion

Before describing the algorithmic details of MOSGWA we will formally introduce the selection criterion mBIC2. Consider a GWAS based on p SNPs and n individuals. For a given model including k_M SNPs our model selection criterion is of the form

$$mBIC2 = -2\log L_M^* + k_M \log(np^2/4) - 2\log(k_M!) \, . \quad (1)$$

Each set of SNPs forms a potential model M, and MOSGWA tries to find that model which minimizes mBIC2. Here L_M^* is the Firth corrected maximum likelihood, which will be discussed in more detail below.

The penalty of the mBIC2 criterion was introduced by Frommlet et al. [21], where its derivation was based on ideas of Abramovich et al. [1]. In particular mBIC2 is closely related to the Benjamini-Hochberg multiple testing procedure [6], and it controls the false discovery rate of detected SNPs. In the context of linear regression certain asymptotic optimality properties of mBIC2 were shown [7,21]. Roughly speaking selection based on mBIC2 minimizes the misclassification error when both p and n are large, while the number of regressors of the correct model is relatively small.

An extensive motivation of mBIC2 can be found in Frommlet et al. [23], where the criterion is applied for linear regression models to analyze GWAS with quantitative traits. In contrast we will focus here on case-control studies, and just like HLASSO [26] and GWASelect [29] we make use of logistic regression to model the disease risk of SNPs. To this end let Y_i denote the disease status of individual $i \in \{1, \ldots, n\}$ ($Y_i = 1$ for a case, $Y_i = 0$ for a control), and let x_{ij} denote the genotype of SNP $j \in \{1, \ldots, p\}$ for individual i. If a model M includes the SNPs $j_1, \ldots, j_k$ then the corresponding logistic regression model can be written as

$$\pi_i := P(Y_i = 1|M,\theta) = \frac{\exp(\beta_0 + \sum_{r=1}^{k} \beta_r x_{ijr})}{1 + \exp(\beta_0 + \sum_{r=1}^{k} \beta_r x_{ijr})}, \quad (2)$$

with the parameter vector $\theta = (\beta_0, \ldots, \beta_k)^T$. These $k+1$ parameters can be routinely estimated by maximizing the corresponding likelihood $L_M(\theta)$, although occasionally the well known problem of separation may occur, where some parameter estimates tend towards infinity [2]. In classical statistical applications, where $p \ll n$, separation typically arises only in case of small sample sizes. For GWAS the sample size is usually very large, but the number of potential regressors is even several orders larger, which results in many combinations of SNPs for which separation occurs. Heinze and Schemper [27] suggested to overcome the problem of separation using a bias corrected version of logistic regression which was originally proposed by Firth [18]. The likelihood of the logistic regression model is multiplied with the corresponding Jeffreys prior, which is just the square root of the determinant of the Fisher information matrix $I(\theta)$. Thus the Firth corrected maximum likelihood from equation (1) is given by

$$L_M^* = \max_\theta L_M(\theta)\sqrt{|I(\theta)|}, \quad (3)$$

and explicit formulas are given for example by Heinze and Schemper [27]. The Firth-corrected log-likelihood $\log L_M^*$ includes the penalty term $\log\sqrt{|I(\theta)|}$, which guarantees that parameter estimates cannot get excessively large. Note that LASSO based procedures like GWASelect do not run into difficulties with separation because the L^1-penalty yields automatically a shrinkage of parameters.

Search strategy

Having defined the model selection criterion (1) the main task is to find the model which minimizes mBIC2. The resulting problem is an extremely challenging mixed integer program, for which one can only attempt to develop heuristic methods which yield an approximate solution. The search algorithm of the software package MOSGWA repeatedly makes use of a strategy called fast stepwise search (FSS).

The aim of FSS is, starting from some initial model, to perform a search heuristic which finds a model with a smaller value of a given selection criterion. The final call of FSS is performed with the target criterion mBIC2, but within the search it is valuable to work with less stringent criteria to avoid getting stuck in local minima corresponding to models which are missing some of the causal SNPs. Specifically we consider the milder criterion

$$mBIC_{60} := -2\log L_M^* + k_M \log(np^2/60).$$

FSS depends on a pre-specified order of all markers not included in the initial model. This order is either based on some marginal test statistics, or on some conditional score tests as described below. We will thus formally write the fast stepwise search as a function

$$M = \mathrm{FSS}(M_{\mathrm{init}}, \mathit{test}, \mathit{criterion}),$$

to emphasize that it depends on the initial model, on the specific order of markers according to *test*, and on the respective *criterion*. Depending on the order of markers two groups are considered: Group G_1 consists of the best m_1 SNPs, and group G_2 of the best m_2 SNPs. Thus $G_1 \subset G_2$, where G_1 is the set of SNPs along which directed forward steps are performed (see below), whereas SNPs within G_2 might enter the model via so called exchange steps (see below). The exact choice of the parameters m_1 and m_2 turns out to be not too important. The default values of MOSGWA which are also used for simulations are $m_1 = 350$ and $m_2 = 5000$ (as long as $p \geq 5000$).

FSS is based on three algorithmic steps which we call directed forward, exchange, and backward step. FSS starts by considering the initial model M_{init} as the current model. The directed forward step repeatedly tests if enhancing the current model with a SNP decreases the *criterion*, where SNPs within G_1 are considered in the order obtained from the *test* (therefore *directed* forward search). The first SNP which improves the current model is added, and an exchange step follows.

In the exchange step all SNPs in the current model are tested whether exchanging them with suitable other SNPs decreases the *criterion*. Suitable candidates for exchanging SNP S_i are all other SNPs within G_2 whose physical distance to S_i on the chromosome is less than d. The default cutoff value of MOSGWA is $d = 50$, that is we only consider the 49 closest neighboring SNPs in both directions. The algorithm starts with the first SNP of the current model, and tries to exchange it with all suitable candidate SNPs. In case of improvement the first SNP is substituted with the best possible alternative. Then exchanges of the second SNP with all corresponding candidates are performed, and so on till each SNP of the model has been considered once. The idea behind this strategy is that in the directed search step it might happen that not the optimal SNP was chosen, but a correlated SNP might further improve the model. Also after several SNPs have been added to the model it can happen that exchanging a particular SNP of the model is beneficial. Limiting the exchange to SNPs close to S_i which themselves have reasonably large test statistic makes this strategy computationally feasible.

The third step of FSS is an extended backward elimination step. First a standard greedy elimination step is performed, which means that all models are considered where one SNP is removed from the current model. If this does not improve the model, greedy elimination is repeated up to three times to look for better models. In other words like in a classical stepwise elimination procedure we first remove the SNP which explains the least, if this does not improve the selection criterion we additionally remove the next SNP which explains the least, and if the resulting model again has larger selection criterion than the original model we try one more time to remove the least explanatory SNP. The resulting best model is then the starting point for another directed forward step. Directed forward, exchange, and backward steps are then performed repeatedly till no further improvement of the *criterion* is achieved.

Starting with the null model M_0 the complete search strategy of MOSGWA can be specified as follows:

1. $M^* = \mathrm{FSS}(M_0$, Cochran Armitage, mBIC_60)
2. $M^{**} = \mathrm{FSS}(M^*$, Score Test, mBIC_60)
3. $M^{\mathrm{final}} = \mathrm{FSS}(M^{**}$, Score Test, mBIC2)

The general strategy of this algorithm can be motivated as follows. In the first round markers are preselected based on their marginal (Cochran Armitage) test statistic. In the second round score tests conditional on the model M^* of the first round are performed over all remaining SNPs (see [26]). Score tests have the benefit of being computationally much less expensive than likelihood ratio tests, and therefore provide a fast way to preselect markers which might be of importance additional to markers within M^*.

The first two rounds are performed with the milder criterion mBIC_60, which is expected to yield models which are too large. In fact when models are getting too large then the value of d from the exchange step is reduced to guarantee reasonable runtime. As mentioned previously the benefit of first working with mBIC_60 is that one reduces the chances of missing out on important SNPs due to local minima. Only in the final round FSS is performed with the target criterion mBIC2, and will then yield a model for which the type I error rate is controlled in terms of FDR.

The software package MOSGWA is available at http://mosgwa.sourceforge.net/. An application note describing the software in more detail is in preparation.

Simulation Studies

Global null hypothesis

Our first set of simulations is concerned with controlling the type I error under the global null hypothesis. Simulations are based on real SNP data from $n = 4077$ individuals from the POPRES sample [34], which are included in the POPRES_Genotypes_QC2 dataset. Individuals are randomly allocated as cases and as controls with equal probability; then MOSGWA, HLASSO and GWASelect are applied to evaluate their ability to control the type I error rate. The random allocation was repeated 200 times, and Table 1 presents the average number of observed false positives to estimate the per-family error rate. A graphical illustration is provided in Figure 1.

To study the influence of the number of SNPs we performed four different simulations using SNPs only from chromosome 1, from the first two, the first four and the first six chromosomes, respectively. The resulting number of SNPs, p, for these four scenarios is given in the first column of Table 1. GWASelect and single marker tests tend to report a large number of correlated SNPs, and thus for these two procedures the number of false positives was obtained by counting clusters of neighboring SNPs [26], where clustering was performed with the algorithm of Frommlet [20]. For HLASSO and MOSGWA no such clustering is necessary, because these algorithms tend to select only one representative for a genomic region anyway.

Table 1 illustrates that MOSGWA controls the type I error under the total null hypothesis irrespective of the number of SNPs. For MOSGWA no parameter needs to be tuned, whereas the latest version of HLASSO allows to choose a parameter α which corresponds to an uncorrected nominal significance level. We consider three Bonferroni-like choices of the form $\alpha \in \{0.3/p, 0.2/p, 0.1/p\}$. The results from Table 1 indicate that the type I error tends to remain below the nominal level, which is not too surprising given the positive correlations between neighboring SNPs due to linkage disequilibrium. Type I error rates for $\alpha = 0.3/p$ are closest to those from MOSGWA, and therefore from now on HLASSO will be used with this parameter setting.

The size of the model selected by GWASelect depends on the stable-selection-threshold ξ, which is defined in the following way; GWASelect reports a SNP as detected when the proportion of random subsamples in which the SNP was selected is larger than ξ. He and Lin [26] recommend a choice between 0.1 and 0.2. However, the results from Table 1 show that for these parameter settings GWASelect completely fails to control the type I error rate under the global null. We therefore considered additionally $\xi = 0.3$, for which the per-family error rate is controlled at least to some extent. Interestingly the type I error from GWASelect decreases when the number of SNPs increases.

The last column of Table 1 provides the results of single marker tests performed with PLINK [36]. We considered logistic regression models for each marker including the first four principle components of all SNP genotypes as covariates to account for population structure. This kind of adjustment is in principle not necessary when simulating under the total null hypothesis, but it becomes important for the simulation of complex traits below. We applied the Benjamini Hochberg procedure to account for multiple testing, and we can see that under the total null hypothesis the single marker tests control the type I error rate pretty much at the nominal level $\alpha = 0.05$.

Complex trait

The second set of simulations is concerned with the power to detect causal SNPs. To this end we consider again the 149478

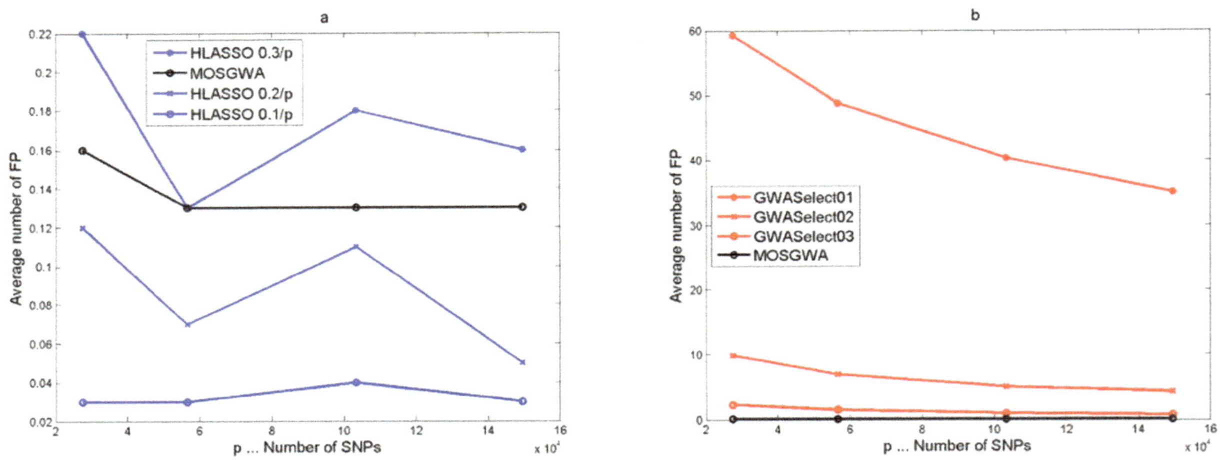

Figure 1. Illustration of the simulation results under the total null hypothesis. The average number of false positives for MOSGWA is compared with HLASSO (Fig 1a) and with GWASelect (Fig 1b), for which false positives were clustered. Simulations were performed for four different numbers of chromosomes, resulting in different numbers of SNPs plotted on the x-axis.

Table 1. False positives under the global null hypothesis.

p	MOS	HLASSO (α)			GWASelect (ξ)			SM
		$.3/p$	$.2/p$	$.1/p$	.1	.2	.3	
27520	0.16	0.22	0.12	0.03	51.1	9.34	2.34	0.04
56629	0.13	0.13	0.07	0.03	43.34	6.73	1.51	0.04
103348	0.13	0.18	0.11	0.04	36.64	4.90	1.06	0.04
149478	0.13	0.16	0.05	0.03	32.22	4.19	0.79	0.06

p refers to the total number of SNPs. The methods analyzed are MOSGWA (MOS), HLASSO with three different choices of the parameter α, GWASelect with three different choices of the stable-selection-threshold ξ, and single marker tests (SM) with Benjamini Hochberg procedure at level $\alpha = 0.05$.

SNPs from the first six chromosomes for the 4077 individuals from the POPRES sample. Simulations are performed for three scenarios, which include 6, 12, and 24 causal SNPs, respectively. All causal SNPs are common (MAF >0.05), equally distributed over the six chromosomes, and with pairwise correlation $\rho < 0.1$ for each pair. Disease risk was computed for each individual according to equation (2), based on which for each scenario 200 case-control data sets were sampled. Effect sizes β_j were ranging in the interval $[0.2, 0.28]$, yielding causal SNPs with intermediate power. The coefficient of the intercept β_0 was chosen such that the number of cases and controls in each simulation run was more or less identical.

Before analyzing the data in each scenario half of the causal SNPs were removed, mimicking the situation where SNPs associated with a trait are not causal themselves, but only in linkage disequilibrium with the cause. SNPs to be removed were selected in such a way that there actually were SNPs in linkage disequilibrium, to make it possible for these signals to be detected. The simulated data were then analyzed with MOSGWA, HLASSO (using parameter $\alpha = 0.3/p$), GWASelect using parameters $\xi \in \{0.1, 0.2, 0.3\}$ and with single marker tests (as previously including the four leading principal components in logistic regression models and applying Benjamini Hochberg procedure at nominal level $\alpha = 0.05$).

Table 2 and Figures 2, 3 and 4 summarize the corresponding results in terms of estimated power (which is just the average number of correctly detected signals divided by the total number of causal SNPs), the average number of false positives, the average number of misclassifications (that is false positives plus missed causal SNPs) and the estimated false discovery rate.

A crucial point in computing all these statistics is the definition of true positives and false positives. Of course we know the SNPs which we used to simulate the data, which we will call causal SNPs or correct SNPs. Now there might be several SNPs in close linkage disequilibrium with a causal SNP, and there is the question whether we count a detected SNP which is strongly correlated with the correct SNP as true positive or as false positive. Furthermore half of the causal SNPs under which we simulated were removed before analyzing the data. Therefore to get reasonable results we actually have to count detections which are strongly correlated with a causal SNP as true positives.

It is quite common in this context to use a threshold value C on the correlation between causal SNPs and any detected SNP to determine whether a detected SNP is a true positive [26,29]. If several detected SNPs are closely correlated to one causal SNP we count all of them as one true positive. Just like for the simulation under the total null we have additionally clustered the false positives of GWASelect and of the single marker analysis. This was performed with the algorithm described in Frommlet [20] which computes so called C-clusters, that is clusters of SNPs where it is guaranteed that within each cluster all SNPs have pairwise correlation larger than C. We used for clustering and for determining true positives always the same constant C. Counting the number of clusters rather than the total number of false positives works in favor of the performance of GWASelect and single marker tests. Both for MOSGWA and HLASSO such clustering appears to be unnecessary, because for a genomic region of closely related SNPs usually these procedures select only one representative.

In Figures 2, 3 and 4 we illustrate the dependence of the different statistics on the threshold values C for correlations which specify true positives via $|R| > C$. Results were computed for $C \in \{0.2, 0.3, 0.4, 0.55, 0.7, 0.9\}$. One can see that within the range of $0.2 \leq C \leq 0.55$ the dependence on the threshold is relatively

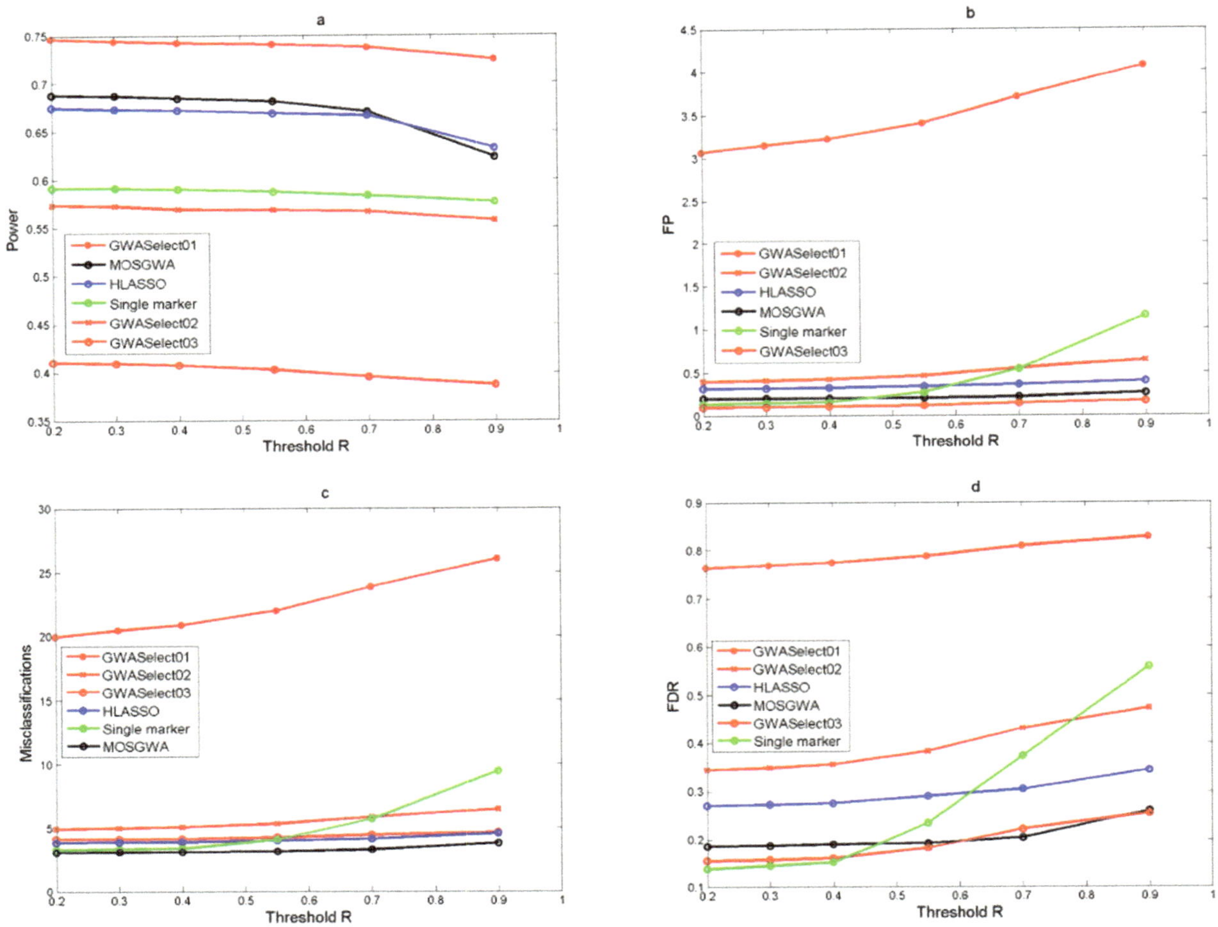

Figure 2. Simulation results under an alternative with $k=6$ causal SNPs. The four panels (Fig 2a, Fig 2b, Fig 2c, Fig 2d) show the average power, number of false positives, misclassification rate and false discovery rate as a function of the threshold value C which determines if a detection is a true or a false positive. The performance of MOSGWA is compared with single marker tests, HLASSO, and with GWASelect using three different parameters for stability selection.

minor for all methods. In general the choice of C has the biggest impact on the results of single marker tests. For those the number of false positives grows much faster than for the other methods, because the number of false positive clusters increases with stricter clustering threshold C. Table 2 specifically reports the results for a threshold $C=0.3$.

For all three scenarios MOSGWA has the lowest number of misclassifications, which is in accordance with theoretical results [21]. Of particular interest is the comparison between MOSGWA and HLASSO. For $k=6$ MOSGWA has slightly larger power and lower Type I error. For $k=12$ and specifically for $k=24$ MOSGWA has much larger power than HLASSO, but also larger Type I error. When the number of causal SNPs is increasing then HLASSO is getting more conservative in comparison with MOSGWA, which is in accordance with the way both algorithms are designed. HLASSO tries to control the FWER at a certain level, whereas MOSGWA tries to control the FDR. According to asymptotic theory [7,24], when aiming at a minimal number of misclassifications in a sparse setting it is preferable to control FDR rather than FWER.

Concerning GWASelect just like under the total null hypothesis the choice of $\xi=0.1$ gives way too large models. The choice of $\xi=0.2$ works slightly better in terms of controlling the Type I error, but is less powerful than MOSGWA and HLASSO. Given the simulation results under the total null hypothesis one actually should use the setting $\xi=0.3$, but then GWASelect is no longer competitive at all in terms of power.

The single marker tests are performing surprisingly well, and the disadvantage compared to the model selection approaches is much less than it was observed by Frommlet et al. [23] for quantitative traits. However, we believe that this is mainly due to the fact that we have added the first four principle components of SNP genotypes. Although we did not specifically simulate scenarios where population structure would play a major role in itself, when testing a specific SNP the principle components in the model help to adjust for the net effect of all the other causal SNPs. Without adding principle components the performance of the single marker tests was extremely poor. Also note that for MOSGWA we did not specifically take any measures to take into account population structure. Still it is much more powerful than single marker tests in all three scenarios, while at the same time controlling FDR at a comparable level.

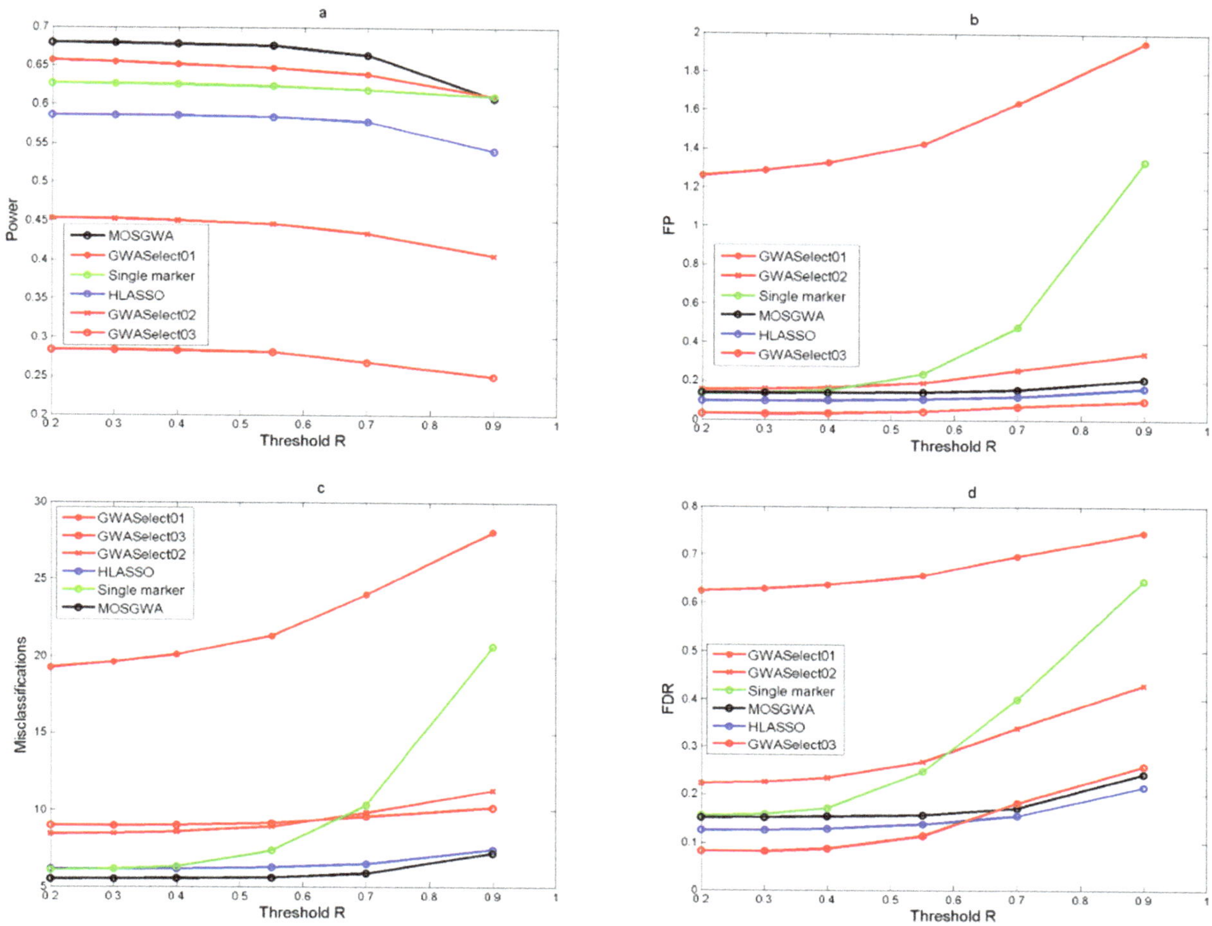

Figure 3. Simulation results under an alternative with $k=12$ causal SNPs. The four panels (Fig 3a, Fig 3b, Fig 3c, Fig 3d) show the average power, number of false positives, misclassification rate and false discovery rate as a function of the threshold value C which determines if a detection is a true or a false positive. The performance of MOSGWA is compared with single marker tests, HLASSO, and with GWASelect using three different parameters for stability selection.

Real Data

The Wellcome Trust data for genome-wide association studies on seven different diseases [41] have become benchmark data sets for comparing different algorithms to analyze GWAS. For each disease approximately 2000 cases were compared with a common set of approximately 3000 controls. More than half a million SNPs were genotyped with the Affymetrix GeneChip 500K, from which less than 400,000 passed quality control. The original analysis from WTCCC was mainly based on single marker tests and identified 24 significant SNPs for the seven diseases.

The analysis of He and Lin [26] using GWASelect resulted in 60 distinct loci. Unfortunately we were not able to completely reproduce their results, which has several reasons. First of all He and Lin [26] did not fully document their preprocessing of data for quality control, and model selection analysis of GWAS data is extremely sensitive with respect to the set of SNPs being studied. Furthermore they seem to have used not always the same parameter ξ for d-GWASelect, but adapted this for different diseases. We provide next a detailed description of the preprocessing steps we performed, and how they differ from [26].

Data preprocessing of WTCCC data

We reanalyzed bipolar disorder (BD), coronary heart disease (CAD), hypertension (HT), Crohn's disease (IBD), rheumatoid athritis (RA), type 1 diabetes (T1D) and type 2 diabetes (T2D). Like in the original article [41] all diseases are compared with the same control group of 3000 individuals. In the following filenames we will denote by <DIS> any of the seven abbreviations for diseases given above. Starting from the already imputed WTCCC data sets we removed individuals for each disease and for the control group according to the files exclusion-list-05-02-2007-<DIS>.txt and exclusion-list-snps-26_04_2007.txt.

After merging cases with controls we removed SNPs with a minimal allelic frequency smaller than 0.01. Furthermore we tested for Hardy Weinberg equilibrium and SNPs with p-values smaller than 0.0001 were also removed. Finally we only considered SNPs for which the genotype calling algorithm from the WTCCC confirmed good clustering, where we took that information from the files WTCCC_summary_data/7_Diseases/<DIS>/basic/snptest_<DIS>_<CHR>.txt. Here <CHR> is the chromosome number ranging from 1 to 22. According to private correspondence with He and Lin they had used the file wtccc_<DIS>_basic_chr_<CHR>.xml for similar purposes. That file must have differed from the file we have used, but is no

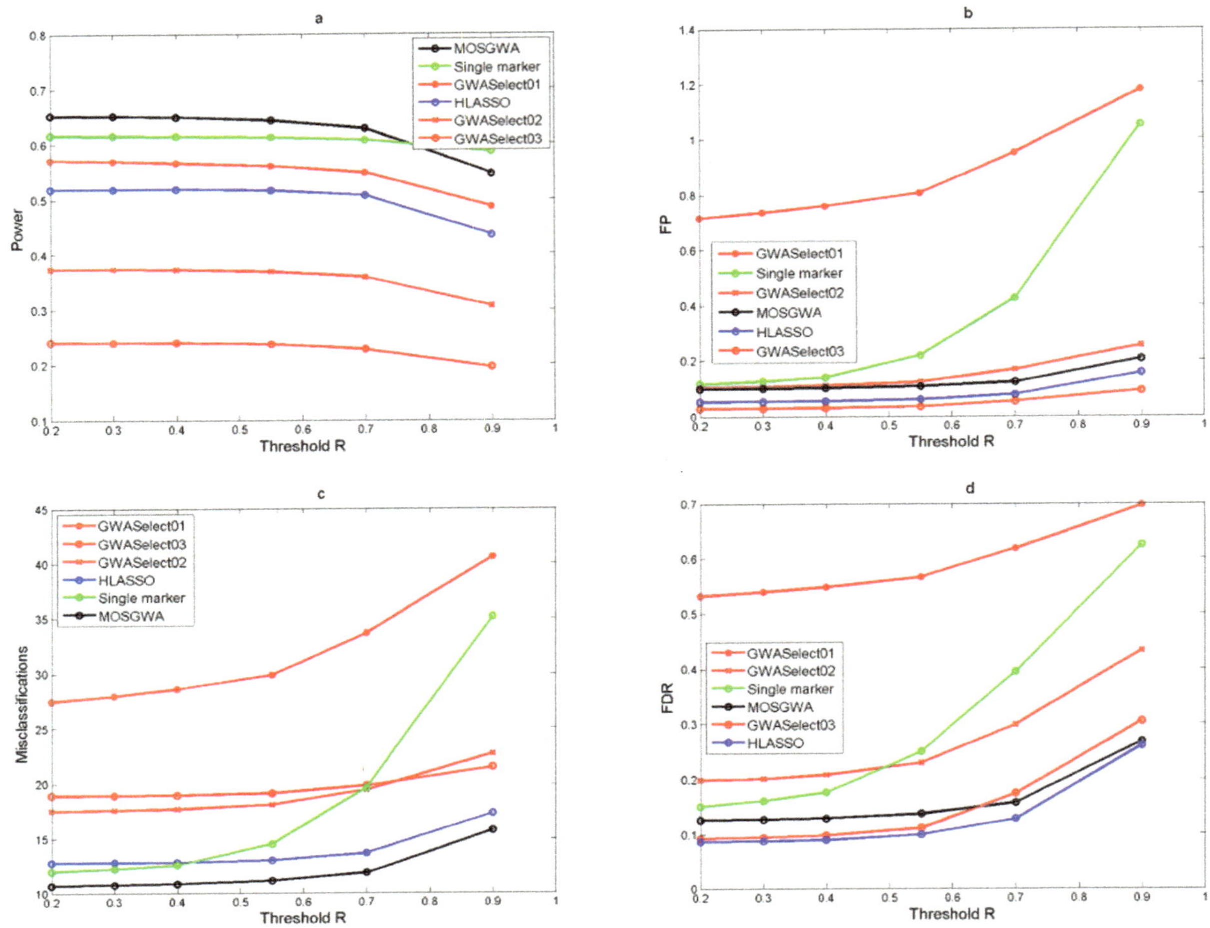

Figure 4. Simulation results under an alternative with $k=24$ causal SNPs. The four panels (Fig 4a, Fig 4b, Fig 4c, Fig 4d) show the average power, number of false positives, misclassification rate and false discovery rate as a function of the threshold value C which determines if a detection is a true or a false positive. The performance of MOSGWA is compared with single marker tests, HLASSO, and with GWASelect using three different parameters for stability selection.

longer available from WTCCC. In summary, after preprocessing we will have ended up with a different set of SNPs than used in [26], and according to email correspondence with the authors it is no longer possible to reconstruct which set of SNPs they had used for their own analysis. Not starting from the same set of SNPs explains why we were not able to completely reproduce the results reported by He and Lin [26].

Summary of results

Like in the simulation study for complex traits HLASSO was applied with parameter $\alpha=0.3$. For GWASelect we present the results again for $\xi\in\{0.1,0.2,0.3\}$, in spite of the fact that we have seen that only $\xi=0.3$ controls the type I error rate under the total null hypothesis. Table 3 gives for each disease the number of detected SNPs (and associated regions) obtained from the original WTCCC analysis, MOSGWA, HLASSO, and GWASelect. A more detailed discussion concerning the detected SNPs follows below.

The first observation is that GWASelect with parameter $\xi=0.1$ is selecting in 6 out of 7 diseases a much larger number of SNPs than the other methods. Given the results from simulations we are forced to conclude that most of those SNPs might be false positives, and we will not give the detailed results for GS 0.1 in the next section except for rheumatoid arthritis, where interestingly GS 0.1 gives quite similar results to MOSGWA and HLASSO (for a detailed explanation see below). For Crohn's disease and Type I diabetes the results for $\xi=0.2$ are relatively close to MOSGWA and HLASSO, whereas for all other diseases $\xi=0.3$ might be the best choice for GWASelect. The general conclusion is that the results of GWASelect heavily depend on the choice of ξ, and it is not really possible to know in advance which choice gives reliable results.

The comparison between MOSGWA and HLASSO is quite interesting. For the four diseases for which only a small number of SNPs was detected (BD, CAD, HT, T2D) MOSGWA finds exactly the same regions as HLASSO, though in two cases one SNP less. Similarly MOSGWA has a tendency to select less representatives of a region than HLASSO for the remaining more complex traits. This might have to do with the fact that the coefficient estimates of MOSGWA suffer from even less shrinkage than the estimates from HLASSO. Hoggart et al. [29] provide a thorough discussion of the fact that in case of shrinkage the regressors which enter a model explain less than they would without shrinkage, which results in a higher chance of including further correlated SNPs in the model. This is the main reason why HLASSO works with the NEG prior, which results in less

Table 2. Summary of simulation results for complex traits.

	MOS	HL	GS 0.1	GS 0.2	GS 0.3	SM
Scenario 1: ($k=6$)						
Size	5.32	5.94	23.36	5.87	3.03	4.40
Power	0.69	0.67	0.74	0.57	0.41	0.59
FP	1.19	1.90	18.90	2.43	0.57	0.85
FDR	0.19	0.27	0.77	0.35	0.16	0.14
Mis	3.07	3.86	20.44	5.00	4.12	3.31
Scenario 2: ($k=12$)						
Size	9.80	8.19	23.35	7.31	3.77	9.17
Power	0.68	0.59	0.65	0.45	0.28	0.63
FP	1.65	1.16	15.49	1.88	0.37	1.65
FDR	0.15	0.17	0.63	0.23	0.08	0.16
Mis	5.49	6.13	19.63	8.46	8.97	6.13
Scenario 3: ($k=24$)						
Size	18.03	13.71	31.29	11.43	6.43	17.76
Power	0.65	0.52	0.57	0.37	0.24	0.62
FP	2.39	1.27	17.63	2.49	0.67	2.99
FDR	0.13	0.09	0.54	0.20	0.09	0.16
Mis	10.75	12.83	27.97	17.56	18.91	12.22

The average over 200 simulation runs is reported for the number of detected associations (Size), the estimated power, the number of false positive detections (FP), the estimated false discovery rate (FDR) and the average number of misclassifications (Mis). GWASelect performed with parameters $\xi \in \{0.1, 0.2, 0.3\}$ is abbreviated as GS ξ, MOSGWA as MOS, HLASSO as HL, and single marker tests as SM.

shrinkage than the double exponential prior corresponding to LASSO.

A second observation is that especially for complex traits MOSGWA tends to select more regions of association than HLASSO. This goes along with the fact that HLASSO is designed to control the FWER, whereas MOSGWA controls the FDR. In case of complex traits MOSGWA is therefore bound to find more SNPs than HLASSO, whereas if there are only few signals both methods behave very similarly. Looking more closely into the results for IBD, RA and T1D, we observe that MOSGWA detects SNPs within all regions which were reported as significant according to the original WTCCC analysis [41]. The same is not true for HLASSO, which misses out one region on chromosome 10 for RA, and another region on chromosome 16 for T1D. On the other hand MOSGWA finds exclusively 7 SNPs for IBD, 4 SNPs for RA, and 6 SNPs for T1D, respectively. We will next provide a thorough discussion on the potential relevance of these SNPs which were exclusively found by MOSGWA.

WTCCC Results in detail

For each disease we provide tables as supporting information which list all SNPs which were detected by different methods. Specifically the first column of these tables gives the reference SNP ID number from dbSNP, followed by the chromosome (Chr) and the position (Pos). The column Gene contains information about the closest lying gene according to the databases dbSNP and ImmunoBase:

Table 3. Summary of real data analysis.

Disease	WTCCC	MOS	HL	GS 0.3	GS 0.2	GS 0.1
BD	(1)	1 (1)	1 (1)	1 (1)	9 (9)	43 (39)
CAD	(1)	2 (2)	3 (2)	3 (2)	4 (2)	29 (21)
HT	(0)	1 (1)	1 (1)	1 (1)	4 (4)	29 (26)
IBD	(9)	17 (16)	12 (8)	12 (5)	15 (6)	32 (19)
RA	(3)	11 (5)	12(2)	1(1)	1(1)	13 (2)
T1D	(7)	25 (11)	22 (4)	12 (2)	20 (2)	33 (2)
T2D	(3)	2 (2)	3 (2)	4 (2)	8 (4)	28 (19)

Number of detected SNPs which are associated to the following seven diseases from WTCCC: Bipolar disorder (BD), coronary artery disease (CAD), hypertension (HT), Crohn's disease (IBD), rheumatoid arthritis (RA), type 1 diabetes (T1D) and type 2 diabetes (T2D). WTCCC refers to the regions reported by the original publication [41] in their Table 3, abbreviations for the other algorithms are just like in Table 2. In brackets we give the number of DNA regions which are covered by the detected SNPs. The whole HLA region on chromosome 6 is counted as only one region.

- dbSNP: http://www.ncbi.nlm.nih.gov/SNP/
- ImmunoBase: http://www.immunobase.org/

The next four columns have bullets whenever a SNP was detected by MOSGWA (M), Hlasso (HL), GWASelect with parameter $\xi=0.3$ (G3) or $\xi=0.2$ (G2). According to our simulation results we believe that the large number of additional SNPs detected by GWASelect with $\xi=0.1$ (G1) will include mainly false positives. Therefore we do not present detailed results for G1, with the exception of rheumatoid arthritis which has a rather particular genetic constellation. If many neighboring SNPs are reported by different methods we consider such groups of SNPs as genetic regions, and we label such groups in the tables using background colors. The crosses in the last column (W) indicate regions which were reported originally in [41].

Bipolar disorder (BD). As illustrated in table S1 SNP rs2837588, which is an intron of DSCAM, was found by all methods, though it was not reported in [41]. On the other hand the only SNP reported by WTCCC, rs4202459, was not detected by any of the algorithms we analyzed here. This can be quite easily explained because all algorithms we study here are based on models incorporating linear trends, and the trend p-value of rs4202459 is quite large (2.19 E-04 according to the WTCCC manuscript). That rs2837588 was not reported by WTCCC might have to do with the large number of missing values for this SNP. Results reported in [41] are not based on imputed data, and imputation changes the marginal p-value for this SNP considerably. More recent research [3] indicates that there actually might be a connection between bipolar disorder and DSCAM, although in general according to a recent large GWAS [37] it appears to be extremely difficult to identify robust and replicable genetic causes for psychiatric disorders. Thus all the other SNPs reported by G2 have a good chance to be false positives.

Coronary artery disease (CAD). Here the original WTCCC study reported only one region, whereas all methods studied here detect two regions (see table S2). Note that MOSGWA selects only one representative of the region reported by WTCCC, whereas HLASSO reports two representatives. This is a pattern we will see again several times, for example in type II diabetes. A possible explanation why HLASSO prefers to choose more representatives of a region than MOSGWA is that MOSGWA is based on model selection criteria which impose less shrinkage on the coefficients than HLASSO does. The effect of shrinkage on the number of selected correlated SNPs is thoroughly described by Hoggart et al. [29].

Hypertension (HT). The original WTCCC study did not report any SNP associated with hypertension, whereas all methods studied here report rs16945811 on chromosome 17 (table S3). The reason for this is again that we work with imputed data, for which the marginal p-value of this SNP is considerably smaller than for the original unimputed data. The other SNPs reported by G2 are again very likely to be false positives.

Crohn's disease (IBD). This is the first disease for which model selection approaches become really interesting, because the trait appears to be a complex one. Note that HLASSO finds one region less (on chromosome 3) than originally reported in [41], whereas MOSGWA finds all regions reported by WTCCC plus seven additional ones which are highlighted in yellow in the table S4. At least five of those have been mentioned meanwhile in the literature on Crohn's disease, which means that based on the WTCCC data MOSGWA would have detected a number of SNPs associated with Crohn's disease which were later confirmed by independent studies.

Let's look at those SNPs in detail. The first SNP rs12035082 is close to rs12037606 which was actually reported in [41] among the SNPs which showed moderate evidence of association, and was later confirmed to be associated with CD [32]. Similarly rs6908425 was reported as being moderately associated in [41], and could later be confirmed in an independent study [4]. rs4263839 was not reported by WTCCC, but it was among the list of confirmed SNPs given in [4]. Furthermore it has later been shown to be associated with irritable bowel syndrome [44]. rs2836753 is in close linkage disequilibrium with rs2836754, which was related to Crohn's disease in [35].

rs6908425 is an intron from the CDKALI gene on chromosome 6 and has been confirmed to be associated to Crohn's disease (see for example snpedia at http://snpedia.com/index.php/Rs6908425). rs9405639 on chromosome 9 lies within the intron of SLC22A23 gene, which is also well known to be related to Crohn's disease (http://www.immunobase.org/page/Overview/display/gene_id/63027).

The only two SNPs detected by MOSGWA based on the WTCCC data which have not been confirmed in the literature are rs11627513 and rs41526044. rs11627513 is relatively close to the IL23R gene which is known to be associated with Crohn's disease (see http://www.immunobase.org/page/Overview/display/gene_id/149233) and it was mentioned in [28] as a potentially associated gene. Up to our knowledge only for rs11627513 nothing is known, and this might well be a false positive. Remember that MOSGWA is designed to control the FDR approximately at a level of 10%, and thus one would actually expect 2 false positive SNPs within this model.

Rheumatoid arthritis (RA). All SNPs detected on chromosome 6 belong to the so called HLA region which has been well known for a long time to be associated with rheumatoid arthritis (see for example [15]). However, HLA genes explain only approximately one-third of the genetic liability of the disease [13], and a great amount of research has been performed to understand genetic causes beyond HLA. For the rheumatoid arthritis data GWASelect performs very poor, for parameters $\xi=0.3$ and $\xi=0.2$ only one SNP in the HLA region is reported. This is quite easy to understand given the way GWASelect works. In the HLA region there are many highly correlated SNPs, and during the stability selection procedure it is very likely that for different samples different representatives of a cluster of SNPs are chosen. Therefore only for the lowest threshold $\xi=0.1$ GWASelect gives results which are more in line with the other methods. This is the reason why He and Lin [26] clustered the HLA region before analyzing that data set, but that appears to be quite an extra effort for the user when applying GWASelect. Neither MOSGWA nor HLASSO did have particular problems with including the HLA region in the analysis, and both find apart from SNPs in the HLA region also rs6679677 on chromosome 1. This SNP was already reported by the WTCCC [41], but according to a recent meta-analysis [13] this region actually could not be confirmed to be associated with rheumatoid arthritis.

Four SNPs were then only detected by MOSGWA which are highlighted in the table S5 in yellow. These detections appear to be rather interesting. rs2104286 lies in the intron of the IL-2RA gene, and according to a recent study [13] this SNP is definitely associated with rheumatoid arthritis. It was reported by WTCCC [41] after pooling data from RA and T1D, but it was not detected when using the standard analysis for data only from the RA population. rs1946518 from chromosome 11 is not mentioned in the meta-analysis, but the GUCY1A2 gene is down regulated in case of rheumatoid arthritis [16]. This indicates that there might be a functional connection between this region and RA.

Finally there remain two SNPs from the GLI3 gene on chromosome 7. Again nothing is said about those in the meta-analysis [13]. However, the GLI3 gene is known to be a member of the Hedgehog signaling pathway which is important for the proper development of embryos, and is also known to play an important role in adults [40]. rs12536071 has a relatively small marginal p-value (5.2E-06), whereas the neighboring SNP rs12531052 has a rather large marginal p-values (0.167944). It is pretty unusual for MOSGWA to select two SNPs which are located so close to each other, which might indicate that actually some epistatic effect could be involved here.

Type I diabetes (T1D). Similarly to rheumatoid arthritis also for type I diabetes the HLA region plays an important role, where approximately half of the genetic risk for T1D is found in the HLA region [10]. GWASelect is handling the situation here slightly better than in case of RA, but still it detects apart from HLA SNPs only rs6679677 on chromosome 1, which is also reported by all other methods. In the original WTCCC publication [41] three more SNPs are found to have strong association with T1D. All of those were found by MOSGWA, whereas HLASSO missed rs12924729 on chromosome 16. MOSGWA reported 6 additional SNPs which are again highlighted in yellow in the table S6.

rs41384747 on chromosome 18 is close to rs2542151 which was already listed among SNPs with moderate association by WTCCC [41]. The region was later confirmed in replication studies (see [5]), and also includes SNP rs478582 listed in the meta-analysis [10]. Similarly the region on chromosome 5 in which rs1025039 lies has been known as a susceptibility locus for T1D. In the same region lies rs6897932 which is associated with T1D [5]. Perhaps the most comprehensive source today for human Type 1 Diabetes loci is the database http://t1dbase.org. There one can find that the region on chromosome 18 is listed as being associated with T1D, but not the region on chromosome 5.

The closest region to rs6928921 on chromosome 6 which is documented in t1dbase is 6q15 with the BACH2 gene, which is 5 MB upstream. Nothing is known about any influence of KIAA1009 on T1D. There is more indication that rs2666236 on chromosome 10 might be associated with T1D, as it is known that the corresponding gene NRP1 is associated with T1D [25]. However, again the region of rs2666236 is not listed in t1dbase. Nothing is known about the other SNPs rs7157296 on chromosome 14 and rs41384747 on chromosome 18, and they might thus be false positives. Remember that MOSGWA is tuned to have an FDR of approximately 10%, and thus 2 or 3 false positive SNPs are to be expected in this model.

Type II diabetes (T2D). With type 2 diabetes a smaller number of genetic regions seems to be associated than with the previous three diseases (table S7). Thus the model selection approach appears to have less benefits compared with the standard analysis. MOSGWA does not report rs9465871 on chromosome 6, but looking at the original WTCCC analysis [41] this SNP has a trend p-value of 1.02 E-6, which is not significant after any standard correction for multiple testing. Apart from that all algorithms report SNPs within the two main regions on chromosome 10 and 16, where MOSGWA chooses again only one representative for gene TCF7L2 on chromosome 10.

Discussion

We have introduced MOSGWA, a new algorithm for GWAS analysis using the FDR controlling model selection criterion mBIC2. We compared its performance with two existing variable selection methods, GWASelect and HLASSO. The first observation was that both MOSGWA and HLASSO are controlling the Type I error rate under the global null hypothesis, whereas GWASelect does not manage to do that when using the recommended parameter setting $\xi \in [0.1, 0.2]$. He and Lin [26] only presented simulation results for scenarios including 10 causal SNPs, for which GWASelect had relatively low FDR. In accordance we observed that GWASelect tends to have lower type I error rate when the true model underlying simulations includes more causal SNPs. However, a method which selects very large models even when we know that there is no genetic cause for the disease status appears to be rather problematic. When increasing the selection threshold to $\xi = 0.3$ then GWASelect more or less controls the type I error under the global null, but then it is no longer competitive in terms of power to detect causal SNPs. One advantage of MOSGWA is that there is actually no parameter tuning necessary at all, because the selection criterion is fixed.

Apart from GWASelect and HLASSO we have also compared the performance of the original LASSO as implemented in glmnet [19], although we decided not to present the corresponding results in this manuscript. LASSO previously has been shown to perform well in GWAS in terms of prediction [30], but here we are only interested in selecting the correct SNPs. For this purpose one has the problem to decide upon the best tuning parameter λ of LASSO. It is well known that cross validation yields too large models, which we also observed in our simulations. As an alternative we tried to search along the LASSO regularization path and find the model which minimizes mBIC2, but that gave too small models. We finally considered a strategy where we searched along the regularization path for that model which minimizes the misclassification rate. This is obviously not feasible in practice when the truth is unknown, but this strategy shows the best possible performance of LASSO that one could achieve at least theoretically. It still turned out that in our simulations even the best possible model along the regularization path could not compete with the models obtained with MOSGWA or HLASSO. We observed that LASSO tends to select too many correlated SNPs with larger effect sizes, and then has difficulties to include causal SNPs with smaller effect size, but rather includes a number of false positives. An explanation of this behavior was given already by Hoggart et al. [29] when motivating the NEG prior.

Our simulation study on complex traits showed that at least for our three scenarios MOSGWA is slightly more powerful than HLASSO, when the parameter α of HLASSO is chosen such that both procedures have similar type 1 error rate. This reflects the theoretical optimality property of mBIC2 to minimize asymptotically the misclassification error under a wide range of sparsity levels [21]. However, this theoretical property holds for the model which actually minimizes the criterion mBIC2. Our heuristic search strategy is attempting to get close to the global minimum, but we know that in most cases it will fail to find the best solution. More involved search strategies will further improve our method, and we are currently exploring the use of memetic algorithms, which have been successfully applied already in the context of QTL mapping [22].

The software architecture of MOSGWA is designed in such a way that it can be quite easily extended in the future to incorporate more advanced features. For example it might be interesting to have a model selection procedure which accounts for population structure. Currently this can be done by adding principle components as covariates to the regression models, but an even better solution would be to add random effects to model population structure. For that reason we are currently working on extending MOSGWA towards mixed models.

Supporting Information

Table S1 Summary of analysis results for Bipolar Disorder.

Table S2 Summary of analysis results for Coronary artery disease.

Table S3 Summary of analysis results for Hypertension.

Table S4 Summary of analysis results for Crohn's disease.

Table S5 Summary of analysis results for Rheumatoid arthritis.

Table S6 Summary of analysis results for Type I diabetes.

Table S7 Summary of analysis results for Type II diabetes.

Acknowledgments

The data set used for simulations in this manuscript was obtained from dbGaP through dbGaP accession number phs000145.v1.p1 at www.ncbi.nlm.nih.gov/projects/gap/cgibin/study.cgi?study_id = phs000145.v1.p1.

The WTCCC data is available at http://www.wtccc.org.uk/.

Author Contributions

Conceived and designed the experiments: ED BB FF. Performed the experiments: ED. Analyzed the data: ED. Contributed reagents/materials/analysis tools: ED BB FF. Contributed to the writing of the manuscript: ED BB FF.

References

1. Abramovich F, Benjamini Y, Donoho DL, Johnstone IM (2006) Adapting to unknown sparsity by controlling the false discovery rate. Ann Stat 34: 584–653.
2. Albert A, Anderson JA (1984) On the existence of maximum likelihood estimates in logistic regression models. Biometrika 71: 1–10.
3. Amano K, Yamada K, Iwayama Y, Detera-Wadleigh SD, Hattori E, et al. (2008) Association study between the Down syndrome cell adhesion molecule (DSCAM) gene and bipolar disorder. Psychiatr Genet 18(1): 1–10. doi: 10.1097/YPG.0b013e3281ac238e.
4. Barrett JC, Hansoul S, Nicolae DL, Cho JH, Duerr RH, et al. (2008) Genome-wide association defines more than 30 distinct susceptibility loci for Crohn's disease. Nat Genet 40(8): 955–962. doi: 10.1038/ng.175.
5. Barrett JC, Clayton DG, Concannon P, Akolkar B, Cooper JD, et al. (2009) Genome-wide association study and meta-analysis find that over 40 loci affect risk of type 1 diabetes. Nat Genet 41(6): 703–707. doi: 10.1038/ng.381.
6. Benjamini Y, Hochberg Y (1995) Controlling the false discovery rate: a practical and powerful approach to multiple testing. J Roy Statist Soc Ser B 57: 289–300.
7. Bogdan M, Chakrabati A, Frommlet F, Ghosh JK (2011) Asymptotic Bayes-Optimality under sparsity of some multiple testing procedures. Ann Stat 39(3): 1551–1579.
8. Bogdan M, Ghosh JK, Doerge RW (2004) Modifying the Schwarz Bayesian information criterion to locate multiple interacting quantitive trait loci. Genetics 167: 989–999.
9. Bogdan M, Żak-Szatkowska M, Ghosh JK (2008) Selecting explanatory variables with the modified version of Bayesian Information Criterion. Qual Reliab Eng Int 24: 627–641.
10. Bradfield JP, Qu HQ, Wang K, Zhang H, Sleiman PM, et al. (2011) A genome-wide meta-analysis of six type 1 diabetes cohorts identifies multiple associated loci. Plos Genet 7(9): e1002293. doi: 10.1371/journal.pgen.1002293.
11. Broman KW, Speed TP (2002) A model selection approach for the identification of quantitative trait loci in experimental crosses. J Roy Statist Soc Ser B 64(4): 641–656.
12. Bühlmann P, van de Geer S (2011) Statistics for High-Dimensional Data: Methods, Theory and Applications. Springer (Heidelberg, London, New York).
13. Chatzikyriakidou A, Voulgari PV, Lambropoulos A, Drosos AA (2013) Genetics in rheumatoid arthritis beyond HLA genes: what meta-analyses have shown? Semin Arthritis Rheu 43(1): 29–38. doi: 10.1016/j.semarthrit.2012.12.003.
14. Chen J, Chen Z (2008) Extended Bayesian Information criteria for model selection with large model spaces. Biometrika 95(3): 759–771.
15. Deighton CM, Walker DJ, Griffiths ID, Roberts DF (1989) The contribution of HLA to rheumatoid arthritis. Clin Genet 36: 178–182.
16. Del Rey MJ, Izquierdo E, Usategui A, Gonzalo E, Blanco FJ, et al. (2010) The transcriptional response of normal and rheumatoid arthritis synovial fibroblasts to hypoxia. Arthritis Rheum 62(12): 3584–3594. doi: 10.1002/art.27750.
17. Fan J, Lv J (2008) Sure independence screening for ultrahigh dimensional feature space. J Roy Statist Soc Ser B 70: 849–911.
18. Firth D (1993) Bias reduction of maximum likelihood estimates. Biometrika 80: 27–38.
19. Friedman J, Hastie T, Tibshirani R (2010) Regularization Paths for Generalized Linear Models via Coordinate Descent. J Stat Softw 33(1): 1–22.
20. Frommlet F (2010) Tag SNP selection based on clustering according to dominant sets found using replicator dynamics. Adv Data Anal Classif 4: 65–83.
21. Frommlet F, Chakrabarti A, Murawska M, Bogdan M (2011) Asymptotic Bayes optimality under sparsity for generally distributed effect sizes under the alternative. Technical report: arXiv:1005.4753.
22. Frommlet F, Ljubic I, Arnardottir HB, Bogdan M (2012) QTL mapping using a memetic algorithm with modifications of BIC as fitness function. Stat Appl Genet Mol Biol 11(4): Article 2. doi: 10.1515/1544-6115.1793.
23. Frommlet F, Ruhaltinger F, Twarog P, Bogdan M (2012) Modified versions of Bayesian Information Criterion for genome-wide association studies. Comput Stat Data An 56(5): 1038–1051.
24. Frommlet F, Bogdan M (2013) Some optimality properties of FDR controlling rules under sparsity. Electronic Journal of Statistics 7: 1328–1368, doi: 10.1214/13-EJS808.
25. Hasan NM, Kendrick MA, Druckenbrod NR, Huelsmeyer MK, Warner TF, et al. (2010) Genetic association of the neuropilin-1 gene with type 1 diabetes in children: Neuropilin-1 expression in pancreatic islets. Diabetes Res Clin Pract 87(3): e29–32. doi: 10.1016/j.diabres.2009.12.016.
26. He Q, Lin D (2011) A variable selection method for genome-wide association studies. Bioinformatics 27(1): 1–8.
27. Heinze G, Schemper M (2002) A Solution to the Problem of Separation in logistic regression. Stat Med 21: 2409–2419.
28. Hoffman GE, Logsdon BA, Mezey JG (2013) PUMA: a unified framework for penalized multiple regression analysis of GWAS data. Plos Comput Biol 9(6): e1003101. doi: 10.1371/journal.pcbi.1003101.
29. Hoggart CJ, Whittaker JC, De Iorio M, Balding DJ (2008) Simultaneous Analysis of All SNPs in Genome-Wide and Re-Sequencing Association Studies. Plos Genet 4(7): e1000130. doi:10.1371/journal.pgen.1000130.
30. Kooperberg C, LeBlanc M, Obenchain V (2010) Risk Prediction Using Genome-Wide Association Studies. Genet Epidem 34: 643–652.
31. Li J, Das K, Fu G, Li R, Wu R (2010) The Bayesian Lasso for Genome-wide Association Studies. Bioinformatics 27(4): 516–523.
32. Weersma RK, Stokkers PC, Cleynen I, Wolfkamp SC, Henckaerts L, et al. (2009) Confirmation of multiple Crohn's disease susceptibility loci in a large Dutch-Belgian cohort. Am J Gastroenterol 104(3): 630–638. doi: 10.1038/ajg.2008.112.
33. Meinshausen N, Bühlmann P (2010) Stability Selection (with discussion) J Roy Statist Soc Ser B 72: 417–473.
34. Nelson MR, Bryc K, King KS, Indap A, Boyko AR, et al. (2008) The Population Reference Sample, POPRES: a resource for population, disease, and pharmacological genetics research. Am J Hum Genet: 83(3): 347–358.
35. Parkes M, Barrett JC, Prescott NJ, Tremelling M, Anderson CA, et al. (2007) Sequence variants in the autophagy gene IRGM and multiple other replicating loci contribute to Crohn's disease susceptibility. Nat Genet 39(7): 830–832. Epub 2007 Jun 6.
36. Purcell S, Neale B, Todd-Brown K, Thomas L, Ferreira MA, et al. (2007) PLINK: a toolset for whole-genome association and population-based linkage analysis. Am J Hum Genet 81: 559–575.
37. Ripke S, Wray NR, Lewis CM, Hamilton SP, Weissman MM, et al. (2013) A mega-analysis of genome-wide association studies for major depressive disorder. Mol Psychiatr 18: 497–511. doi:10.1038/mp.2012.21.
38. Schwarz G (1978) Estimating the dimension of a model. Ann Stat 6, 461–464.
39. Tibshirani R (1996) Regression shrinkage and selection via the lasso. J Roy Statist Soc Ser B 58(1): 267–288.
40. Villavicencio EH, Walterhouse DO, Iannaccone PM (2000) The sonic hedgehog-patched-gli pathway in human development and disease. Am J Hum Genet 67(5): 1047–1054.
41. Wellcome Trust Case Control Consortium (2007) Genome-wide association study of 14,000 cases of seven common diseases and 3,000 shared controls. Nature 447: 661–678.

42. Wu TT, Chen YF, Hastie T, Sobel E, Lange K (2011) Genome-wide association analysis by lasso penalized logistic regression. Bioinformatics 25(6): 714–721.
43. Yang J, Benyamin B, McEvoy BP, Gordon S, Henders AK, et al. (2010) Common SNPs explain a large proportion of the heritability for human height. Nat Genet 42(7): 565–608.
44. Zucchelli M, Camilleri M, Andreasson AN, Bresso F, Dlugosz A, et al. (2011) Association of TNFSF15 polymorphism with irritable bowel syndrome. Gut 60(12): 1671–1677. doi: 10.1136/gut.2011.241877.
45. Żak-Szatkowska M, Bogdan M (2011) Modified versions of Bayesian Information Criterion for sparse Generalized Linear Models. Comput Stat Data An 55: 2908–2924.

6

Identification of Autoantibodies against Transthyretin for the Screening and Diagnosis of Rheumatoid Arthritis

Saurabh Sharma[1,2], Sreejoyee Ghosh[1], Lalit Kumar Singh[1], Ashish Sarkar[1], Rajesh Malhotra[4], Onkar Prasad Garg[3], Yogendra Singh[1], Radhey Shyam Sharma[2], Darshan Singh Bhakuni[3], Taposh Kumar Das[5], Sagarika Biswas[1]*

1 Department of Genomics & Molecular Medicine, CSIR-Institute of Genomics and Integrative Biology, Delhi, India, **2** Department of Environmental Studies, Delhi University, Delhi, India, **3** Department of Clinical Immunology and Rheumatology, Army Hospital (Research and Referral), New Delhi, India, **4** Department of Orthopaedic, All India Institute of Medical Sciences, New Delhi, India, **5** Department of Anatomy, All India Institute of Medical Sciences, New Delhi, India

Abstract

Rheumatoid arthritis (RA) is a chronic, autoimmune, systemic and inflammatory rheumatic disease that leads to inflammation of the joints and surrounding tissues. Identification of novel protein(s) associated with severity of RA is a prerequisite for better understanding of pathogenesis of this disease that may also have potential to serve as novel biomarkers in the diagnosis of RA. Present study was undertaken to compare the amount of autoantigens and autoantibodies in the plasma of RA patients in comparison to healthy controls. Plasma samples were collected from the patients suffering from RA, Osteoarthritis (OA), Systemic lupus erythematosus (SLE) and healthy volunteers. The screening of plasma proteins were carried out using 2-dimensional gel electrophoresis followed by identification of differentially expressed protein by MALDI-TOF MS/MS. Among several differentially expressed proteins, transthyretin (TTR) has been identified as one of the protein that showed significantly up regulated expression in the plasma of RA patients. The results were further validated by Western blot analysis and ELISA. In comparison to OA synovium, an exclusive significantly high expression of TTR in RA has been validated through IHC, Western blotting and IEM studies. Most importantly, the increase in expression of TTR with the progression of severity of RA condition has been observed. The autoantibodies against TTR present in the RA plasma were identified using immunoprecipitation-Western methods. The significant production of autoantibodies was validated by ELISA and Western blot analysis using recombinant pure protein of TTR. Hence, these novel observations on increase in TTR expression with the increase in severity of RA conditions and significant production of autoantibodies against TTR clearly suggest that a systematic studies on the role TTR in the pathogenesis of RA is immediately required and TTR may be used as a serum diagnostic marker together with other biochemical parameters and clinical symptoms for RA screening and diagnosis.

Editor: Anthony W.I. Lo, The Chinese University of Hong Kong, Hong Kong

Funding: Financial assistance was partly provided by Indian Council of Medical Research (ICMR) and Council of Scientific and Industrial Research (CSIR), New Delhi, India. The funders had no role in study design, data collection and analysis, decision to publish, or preparation of the manuscript.

Competing Interests: The authors have declared that no competing interests exist.

* E-mail: sagarika.biswas@igib.res.in

Introduction

Rheumatoid arthritis (RA) is a complex, multifactorial, inflammatory autoimmune disease with the anonymous etiology that leads to cartilage destruction, joint deformation and subsequent loss of multiple joints functions which affects 0.5–1% of population [1], [2]. The disease severity depends on the degree of the inflammation that is characterized by the increase in number of immune cells such as lymphocytes, monocytes and macrophages leading to the production of different immune mediators [3], [4]. Thus, an effective assessment of disease severity is a difficult process in an efficient clinical management of the disease [5]. Diagnosis criteria developed by American College of Rheumatology and European League against Rheumatism are primarily based on clinical symptoms. In the last few years, autoantibody reactivity against autoantigens had been described in RA diagnosis. Anti-cyclic citrullinated peptide (anti-CCP), anti citrullinated protein antibodies (ACPA) and RF factor in the serum of RA patients have been extensively studied [6]. Autoantibodies have been used as a diagnostic tool for RA, however they lack specificity and sensitivity. So there is an urgent need to investigate more specific disease associated proteins and autoantibodies, which would aid in better understanding of the disease.

Although a great improvement has been made in the management of RA, the mechanism associated with pathology is still remains undefined [7]. In spite of availability of several RA biomarkers, a large number of atypical RA patients dissociate from timely diagnosis and treatment due to limited specificity and sensitivity of the biomarkers. Therefore, identification of specific disease associated protein or specific autoantibodies will be useful in rapid diagnosis of the disease. Thus, the main focus of our study was to identify new proteins, autoantigens and autoantibodies in the sera of RA patients for the better assessment of severity of RA condition that can serve as specific and sensitive biomarker for RA.

Table 1. Demographics and clinical assessment scores for the RA, OA, SLE patients and healthy controls.

S.N.	Characterstics	RA (n = 60)		OA (n = 34)	SLE (n = 10)	Healthy Control (n = 60)
		Non severe RA (n = 22)	Severe RA (n = 38)			
1	Mean AGE ± SD	25±11	49±10	67±8	34±4	35±10
2	Mean weight±SD	54±10	55±10	60 ±15	40±10	55±5
3	SEX	16F+6M	32F+6M	26F+8M	10F	30F+30M
4	Mean Disease Duration(Y)	3±1	10±5	8±5	7±5	-
5	Mean Serum CRP (mg/liter) ± SD	35±5	80±5	30±2	15±1	10±5
6	Mean Tender joint	2±1	10±5	3 ± 2	3±1	-
7	Mean Swollen joints±SD	2±1	10±5	3±2	2±1	-
8	RF (IU/ml)	30±10	80±20	25±5	20±5	15±5
9	Mean ESR (mm/hr)	20±5	85±20	45±5	40±5	10±5
10	DAS 28 score±SD	3±2	6.5±2	-	-	-
11	Medicines	Mtx, HCQS, Tcz, Aba, Anti TNF-Etn, Anti TNF- Ifx	Mtx, HCQS, Tcz, Aba, Anti TNF-Etn, Anti TNF- Ifx	NSAIDs	HCQC, Prednisone, Azathiprine, Cyclophospha- mide	-

RA – Rheumatoid Arthritis, OA – Osteoarthritis, SLE – Systemic lupus erythematosus, SD – Standard Deviation, RF – Rheumatoid Factor, ESR – Erythrocyte Sedimentation Rate, CRP – C Reactive Protein, IU – International Unit, ml – Milliliter, mm – Millimeter, hr – Hour, DAS 28 – Disease Activity Score (maximum 28 joints), F – Female, M- Male, NSAIDs - Nonsteroidal anti-inflammatory drugs. Mtx-Methotrexate, HCQS -Hydroxychloroquine,TCZ- tocilizumab, Aba- Abatacepr, Etn-Etanercept, Ifx- Infliximab.

In the recent years, proteomic techniques like two dimensional gel electrophoresis (2-DE) and matrix-assisted laser desorption/ ionization time-of-flight mass spectrometry (MALDI-TOF-MS/ MS) are increasingly gaining importance in the field of biomarker discovery and have been used for analyzing serum proteomic spectra [8], [9]. In this study, we compared the serum protein profiles of RA patients and healthy volunteers with an aim to identify RA-associated proteins which can be used for diagnosis of RA. Using 2-DE followed by MALDI-TOF-MS/MS, we observed that TTR was highly expressed protein in the plasma of RA patients. TTR is a major serum thyroid hormone binding protein with a molecular mass of 14 kDa [10] which was formerly known as thyroxine-binding prealbumin protein. It was first recognized to bind thyroxine (T4) in 1958 [11] and subsequently shown that TTR also binds to retinol-binding protein and thus plays a role in the transport of vitamin A [12], [13].Thus, the name was changed to transthy(roxin)retin(ol) for denoting its dual transport function [14]. Plasma TTR is synthesized by the hepatic parenchymal cells while in fetal life it is synthesized by the yolk sac of endothelium [15]. Further, correlation of TTR expression with the clinical parameters of disease severity in RA patients was carried out. Immunohistochemistry (IHC) and immune electron-microscopy (IEM) were performed to validate the expression of TTR in synovium during the disease conditions.TTR expression profiling was also carried out in the plasma samples of other joint disorders and autoimmune diseases to confirm that TTR is a specific marker for RA.

Materials and Methods

Ethics statement

The study protocols were approved by medical ethics committee of Institute of Genomics and Integrative Biology, Delhi University Campus, Mall Road, Delhi, India and Department of Orthopaedic, All India Institute of Medical Sciences (AIIMS), New Delhi, India.

Sample Collection

In this study, 60 RA, 34 OA and 10 SLE patients showing active disease were enrolled together with sixty healthy control of similar age. Plasma samples from RA (n = 60, Male 12, Female 48), OA (n = 34, Male 8, Female 26), SLE (n = 10, Female 10) and healthy individuals (n = 60, Male 30, Female 30) (Table 1); synovial fluid from RA (n = 6, Male 3, female 3) and OA (n = 6, Male 3, female 3); synovium from RA (n = 7, Male 3, female 4), OA(n = 7, Male 3, female 4) were collected from Indian population in the age range of 25–70 years from AIIMS, New Delhi, India. A detailed medical history of each patient was recorded. Clinical examinations including early morning stiffness along with swelling, tenderness of joints and radiographs depicting erosions and deformities of small and big joints, bilateral pain were recorded under the supervision of rheumatologist. Diagnosis of RA was based on the established criteria given by The American College of Rheumatology/European league, that includes disease activity score (DAS) calculated from online DAS28 tool based on 28 joints count. In this study, all the patients were classified as non severe (DAS score $\leq$ 2.6) or severe (DAS score $\geq$5.1) (Table 1). Except for a few non severe cases, all patients were being treated with disease modifying anti-rheumatic drugs (Table 1). Anti-TNF treatment were given to 18 severe patients and 4 non severe patients. Pregnant women, alcoholic patients and patient's having other disease such as diabetes, cardiovascular disease or any other inflammatory disease were excluded from the study. None of the healthy volunteers had previous history of arthralgia, any other chronic diseases or acute infections during the last three months before enrollment. All participants had signed written informed consent before their enrollment.

Sample preparation

Blood was collected into tubes containing ethylene diamine tetraacetic acid (EDTA). The tubes were centrifuged at 2,000 rpm for 15 min at 4°C, plasma were collected and stored at –80°C.

The biopsy samples of synovium (RA, OA) were collected in Dulbecco's Modified Eagle's Medium (DMEM) having 10% FBS and 1% antibiotics. The synovium were washed several time with PBS and lysed by lysis buffer containing 25 mM tris (pH 8), 1% nonidet P-40, 150 mM NaCl, 1.5 mM EDTA, 0.5% SDS, 1 mM PMSF, 10 mM sodium orthovanadate, 3 mg/ml Aprotonin [16]. The lysed tissue samples were centrifuged at 11,000 rpm for 1 h, supernatant was collected and stored at –80°C until use.

Synovial fluids were centrifuged at 13,000 rpm for 15 min at 4°C to remove blood contamination. The clear supernatants were treated with hyaluronidase enzyme (Sigma- Aldrich, USA) and the mixture was digested by incubating at 37°C for 4 h. After centrifugation, clear supernatant was stored at –80°C till further use. The protein concentrations were estimated by the Bradford method (Bio-Rad, USA).

Two-dimensional gel electrophoresis and gel image analysis

Plasma proteins (150 μg) were added to the rehydration solution (7 M urea, 2 M thiourea, 2% CHAPS) containing 50 mM DDT and 0.2% ampholyte and applied to the first dimension immobilized pH gradient (IPG) strips (17 cm, pH 4-7, Bio-Rad, USA). First dimension isoelectric focusing (IEF) of the above strips were carried out using Protean IEF cell (Bio-Rad, USA) according to the following protocol: 200 V for 1 h, 500 V for 1 h followed by ramping at 1000 V for 1 h and final focusing at 8000 V for 5 h for a total of 13000 VH (Bio-Rad, USA). After being focused, strips were equilibrated for 20 min in equilibration buffer (50 mM Tris-HCl, pH 8.8, 6 M urea, 4% (w/v) SDS, and 20% (w/v) glycerol) containing 10 mg/ml dithiothreitol (DTT) and then for 20 min in the same equilibration buffer containing 40 mg/ml iodoacetamide (IAA) instead of DTT. Second dimension sodium dodecyl sulfate polyacrylamide gel (12%) electrophoresis (SDS-PAGE) was performed to resolve the proteins on the basis of molecular mass along with broad range pre-stained markers (Biolinkk India, New Delhi). Similarly, samples were prepared and separated from blood obtained from healthy control subjects. Gels were stained using ammonical silver nitrate (Merck Chemicals, Germany) and stained gels were scanned in 16 bit grey scale Tiff-images with an Alpha Digidoc 1201 scanner [17].

In gel digestion of proteins and extraction of peptides

Proteins were extracted by digesting the gel spots using trypsin gold (Promega, USA), washed with distilled water, excised in 1 mm cubes and destained with 50 μl of 1:1 solution of 30 mM potassium ferricyanide (Sigma-Aldrich, USA) and 100 mM sodium thiosulphate (Sigma-Aldrich, USA). The gel pieces were washed and dehydrated by incubation with 40 μl of 1:1 acetonitrile (ACN)/water for 15 min followed by washing with 40 μl of ACN until they become white and sticky. The gel pieces were then equilibrated for 5 min by adding 50 μl of 100 mM ammonium bicarbonate followed by addition of 50 μl ACN (Sigma-Aldrich, USA). The solutions were discarded after 15 min. Gel pieces were dehydrated in a vacuum centrifuge, digested by adding 10 μl of trypsin (0.1 μg/μl trypsin, Promega, USA) in trypsin digestion buffer and incubated for 45 min in ice. The solutions were discarded after incubation and 25-60 μl of trypsin digestion buffer (5 μl of 1 M $CaCl_2$, 25 μl of 1 M NH_4CO_3 and 970 μl distilled water) was added and incubated overnight at 37°C. The supernatants were collected and dried in vacuum centrifuge. The peptides were extracted from gel pieces by varying the concentration of ACN and trifluoroacetic acid (TFA, Sigma-Aldrich, USA), sonicated in a water bath for 30 min, dried in speed-vac to remove TFA/ACN and stored at –20°C till further use [18].

Matrix-assisted laser desorption ionization-MS/MS

MALDI-TOF MS/MS (Applied Biosystems, Life Technologies, USA) was utilized to determine the molecular masses of polypeptides. ZipTip C4 was used for the desalting and purification of extracted peptides. One microliter of peptide extract was mixed with 1 μl sinapinic acid matrix onto the MALDI target plate and allowed to air dry. MS/MS spectra were acquired across the mass range of 10,000–20,000 Da in reflector positive mode with 5600 laser shots intensity (25 Shots/Sub-Spectrum for 500 total Shots/Spectrum). The internal calibration was performed using standard calibration mix 5 (Applied Biosystems). For the MS/MS precursor selection, minimum S/N (signal/noise) filter was set at 25 with an exclusion list for α-Cyano-4-hydroxycinnamic acid (CHCA) matrix peaks. Protein identifications were accepted with a statistically significant probability based Mowse score ($p \leq 0.05$). Proteins with at least 2 peptides that were unique to the specific protein were only considered.

Western blot analysis

Hundred micrograms of plasma protein from RA ($n = 12$) and control ($n = 12$) was subjected to 12% SDS–PAGE. Proteins were transferred to the nitrocellulose membrane (Millipore, USA) using Western-Blot technique followed by blocking using 5% bovine serum albumin (BSA, Sigma-Aldrich, USA) for 1 h at room temperature (RT) with gentle shaking. The membranes were then incubated with anti-TTR (ProSci, USA) antibody (1:1000 dilutions) for 1 h followed by the incubation of membranes with HRP conjugated anti-mouse antibody at RT with mild shaking. Enhanced chemiluminescence assay (ECL) (Thermo Scientific, Pierce, USA) was used to develop the membrane and autoradiographed on high performance chemiluminescence film (GE Healthcare) according to the manufactures guidelines. After each step the membrane was washed with 1X PBS [19].

Similar experiment was carried out using synovium (RA, $n = 7$) (OA, $n = 7$) and synovial fluid (RASF, $n = 6$) (OASF, $n = 6$) of RA and OA patients. Proteins (50 μg) of synovium homogenate and synovial fluid were loaded separately in SDS-PAGE and transferred on to nitrocellulose membrane. The anti-TTR and anti-mouse antibodies were used as a primary and secondary antibody respectively.

ELISA validation

ELISA was carried out using commercially available anti-TTR monoclonal antibody (ProSci Antibody, USA). For comparison between patient and control group, 60 plasma samples from each group were taken. Individual plasma samples from the enrolled participants were diluted (1 μl/200 μl) in a coating buffer (0.01 M Na_2CO_3 and 0.035 M $NaHCO_3$, pH 9.6), coated on 96 well plates (Thermo Scientific, Nunc, USA) and incubated overnight at 4°C. Next day the plates were washed three times with 100 μl PBST and incubated with 100 μl blocking buffer (1% BSA in 1X PBS) for 1 h at RT. The blocking buffer was extracted, plates were washed and incubated with 100 μl of anti-TTR as a primary antibody (1:2000 dilution) for 2 h at RT. The plates were then washed three times and incubated with 100 μl of anti-mouse HRP conjugate (1:1000 dilution) for 1 h and developed with ortho phenylene diamine (1 mg/ml in 0.05 M citrate buffer and 5 μl/ml H_2O_2, Sigma-Aldrich, USA). The reactions were stopped by adding 2N H_2SO_4 in each well and binding efficiency was checked by reading absorbance at 492 nm in an ELISA reader (Spectramax Plus; Molecular Devices, USA) [20]. Plasma levels of TTR in RA patients was also compared from patients of different diseases.

Immunohistochemistry of synovial tissue

To validate the expression of TTR in synovial tissue (RA, n = 3 and OA, n = 3), the tissues were fixed in formalin (10%) and subjected to immunohistochemical analysis. Briefly, the tissue sections were paraffin-embedded and cut into a desired thickness (5 μm) using microtome. The slides were placed in a container, submerged in citrate buffer (pH 6.0) and incubated at 40°C for 2 min periods repeatedly for three times and then finally kept for 20 min in microwave. The sections were then allowed to equilibrate at RT in the buffer, and rinsed with distilled water. The anti-TTR antibody (ProSci, USA) was applied to the sections at a 1:400 dilution for overnight incubation at 4°C. Anti-mouse HRP conjugated was used as a secondary antibody (1:200 dilutions) for 2 h. The sections were counterstained in hematoxylin followed by freshly prepared 3,3′-diaminobenzidine (DAB, Sigma-Aldrich, USA). The slides were then mounted with cover slip and observed under microscope [21].

Immuno-electron microscopy

To further validate the expression of TTR in synovial tissues, the ultrathin sections of the tissues were subjected to immune-electronmicroscopy analysis.The RA (n = 3) and OA (n = 3) tissue samples were fixed in 0.5% glutaraldehyde and 2% paraformaldehyde solution for 8 h at 4°C. After three times washing with 0.1 M phosphate buffer, the tissue samples were gradually dehydrated, in-filtered and embedded in London Resin White (TAAB, UK). Blocks were cured at 65°C for 72 h and made ultra-thin sections (ranges 60-90 nm) with Leica Ultra-cut UC6 ultra microtome (Leica-Microsystems, USA). Sections were incubated for 1 h with 2% skimmed milk and intermittent washing was done with distilled water. Sections containing grids were incubated with primary anti-TTR antibody (1:200 dilutions, ProSci Antibody, USA) at 4°C overnight. Finally sections were washed with 1% fish gelatin in sodium phosphate buffer and incubated with 1:100 dilutions gold conjugated secondary antibody (TAAB, UK) at RT for 2 h. The grids were stained with 2% aqueous uranyl acetate (Merck Chemical, Germany) and analyzed under electron microscope (FEI Tecnai G^2 Spirit) at 200 kV [22],[23].

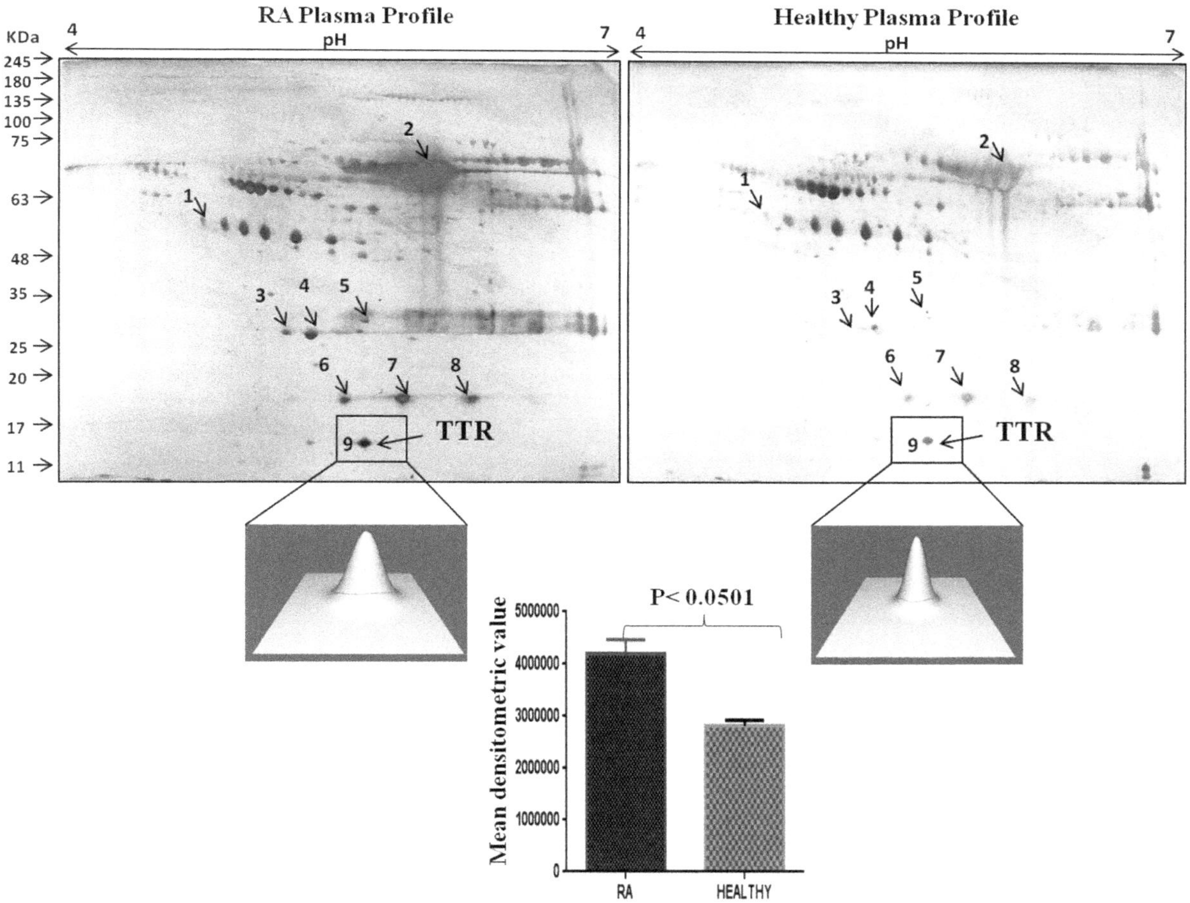

Figure 1. Two dimensional gel electrophoresis of plasma proteins. A representative silver stained 2-DE gel image of plasma proteins from three sets of samples from RA and controls patients. The gels were analyzed for differential expression of proteins using PD-Quest software. The lower panel showed 3D view of TTR expression and their densitometric analysis demonstrated 1.4 fold elevated expression of TTR in RA as compared to healthy control.

Table 2. List of differentially expressed proteins in plasma of RA patients with respect to healthy control.

Spot No.	Protein identified	Accession No.	M.W.(Da)/PI calculated	Peptide matched	Biological Functions
1	Haptoglobin beta chain	P00738	45,205/6.13	11	Cellular iron ion homeostasis, Defence response to bacterium, Intestinal permeability
2	Human Serum Albumin	P02768	69,366/5.92	12	Regulation of the colloidal osmotic pressure of blood, Bile salts transport, Lipid metabolism
3	Serum amyloid protein	P02743	26,246/5.97	6	Acute phase inflammation, Transport of cholesterol
4	Apolipoprotein A 1	P02647	30,778/5.56	11	Cholesterol transport, Fat efflux from tissue
5	Alpha-1 Microglobulin	P02760	38,999/5.95	9	Cell adhesion, Heme Catabolism, Regulation of Immune response
6	HP alpha 2 chain	P00738	16,330/6.1	6	Associated with higher serum iron, Decreased antimicrobial and antioxidant capability, Antigen binding
7	HP alpha 2 chain	P00738	16,330/6.1	12	Antigen binding, Defence response
8	HP alpha 2 chain	P00738	16,330/6.1	12	Intestinal permeability, allowing intercelllular tight junction disassembly
9	Transthyretin	P02766	15,887/5.49	9	Transport, Retinol metabolic process, Phototransduction, extracellulal matrix organization

M.W. – Molecular Weight, PI - Isoelectric Point.

Detection of autoantibodies by immunoprecipitation-Western blotting

To ascertain the significance of increase level of TTR in the diagnosis of RA, autoantibodies in the plasma of RA patients and healthy individuals were detected using immunoprecipitation-Western blotting methods. Immunoprecipitation (IP) was performed using Catch and Release v2.0 reversible immunoprecipitation system (Millipore, USA) as per manufacturer's instructions. Briefly, plasma proteins (500 µg) of individual RA patients was incubated for 2 h in mild shaking condition at RT with anti-TTR antibody separately along with 10 µl antibody capture affinity ligand buffer. The antigen-antibody complexes were eluted with 70 µl elution buffer and separated on 12% SDS-PAGE. Proteins were transferred to nitrocellulose membrane (Millipore, USA) and blocking was carried out using 5% bovine serum albumin (BSA) for 1 h at RT with gentle shaking. Plasma of RA and healthy individuals was added to the membrane as a primary antibody for overnight incubation at 4°C. After each step, the membrane was washed with PBST. The membrane was then incubated with HRP conjugated anti-human antibody for 1 h at RT with mild shaking. Enhanced chemiluminescence assay (ECL) (Thermo-Scientific, Pierce, USA) was used to develop the membrane and autoradiographed on high performance chemiluminescence film (GE Healthcare).

Validation of autoantibodies against transthyretin in the plasma of RA, OA and healthy individuals by ELISA using recombinant pure protein

Each well of the 96 well microtiter plates (Thermo-Scientific, Nunc, USA) were coated with purified recombinant TTR protein having concentration (0.20 µg/100 µl buffer containing 0.01 M Na_2CO_3 and 0.035 M $NaHCO_3$, pH 9.6). The plates were kept at 4°C for 24 h, washed three times with 200 µl PBST and incubated with 200 µl blocking buffer (2% BSA in PBS) for 2 h. The blocking buffer was discarded, washed and incubated with 100 µl plasma of RA, OA and healthy individuals (1:250 dilution) for 3 h at RT. The plates were then washed (three times) and incubated with 100 µl of anti-human HRP conjugate for 1 h and developed with ortho-phenylene diamine (1 mg/ml in 0.05 M citrate buffer and 5 µl/ml H_2O_2) for 30 min. The reactions were stopped by adding 2N H_2SO_4 to each well and the binding efficiency was checked by reading absorbance at 492 nm in an ELISA reader (Spectramax Plus; Molecular Devices, USA).

Invitro validation

To validate the increased level of TTR in vitro conditions, the hepatocellular carcinoma (HepG2) cell lines were challenged with *E. coli* LPS for inflammation and level of TTR expression was determined. HepG2 cell line was maintained as sub confluent monolayer in Dulbecco's modified eagles's medium (DMEM, Invitrogen, USA) with 10% fetal bovine serum (HyClone, Logan, USA) and 100 units/ml penicillin plus 100 µg/ml streptomycin (Life Technology, Invitrogen, USA) in humidified chamber at 37°C with 5% CO_2. The culture was allowed to grow to confluence and used for further experiments. Viability of the cells was determined by the Trypan blue (0.4% Trypan blue in PBS) exclusion method. The cells were challenged with different concentrations of lipopolysaccharide (LPS, Sigma-Aldrich, USA) of *Escherichia coli* and LPS concentration was optimized for inducing measurable concentration of nitrite with minimum cytotoxicity.

The MTT assay was performed to check the cell viability in a 96 well plate. The cells were treated with different concentrations of LPS. At the end of each experiment, the cells were incubated with MTT (20 µl of 5 mg/ml per well, Sigma-Aldrich, USA) at 37°C for 4 h. The formazan product was solubilized by the addition of 100 µl of 0.1N HCl in isopropanol. Cell viability was estimated by recording the absorbance at 595 nm in an ELISA plate reader (data not shown).

Statistical Analysis

Statistical analysis was performed using Windows GraphPad Prism 5 (GraphPad Software, La Jolla, California, USA). Comparisons in expression TTR between healthy control and diseased groups were performed using the two tailed paired *t*-test, and for comparison between more than two groups two tailed

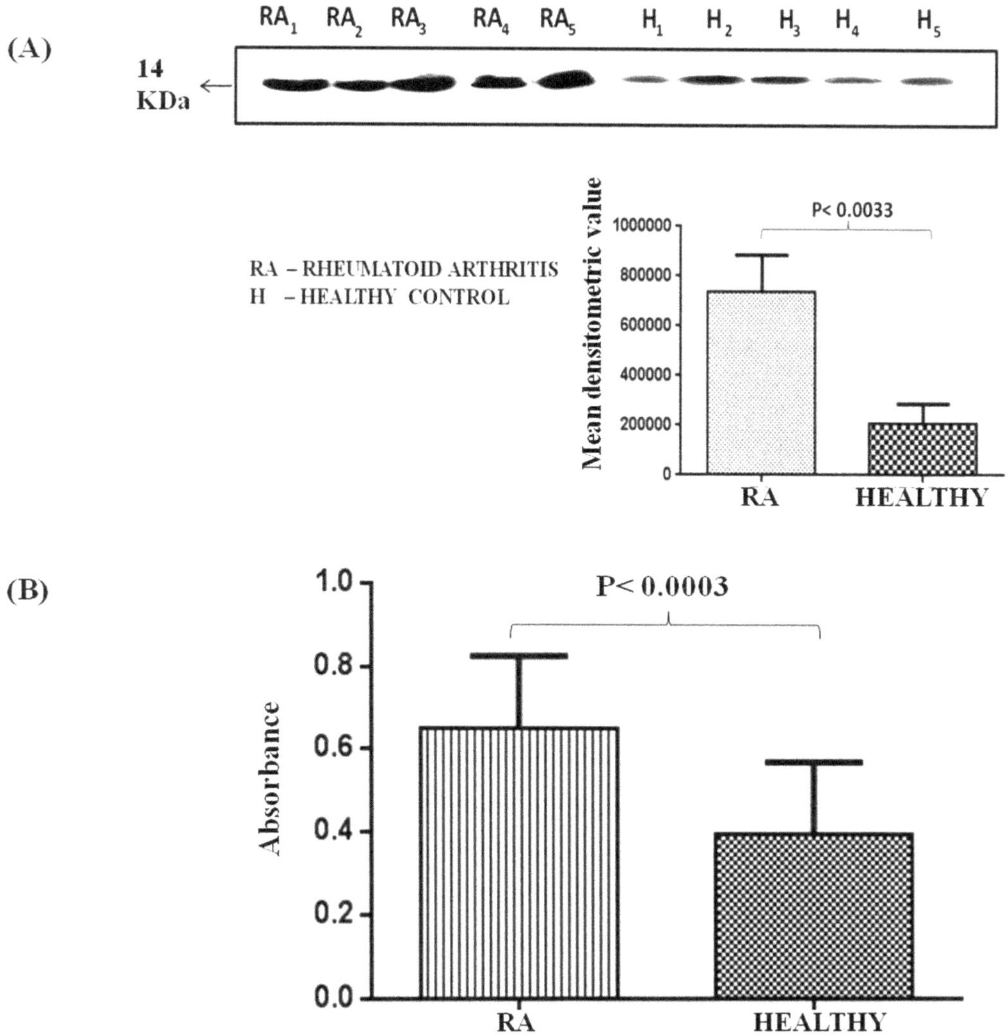

Figure 2. Expression analysis of TTR in the plasma of RA. (**A**) Western blot was performed using plasma proteins of RA patients (n = 12) and healthy controls (n = 12). Densitometric analysis of band developed for TTR followed by statistical analysis using paired two tailed *t*-test showed 3.6 fold elevated expression of TTR in RA as compared to healthy controls. (**B**) ELISA of TTR in the plasma of RA patients (n = 60) and controls (n = 60) indicated 1.6 fold increased expression of TTR in the plasma of RA.

unpaired one-way ANOVA were used. Results were considered statistically significant if $p<0.05$.

Results

Identification of differentially expressed proteins

Two-dimensional gel electrophoresis coupled with MALDI-TOF MS/MS analysis was carried out to identify the differentially expressed proteins in RA patients. The PD-Quest software analysis of 2-DE gels displayed 119 spots in RA sera and 96 spots in healthy sera. Out of 23 differential protein spots, 9 protein spots were successfully identified by MALDI-TOF MS/MS [Table 2].The identified proteins included haptoglobin (β-chain), haptoglobin alpha 2 chain, alpha 1 microglobulin, serum amyloid, albumin and apolipoprotein which were upregulated in the sera of RA patients as compared to healthy control. One of the protein, identified as TTR also exhibited elevated levels in sera of RA patients as compared to other proteins. PD-Quest and densitometry analysis showed 1.4 fold higher expression of TTR in RA patients as compared to healthy volunteers (Figure 1 and S1).

Validation of elevated expression of TTR in plasma, synovium and synovial fluid

The significant increase in expression of TTR in plasma, synovium and synovial fluid has been validated using Western blotting, ELISA, immune-histochemical and immuno-electronmicrosocpic analysis. Among all the identified proteins in plasma of RA patients, TTR was found to be associated with inflammation [24] and was validated in healthy controls and RA patients using Western blot analysis.The densitometric analysis of Western blots performed (Figure 2A) with plasma of severe RA patients (n = 12) showed 3.6 fold higher TTR levels in RA patients as compared to healthy control (n = 12). Levels of TTR was also analyzed by ELISA and found to be elevated (1.6 fold) in RA patients (n = 60) as compared to the healthy controls (Figure 2B).

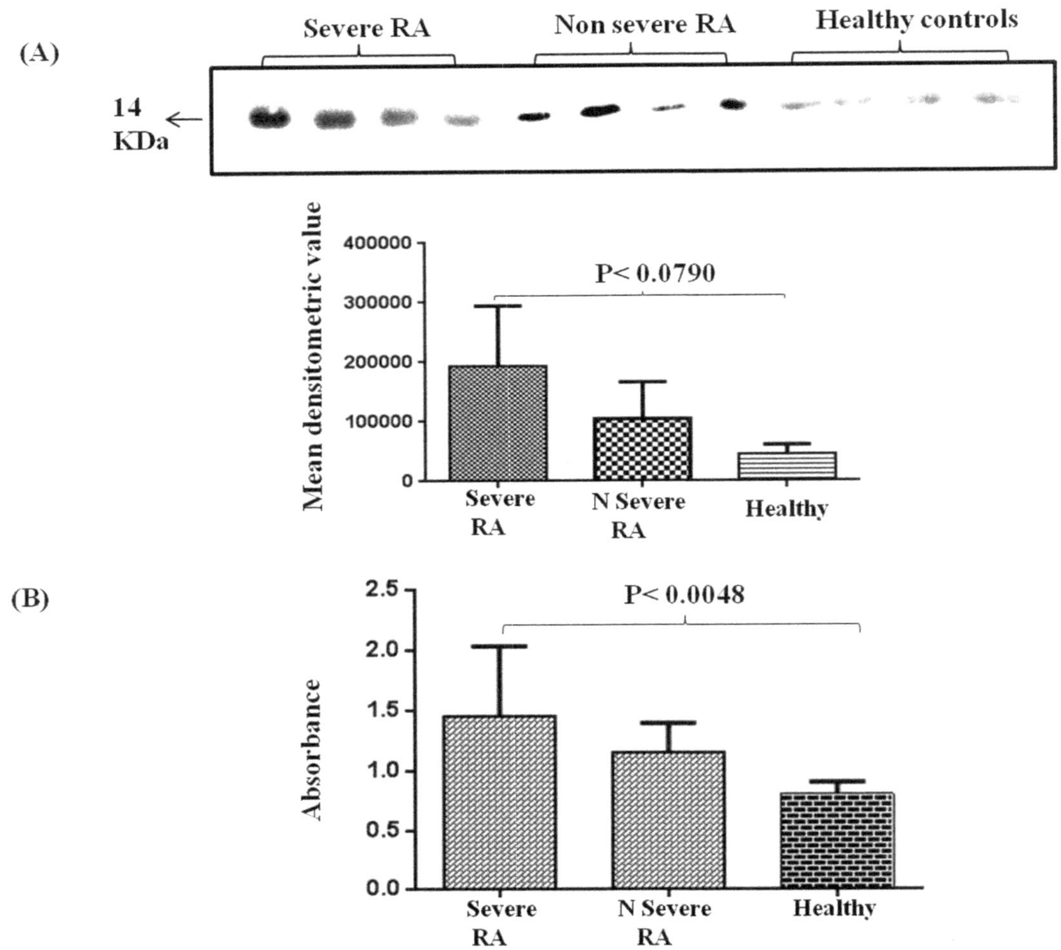

Figure 3. Expression of TTR in plasma of severe and non severe RA and healthy control. (**A**) Western blot analysis of plasma obtained from severe (n = 28), non severe (n = 22) and healthy control (n = 25) revealed 4.75 fold and 2.5 fold increased expression of TTR in severe and non severe RA patients respectively as compared to healthy controls. (**B**) ELISA of TTR in severe and non severe samples was performed and compared with healthy controls. TTR expression was significantly up regulated ($p<0.0048$) in severe and non severe RA patients as compared to healthy control (2.0 fold and 1.5 fold respectively).

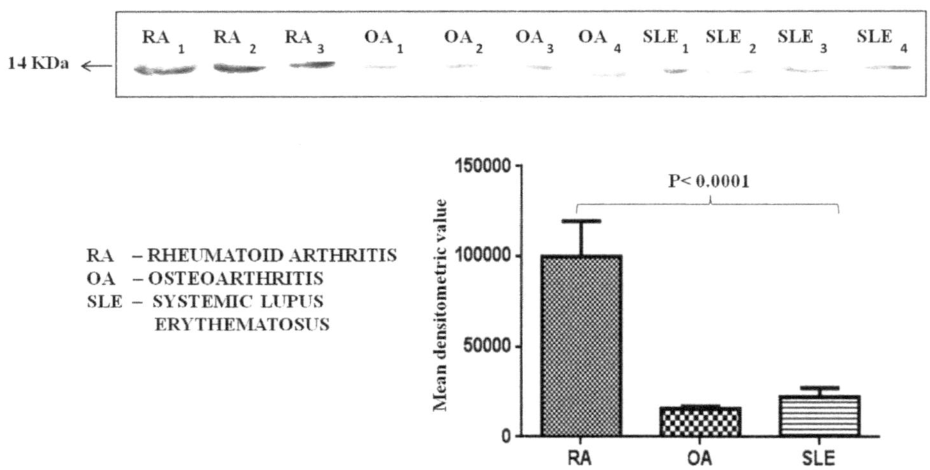

Figure 4. Expression of TTR in RA, Osteoarthritis and Systemic lupus erythematosus patients. TTR expressions were examined in other joint disease and autoimmune disease such as OA and SLE. Western blot analysis showed that TTR level was significantly down regulated ($p<0.0001$) in the plasma of OA and SLE patients as compared to the RA patients. Densitometric analysis indicated 6.6 and 5 fold higher expression of TTR in RA (n = 9) as compared to OA (n = 12) and SLE (n = 12) respectively.

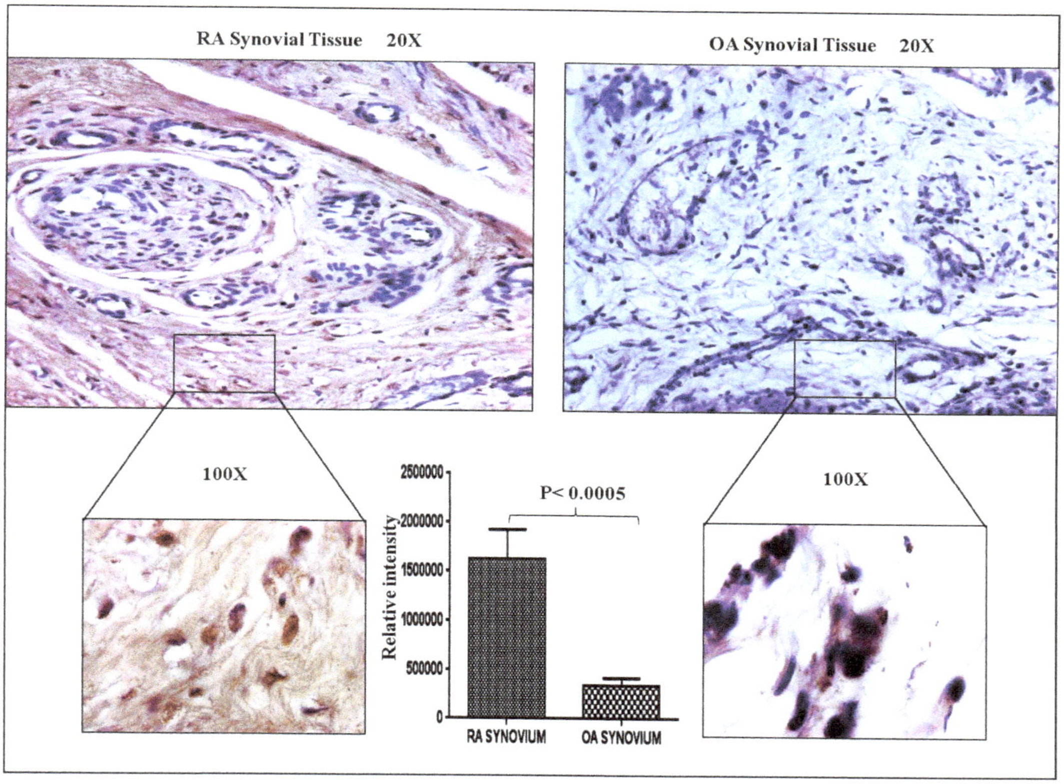

Figure 5. Immunohistochemistry of synovium. To observe the expression of TTR in synovium (RA, n = 3 and OA, n = 3), IHC were performed. Tissue samples were fixed, processed and stained with DAB. Brown colour indicates the presence of autoantigen in synovium. Upper panel shows the image of synovial tissue at 20X and lower panel shows the image at 100X magnification. TTR expression was predominantly high in RA as compared to OA synovium. Densitometric analysis revealed approximately 5 fold up regulation of TTR expression in RA synovium as compared to OA.

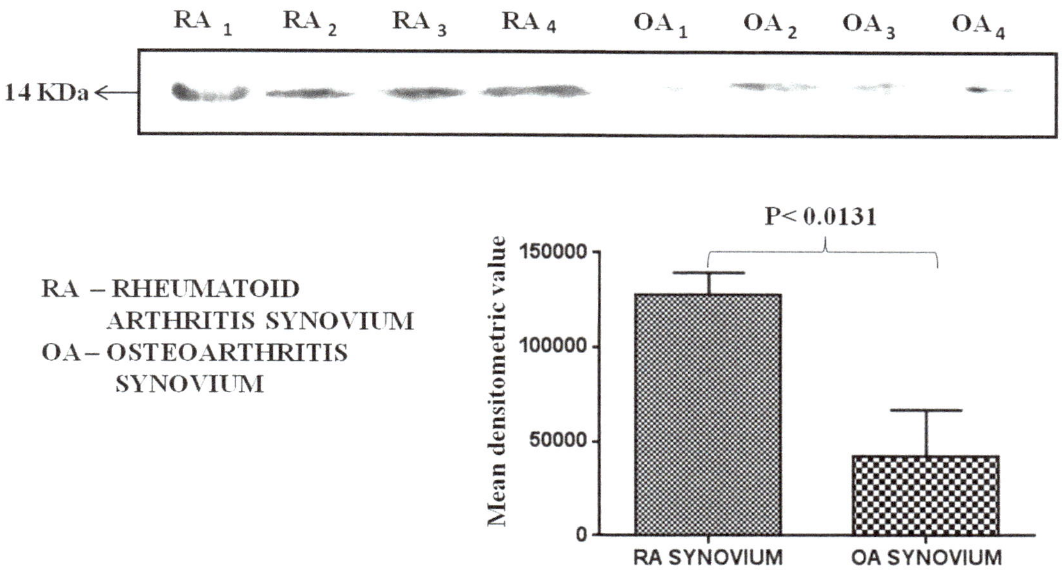

Figure 6. Quantitation of TTR in synovium by Western blotting. Protein (50 µg) of RA synovium (n = 7) and OA synovium (n = 7) was loaded in SDS-PAGE gels, the proteins were separated and transferred onto nitrocellulose. Western blot results revealed 3.2 fold higher expression (p< 0.0131) of TTR in RA synovium as compared to OA synovium.

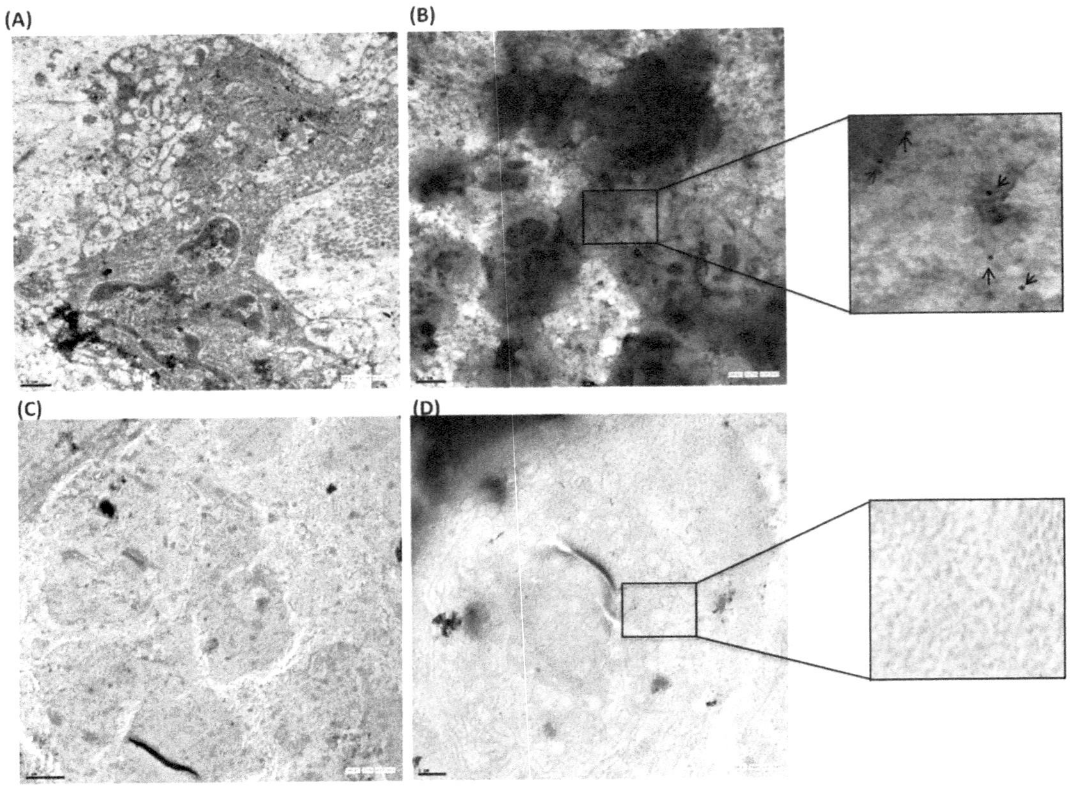

Figure 7. Quantitation of TTR in synovium by immunoelectron microscopy. RA (n = 3) and OA (n = 3) synovium were surgically removed in aseptic condition, fixed and processed for electron microscopy. Ultrathin sections were labelled with 20 nm gold conjugated secondary antibody. Upper panel (**A**) shows evenly distributed gold label in RA synovium (**B**) Selected area has been magnified and marked with arrows to show the gold labelling. Lower panel (C, D) shows the negligible level of TTR expression in OA synovium (Scale bar A, B, D 1 μm, C 2 μm).

The expression analysis among the RA population suggested that 71% patients exhibit statistically significant upregulation of TTR in RA patients, whereas, 15% patient population showed similar levels of TTR as observed in healthy controls (Figure S2) These results suggest that TTR may be a disease associated protein. This data led us to analyze if the TTR expression is dependent on the disease severity as well. To answer this, we segregated the patient population in terms of their respective disease severity and then analyzed the TTR expression in the patient groups.

Based on DAS score, the RA patient population was segregated into two groups, severe (DAS score$\geq$5.1) and non-severe (DAS score$\leq$2.6) population. Interestingly, both Western blotting and ELISA analysis confirmed that there is a significant increase in expression of TTR in the plasma as per increase in severity of RA conditions of patients. TTR expression was analyzed in plasma of severe (n = 28), non-severe (n = 22) RA and healthy control (n = 25) groups by Western blot. Densitometry analysis revealed that TTR expression was 4.75 fold and 2.5 fold higher in severe and non-severe RA patients respectively in comparison to healthy controls (Figure 3A). The observation was then validated by ELISA that showed TTR expression increases with the progression of disease severity. ELISA result demonstrated that TTR expression in severe RA condition was up regulated by 2.0 fold and 1.5 fold in severe and non-severe RA patients ($p<0.0048$) in comparison to healthy control (Figure 3B).

To prove the specificity of TTR for RA diagnosis, it was necessary to measure the TTR levels in patients of other joint disease and autoimmune diseases such as OA and SLE. It was interesting to note that the levels of TTR was 6.6 fold and 5 fold more in the plasma of RA patients as compared to OA and SLE respectively (Figure 4).

We observed that TTR protein was up regulated in plasma samples of RA patients. Therefore, it was intriguing to investigate the status of TTR expression in RA synovium and synovial fluid. Immunohistochemistry, Western blotting and IEM were performed to check the level of TTR in RA synovium as compared to OA synovium. As shown in Figure 5, TTR was predominantly expressed ($p<0.0005$) in RA synovium, whereas, TTR amount was negligible in OA synovium. The relative intensity as calculated by using Alpha Digidoc 1201 software that showed significantly higher expression (~5 fold) of TTR in RA synovium as compared to OA synovium. To further validate the IHC result, Western blotting was carried out using RA and OA synovium. The results indicated 3.2 fold elevated expression of TTR in RA synovium as compared to OA (Figure 6) and these observations were similar to the results we observed with the plasma of RA patients. We also measured the TTR expression in synovial fluid of RA and OA samples (control) and found the similar trend showing up regulation of TTR in RA synovial fluid (Figure S4) which confirmed the significance of such an increase in TTR expression especially in RA conditions.

Immunoelectron microscopy analysis confirmed that as compared to synovium of OA patients, there is significantly high global expression of TTR in synovium of RA patients. Immunoelectron microscopy using gold labelled anti-TTR antibodies (20 nm)

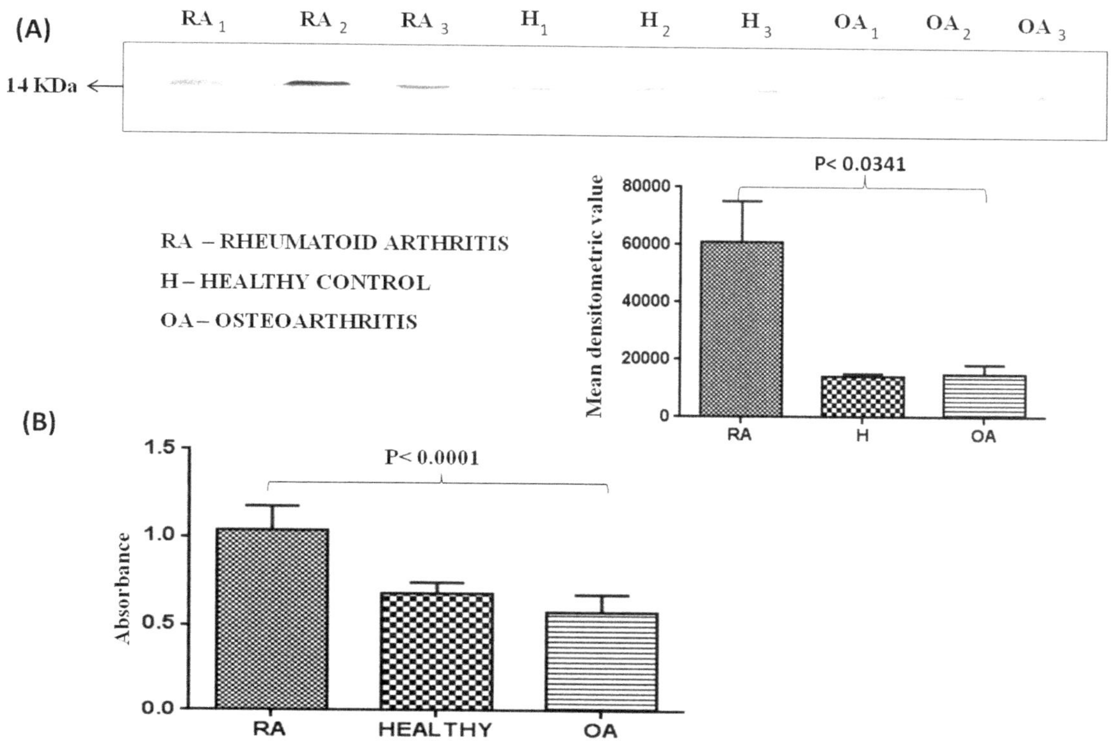

Figure 8. Quantitation of autoantibodies against TTR in plasma of RA, OA patients and healthy controls. (**A**) TTR was immunoprecipitated using anti-TTR antibody and separated on SDS-PAGE and Western blotting was performed. Autoantibodies against TTR in RA (n = 30) were approximately 5 fold higher as compared to healthy control (n = 30) and OA (n = 34) patients. Each bar represents the mean ± SD of values obtained from densitometeric analysis of bands. (**B**) Expression of autoantibodies against TTR in RA was further confirmed by ELISA and analysis showed 1.6 and 2 fold higher levels of autoantibodies in RA as compared to healthy control and OA respectively.

showed that TTR was predominantly present in RA synovium as compared to OA synovium (Figure 7). The expression of TTR was observed in extra-cellular matrix as well as inside the synovial cells of RA patients. The TTR labeling demonstrates higher expression in the RA synovium, while it was not detected in OA patient's synovium.

Invitro experiment was performed to see the effect of inflammation on TTR level and the inflammation was induced in HepG2 cells by LPS of *E.coli.* TTR level was analyzed in the LPS stimulated culture supernatant and compared with the supernatant obtained from unstimulated cells. TTR level was found to be higher in the LPS treated supernatant as compared to the untreated cells (Figure S3).

Identification of autoantibodies against TTR

As compared to health individuals, there has been a several fold high induction of autoantibodies production in RA plasma. Antibodies against TTR were assayed in the plasma of RA (n = 30), OA (n = 34) and healthy control (n = 30) groups using the immunoprecipitation method followed by Western blotting (Figure 8A). It was found that autoantibodies against TTR were 5 fold higher in RA plasma as compared to OA and healthy subjects. Autoantibodies against TTR were also found using recombinant pure protein of TTR in Western blot analysis (data not shown). The quantification of autoantibodies against TTR was done by ELISA which indicated that the level of autoantibodies was 1.6 fold and 2 fold higher ($p<0.0001$) in RA sera as compared to healthy control and OA respectively (Figure 8B).

Discussion

The key to early recognition of autoimmune disease lies within the humoral system. To date, a variety of candidate disease-associated proteins (autoantigen) and autoantibodies have been found to play an important roles in the pathogenesis of RA [25], [26], [27]. Proteomic pattern analysis is one of the most promising approaches for the discovery and identification of proteins associated with diseases[28], [29], [30], [31], [32]. Therefore, the present study was based on the screening of proteins present in the sera of RA patients for the identification of proteins associated with severity of diseases and have potential for diagnosis. Proteomic approach is used to investigate differentially expressed proteins in the plasma of RA patients. In this study, nine differentially expressed proteins were identified in RA patients in comparison to healthy control using MALDI TOF-MS/MS suggesting that many proteins are associated with RA. Some of these proteins such as apolipoprotein, albumin, heptoglobulin beta chain are already known to be involved in the development of RA [8], [33], [34]. Recently, significantly higher level ($p<0.05$) of TTR in RA plasma compared to healthy control has been reported, however, their role in the pathogenesis of RA is not understood. In addition, no statistical significant expression of TTR between OA and healthy control ($p>0.05$) has been reported [35].

In the present study, among all the identified proteins TTR autoantigen was found to be over expressed in the plasma, synovium and synovial fluid of RA patient.TTR protein has also been suggested as a possible biomarker in other diseases such as ovarian cancer [36], hepatocellular carcinoma [37], malnutrition [38] and mycosis fungoides [39].

To assess the TTR expression profile for joint diseases, OA and SLE in addition to RA patients were included in this study. Plasma TTR expression was significantly down regulated in OA and SLE patients as compared to RA patients. Thus, it can be conveniently considered that expression of TTR protein is not affected in all the joint diseases and due to inflammation in general except in RA. One of the important observations of this study includes demonstration of increase in expression of TTR with the increase in severity of RA. Such an association of TTR with severity of RA has not been previously shown. Although very recently there has been a report on elevated expression of TTR in RA sera samples [35] but no information is available on the expression of TTR with severity of RA conditions. We found that TTR level was influenced with the severity of the disease (Figure 3). In addition, our study further demonstrated that the TTR expression profiling in RA and OA synovium samples using IHC and Western blotting that was further confirmed by IEM. These findings revealed that TTR was significantly over expressed in RA synovium whereas moderate expression has been observed in OA synovium. The IEM study demonstrated the higher levels of TTR in RA synovium and it showed both cytosolic and nuclear localization. The study was extended by performing an *invitro* experiment using HepG2 cell line in which the inflammation was induced by bacterial LPS and the TTR levels were measured in the medium. Such a comprehensive study on expression of proteins involving plasma, synovium and synovial fluid was lacking. Therefore, the observation on increase in expression of TTR with the increase in severity of RA has a merit in RA pathogenesis and etiology.

The present study has also demonstrated that the autoantibodies against TTR are over expressed in RA patients. This over expression was demonstrated using Western blotting and subsequently confirmed in the population of RA patients using ELISA. Most importantly, ELISA and Western blot results showed entirely consistent results. The autoantibodies against TTR were observed to be higher in RA patients which was not seen in the samples obtained from OA patients. In this context, our study opens a new door to further carry out the systematic investigation on the role of TTR in the pathogenesis of RA and the potential of TTR to serve as a novel biomarker in addition to the existing battery of biomarkers.

In conclusion, this study identified that TTR is a differentially expressed protein in the plasma, synovium and synovial fluid of RA patients. We also report that the TTR expression level is predominantly associated with the progression of severity of the disease. In addition, autoantibodies against TTR were present in the sera of RA patients. We propose that autoantibodies against TTR can be used as diagnostic tool for RA and its progression along with other tests. A systematic investigation on the role of TTR may help in better understanding of the pathogenesis of RA.

Supporting Information

Figure S1 **MALDI TOF MS/MS spectrum of Transthyretin (TTR).**

Figure S2 **Pie chart shows the severity of disease in RA patients based on TTR levels.**

Figure S3 ***Invitro* validation of TTR expression.** Inflammation was induced by *E.coli* LPS in HepG2 cell line. TTR expression was found to be higher in treated supernatant as compared to untreated.

Figure S4 **TTR expression in synovial fluid.** Western blot analysis of synovial fluid demonstrated higher expression ($p < 0.0019$) of TTR in RA patients ($n = 6$) as compared to OA ($n = 6$).

Acknowledgments

We would like to acknowledge Dr. Shivender Kumar Srivastava, Orthropaedic Department, AIIMS, New Delhi for providing us RA and OA samples. We thank to Dr U. Mabalirajan, Trayambak Basak and Sandip Kumar Dash, Institute of Genomics and Integrative Biology, Delhi University Campus, Mall Road, Delhi for their support. We would like to thank Indian Council of Medical Research (ICMR), Ramalingaswami Bhawan, New Delhi, India for providing the financial support to carry out the research work.

Author Contributions

Conceived and designed the experiments: SB SS SG. Performed the experiments: SS SG. Analyzed the data: SS SB SG LKS AS DSB RM OPG TKD. Contributed reagents/materials/analysis tools: SB SS LS. Wrote the paper: SS SB LKS YS RSS.

References

1. Smolen JS, Steiner G (2003) Therapeutic strategies for rheumatoid arthritis. Nat Rev Drug Discov 2: 473–488.
2. Gay S, Gay RE, Koopman WJ (1993) Molecular and cellular mechanisms of joint destruction in rheumatoid arthritis: two cellular mechanisms explain joint destruction? Ann Rheum Dis 52: S39–S47.
3. Mittler RS (2004) Suppressing the self in rheumatoid arthritis. Nat Med 10: 1047–1049.
4. Bromberg J (2013) TNFα trips up Treg cells in rheumatoid arthritis. Nat Med 19: 269–270.
5. Wolfe F (1997a) The prognosis of rheumatoid arthritis: assessment of disease activity and disease severity in the clinic. Am J Med 103: 12–18.
6. Snir O, Widhe M, Hermansson M, VonSpee C, Linderberg J, et al. (2010) Antibodies to several citrullinated antigens are enriched in the joints of rheumatoid arthritis patients. Arthritis Rheum 62: 44–52.
7. Ziff M (1990) Rheumatoid arthritis-its present and future. J Rheumatol 17: 127–133.
8. Liao H, Wu J, Kuhn E, Chin W, Chang B, et al. (2004) Use of mass spectrometry to identify protein biomarkers of disease severity in the synovial fluid and serum of patients with rheumatoid arthritis. Arthritis Rheum 50: 3792–3803.
9. Wang J, Zhou N, Xu B, Hao H, Kang L, et al. (2012) Identification and Cluster Analysis of *Streptococcus pyogenes* by MALDI-TOF Mass Spectrometry. PloS One 7: e0047152.
10. Marchi N, Fazio V, Cucullo L, Kight K, Asaryk T, et al. (2003) Serum transthyretin monomer as a possible marker of blood-to-CSF barrier disruption. J Neurosci 23: 1949–1955.
11. Davis PJ, Handwerger BS, Gregerman RI (1972) Thyroid hormone binding by human serum prealbumin (TBPA) electrophoretic studies of triiodothyronine-TBPA interaction. J Clin Invest 51: 515–521.
12. Kanai M, Raz A, Goodman DS (1968) Retinol-binding protein: the transport protein for vitamin A in human plasma. J Clin Invest 47: 2025–2044.
13. Peterson PA (1971) Characteristics of a vitamin A-transporting protein complex occurring in human serum. J Biol Chem 246: 34–43.
14. Berry DC, Croniger CM, Ghyselinck NB, Noya (2012) Transthyretin Blocks Retinol Uptake and Cell Signaling by the Holo-Retinol-Binding Protein Receptor STRA6. Mol Cell Biol 19: 3851–3859.
15. Gitlin D, Perricelli A (1970) Synthesis of serum albumin, prealbumin, alpha-fetoprotein, alpha-1-antitrypsin and transferrin by the human yolk sac. Nature 228: 995–997.
16. Chang X, Zhao Y, Wang Y, Chen Y, Yan X (2013). Screening citrullinated proteins in synovial tissues of rheumatoid arthritis using 2-dimensional western blotting. J Rheumatol 40: 219–27.
17. Saroha A, Kumar S, Chatterjee BP, Das HR (2012) Jacalin bound plasma O-glycoproteome and reduced sialylation of alpha 2-HS glycoprotein in rheumatoid arthritis patients. PloS One 7: e46374.

18. Biswas S, Sharma S, Saroha A, Bhakuni DS, Malhotra R, et al. (2013) Identification of novel autoantigen in the synovial fluid of rheumatoid arthritis patients using an immunoproteomics approach. PloS One 8: e56246.
19. Bo GP, Zhou LN, He WF, Luo GX, Jia XF, et al. (2009) Analyses of differential proteome of human synovial fibroblasts obtained from arthritis. Clin Rheumatol 28: 191–199.
20. Hueber W, Tomooka BH, Batliwalla F, Li W, Monach PA, et al. (2009) Blood autoantibody and cytokine profiles predict response to anti-tumor necrosis factor therapy in rheumatoid arthritis. Arthritis Res Ther 11: R76.
21. Ahmad A, Mukherjee S, Pattnaik B, Kumar M, Singh S, et al. (2014) Miro1 regulates intracellular mitochondrial transport and enhances mesenchymal stem cell rescue efficacy. EMBO J "In press".
22. Smith RM, Charron MJ, Shah N, Lodish HF (1991) Immunoelectron microscopic demonstration of insulin-stimulated translocation of glucose transporters of plasma membrane of isolated rat adipocytes and masking of carboxy-terminal epitope of intracellular GLUT-4. Proc Natl Acad Sci U S A 88: 6893–6897.
23. Riveraa J, Cordeora RB, Nakouzia AS, Frasesb S, Nicolaa A, et al. (2010) *Bacillus anthracis* produces membrane-derived vesicle containing biologically active toxins. Proc Natl Acad Sci, U S A 107: 19002–19007.
24. Johnson AM, Merlini G, Sheldon J, Ichihara K (2007) Clinical indications of plasma protein assays: transthyretin (prealbnumin) in inflammation and malnutrition. Clin Chem Lab Med 47: 419–426.
25. Sekine T, Masuko-Hongo K, Matsui T, Asahara H, Takigawa M, et al. (2001) Recognition of YKL-39, a human cartilage related protein, as a target antigen in patients with rheumatoid arthritis. Ann Rheum Dis 60: 49–54.
26. Tsuruha J, Masuko-Hongo K, Kato T, Sakata M, Nakamura H, et al. (2001) Implication of cartilage intermediate layer protein in cartilage destruction in subsets of patients with osteoarthritis and rheumatoid arthritis. Arthritis Rheum 44: 838–845.
27. Iwaki-Egawa S, Matsuno H, Yudoh K, Nakazawa F, Miyazaki K, et al. (2004) High diagnostic value of anticalpastatin autoantibodies in rheumatoid arthritis detected by ELISA using human erythrocyte calpastatin as antigen. J Rheumatol 31: 17–22.
28. Westhoff CM (2007) The structure and function of the Rh antigen complex. Semin Hematol 44: 42–50.
29. Drake RR, Cazares LH, Semmens OJ, Wardsworth JT (2005) Serum, salivary and tissue proteomics for discovery of biomarkers for head and neck cancers. Expert Rev Mol Diagn 5: 93–100.
30. Karpova MA, Moshkovskii SA, Toropygin IY, Archakov AI (2010) Cancer specific MALDI-TOF profile of blood serum and plasma: Biological meaning and perspectives. J Proteomics 73: 537–551.
31. Howard BA, Wang MZ, Campa MJ, Corro C, Fitzgerald MC, et al. (2003) Identification and validation of a potential lung cancer serum biomarker detected by matrix-assisted laser desorption/ionization- time of flight spectra analysis. Proteomics 9: 1720–1724.
32. Zheng Y, Xu Y, Ye B, Lei J, Weinstein MH (2003) Prostate carcinoma tissue proteomics for biomarker discovery. Cancer 15: 2576–2582.
33. Trocme C, Marotee H, Baillet A, Pallot-Prades B, Garin J, et al. (2009) Apolipoprotein A-I and platelet factor 4 are biomarkers for infliximab response in rheumatoid arthritis. Ann Rheum Dis 68: 1328–1333.
34. Niu Q, Huang Z, Shi Y, Wang L, Pan X, et al. (2010) Specific serum protein biomarkers of rheumatoid arthritis detected by MALDI-TOF-MS combined with magnetic beads. Int Immunol 22: 611–618.
35. Ni M, Wei W, Feng Q, Sun XG, Wang YC, et al. (2013) Transthyretin as a potential serological marker for the diagnosis of patients with early rheumatoid arthritis. Clin Exp Rheumatol 31: 394–399.
36. Kozak KR, Su F, Whitelegge JP, Faull K, Reddy S, et al. (2005) Characterization of serum biomarkers for detection of early stage ovarian cancer. Proteomics 5: 4589–4596.
37. Feng JT, Liu YK, Song HY, Dai Z, Qin LX, et al. (2005) Heat-shock protein 27: a potential biomarker for hepatocellular carcinoma identified by serum proteome analysis. Proteomics 5: 4581-4588.
38. Marten NW, Sladek FM, Straus DS (1996) Effect of dietary protein restriction on liver transcription factors. Biochem J 317: 361–370.
39. Escher N, Kaatzy M, Melle C, Hiplery C, Ziemery M, et al. (2007) Posttranslational modifications of Transthyretin are serum markers in patients with Mycosis Fungoides. Neoplasia 9: 254–259.

7

Cellular Adhesion Gene *SELP* Is Associated with Rheumatoid Arthritis and Displays Differential Allelic Expression

Jana Burkhardt[1*❡], Mechthild Blume[2❡], Elisabeth Petit-Teixeira[3], Vitor Hugo Teixeira[4], Anke Steiner[2], Elfi Quente[5], Grit Wolfram[1], Markus Scholz[6], Céline Pierlot[3], Paola Migliorini[7], Stefano Bombardieri[7], Alejandro Balsa[8], René Westhovens[9], Pilar Barrera[10], Timothy R. D. J. Radstake[11], Helena Alves[12], Thomas Bardin[13], Bernard Prum[14], Frank Emmrich[1,2,5], François Cornelis[15], Peter Ahnert[6,16❡], Holger Kirsten[5,6,16❡]

1 Translational Centre for Regenerative Medicine (TRM), Universität Leipzig, Leipzig, Germany, **2** University Leipzig, Institute for Clinical Immunology and Tranfusion Medicine (IKIT), Universität Leipzig, Leipzig, Germany, **3** Genhotel-EA 3886, Université d'Evry-Val d'Essonne, Evry, France, **4** Centre for Respiratory Research, University College London, London, United Kingdom, **5** Fraunhofer Institute for Celltherapy and Immunology (IZI), Leipzig, Germany, **6** LIFE – Leipzig Research Center for Civilization Diseases, Universität Leipzig, Leipzig, Germany, **7** Pisa University, Pisa, Italy, **8** La Paz Hospital, Madrid, Spain, **9** Rheumatology KU Leuven, Leuven, Belgium, **10** Nijmegen University, Nijmegen, the Netherlands, **11** University Medical Center Utrecht, Utrecht, the Netherlands, **12** Porto San Joao Hospital, Porto, Portugal, **13** Fédération de Rhumatologie, Lariboisière Hospital, Paris, France, **14** Laboratoire Statistique & Génome, Université d'Evry-Val d'Essonne, Evry, France, **15** GenHotel-Auvergne, Université d'Auvergne, Clermont-Ferrand, France, **16** Institute for Medical Informatics, Statistics and Epidemiology (IMISE), Universität Leipzig, Leipzig, Germany

Abstract

In rheumatoid arthritis (RA), a key event is infiltration of inflammatory immune cells into the synovial lining, possibly aggravated by dysregulation of cellular adhesion molecules. Therefore, single nucleotide polymorphisms of 14 genes involved in cellular adhesion processes (*CAST, ITGA4, ITGB1, ITGB2, PECAM1, PTEN, PTPN11, PTPRC, PXN, SELE, SELP, SRC, TYK2, and VCAM1*) were analyzed for association with RA. Association analysis was performed consecutively in three European RA family sample groups ($N_{families} = 407$). Additionally, we investigated differential allelic expression, a possible functional consequence of genetic variants. *SELP* (selectin P, CD62P) SNP-allele rs6136-T was associated with risk for RA in two RA family sample groups as well as in global analysis of all three groups ($p_{total} = 0.003$). This allele was also expressed preferentially ($p < 10^{-6}$) with a two- fold average increase in regulated samples. Differential expression is supported by data from Genevar MuTHER ($p_1 = 0.004$; $p_2 = 0.0177$). Evidence for influence of rs6136 on transcription factor binding was also found *in silico* and in public datasets reporting *in vitro* data. In summary, we found SELP rs6136-T to be associated with RA and with increased expression of SELP mRNA. SELP is located on the surface of endothelial cells and crucial for recruitment, adhesion, and migration of inflammatory cells into the joint. Genetically determined increased SELP expression levels might thus be a novel additional risk factor for RA.

Editor: Masataka Kuwana, Keio University School of Medicine, Japan

Funding: The work presented in this paper was made possible by funding from the German Federal Ministry of Education and Research (BMBF, PtJ-Bio, 1315883, www.bmbf.de). This project was also supported by grant no. 7692/1187 from the Sächsische Aufbaubank–Förderbank (www.sab.sachsen.de), by grant no. 4212/04-04 from the European Fund for Regional Development (EFRE, ec.europa.eu), by the German Federal Ministry for Education and Research (Hochschul- und Wissenschaftsprogramm; "Kompetenznetz Rheuma" 01GI9949 to IM), by the Rosa-Luxemburg-Stiftung (www.rosalux.de) and by the Foundation for Science and Technology, Portugal (grant SFRH/BD/23304/2005, www.fct.pt). PA, MS and HK were also supported by LIFE – Leipzig Research Center for Civilization Diseases (life.uni-leipzig.de), Universität Leipzig. LIFE is funded by means of the European Union, by the European Regional Development Fund (ERDF) and by means of the Free State of Saxony within the framework of the excellence initiative. The funders had no role in study design, data collection and analysis, decision to publish, or preparation of the manuscript.

Competing Interests: The authors have declared that no competing interests exist.

* Email: jana.burkhardt@trm.uni-leipzig.de

❡ These authors contributed equally to this work.

Introduction

Rheumatoid Arthritis (RA) is a chronic inflammatory disease with features of an autoimmune disease [1]. There is ample evidence for genetic influences on RA and heritability is estimated to be about 60% [2]. It is estimated that risk alleles identified up to now explain about 17% of seropositive RA [3]. One hallmark of RA pathogenesis is infiltration of synovial fluid by autoreactive immune cells. These cells release inflammatory cytokines, immunoglobulins, and rheumatoid factor (RF). Macrophages ingest these RF immune complexes and release additional cytokines (e.g. IL1, IL6), leading to activation of the complement system and release of more inflammatory mediators and cartilage degrading enzymes. Macrophages as well as proliferating fibroblast-like cells induce typical joint swelling and pannus formation in the inflamed synovial membrane. This cycle of activation and infiltration of inflammatory cells, release of inflammatory mediators and action of aggressive cartilage degrading enzymes finally causes destruction of cartilage and joints. Hence, in the pathogenesis of RA, infiltration of inflammatory cells into the synovial lining plays an important role and may be modulated by dysregulation of cellular adhesion molecules [4,5]. Adhesion molecules are expressed on the surface of cells and mediate adhesion of cells to other cells or to the extracellular matrix [6]. They can be divided into three superfamilies: selectins, integrins, and the Ig-superfamily. Adhesion molecules regulate leukocyte circulation, lymphoid cell homing to tissues and inflammatory sites, and transendothelial migration. They also participate in lymphocyte co-stimulation, cytotoxicity, lymphohemopoiesis, and B cell apoptosis. In RA, gene expression of integrins and their ligands were found to be up-regulated [7] and studies even suggest correlations with prognosis and disease activity for adhesion gene products such as selectin P which is encoded by the gene *SELP* [8,9]. Therefore, genes involved in cellular adhesion processes are highly relevant candidate genes for studying genetic association with RA.

To identify genes involved in cellular adhesion relevant in RA, we performed a thorough literature and database analysis. We favored genes that are located in genomic regions identified in genome-wide linkage scans in RA families [10] and genes with polymorphisms known to be associated with autoimmune disorders. Table 1 displays relevant information on all 14 genes selected. In brief, some properties and functions of these genes are as follows: Integrin: Integrin ITGA4 is the alpha-4 subunit of integrin VLA-4, ITGB1 is the beta-1 subunit of the same molecule. VLA-4 is a cell surface receptor on activated lymphocytes and monocytes that binds the ligand VCAM1 on endothelial cells. It is particularly involved in firm adhesion prior to migration. ITGB2 is the beta-2 subunit of the integrin LFA-1, which is also expressed on lymphocytes, especially leukocytes. Ligands of LFA-1 are ICAM1, ICAM2, and VCAM1 on endothelial cells. TYK2 is a tyrosine kinase belonging to the group of Janus kinases. The molecule is part of the regulatory network of integrin mediated adhesion and migration by activating negative regulators upon signaling [11]. The *PXN* (*paxillin*) gene is located in an RA linkage region and part of the focal adhesion process. Its protein product, PXN is in direct contact with the focal adhesion kinase (FAK). PXN is part of growth factor and adhesion mediated cell signaling processes including migration, proliferation, and gene expression activation [12]. SRC is a kinase and part of the integrin signaling network. Its gene is highly regulated by multiple binding partners such as FAK. PTPRC is a binding partner and regulator of SRC. During integrin mediated adhesion, PTPRC is bound to the tyrosine kinase complex and inhibits SRC mainly via the kinase domain [13]. There are several association studies published for *PTPRC* with autoimmune diseases [14,15]. *PTEN* and *PTPN11* both are tumor suppressor genes involved in migration processes. FAK is a substrate for PTEN and the FAK pathway influences organization of actin filaments during cellular migration [16]. PTPN11 is involved in Rho signaling, which is part of cellular adhesion processes. It is also a positive regulator of the SRC mediated integrin pathway [17]. Calpastatin (CAST) is an inhibitor of calpain, a protease involved in apoptosis, proliferation, and migration. This molecule is part of the regulatory network of integrin mediated cellular adhesion via RhoA and FAK signaling pathways as well as via direct binding to the beta subunit of integrins,. Additionally, calpain regulates integrin activation via talin, a prerequisite for firm adhesion. Inhibition of calpain has been shown to reduce cellular migration [18]. PECAM1 and VCAM1 belong to the Ig superfamily and are widely expressed on hematopoietic cells. The blocking of PECAM1 with specific antibodies reduces 90% of leukocyte migration. In combination with CD99 blocking, diapedesis is nearly completely inhibited [19]. SELE and SELP are adhesion proteins belonging to the selectin class and are expressed on the surface of activated endothelial cells. SELP (selectin P, CD62P) can be activated immediately due to its location in Weibel-Palade bodies, where it is stored along with von Willebrand factor. The function of selectins is the binding of blood-leukocytes on activated endothelial cells prior to migration in inflamed tissue and therefore it is relevant for autoimmune diseases and RA in particular. Circulating SELE is found to be increased in RA patients and correlates with disease progression [20]. SELP is up-regulated in atherosclerotic plaque and in patients with angina pectoris. The non-synonymous single nucleotide polymorphisms (SNP) rs6136 in SELP has previously been associated with myocardial infarction with the A allele representing a risk factor [21,22]. RA patients may also carry a higher risk for myocardial infarction [23].

Our aim was to investigate genetic variants in these 14 genes for association with RA. We applied a multi-step approach, including two consecutively genotyped French RA family trio sets for discovery and replication. An additional set of 207 European RA family trios was analyzed to assess broader applicability of detected association effects in different populations. Overall, $N_{families} = 407$ family trios were genotyped. Possible functional aspects of identified associated SNPs were assessed by analysis of differential allelic expression (DAE) and respective eQTLs (expression quantitative trait loci). Losses and gains of possible transcription factor binding sites (TFBS) due to presence of SNPs was analyzed *in silico* and functional *in vitro* studies publicly available from the ENCODE project were reviewed [24].

Materials and Methods

Gene and marker selection

We selected genes in cellular adhesion processes following a thorough analysis of literature and databases at the time of candidate selection. For this purpose we used MeSH (medical subject headings) search terms in the PubMed database, available information on biological pathways (e.g. KEGG pathways, http://www.genome.jp/kegg/), gene ontology terms (http://www.geneontology.org/), and genetic databases such as OMIM (Online Mendelian Inheritance in Man, http://www.omim.org/), GDPinfo (genomics and disease prevention information system, currently accessible at http://hugenavigator.net/HuGENavigator/home.do), and GAD (genetic association database, http://geneticassociationdb.nih.gov/). Genes associated with autoimmunity and genes located in genomic regions linked to RA in genome-wide linkage analysis were preferred [10]. We note that our selection of genes must be considered essentially subjective. It represents a subset of genes for each of which a plausible link to cellular adhesion processes and to immune diseases is given.

Haplotype structure of each gene was analyzed by Haploview [25] and SNPs located in different LD (linkage disequilibrium) blocks were selected. SNPs with previously published disease associations or known functional consequences (e.g. non-synonymous coding SNPs) if existent were preferred. Information on SNPs was retrieved from databases EnsMart (http://www.ensembl.org/), PupaSNP [26], UCSC (http://genome.ucsc.edu), HapMap (www.hapmap.org), and dbSNP (http://www.ncbi.nlm.nih.gov/SNP/).

Probands

Three sets of family-trios, each trio comprising an RA patient (=affected individual) and both parents, were genotyped. Detailed characteristics of the first (French discovery set), second (French replication set), and third (multinational European replicaton set)

Table 1. Adhesion genes and SNPs selected for association study with RA.

Hugo gene ID	Gene name	RA linkage region*	Known associations	position	SNP IDs	Involvement in cellular adhesion	reference
CAST	Calpastatin	Yes	RA	5q15	rs27433; rs31250; rs754615; rs9667	Focal adhesion	[18,57]
ITGA4	VLA-4, integrin alpha 4	-	-	2q31.3	rs12690517; rs155095; rs3770138; rs4667319	Adhesion molecule	[58,59]
ITGB1	VLA-4, integrin beta 1	-	-	10p11.2	rs11009157; rs2153875; rs3780871;	Adhesion molecule	[7]
ITGB2	LFA 1, integrin beta 2	-	LAD	21q22.3	rs11559271; rs235326; rs7283236	Adhesion molecule	[60]
PECAM1	Platelet/endothelial cell adhesion molecule (CD31)	-	CP	17q23	rs1131012; rs13306812; rs6808	Adhesion molecule	[19,61]
PTEN	phosphatase and tensin homolog	-	DM2, Cancer	10q23.3	rs10490920; rs2299939; rs2673836; rs532678	Negative regulator	[62]
PTPN11	protein tyrosine phosphatase, non-receptor type 11	Yes	-	12q24	rs11066320; rs11066323; rs7977332	Negative regulator	[63,64]
PTPRC	protein tyrosine phosphatase, receptor type, C	-	MS, AIH	1q31-q32	rs10800584; rs1326269; rs17612648; rs1998843	Focal adhesion	[13–15,65]
PXN	Paxillin	Yes	-	12q24.31	rs1634815; rs3742039; rs4767884	Focal adhesion	[12]
SELE	selectin E	-	SLE, RA	1q22-q25	rs5361	Adhesion molecule	[20]
SELP	selectin P (CD62P)	-	CP	1q22-q25	rs3917647; rs6131; rs6136	Adhesion molecule	[21,22]
SRC	v-src sarcoma viral oncogene homolog	-	-	20q12-q13	rs6018199; rs6018257	Focal adhesion	[66]
TYK2	tyrosine kinase 2	-	SLE	19p13.2	rs12720214; rs2304256; rs280519	Activation of integrins	[11]
VCAM1	vascular endothelial adhesion molecule-1 (CD106)	-	Joint destruction	1p32-p31	rs3176878; rs3181088; rs3176860	Adhesion molecule	[67]

* Linkage regions according to Osorio et al. [5].
LAD = leukocyte adhesion defect; SLE = systemic lupus erythematodes; DM = diabetes mellitus; AIH = autoimmune hepatitis; CP = cardiopathy.

cohort are described elsewhere [27,28]. Briefly, the French discovery and French replication set each consisted of 100 family trios of French Caucasian origin with mostly similar characteristics. The third set consisted of 207 additional European Caucasian families, originating from France, Italy, Portugal, Spain, the Netherlands, and Belgium. Table 2 displays clinical information on all three cohorts as published previously [28]. All affected individuals fulfilled the American College of Rheumatology 1987 revised criteria for RA [29].

Ethics Statement

All individuals provided written informed consent and the study was approved by the Ethics Committee of Hôpital Kremlin-Bicêtre (Paris, France) according to the principles expressed in the Declaration of Helsinki.

Analysis strategy and power calculation

In our multi-step approach all SNPs were genotyped in the first sample set, the French discovery set. Markers with a significant association with RA (uncorrected p value<0.05) were then genotyped in the second sample set of the same homogeneous population origin, the French replication set. As the replication set was highly similar to the discovery set regarding ethnicity, phenotyping procedure, and clinical characteristics, association in the replication set can be considered a successful replication of associations. When evidence increased in favor of an association, i.e. the p-value of the association decreased in the combined analysis of both sets, markers were genotyped in the third sample set, the multinational European replication set. As the third set is more heterogeneous due to its multiethnic origin, additional association in set three can be considered informative for the general relevance of an identified association.

For a marker with 35% minor allele frequency, we had 80% power to identify a genotype relative risk of 1.66, 1.44, and 1.29 within 100, 200, and 407 trio families in the TDT test, respectively. For a marker with 10% minor allele frequency, we had the same power to identify a genotype relative risk of 2.06, 1.7, and 1.47 within 100, 200, and 407 trio families in the TDT test, respectively. Power calculation was done using the R add-on package "powerpkg" using formula as described [30].

Extraction of DNA and RNA

Genomic DNA and/or RNA were purified from fresh peripheral blood leukocytes or from Epstein-Barr virus (EBV) transformed cell lines for differential allelic expression analysis using standard methods.

Genotyping

Genotyping was carried out using the Genosnip technique by Bruker Daltonics [31]. PCR primers were designed using MuPlex Vs 2.2 [32]. Primer design for SBE (single base extension) was carried out using PrimExtend, an in-house software tool based on CalcDalton [33]. Primer-sequences are shown in Table S1. Samples of the third set were genotyped by TaqMan 5′ allelic discrimination assays (Applied Biosystems, Foster City, CA, USA) following manufacturer's protocols. In quality control Mendel's 1st law of inheritance had to be fulfilled in at least 95% of all children. Hardy-Weinberg Equilibrium (HWE) in non-transmitted controls had not to be violated in a chi-square test with 1 degree of freedom ($p>0.01$), all SNPs fulfilled these criteria. Non-transmitted controls refer to a genotype comprising of the two alleles that were not transmitted from the parents to the child. Individual-wise genotype call-rate in any set of family trios was always at least 94%.

Association analysis

Linkage and association analyses were performed using the Transmission Disequilibrium Test (TDT) [34]. The TDT compares the transmission of SNP alleles from heterozygous parents to affected offspring with a transmission ratio of 50% as expected by Mendel's 1st law. The allelic odds ratio (OR) compares differences in genotype distribution between RA cases and 'virtual controls' reconstructed from non-transmitted parental alleles. For gene-wide haplotype analysis the software Haploview 4.1 was used [25].

Differential allelic expression (DAE) analysis

Complementary genomic DNA (gDNA) was derived from EBV immortalized B cells of individual probands (N = 52) and screened for individuals heterozygous for rs6136 applying Genosnip (see genotyping for details and Table S1 for primers). Total RNA of samples (N = 7) was extracted and reverse transcribed using standard protocols. Three of these samples (tagged with prefix "RA") were derived from RA patients, which was not the case for samples termed 1–4. cDNA was genotyped applying Genosnip technology similar to gDNA with PCR primers designed to span exons (for-CTTCAGGACAATGGACAGCAGTA, rev-TCTTAGCAAAG-CCAGGAGCG). Such primers make efficient co-amplification of gDNA unlikely. Correct PCR product size was controlled by agarose gel electrophoresis. For each cell line, three replicates were analyzed. Each single replicate was quantified at least in triplicates applying Genosnip and averaged. As the Genosnip method results in quantitative signals for the genotyped alleles, data from genotyping heterozygous cDNA can be used to quantify gene expression in an

Table 2. Characteristics of rheumatoid arthritis (RA) index cases from the investigated samples.

	discovery set (N = 100)	replication set (N = 100)	multinational replication set 3 (N = 207)
Population	French Caucasian	French Caucasian	European Caucasian
Females (%)	87	90	86
Mean age of disease onset (y)	32 (±10)	31 (±6)	30 (±9)
Mean disease duration (y)	18 (±7)	16 (±8)	8 (±7)
patients with bone erosions (%)	90	79	70
RF+ patients (%)	81	76	73
Patients carrying >1 HLA-DRB1 shared epitope allele (%)	78	80	Not available

N = number of families; RF+ = rheumatoid factor positive.

Table 3. Results of genetic association analysis for rs754615 – *CAST* (minor allele C).

	discovery set	replication set	joined discovery & replication set
# informative parents	98/200	87/200	185/400
minor allele transmission	61:37	42:41	103:78
Estimated Genotyping Accuracy (Mendel Errors)	**100% (0)**	**100% (0)**	**100% (0)**
TDT p-value	**0.017**	0.94	0.07
Minor allele frequency	34%	40%	37%
allelic OR (CI)	1.7 (1.1–2.5)	1.02 (0.7–1.6)	1.34 (1–1.8)

Shown are results in all samples in a given sample set; Minor allele transmissions (transmitted alleles/untransmitted alleles) are shown. Informative parents: Number of parental individuals carrying a heterozygous genotype TDT: Transmission disequilibrium test considering informative parents, only. OR (CI) allelic odds ratio and 95% confidence interval of the minor allele when considering all parents (transmitted vs. non-transmitted alleles). Minor allele frequency relates to controls (non-transmitted alleles).

allele specific manner. To identify DAE, the allelic ratio of genotyped cDNA is compared with the allelic ratio found in gDNA, which is expected to be around one. For robust quantification, signal to noise ratios were used and the natural logarithm of the ratios was calculated. We applied ANOVA to globally identify if allelic ratios differed in cDNA from cell lines and gDNA (implemented in the statistical software R (http://www.R-project.org) applying the R add-on package "car"). Then, we used Dunnett's test to identify "regulated cell lines", i.e. cell lines where DAE is present. This was defined to be the case when the allelic ratios of cDNA was statistically significant different from the allelic ratios of gDNA according to Dunnett's test (applying the R add-on package "multcomp" [35]). In the context of this manuscript, "cis-regulation" refers to DAE where regulated samples showed increased expression of always the same allele [36]. This might result from some direct mechanism which is not influenced much by other aspects of the state of a cell.

For verification of DAE by an independent method, purified PCR products (PCR-Purifying-Kit, Seqlab, Göttingen, Germany) originating from cDNA and genomic DNA of selected samples were analyzed by eurofins-MWG/operon (Ebersberg, Germany) with fluorescence-based sequencing (cycle sequencing technology with dideoxy chain termination using an Applied Biosystems ABI 3730XL-sequencer). In this analysis, relative peak height in sequencing traces was analyzed for evidence of DAE in an analogous fashion.

eQTLs and gene expression analysis

Evidence for eQTL from public databases may be considered corroborative evidence for DAE. Therefore, eQTLs were assessed by comparing microarray expression data and genotyping data available via Genevar database (Version 3.5.0). Specifically, we used data from the pilot phase of The MuTHER Study [37] measured in lymphoid, skin, and adipose tissues derived from healthy female twin pairs.

Supplemental microarray gene expression data was accessed through the Gene Expression Atlas 2.0.7.5 05/11 (http://www-test.ebi.ac.uk/gxa/).

Evaluation of allele effects on transcription factor binding sites

Genomatix SNPinspector software suite (v2.1, matrix library 8.3) was used to evaluate potential effects of SNP alleles on loss or gain of potential transcription factor binding sites (TFBS). Two scores, core similarity and matrix similarity, were analyzed. These scores are based on similarities between the highest conserved nucleotides of a predicted TFBS or a TFBS family matrix. Putative gains or losses of TFBS were deemed relevant for scores >0.8 [38].

Additionally, we reviewed *in vitro* data on TFBS at the genomic location of rs6136. Data are publicly available from the ENCODE project and accessible via the UCSC genome browser [24].

Table 4. Results of genetic association analysis for rs6136 – *SELP* (minor allele G).

	discovery set	replication set	joined discovery & replication set	multinational replication set	all sets combined
# informative parents	34/200	32/200	66/400	80/412	146/812
minor allele transmission	11:23	9:23	20:46	35:45	55:91
Estimated Genotyping Accuracy (Mendel Errors)	**100% (0)**	**99.1% (1)**	**99.6% (1)**	**100% (0)**	**99.8% (1)**
TDT p-value	**0.042**	**0.015**	**0.002**	0.26	**0.003**
Minor allele frequency	13%	12%	13%	12%	12%
OR (CI)	0.54 (0.3–1.1)	0.38 (0.2–0.8)	0.47 (0.3–0.8)	0.77 (0.5–1.2)	0.62 (0.4–0.9)

Shown are results in all samples in a given sample set; Minor allele transmissions (transmitted alleles/untransmitted alleles) are shown. Informative parents: Number of parental individuals carrying a heterozygous genotype TDT: Transmission disequilibrium test considering informative parents, only. OR (CI) allelic odds ratio and 95% confidence interval of the minor allele when considering all parents (transmitted vs. non-transmitted alleles). Minor allele frequency relates to controls (non-transmitted alleles).

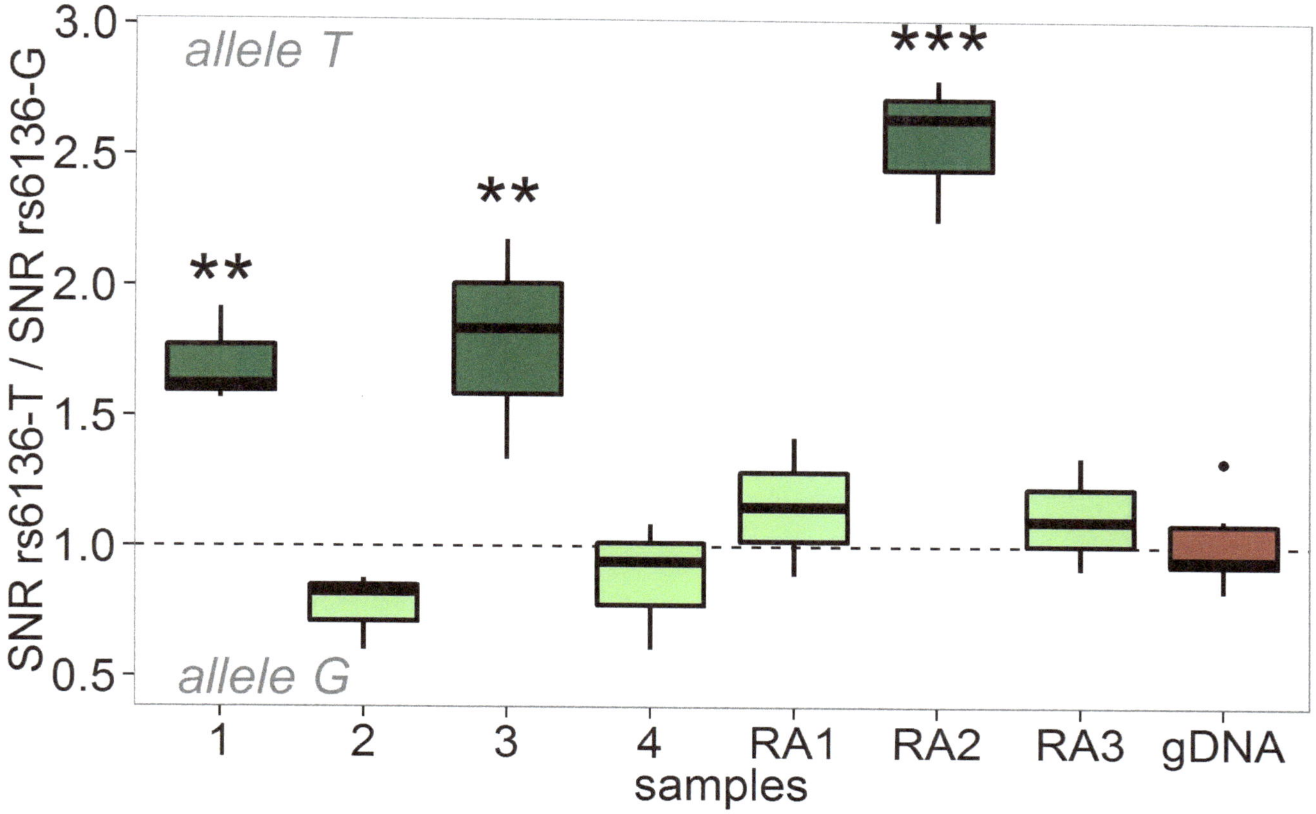

Figure 1. Cis-directed DAE pattern of rs6136 in the *SELP* gene. Green boxplots indicate samples resulting from allele specific expression analysis of cDNA. Samples tagged "RA" were derived from RA patients, which was not the case for samples 1–4; gDNA = allelic ratios of gDNA samples which served as reference. SNR = signal to noise ratio. Stars indicate cDNA samples with increased expression of transcripts carrying variant rs6136-T. ** = p-val<0.01, *** = p-value<0.001.

Results

Association study

Of 14 selected genes comprising 43 SNPs, two SNPs in genes *SELP* and *CAST* showed nominally significant association with RA in the discovery set of French RA family trios (Table S2). We also analyzed the association of gene-wide haplotypes in that sample set, but did not find significant haplotype associations after Bonferroni correction for the number of haplotypes found within the gene. We then genotyped SNPs rs754615 (*CAST*, p_{TDT} = 0.017) and rs6136 (*SELP*, p_{TDT} = 0.042) in the replication set of French RA family trios. *CAST* SNP rs754615 did not achieve significance in the replication set alone (Table 3). In contrast, SNP rs6136 was successfully replicated (p_{TDT} = 0.015, Table 4). As the direction of the association was the same in the discovery and replication sets, association of SNP rs6136 with RA was even stronger (p_{TDT} = 0.002) when analyzed in joined data from both sets. In consequence, SNP rs6136 qualified for genotyping in the European RA family trio set for evaluation of broader relevance. Here again rs6136 showed over-transmission of the major T-allele, but significance was only reached if analyzed in combination with the other two sets (pTDT = 0.003, Table 4). The power to detect the association of rs6136 with RA as reported in Table 4 for all sets combined was >95%. In subgroup analysis, the observed association for rs6136 was stronger in females (OR 0.58; 95%CI 0.4–0.8) than in males (OR 0.9; 95%CI 0.4–2.2) and stronger in patients with radiographic erosion (OR 0.71; 95%CI 0.4–1.4) than in those without erosion (OR 0.9; 95%CI 0.4–2.2). However, differences in odds ratios between subgroups were not statistically significant (p>0.3).

Table 5. DAE pattern of *SELP* SNPs for selected samples.

SNP	Sample	Allelic expression ratio genotyping	Allelic expression ratio sequencing	p-val
rs6136 (T vs. G)	1	1.78	1.36	0.0037
	RA2	2.51	6.18	<0.001
	RA3	1.12	1.65	0.97

Samples were measured with mass spectrometry-based genotyping and fluorescence-based sequencing; p-values refer to data from genotyping and are calculated by Dunnett's test analyzing significant differences between allelic fold changes between cDNA and gDNA.

Differential allelic expression

As *SELP* rs6136 was associated with RA in our multi-step RA family trio study we analyzed SNP rs6136 for differential allelic expression. We observed a cis-effect on expression levels of SELP for rs6136 (ANOVA $p<10^{-6}$, figure 1). Dunnett's test revealed that three of the seven samples heterozygous for rs6136 individually showed significant DAE, always with the T-allele

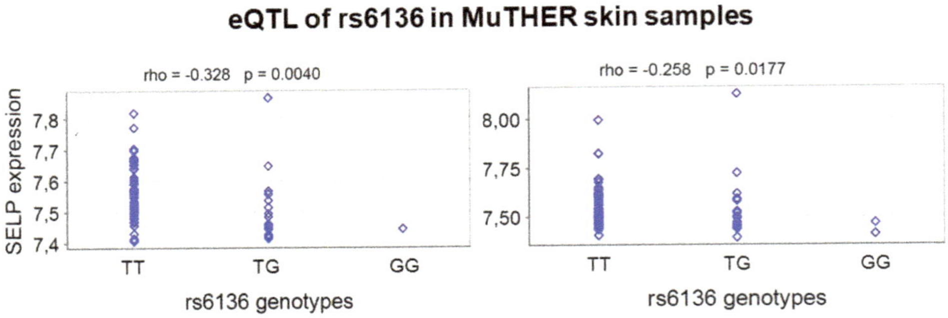

Figure 2. Cis-eQTL for rs6136 in the *SELP* gene in skin tissue from two sets of twins. Data were derived from The MuTHER Study [37] and analyzed by applying Genevar 3.5.0. These data successfully replicated DAE for rs6136. The two diagrams represent results from two skin sample groups derived from 76 and 84 female twins.

being higher expressed than the C-allele. The average fold change in regulated samples was 2. Direction of allelic expression fold changes was verified by Sanger sequencing (Table 5).

To further evaluate our finding of overexpression of the rs6136-T allele, we compared microarray expression data and genotype data available via the Genevar database. Within data from the pilot phase of The MuTHER Study [37] we observed a consistent cis-eQTL with overexpression of the rs6136-T allele (*SELP* probe: ILMN_1715417) in both ($p_1 = 0.004$; $p_2 = 0.0177$; figure 2). The rs6136 variant was the strongest cis-eQTL hit within available Genevar expression data in a region of at least 200 kbp up- and downstream of *SELP*. For the closest neighbouring gene *F5* (coagulating factor 5) no cis-eQTLs were detected.

The Genomatix SNPinspector software suite [38] was applied to calculate possible gains or losses of transcription factor binding sites (TFBS) for rs6136 and a SNP, rs9332575. SNP rs9332575 is in perfect LD ($D' = 1$, $r^2 = 1$) with exonic rs6136 within the Caucasian HapMap population, but located 40 kbp upstream of it (Table 6). The A-allele of rs9332575 corresponds to the T-allele of rs6136. Higher similarity values predict higher probability of transcription factor (TF) binding at this site. Table 6 shows several identified possible losses or gains of TFBS for rs6136 and rs9332575.

We also reviewed functional *in vitro* data on TF occupation near rs6136. Such data is publicly available via the ENCODE project [24]. For the genomic position of rs6136 we found an NFKB TFBS with the highest possible score in an assay based on chromatin immunoprecipitation (ChIP) followed by genome-wide sequencing in lymphocytes. Additionally, the locus appeared to be an open chromatin region as revealed through DNase I hypersensitivity assay, indicating that the locus would be accessible for TF.

Discussion

Adhesion molecules are potential candidate genes for involvement in the complex immune disease Rheumatoid Arthritis. We selected 14 genes involved in cellular adhesion processes and investigated possible association with RA. Two of these genes, *CAST* (encoding calpastatin) and *SELP* (encoding P selectin), were associated with RA in our discovery set of French RA family trios. Association of SNP rs6136 in *SELP* with RA could be successfully independently replicated in our replication set of French family trios and was still significant when including a larger European Caucasian family trio cohort ($p_{Total} = 0.003$). Within all three sets, the major T-allele was over-transmitted to RA patients in TDT, which is robust against ethnic heterogeneity [39].

We compared our findings with data of a large meta-analysis of genome-wide association studies (GWAS) for RA [40]. Although rs6136 itself was not associated with RA ($p = 0.86$), several nominal associations ($p = 0.023$ to $p = 0.043$) were found within a range of +/−75 kb of the SNP. However, LD was rather low with those markers ($R^2 < 0.1$). As association of rs6136 within our

Table 6. Possible losses or gains of transcription factor binding sites for rs6136 and rs9332575.

SNP	alleles	loss/gain	TF family/gene	TF name	Core sim.	Matrix sim.
rs6136	T→G	loss	HNF1/HMBOX	Homeobox containing 1	0.77	**0.831**
rs6136	T→G	gain	SNAP/PSE	Proximal sequence element	**0.967**	0.756
rs6136	T→G	gain	E2FF/E2F	E2F transcription factor 1	0.785	**0.852**
rs9332575	A→G	loss	GATA	globin transcription factor 1	1	**0.938**
rs9332575	A→G	loss	HNF1	Hepatocyte nuclear factor 1 alpha	1	**0.841**
rs9332575	A→G	loss	EVI1	Ecotropic viral integration site 1 encoded factor	0.75	**0.819**
rs9332575	A→G	gain	ZFHX/AREB6	Atp 1a1 regulatory element binding factor 6	1	**0.984**

Prediction of altered transcription factor binding sites due to alleles of rs6136 and rs9332575. rs9332575 is a neighboring variant for rs6136 which is in perfect linkage disequilibrium. Core sim.: score for highest conserved nucleotides of a known TFBS. Matrix sim.: score for highest conserved nucleotides of a known TFBS family matrix. Similarity scores >0.8 indicate relevant predictions [38].

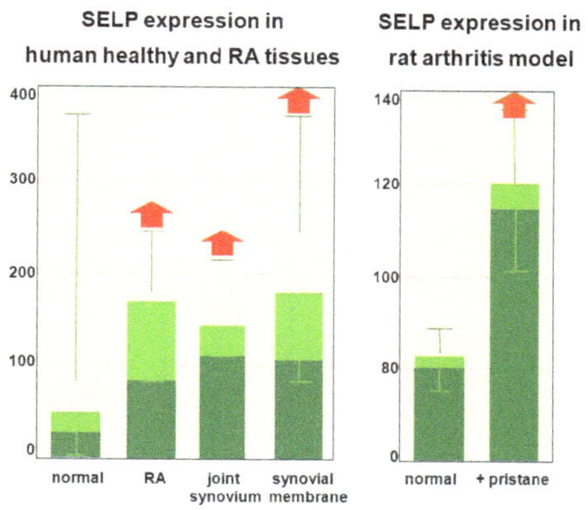

Figure 3. *SELP* expression profiles for human RA compared to healthy tissue and pristane induced arthritis in rat. Data derived from Gene Expression Atlas (E-GEOD-7307). $N_{normal} = 679$ (including healthy joint synovium and synovial membrane samples), $N_{RA} = 5$, $N_{joint\ synovium} = 3$ (all healthy), $N_{synovial\ membrane} = 11$ ($N_{normal} = 6$, $N_{RA} = 5$). $N_{rats\text{-}untreated} = 5$, $N_{rats+pristane} = 5$.

European Caucasian family trio cohort alone showed the same direction but did not reach significance, *SELP*-rs6136 might be of specific relevance in subgroups of RA patients with characteristics similar to our French discovery and replication cohorts. In particular, these two patient cohorts are known to be enriched for early onset RA and more severe phenotypes [41]. This should be considered when planning replication of the association of rs6136 in additional populations in addition to the power issues resulting from the relatively low minor allele frequency of rs6136 (Table 2).

We investigated SNP rs6136 for preferential expression of one of its alleles. Indeed, we observed preferential overexpression of the rs6136-T allele in three samples with an average fold change of 2.0 in regulated samples. Note, that there is a very high probability that DAE identified in at least three heterozygous individuals represents a true biological phenomenon [42]. However, not all samples heterozygous for rs6136 showed DAE, some appeared unregulated. This might indicate that in addition to the rs6136-T allele additional factors are necessary for upregulated SELP expression. Sampling effects might also offer an explanation. Alternatively, a SNP in non-perfect LD with rs6136 may be the true causative variant. However, we did not find any other polymorphism in or near the *SELP* gene which correlates with SELP expression more strongly than rs6136, even when accounting for common haplotype tagging SNPs. Interestingly, the highest differential expression was found in a cell line from an RA patient. However, overall, the pattern of DAE appeared to be rather similar between RA patients and non-RA patients (figure 1). Upregulation of SELP expression for carriers of rs6136-T was successfully replicated using data of The MuTHER Study [37] (figure 2). An association between rs6136 and SELP protein levels was also reported by the CHARGE consortium [43]. As this data is from different tissue and from different populations, this might hint at a general relevance of rs6136-T for increased gene expression of SELP.

Several TFBS were predicted to be changed either by variants of rs6136 or rs9332575, the latter a SNP in perfect linkage disequilibrium with rs6136. The highest scored (similarity score) loss of a TFBS was that of a GATA1 binding site for rs9332575 and the highest scored gain that of AREB6. While no RA relevant function is known for AREB6, GATA1 (globin transcription factor 1) plays a role in erythroid development and differentiation, but is also expressed in various cells, especially of hematopoietic lineage. GATA1 is reported to play a role in maturation of dendritic cells, an antigen presenting cell population able to activate naïve T cells during immune response [44].

We also found an NFKB TFBS by reviewing ENCODE *in vitro* data originally acquired by ChIP followed by genome-wide sequencing. An open chromatin structure at the site of rs6136 was found, indicating accessibility for TF binding. As NFKB is a TF predominantly activated during inflammatory processes and found to be especially relevant for RA pathology, NFKB might also be involved in increased selectin P expression levels in genetically predestined patients [45].

Within the Gene Expression Atlas (experiment E-GEOD-7307), *SELP* mRNA expression was found increased in two tissues most relevant for RA pathogenesis: joint synovium ($p = 0.007$, $N = 3$) and synovial membrane ($p = 4 \times 10^{-10}$, $N = 11$) (figure 3). *SELP* expression was also increased in RA patients ($p = 0.033$, $N = 5$) and in a rat model of pristane induced arthritis (experiment E-MEXP-782) ($p = 0.047$). Functional studies focusing on cis-regulation of *SELP* expression would be required to further corroborate our findings and possibly reveal the mechanism and consequences of *SELP* DAE.

The relevance of SELP in RA and other diseases is underlined by the finding of increased soluble SELP levels for many diseases, including atherosclerosis, in which soluble SELP is derived mostly from endothelial cells [44], and RA [46]. RA shows considerable comorbidity with cardiovascular diseases [23]. Soluble SELP correlates with RA disease activity [9,47] and lower SELP levels are found during RA remission [48]. High levels of soluble SELP are predictive of future cardiovascular events [49–51]. Supporting this, Lee et al. reported SNP rs6136 being linked to high serum SELP levels within the Framingham Heart Study [52]. After adjustment for clinical factors such as hormone therapy, about 10% of altered SELP concentration in serum of participants is explained by the rs6136 variant. Individuals carrying the TT genotype display about double the SELP concentrations compared to individuals carrying the GG variant. These findings corroborate our own findings that rs6136 may be a functional SNP.

SELP is essential for recruitment, adhesion and migration of inflammatory cells into joint tissue and synovial membrane. Blocking of SELP expression with specific antibodies resulted in blocked adhesion [53], as well as reduced neutrophil recruitment [54]. In a *SELP* deficient mouse model of antigen-induced arthritis leukocyte-endothelial cell interaction was decreased [55]. Additionally, a chemical compound acting as SELP antagonist efficiently reduced inflammation in the rat adjuvant induced arthritis model [56].

The RA-associated major T-allele of rs6136 was linked to increased *SELP* expression. As a possible mechanism, we suggest that increased *SELP* expression might promote the increased recruitment of leukocytes to a site of inflamed tissue such as the synovial lining in RA. Subsequently, the inflammation may be prolonged or elevated, which might influence disease activity and severity. These processes related to *SELP* expression should be studied in more detail in the future.

In summary, we found *SELP* rs6136-T to be associated with RA and with increased expression of *SELP* mRNA. Genetically determined increased SELP expression levels might thus be a novel additional risk factor for RA.

Supporting Information

Table S1 PCR and SBE Primer for Genotyping of adhesion genes. PCR primer designed with MuPlex 2.2, SBE primers designed with PrimeExtend (in house, request at peter.ahnert@gmx.net).

Table S2 Results of Genotyping in French RA family trio set 1.

Acknowledgments

We like to thank the patients and their families for participating in our study. Material was collected by ECRAF (European Consortium on Rheumatoid Arthitis Families: Paola Migliorini, Alejandro Balsa, René Westhovens, Pilar Barrera, Helena Alves, Carlos Vaz, Manuela Fernandes, Dora Pascuale-Salcedo, Stefano Bombardieri, Jan Dequeker, Timothy R Radstake, Piet Van Riel, Leo van de Putte, Antonio Lopes-Vaz, and François Cornélis) with support of the Association Française des Polyarthritiques, Association Rhumatisme et Travail, Societe Francaise de Rhumatologie, Association Polyarctique, Groupe Taitbout, Genopole and European Union AutoCure.

Author Contributions

Conceived and designed the experiments: JB MB EPT VHT AS FC PA HK. Performed the experiments: JB MB VHT AS EQ GW HK. Analyzed the data: JB MB MS PA HK. Contributed reagents/materials/analysis tools: EPT CP PM SB AB RW PB TR HA TB BP FE FC. Wrote the paper: JB MB EPT FC PA HK.

References

1. Seldin MF, Amos CI, Ward R, Gregersen PK (1999) The genetics revolution and the assault on rheumatoid arthritis. Arthritis Rheum 42: 1071–1079. doi:10.1002/1529-0131(199906)42:6<1071::AID-ANR1>3.0.CO;2-8.
2. MacGregor AJ, Snieder H, Rigby AS, Koskenvuo M, Kaprio J, et al. (2000) Characterizing the quantitative genetic contribution to rheumatoid arthritis using data from twins. Arthritis Rheum 43: 30–37. doi:10.1002/1529-0131(200001)43:1<30::AID-ANR5>3.0.CO;2-B.
3. Diogo D, Okada Y, Plenge RM (2014) Genome-wide association studies to advance our understanding of critical cell types and pathways in rheumatoid arthritis: recent findings and challenges. Curr Opin Rheumatol 26: 85–92. doi:10.1097/BOR.0000000000000012.
4. Sidiropoulos PI, Goulielmos G, Voloudakis GK, Petraki E, Boumpas DT (2008) Inflammasomes and rheumatic diseases: evolving concepts. Ann Rheum Dis 67: 1382–1389. doi:10.1136/ard.2007.078014.
5. Davis LS (2003) A question of transformation: the synovial fibroblast in rheumatoid arthritis. Am J Pathol 162: 1399–1402. doi:10.1016/S0002-9440(10)64272-1.
6. McMurray RW (1996) Adhesion molecules in autoimmune disease. Semin Arthritis Rheum 25: 215–233.
7. Lowin T, Straub RH (2011) Integrins and their ligands in rheumatoid arthritis. Arthritis Res Ther 13: 244. doi:10.1186/ar3464.
8. Gasparyan AY, Stavropoulos-Kalinoglou A, Mikhailidis DP, Douglas KMJ, Kitas GD (2011) Platelet function in rheumatoid arthritis: arthritic and cardiovascular implications. Rheumatol Int 31: 153–164. doi:10.1007/s00296-010-1446-x.
9. Littler AJ, Buckley CD, Wordsworth P, Collins I, Martinson J, et al. (1997) A distinct profile of six soluble adhesion molecules (ICAM-1, ICAM-3, VCAM-1, E-selectin, L-selectin and P-selectin) in rheumatoid arthritis. Br J Rheumatol 36: 164–169.
10. Osorio Y Fortéa J, Bukulmez H, Petit-Teixeira E, Michou L, Pierlot C, et al. (2004) Dense genome-wide linkage analysis of rheumatoid arthritis, including covariates. Arthritis Rheum 50: 2757–2765. doi:10.1002/art.20458.
11. Ingley E, Klinken SP (2006) Cross-regulation of JAK and Src kinases. Growth Factors Chur Switz 24: 89–95. doi:10.1080/08977190500368031.
12. Turner CE (1998) Paxillin. Int J Biochem Cell Biol 30: 955–959.
13. Thomas ML, Brown EJ (1999) Positive and negative regulation of Src-family membrane kinases by CD45. Immunol Today 20: 406–411.
14. Jacobsen M, Schweer D, Ziegler A, Gaber R, Schock S, et al. (2000) A point mutation in PTPRC is associated with the development of multiple sclerosis. Nat Genet 26: 495–499. doi:10.1038/82659.
15. Vogel A, Strassburg CP, Manns MP (2003) 77 C/G mutation in the tyrosine phosphatase CD45 gene and autoimmune hepatitis: evidence for a genetic link. Genes Immun 4: 79–81. doi:10.1038/sj.gene.6363918.
16. Yamada KM, Araki M (2001) Tumor suppressor PTEN: modulator of cell signaling, growth, migration and apoptosis. J Cell Sci 114: 2375–2382.
17. Roskoski R Jr (2005) Src kinase regulation by phosphorylation and dephosphorylation. Biochem Biophys Res Commun 331: 1–14. doi:10.1016/j.bbrc.2005.03.012.
18. Perrin BJ, Huttenlocher A (2002) Calpain. Int J Biochem Cell Biol 34: 722–725.
19. Muller WA (2003) Leukocyte-endothelial-cell interactions in leukocyte transmigration and the inflammatory response. Trends Immunol 24: 327–334.
20. Cobankara V, Ozatli D, Kiraz S, Oztürk MA, Ertenli I, et al. (2004) Successful treatment of rheumatoid arthritis is associated with a reduction in serum sE-selectin and thrombomodulin level. Clin Rheumatol 23: 430–434. doi:10.1007/s10067-004-0915-6.
21. Herrmann SM, Ricard S, Nicaud V, Mallet C, Evans A, et al. (1998) The P-selectin gene is highly polymorphic: reduced frequency of the Pro715 allele carriers in patients with myocardial infarction. Hum Mol Genet 7: 1277–1284.
22. Kee F, Morrison C, Evans AE, McCrum E, McMaster D, et al. (2000) Polymorphisms of the P-selectin gene and risk of myocardial infarction in men and women in the ECTIM extension study. Etude cas-temoin de l'infarctus myocarde. Heart Br Card Soc 84: 548–552.
23. Turesson C, Jarenros A, Jacobsson L (2004) Increased incidence of cardiovascular disease in patients with rheumatoid arthritis: results from a community based study. Ann Rheum Dis 63: 952–955. doi:10.1136/ard.2003.018101.
24. ENCODE Project Consortium, Birney E, Stamatoyannopoulos JA, Dutta A, Guigó R, et al. (2007) Identification and analysis of functional elements in 1% of the human genome by the ENCODE pilot project. Nature 447: 799–816. doi:10.1038/nature05874.
25. Barrett JC, Fry B, Maller J, Daly MJ (2005) Haploview: analysis and visualization of LD and haplotype maps. Bioinforma Oxf Engl 21: 263–265. doi:10.1093/bioinformatics/bth457.
26. Conde L, Vaquerizas JM, Santoyo J, Al-Shahrour F, Ruiz-Llorente S, et al. (2004) PupaSNP Finder: a web tool for finding SNPs with putative effect at transcriptional level. Nucleic Acids Res 32: W242–248. doi:10.1093/nar/gkh438.
27. Burkhardt J, Petit-Teixeira E, Teixeira VH, Kirsten H, Garnier S, et al. (2009) Association of the X-chromosomal genes TIMP1 and IL9R with rheumatoid arthritis. J Rheumatol 36: 2149–2157. doi:10.3899/jrheum.090059.
28. Jacq L, Garnier S, Dieudé P, Michou L, Pierlot C, et al. (2007) The ITGAV rs3738919-C allele is associated with rheumatoid arthritis in the European Caucasian population: a family-based study. Arthritis Res Ther 9: R63. doi:10.1186/ar2221.
29. Arnett FC, Edworthy SM, Bloch DA, McShane DJ, Fries JF, et al. (1988) The American Rheumatism Association 1987 revised criteria for the classification of rheumatoid arthritis. Arthritis Rheum 31: 315–324.
30. Abel L, Müller-Myhsok B (1998) Maximum-likelihood expression of the transmission/disequilibrium test and power considerations. Am J Hum Genet 63: 664–667. doi:10.1086/301975.
31. Wenzel T, Elssner T, Fahr K, Bimmler J, Richter S, et al. (2003) Genosnip: SNP genotyping by MALDI-TOF MS using photocleavable oligonucleotides. Nucleosides Nucleotides Nucleic Acids 22: 1579–1581. doi:10.1081/NCN-120023038.
32. Rachlin J, Ding C, Cantor C, Kasif S (2005) MuPlex: multi-objective multiplex PCR assay design. Nucleic Acids Res 33: W544–547. doi:10.1093/nar/gki377.
33. Kirsten H, Dienst S, Emmrich F, Ahnert P (2006) CalcDalton: a tool for multiplex genotyping primer design for single-base extension reactions using cleavable primers. BioTechniques 40: 158, 160, 162.
34. Spielman RS, McGinnis RE, Ewens WJ (1993) Transmission test for linkage disequilibrium: the insulin gene region and insulin-dependent diabetes mellitus (IDDM). Am J Hum Genet 52: 506–516.
35. Hothorn T, Bretz F, Westfall P (2008) Simultaneous inference in general parametric models. Biom J Biom Z 50: 346–363. doi:10.1002/bimj.200810425.
36. Antoun GR, Re GG, Terry NH, Zipf TF (1991) Molecular genetic evidence for a differentiation-proliferation coupling during DMSO-induced myeloid maturation of HL-60 cells: role of the transcription elongation block in the c-myc gene. Leuk Res 15: 1029–1036.
37. Nica AC, Parts L, Glass D, Nisbet J, Barrett A, et al. (2011) The architecture of gene regulatory variation across multiple human tissues: the MuTHER study. PLoS Genet 7: e1002003. doi:10.1371/journal.pgen.1002003.
38. Cartharius K, Frech K, Grote K, Klocke B, Haltmeier M, et al. (2005) MatInspector and beyond: promoter analysis based on transcription factor binding sites. Bioinforma Oxf Engl 21: 2933–2942. doi:10.1093/bioinformatics/bti473.
39. Risch N, Teng J (1998) The relative power of family-based and case-control designs for linkage disequilibrium studies of complex human diseases I. DNA pooling. Genome Res 8: 1273–1288.
40. Stahl EA, Raychaudhuri S, Remmers EF, Xie G, Eyre S, et al. (2010) Genome-wide association study meta-analysis identifies seven new rheumatoid arthritis risk loci. Nat Genet 42: 508–514. doi:10.1038/ng.582.
41. Teixeira VH, Pierlot C, Migliorini P, Balsa A, Westhovens R, et al. (2009) Testing for the association of the KIAA1109/Tenr/IL2/IL21 gene region with rheumatoid arthritis in a European family-based study. Arthritis Res Ther 11: R45. doi:10.1186/ar2654.
42. Serre D, Gurd S, Ge B, Sladek R, Sinnett D, et al. (2008) Differential allelic expression in the human genome: a robust approach to identify genetic and

epigenetic cis-acting mechanisms regulating gene expression. PLoS Genet 4: e1000006. doi:10.1371/journal.pgen.1000006.
43. Barbalic M, Dupuis J, Dehghan A, Bis JC, Hoogeveen RC, et al. (2010) Large-scale genomic studies reveal central role of ABO in sP-selectin and sICAM-1 levels. Hum Mol Genet 19: 1863–1872. doi:10.1093/hmg/ddq061.
44. Kozma GT, Martelli F, Verrucci M, Gutiérrez L, Migliaccio G, et al. (2010) Dynamic regulation of Gata1 expression during the maturation of conventional dendritic cells. Exp Hematol 38: 489–503.e1. doi:10.1016/j.exphem.2010.03.006.
45. Makarov SS (2001) NF-kappa B in rheumatoid arthritis: a pivotal regulator of inflammation, hyperplasia, and tissue destruction. Arthritis Res 3: 200–206.
46. Ertenli I, Kiraz S, Arici M, Haznedaroglu IC, Calgüneri M, et al. (1998) P-selectin as a circulating molecular marker in rheumatoid arthritis with thrombocytosis. J Rheumatol 25: 1054–1058.
47. Nasonov EL, Samsonov MI, Tilz GP, Nikiforova EL, Chichasova NV, et al. (1999) [Soluble adhesion molecules (P-selectin, ICAM-1 and ICAM-3) in rheumatoid arthritis]. Ter Arkhiv 71: 17–20.
48. Sfikakis PP, Charalambopoulos D, Vaiopoulos G, Mavrikakis M (1999) Circulating P- and L-selectin and T-lymphocyte activation and patients with autoimmune rheumatic diseases. Clin Rheumatol 18: 28–32.
49. Ay C, Jungbauer LV, Kaider A, Koder S, Panzer S, et al. (2008) P-selectin gene haplotypes modulate soluble P-selectin concentrations and contribute to the risk of venous thromboembolism. Thromb Haemost 99: 899–904. doi:10.1160/TH07-11-0672.
50. Hillis GS, Terregino C, Taggart P, Killian A, Zhao N, et al. (2002) Elevated soluble P-selectin levels are associated with an increased risk of early adverse events in patients with presumed myocardial ischemia. Am Heart J 143: 235–241.
51. Ridker PM, Buring JE, Rifai N (2001) Soluble P-selectin and the risk of future cardiovascular events. Circulation 103: 491–495.
52. Lee DS, Larson MG, Lunetta KL, Dupuis J, Rong J, et al. (2008) Clinical and genetic correlates of soluble P-selectin in the community. J Thromb Haemost JTH 6: 20–31. doi:10.1111/j.1538-7836.2007.02805.x.
53. Grober JS, Bowen BL, Ebling H, Athey B, Thompson CB, et al. (1993) Monocyte-endothelial adhesion in chronic rheumatoid arthritis. In situ detection of selectin and integrin-dependent interactions. J Clin Invest 91: 2609–2619. doi:10.1172/JCI116500.
54. Lally F, Smith E, Filer A, Stone MA, Shaw JS, et al. (2005) A novel mechanism of neutrophil recruitment in a coculture model of the rheumatoid synovium. Arthritis Rheum 52: 3460–3469. doi:10.1002/art.21394.
55. Schmitt-Sody M, Metz P, Gottschalk O, Birkenmaier C, Zysk S, et al. (2007) Platelet P-selectin is significantly involved in leukocyte-endothelial cell interaction in murine antigen-induced arthritis. Platelets 18: 365–372. doi:10.1080/09537100701191315.
56. Kaila N, Janz K, DeBernardo S, Bedard PW, Camphausen RT, et al. (2007) Synthesis and biological evaluation of quinoline salicylic acids as P-selectin antagonists. J Med Chem 50: 21–39. doi:10.1021/jm0602256.
57. Mimori T, Suganuma K, Tanami Y, Nojima T, Matsumura M, et al. (1995) Autoantibodies to calpastatin (an endogenous inhibitor for calcium-dependent neutral protease, calpain) in systemic rheumatic diseases. Proc Natl Acad Sci U S A 92: 7267–7271.
58. Ghosh S, Goldin E, Gordon FH, Malchow HA, Rask-Madsen J, et al. (2003) Natalizumab for active Crohn's disease. N Engl J Med 348: 24–32. doi:10.1056/NEJMoa020732.
59. Miller DH, Khan OA, Sheremata WA, Blumhardt LD, Rice GPA, et al. (2003) A controlled trial of natalizumab for relapsing multiple sclerosis. N Engl J Med 348: 15–23. doi:10.1056/NEJMoa020696.
60. Roos D, Law SK (2001) Hematologically important mutations: leukocyte adhesion deficiency. Blood Cells Mol Dis 27: 1000–1004. doi:10.1006/bcmd.2001.0473.
61. Elrayess MA, Webb KE, Bellingan GJ, Whittall RA, Kabir J, et al. (2004) R643G polymorphism in PECAM-1 influences transendothelial migration of monocytes and is associated with progression of CHD and CHD events. Atherosclerosis 177: 127–135. doi:10.1016/j.atherosclerosis.2004.06.009.
62. Ishihara H, Sasaoka T, Kagawa S, Murakami S, Fukui K, et al. (2003) Association of the polymorphisms in the 5′-untranslated region of PTEN gene with type 2 diabetes in a Japanese population. FEBS Lett 554: 450–454.
63. Legius E, Schrander-Stumpel C, Schollen E, Pulles-Heintzberger C, Gewillig M, et al. (2002) PTPN11 mutations in LEOPARD syndrome. J Med Genet 39: 571–574.
64. Mohi MG, Williams IR, Dearolf CR, Chan G, Kutok JL, et al. (2005) Prognostic, therapeutic, and mechanistic implications of a mouse model of leukemia evoked by Shp2 (PTPN11) mutations. Cancer Cell 7: 179–191. doi:10.1016/j.ccr.2005.01.010.
65. Lynch KW, Weiss A (2001) A CD45 polymorphism associated with multiple sclerosis disrupts an exonic splicing silencer. J Biol Chem 276: 24341–24347. doi:10.1074/jbc.M102175200.
66. Irby RB, Mao W, Coppola D, Kang J, Loubeau JM, et al. (1999) Activating SRC mutation in a subset of advanced human colon cancers. Nat Genet 21: 187–190. doi:10.1038/5971.
67. Ilgner S, Stiehl P (2002) Strong LFA-1 and VCAM-1 expression in histological type II of rheumatoid arthritis. Cell Mol Biol Noisy-Gd Fr 48 Online Pub: OL243–249.

8

B Cell Receptor Signaling-Based Index as a Biomarker for the Loss of Peripheral Immune Tolerance in Autoreactive B Cells in Rheumatoid Arthritis

Taras Lyubchenko[1]*, Gary O. Zerbe[2]

1 Division of Rheumatology, University of Colorado School of Medicine, Aurora, Colorado, United States of America, 2 Department of Biostatistics and Informatics, University of Colorado School of Public Health, Aurora, Colorado, United States of America

Abstract

This study examines the loss of peripherally induced B cell immune tolerance in Rheumatoid arthritis (RA) and establishes a novel signaling-based measure of activation in a subset of autoreactive B cells - the *Induced tolerance status index* (ITSI). Naturally occurring naïve autoreactive B cells can escape the "classical" tolerogenic mechanisms of clonal deletion and receptor editing, but remain peripherally tolerized through B cell receptor (BCR) signaling inhibition (postdevelopmental "receptor tuning" or anergy). ITSI is a statistical index that numerically determines the level of homology between activation patterns of BCR signaling intermediaries in B cells that are either tolerized or activated by auto antigen exposure, and thus quantifies the level of peripheral immune tolerance. The index is based on the logistic regression analysis of phosphorylation levels in a panel of BCR signaling proteins. Our results demonstrate a new approach to identifying autoreactive B cells based on their BCR signaling features.

Editor: Oliver Frey, University Hospital Jena, Germany

Funding: This work was supported by grants from the National Institutes of Health (5K01AR056023 and 3U19AI050864). The funders had no role in study design, data collection and analysis, decision to publish, or preparation of the manuscript.

Competing Interests: The authors have declared that no competing interests exist.

* Email: Taras.Lyubchenko@ucdenver.edu

Introduction

We recently reported about changes in B cell antigen receptor signaling profiles associated with the loss of postdevelopmentally induced peripheral immune tolerance (anergy) in a subset of autoreactive B cells in patients with Rheumatoid arthritis [1,2]. This follow-up study further examines the loss of B cell immune tolerance in RA and proposes a novel BCR signaling-based measure of autoimmune activation in the autoreactive B cell subset - the *Induced Tolerance Status Index* (ITSI).

Significant evidence supports the pathogenic role of autoreactive B cells in Rheumatoid arthritis (RA) [3,4,5,6,7,8]. B cell targeted therapies are effective in RA (reviewed in [6,9,10]). B cells accumulating in the joints of RA patients produce autoreactive antibodies [11] and elevated B cell antigen receptor (BCR) signaling activity positively correlates with RA assessment scores [12]. The loss of B cell immune tolerance has been recognized as an important factor in the onset of RA [7,8,13].

BCR signaling regulation mechanisms involved in the control of peripheral immune tolerance have been under investigation from the autoimmunity perspective since the development of suitable transgenic mouse models in the 1990's [14,15,16]. The post-developmentally induced peripheral immune tolerance is attained through selective BCR signaling inhibition (receptor tuning, anergy [17,18,19]) in naturally occurring autoreactive B cells that have escaped the "classical" tolerogenic mechanisms of clonal deletion and receptor editing [20,21] earlier in the development. These B cells recognize self-antigens and have the capacity to produce autoreactive antibodies, but under normal conditions are prevented from autoimmune activation by selective intrinsic BCR signaling inhibition [22]. However, this potentially autoreactive B cell subset remains vulnerable to activation by crossreactive autoantigens [23]. Peripheral induced immune tolerance is a signaling phenomenon, and the tolerogenic balance between activatory and inhibitory BCR signaling inputs is reversible [24,25].

Despite the landmark studies in mouse models [23,26], a distinct subset of naturally occurring autoreactive B cells with postdevelopmentally induced tolerance (**PIT** for short) has been identified in humans only recently [27]. These naïve $CD19^{+}CD27^{-}IgD^{+}IgM^{low/-}$ peripheral blood B cells (termed $\mathbf{B_{ND}}$ [27]) retain a degree of autoreactivity after receptor editing, are hyporesponsive to BCR stimulation *in vitro* and produce autoreactive Abs (anti-dsDNA and anti-HEp-2). This autoreactivity appears innate, as variable *Ig* genes show no evidence of somatic hypermutation, indicating that it was not generated during an adaptive immune response. Two major signaling properties distinguish cells with PIT from other B cell types: reduced amplitude of protein phosphorylation and Ca^{2+} responses to antigen receptor ligation, and elevated BCR-related baseline protein phosphorylation activity in intact cells. These signaling features, described in both humans and mice [17,23,27], reflect chronic stimulation with crossreactive autoantigens paralleled by the continuous inhibition of intracellular BCR signaling through downregulatory mechanisms, and represent an important mechanism that prevents autoimmunity (Figure 1).

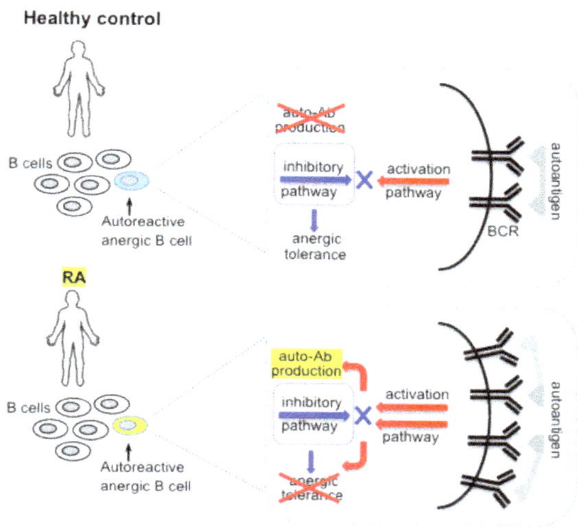

Figure 1. Normal (tolerance in healthy controls) and pathological (broken tolerance in RA) BCR signaling in autoreactive B cells with induced peripheral immune tolerance.

After the recent definitive reports on the postdevelopmantally tolerized autoreactive B_{ND} cell subset in humans [2,27,28], new evidence has emerged suggesting that PIT sustained via tolerogenic BCR signaling inhibition is present in a much larger fraction of human B cells than previously thought, and this reflects a state of peripheral immune tolerance induced by the chronic autoantigen stimulation [28]. Recent studies in RA patients also revealed the increased frequency of B cells with PIT producing germline autoreactive antibodies, which recognize nuclear and cytoplasmic structures [29]. Elevated numbers of highly autoreactive B cells with PIT found in the blood of RA patients are not being eliminated, and remain in circulation for extended periods, which creates a favorable environment for breaking the tolerance in this B cell subset [29]. Furthermore, it has been demonstrated that in contrast to T cells, immune tolerance attained through BCR signaling inhibition, rather than clonal deletion, accounts for a very significant part of B cell tolerance, and that antigen exposure "tunes" the responsiveness of BCR signaling in B cells by downmodulating the expression of surface IgM and by modifying basal Ca^{2+} levels, and that a continuum of functional PIT persists in the mature naïve B cell repertoire [30]. According to recent assessments, it is clear that postdevelopmental B cell tolerogenic mechanisms of selective BCR signaling inhibition are compromised in the onset of autoimmunity (reviewed in [31]).

Studies in our laboratory have established the loss of PIT in autoreactive B_{ND} cells as a contributing factor in the development of RA and demonstrated that inhibitory BCR signaling cascades involved in the maintenance of PIT are altered in human RA [2], as well as in the mouse model of experimentally induced arthritis [32]. Major biological effects associated with the loss of tolerogenic BCR signaling inhibition in human B_{ND} cells in RA are illustrated in Figure 2 in the context of signaling pathways. In addition, our studies in human subjects discovered significant positive correlations between BCR signaling activity in B_{ND} cells and RA Clinical Disease Activity Index (CDAI) [33], and established phosphorylation levels of specific BCR signaling intermediaries as predictors of RA through linear regression analysis [2]. These findings demonstrated a link between phosphoprotein signaling activity in autoreactive anergic B cells and clinical manifestations of RA. Noteworthy, RA-related phosphoprotein profile changes are unique to the $CD19^{+}CD27^{-}IgD^{+}IgM^{low/-}$ subset of autoreactive B_{ND} cells: nominal logistic fit demonstrated that RA predictive value of the combined phosphorylation profile of several major BCR signaling proteins and Ca^{2+} levels in response to BCR stimulation [2] in B_{ND} cells was highly significant ($R^2 = 1.0$, $p = 0.0002$), while in mature naïve $CD19^{+}IgM^{+}$ B cells this predictive value was substantially less evident ($R^2 = 0.505$, $p = 0.053$). This moderate effect in $CD19^{+}IgM^{+}$ cells may be related to the recently recognized immunoregulatory role of B cells with PIT [34].

Linear regression analysis of the combined group of RA patients and normal controls, adjusted for the subject's age and gender, demonstrated a modest trend toward a lower total tyrosine phosphorylation activity in response to BCR cross-linking with age ($R^2 = 0.12$, $p = 0.0518$). However, RA subjects exhibited substantially increased phosphoprotein responses to BCR stimulation in the $CD19^{+}CD27^{-}IgD^{+}IgMl^{low/-}$ B cell subset, as compared to normal controls (total pTyr mean±SE % increase of 121.4±30.6 vs. 22.5±31.0 in RA and control groups, respectively ($p = 0.05$)), suggesting that the breach of PIT in RA patients occurs regardless of the age (data previously reported [2]).

Results and Methods

Inhibitory signaling features that maintain PIT in B_{ND} cells of healthy controls are reversed/altered in RA and B_{ND} cells isolated from RA patients exhibit distinctly different phosphorylation (activation) patterns of major BCR signaling intermediaries [2]. These findings are based on the analysis of BCR signaling protein phosphorylation profiles of 32 healthy controls (mean age 35.7; male/female ratio 0.68) and 20 RA patients (mean age 55.9; male/female ratio 0.54) recruited at the University of Colorado Rheumatology Clinic. RA subjects have been diagnosed in recent years, were RF/anti-CCP positive, treated with DMARDs and have not undergone steroid or B cell targeted treatments. Subjects were recruited according to the Colorado Institutional Review Board approved protocol (#10-0250) with a written informed consent agreement. PBMC were isolated from freshly collected blood samples (IV 20 mL). Phosphorylation levels of BCR signal transduction proteins were measured with BD Phosflow assay in $CD19^{+}CD27^{-}IgD^{+}IgM^{low/-}$ B_{ND} cells as described in [2]; cells were stimulated (or not) with anti-BCR (polyclonal goat F(ab')2 anti-human Ig(H+L) purchased from Southern Biotech) *in vitro* for 10 min and baseline and phospho-response amplitude levels of individual BCR signal transduction proteins were compared between RA patients and healthy controls [2]. Figure 3 compares phosphorylation levels of major BCR signal transduction proteins and total tyrosine phosphorylation levels (pTyr) in $CD19^{+}CD27^{-}IgD^{+}IgM^{low/-}$ B_{ND} cells of RA patients (red) and healthy control subjects (blue) at baseline and in response to anti-BCR stimulation *in vitro* (as described in [2]). The integrated pattern of relative distances between blue and red dots for each BCR signaling protein illustrates differences in phosphoprotein activation levels for each group (i.e. red/blue dots would overlap if phosphoprotein activation levels were identical). These patterns appear different in unmanipulated B_{ND} cells (Figure 3, left panel), as well as in cells stimulated with anti-BCR (Figure 3, right panel).

Induced Tolerance Status Index (ITSI)

To quantify the BCR signaling patterns (Figure 3) in order to establish a signaling-based measure of autoimmune activation in autoreactive B_{ND} cells, we propose the *Induced tolerance status index* (ITSI). This statistical parameter numerically determines the level of homology between BCR phosphoprotein activation

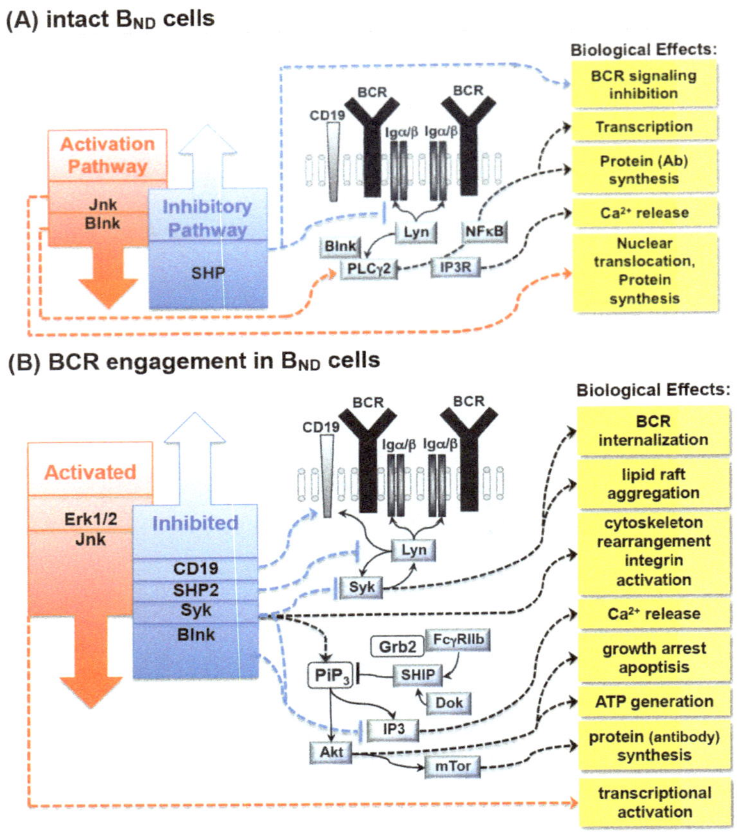

Figure 2. BCR signaling pathways associated with the loss of peripheral induced tolerance in autoreactive B_{ND} cells of RA patients [2]. (A) Unmanipulated B_{ND} cells: increased baseline activity Blnk, SHP and Jnk. **(B)** Response to BCR engagement in B_{ND} cells: decreased phosphorylation of Blnk, Syk, SHP2, CD19 and increased activation of Erk1/2, Jnk.

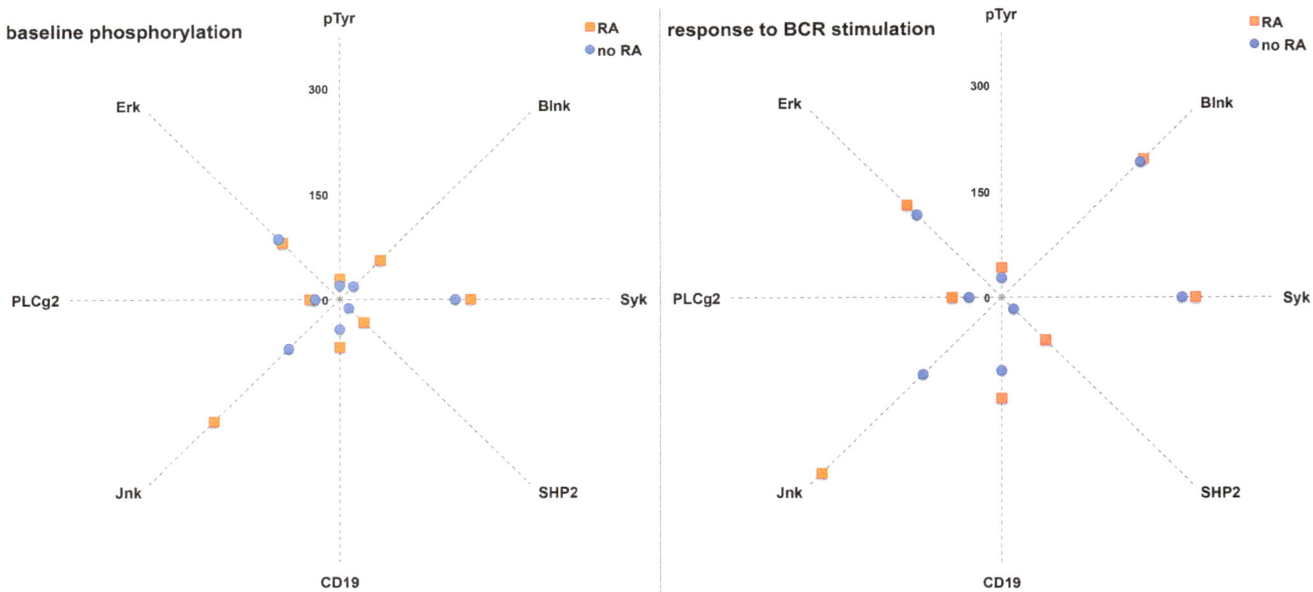

Figure 3. Phosphorylation levels of major BCR signal transduction proteins and total tyrosine phosphorylation levels (pTyr) in $CD27^{-}IgD^{+}IgM^{low/-}$ B cells of RA patients (red) and healthy control subjects (blue) at baseline and in response to anti-BCR stimulation *in vitro*.

patterns in B_{ND} cells ($CD19^+CD27^-IgD^+IgM^{low/-}$) with intact PIT (healthy controls) vs. the cells with compromised PIT (RA patients), and thus quantifies the level of PIT. The index is based on the logistic regression analysis of phosphorylation levels in the panel of B cell signaling proteins in individual subjects. Phosphorylation of specific BCR signaling proteins was assessed with BD Phosflow assay as mean fluorescence intensity (MFI) of protein-specific phospho-Ab staining as described [2]. BCR protein phosphorylation patterns (those exemplified in Figure 3) were analyzed by logistic regression in cross-referenced datasets of B_{ND} cells that were unmanipulated or stimulated with anti-BCR, and obtained from either RA patients or healthy control subjects [2].

Statistical Analysis

This type of statistical approach (i.e. logistic regression) has been successfully used in another study in our laboratory to compute the Cytokine Score [35] in order to address a mathematically similar task of analyzing complex associations between cytokine production patterns and the risk of RA [35].

The current study compares ITSI parameters between human subjects with RA and healthy controls through the logistic regression analysis of our recently reported data [2] on 7 signaling proteins (Blnk, Syk, SHP2, CD19, Jnk, PLCγ2, Erk1/2) and total pTyr in B_{ND} cells with assumed dichotomous type of dependant variable (i.e. RA = Yes/No). Because the logistic regression analysis requires complete datasets, some subjects with missing data points for at least one of the phosphoproteins had to be excluded altogether (15 subjects with RA and 12 controls had complete datasets). We designed an algorithm (Appendix 1) to calculate logistic regression coefficients and to construct a composite index that could discriminate RA from healthy control subjects with sensitivity of 88.7% and specificity of 83.3% based on the phosphorylation pattern changes in response to anti-BCR stimulation, and with sensitivity of 73.3% and specificity of 83.3% based on the baseline protein phosphorylation levels. In both instances, the ITSI index predictably distinguished between RA and healthy control groups based on their B_{ND} BCR signaling profiles (Figure 4). ITSI ranged between −2.16 and 10.92 (RA) and −9.95 and 1.06 (no RA) for anti-BCR-stimulated B_{ND} cells, and from −1.82 to 11.42 (RA) and from −3.19 to 0.20 (no RA) for baseline MFI phosphorylation values. The mean value of the index ± standard error was 3.37±0.85 (RA) and −2.81±0.99 (no RA) for anti-BCR-stimulated B_{ND} cells, and 2.34±0.85 (RA) and −0.91±0.32 (no RA) for baseline MFI phosphorylation values (Figure 4). Data analysis algorithm (SAS code) is shown in Appendix 1.

Supplemental data in Data S1 and Data S2 show individual subject datapoins with spreads and further statistical analysis, and a detailed description of the logistic regression algorithm, including the model fit statistics, analysis of maximum likelihood estimates for each individual phosphoprotein in the pattern, sensitivity and specificity calculation tables, odds ratio estimates and associations of predicted probabilities with observed responses.

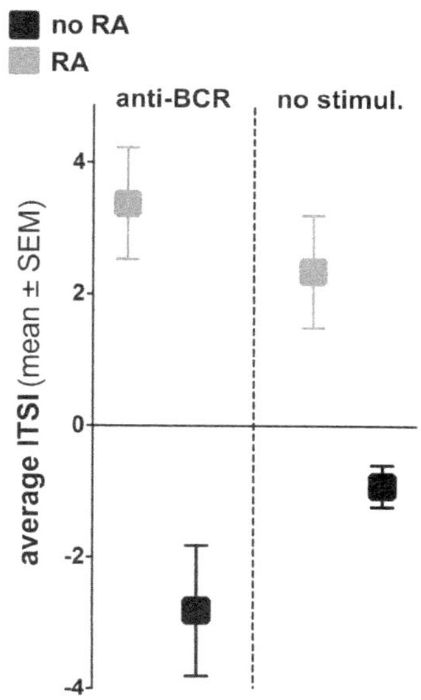

Figure 4. Induced tolerance status index (ITSI) discriminates between autoreactive B_{ND} cells from healthy controls and RA subjects based on BCR phosphoprotein activation patterns.

Discussion

In RA, chronic exposure to the omnipresent autoantigens can set off B cell activation and production of pathogenic autoreactive Abs [36]. Our study examines statistical distributions of BCR phosphoprotein signaling patterns in autoreactive B_{ND} cells in patients with RA. Our recent studies identified unique BCR signaling features associated with the loss of immune tolerance in a subset of $CD19^+CD27^-IgD^+IgM^{low/-}$ anergic B cells (B_{ND}) in RA patients [2]. Autoreactive properties of this naturally occurring B cell subset were recently discovered [27]. B_{ND} cells exhibit a specific type of reversible immune tolerance – the post-developmentally induced peripheral tolerance (PIT), which is attained through selective BCR signaling inhibition (receptor tuning, anergy [17,18,19]) in a subset of autoreactive cells that escaped the central tolerogenic mechanisms of clonal deletion and receptor editing [20,21] earlier in their development.

We have established the loss of PIT in autoreactive B_{ND} cells as a contributing factor in the development of RA and demonstrated that inhibitory BCR signaling cascades involved in the maintenance of PIT are altered in RA [2]. According to the central hypothesis of our study (Figure 1), in healthy individuals, autoreactive B_{ND} cells that have escaped the mechanisms of central tolerance maintain the peripheral immune tolerance (PIT) to ubiquitous autoantigens through continuous receptor tuning and BCR signaling inhibition, and our results demonstrate that this tolerogenic mechanism is compromised in RA.

PIT is a signaling phenomenon occurring late in the development cycle of B cells. However, the signaling aspects of this tolerogenic BCR signaling inhibition mechanism have not been studied in detail beyond the general features such as BCR-mediated Ca^{2+} influx and total protein phosphorylation activity (pTyr), particularly in human B cells. The novelty of our study is in addressing the signaling pathways involved in the maintenance and pathological alterations of PIT in RA with a quantitative approach. ITSI values provide a scale to measure the level of BCR signaling inhibition which sustains the postdevelopmentally induced peripheral immune tolerance and enables future studies of correlations between ITSI and clinical RA scores in large datasets generated by comprehensive phosphoprotein microarrays. Our preliminary findings in a relatively small 8-phosphoprotein panel are encouraging. Furthermore, although murine models of autoimmunity provided important insights into peripheral tolerogenic mechanisms in B cells and suggested that the loss of PIT has clinical significance in autoimmunity, human autoreactive B cells with PIT have not been well studied due to the difficulty of identifying this subset. Recent discovery of the B_{ND} subset in humans [27] provided an opportunity to study the role of PIT in RA (and other inflammatory autoimmune diseases where B cells play a pathogenic role). To our knowledge, our study is [among] the first to address the tolerogenic/inhibitory BCR signaling mechanisms in human B cells and investigate the loss of peripherally induced immune tolerance in RA with statistical analysis of BCR signaling patterns.

In our previous studies of RA, the conclusions about specific BCR signaling pathways involved in the alterations of PIT were based on direct comparisons of baseline phosphoprotein activation levels and normalized anti-BCR response amplitudes in the context of signaling cascades in RA vs. control groups and on the empirical analysis of phosphorylation/activation levels of specific BCR signaling proteins based on their known functions in the BCR pathways (i.e. Figure 2), as well as on pairwise correlation matrices of the activation of levels of phosphoproteins involved in BCR signal transduction, and on correlations between the BCR signaling activity in B_{ND} cells and severity of RA clinical manifestations [2]. These approaches are summarized in Table 1A–C. ITSI, however, enables the integrative quantification of these differences between BCR phosphoprotein activation patterns through logistic regression analysis (Table 1D). ITSI predictably discriminates between autoreactive B_{ND} cells that either have (control group) or do not have (RA group) the PIT. Authors believe this report will be of interest as it demonstrates a new approach to identify autoreactive B cells based on their BCR signaling features, and introduces a novel signaling-based biomarker associated with the loss of B cell immune tolerance in inflammatory autoimmune diseases such as Rheumatoid arthritis.

The association of the HLA region with RA was noted when the frequency of individuals with the HLA-Dw4 serotype was found to be increased among RA patients compared with healthy controls [37]. This particular serotype links a set of alleles at the HLA-DR gene. Many studies have examined and expanded these associations in order to better elucidate the genetic underpinnings of rheumatoid arthritis. Both linkage and association studies of the HLA-DR gene have confirmed that it is a genetic susceptibility locus for RA and provided an important clue to pathogenesis. Subsequent discoveries using high-throughput genotyping have identified over 40 additional loci outside of the HLA locus that also play roles in RA risk and implicate various pathways in pathogenesis. However, the issue of clinical utility of genotyping in patients with RA remains unresolved (reviewed in [38,39,40,41,42]). HLA genotyping/matching of control and RA groups were not performed in our study because we have no direct evidence that known HLA polymorphisms that may (or may not) be involved in antigen-specific signaling in T cells, can have an effect on intrinsic BCR signaling events that are not the result of adaptive (antigen specific) B cell immune response [27], which is the major focus of our study. While the subjects in our study were not HLA-matched, the ITSI score clearly discriminated between RA vs. non-RA groups based on BCR phosphoprotein activation patterns that reflect the loss of peripherally induced immune tolerance. However, the importance of HLA-related genetic susceptibility factors in RA should not be underestimated, as little is known about the role of these factors in the peripherally induced B cell tolerance. Although beyond the focus of this report, potential associations between specific HLA phenotypes and B cell

Table 1. Strategies for BCR phosphoprotein data analysis in autoreactive B_{ND} cells.

Data analysis approach			
Phosphoprotein activation patterns in B_{ND} cells with postdevelopmentally induced tolerance (PIT)			**D.** BCR signaling-based ***Induced Tolerance Status Index*** (ITSI) as a functional biomarker of autoimmune activation.
A. Direct comparison of normalized anti-BCR response amplitudes in the context of signaling cascades in RA vs. control groups.	**B.** Pairwise correlation matrix of the activation levels of phosphoproteins involved in BCR signal transduction.	**C.** Correlation between BCR signaling activity in B_{ND} cells and severity of RA.	
in vitro B cell responses to anti-BCR calculated as % increase over corresponding non-stimulated controls separately for B_{ND} and $CD19^+IgM^+$ B cell subsets for each subject, followed by the calculation of relative differences between % response amplitudes of B_{ND} and $CD19^+IgM^+$ B cells within RA and control groups independently.	Spearman's multivariate analysis to establish correlation-based pairwise relationships among BCR signaling intermediaries in B_{ND} cells. Correlation matrices for phosphoprotein activation levels in control and RA groups.	1) Logistic fit model to establish the overall signaling activity in B_{ND} cells as a predictor of RA. 2) Linear regression model to correlate the activity of individual BCR signal transduction proteins with RA severity score (CDAI, DAS28crp).	Logistic regression analysis computes ITSI - a statistical parameter that numerically determines the level of homology between BCR phosphoprotein activation patterns in B_{ND} vs. naïve $CD19^+IgM^+$ B cells, and thus quantifies the level of PIT.
Results and interpretation			
1) Determine changes in phospho-rylation of each BCR signaling protein associated with RA. 2) Direct comparison between phosphoprotein signaling patterns in B_{ND} cells in control and RA subjects. 3) Empirical conclusions on the balance of stimulatory and inhibitory BCR signaling pathways in B_{ND} cells based on the known functions of these proteins in BCR pathways. 4) Predictions on the physiological outcomes of B cell activation based on the known BCR pathway roles.	1) Statistically significant correlation values indicate that increases/decreases in the phosphorylation of each protein pair are pairwise linked and therefore the two proteins are functionally involved in the same signaling pathway. 2) Correlations between proteins involved in multiple or different signaling pathways reveal the interpathway crosstalk. 3) Establish a detailed PIT-specific phosphorylation pattern for proteins involved in BCR signaling inhibition in B_{ND} cells, and thus define the relationship between stimulatory and inhibitory signaling pathways.	1) Association between the global BCR signaling activity in B_{ND} cells and severity of RA. 2) Determine that RA-related BCR phospho-protein profile changes are unique to the B_{ND} cell subset. 3) Signaling-based biomarker approach to identify phosphoprotein predictors of RA based on the activation of autoreactive B_{ND} cells.	1) Lower ITSI values reflect increased levels of immune tolerance (PIT) and suppressed responses to autoantigens in B_{ND} cells. 2) ITSI discriminates between control and RA groups based on B_{ND} BCR signaling patterns. 3) Propose the ITSI as a signaling-based diagnostic biomarker for the loss of peripheral tolerance in autoreactive B_{ND} cells.

immune tolerance in RA patients are a promising subject for future studies.

Our initial findings strongly support the prospective use of ITSI as a clinically relevant diagnostic measure of the humoral immunity/B cell component in RA, particularly in light of the recent evidence suggesting that peripherally induced immune tolerance in response to the chronic autoantigen stimulation is present in a major fraction of human naive B cells, and the scale of this tolerogenic mechanism is unique to B cells, and that peripheral tolerogenic mechanisms of selective BCR signaling inhibition are compromised in the onset of autoimmunity [28,30,31]. Building up on our initial findings in the relatively small 8-phosphoprotein panel used in our pilot study [2], clinical relevance of the ITSI score will benefit from further validation in additional RA patient subgroups with the use of a comprehensive B cell phosphoprotein array. Results of our studies in RA patients indicate that BCR signal inhibitory pathways that maintain peripherally induced B cell tolerance are altered in RA and provide the rationale for future studies to investigate the loss of B cell anergic tolerance as a contributing factor in the pathigenesis of the disease. This approach will likely identify BCR signaling proteins that can be targeted for pharmacological interference, and used as signaling-based functional biomarkers associated with the loss of peripheral B cell tolerance in RA. The results will provide new insights into the role of B cell tolerance in the pathology and early diagnosis of RA.

In addition to the $CD19^{+}CD27^{-}IgD^{+}IgM^{low/-}$ subset of autoreactive B_{ND} cells, recent reports suggest that another B cell subset with anergic features – $IgM^{+}CD21^{low}$ may also play a role in autoimmunity. According to recent reports [29,43], this subset comprises a minor fraction (under 1%) of the "bulk" of mature naïve $CD19^{+}CD27^{-}IgM^{+}CD21^{+}$ peripheral blood B cells, but may expand by a few percentage points in some (but not all) RA patients [29]. However, the pathogenic role the $IgM^{+}CD21^{low}$ B cell subset has not been definitively characterized after the initial reports that indicated its potential involvement in RA and in hepatitis C virus infection-related autoimmunity. $IgM^{+}CD21^{low}$ anergic B cells are phenotypically different from the $IgM^{-/low}$ B_{ND} subset. Recent evaluations suggest that RA is best considered as a clinical syndrome spanning several disease subsets [36]. These different subsets involve a number of inflammatory cascades that all lead towards a final common pathway with persistent synovial inflammation and associated damage to the cartilage, and engage multiple B cell subsets that may include more than one type of anergic B cells. $IgM^{+}CD21^{low}$ anergic B cells are a promising target for the investigation of their pathogenic role in RA, however, such studies constitute a separate research direction and are beyond the main focus of this study - the $IgM^{-/low}$ B_{ND} cells.

Conclusions

1) Our results demonstrate a novel approach for identifying autoreactive B cells based on intrinsic BCR signaling features and introduce the ITSI score as signaling-based biomarker associated the loss of peripheral immune tolerance in the autoreactive B cell subset in RA.
2) ITSI discriminates between control and RA groups based on the inhibitory BCR phosphoprotein signaling patterns in autoreactive B cells, and thus confirms the loss of induced peripheral immune tolerance as a pathogenic factor in RA.
3) Lower ITSI values reflect increased levels of peripheral immune tolerance and suppressed responses to autoantigens in B_{ND} cells.
4) We recommend ITSI as a potential diagnostic measure of activation for innately autoreactive B_{ND} cells in RA.

Supporting Information

Appendix S1 Logistic regression algorythm (SAS code).

Data S1 Individual subject datapoins with spreads and basic statistical analysis.

Data S2 Detailed description of the logistic regression analysis with model fit statistics, maximum likelihood estimates for each individual phosphoprotein in the pattern, sensitivity and specificity calculation tables, odds ratio estimates and associations of predicted probabilities with observed responses.

Acknowledgments

Authors thank Dr. Michael Holers (University of Colorado School of Medicine) for his support of this study, Drs. Christopher Striebich, Kevin Deane and Jason Kolfenbach for assistance with recruiting research subjects at the University of Colorado Hospital, and Janet Siebert (CytoAnalytics, Denver, CO) for helpful discussions on the statistical analysis.

Author Contributions

Conceived and designed the experiments: TL. Performed the experiments: TL. Analyzed the data: TL GZ. Contributed reagents/materials/analysis tools: TL. Wrote the paper: TL. Software analysis: GZ.

References

1. (2012) ACR Meeting. Arthritis & Rheumatism 64: S755.
2. Liubchenko GA, Appleberry HC, Striebich CC, Franklin KE, Derber LA, et al. (2013) Rheumatoid arthritis is associated with signaling alterations in naturally occurring autoreactive B-lymphocytes. J Autoimmun 40: 111–121.
3. Marino E, Grey ST (2012) B cells as effectors and regulators of autoimmunity. Autoimmunity 45: 377–387.
4. Finnegan A, Ashaye S, Hamel KM (2012) B effector cells in rheumatoid arthritis and experimental arthritis. Autoimmunity 45: 353–363.
5. Luckey D, Medina K, Taneja V (2012) B cells as effectors and regulators of sex-biased arthritis. Autoimmunity 45: 364–376.
6. Nakken B, Munthe LA, Konttinen YT, Sandberg AK, Szekanecz Z, et al. (2011) B-cells and their targeting in rheumatoid arthritis—current concepts and future perspectives. Autoimmun Rev 11: 28–34.
7. Meffre E, Wardemann H (2008) B-cell tolerance checkpoints in health and autoimmunity. Curr Opin Immunol 20: 632–638.
8. Mandik-Nayak L, Ridge N, Fields M, Park AY, Erikson J (2008) Role of B cells in systemic lupus erythematosus and rheumatoid arthritis. Curr Opin Immunol 20: 639–645.
9. Leandro MJ, Becerra-Fernandez E (2011) B-cell therapies in established rheumatoid arthritis. Best Pract Res Clin Rheumatol 25: 535–548.
10. Keystone E, Burmester GR, Furie R, Loveless JE, Emery P, et al. (2008) Improvement in patient-reported outcomes in a rituximab trial in patients with severe rheumatoid arthritis refractory to anti-tumor necrosis factor therapy. Arthritis Rheum 59: 785–793.
11. Amara K, Steen J, Murray F, Morbach H, Fernandez-Rodriguez BM, et al. (2013) Monoclonal IgG antibodies generated from joint-derived B cells of RA patients have a strong bias toward citrullinated autoantigen recognition. J Exp Med 210: 445–455.
12. Galligan CL, Siebert JC, Siminovitch KA, Keystone EC, Bykerk V, et al. (2009) Multiparameter phospho-flow analysis of lymphocytes in early rheumatoid arthritis: implications for diagnosis and monitoring drug therapy. PLoS One 4: e6703.
13. Menard L, Samuels J, Ng YS, Meffre E (2011) Inflammation-independent defective early B cell tolerance checkpoints in rheumatoid arthritis. Arthritis Rheum 63: 1237–1245.

14. Adams E, Basten A, Goodnow CC (1990) Intrinsic B-cell hyporesponsiveness accounts for self-tolerance in lysozyme/anti-lysozyme double-transgenic mice. Proc Natl Acad Sci U S A 87: 5687–5691.
15. Goodnow CC, Adelstein S, Basten A (1990) The need for central and peripheral tolerance in the B cell repertoire. Science 248: 1373–1379.
16. Goodnow CC, Crosbie J, Adelstein S, Lavoie TB, Smith-Gill SJ, et al. (1988) Altered immunoglobulin expression and functional silencing of self-reactive B lymphocytes in transgenic mice. Nature 334: 676–682.
17. Cambier JC, Gauld SB, Merrell KT, Vilen BJ (2007) B-cell anergy: from transgenic models to naturally occurring anergic B cells? Nat Rev Immunol 7: 633–643.
18. Goodnow CC (1996) Balancing immunity and tolerance: deleting and tuning lymphocyte repertoires. Proc Natl Acad Sci U S A 93: 2264–2271.
19. Singh NJ, Schwartz RH (2006) Primer: mechanisms of immunologic tolerance. Nat Clin Pract Rheumatol 2: 44–52.
20. Nemazee D, Hogquist KA (2003) Antigen receptor selection by editing or downregulation of V(D)J recombination. Curr Opin Immunol 15: 182–189.
21. Casellas R, Shih TA, Kleinewietfeld M, Rakonjac J, Nemazee D, et al. (2001) Contribution of receptor editing to the antibody repertoire. Science 291: 1541–1544.
22. Healy JI, Goodnow CC (1998) Positive versus negative signaling by lymphocyte antigen receptors. Annu Rev Immunol 16: 645–670.
23. Merrell KT, Benschop RJ, Gauld SB, Aviszus K, Decote-Ricardo D, et al. (2006) Identification of anergic B cells within a wild-type repertoire. Immunity 25: 953–962.
24. Gauld SB, Benschop RJ, Merrell KT, Cambier JC (2005) Maintenance of B cell anergy requires constant antigen receptor occupancy and signaling. Nat Immunol 6: 1160–1167.
25. Kilmon MA, Rutan JA, Clarke SH, Vilen BJ (2005) Low-affinity, Smith antigen-specific B cells are tolerized by dendritic cells and macrophages. J Immunol 175: 37–41.
26. Allman D, Lindsley RC, DeMuth W, Rudd K, Shinton SA, et al. (2001) Resolution of three nonproliferative immature splenic B cell subsets reveals multiple selection points during peripheral B cell maturation. J Immunol 167: 6834–6840.
27. Duty JA, Szodoray P, Zheng NY, Koelsch KA, Zhang Q, et al. (2009) Functional anergy in a subpopulation of naive B cells from healthy humans that express autoreactive immunoglobulin receptors. J Exp Med 206: 139–151.
28. Quach TD, Manjarrez-Orduno N, Adlowitz DG, Silver L, Yang H, et al. (2011) Anergic responses characterize a large fraction of human autoreactive naive B cells expressing low levels of surface IgM. J Immunol 186: 4640–4648.
29. Isnardi I, Ng YS, Menard L, Meyers G, Saadoun D, et al. (2010) Complement receptor 2/CD21- human naive B cells contain mostly autoreactive unresponsive clones. Blood 115: 5026–5036.
30. Zikherman J, Parameswaran R, Weiss A (2012) Endogenous antigen tunes the responsiveness of naive B cells but not T cells. Nature 489: 160–164.
31. Papatriantafyllou M (2012) B cell signalling: Discouraging encounters. Nat Rev Immunol 12: 680–681.
32. Liubchenko GA, Appleberry HC, Holers VM, Banda NK, Willis VC, et al. (2012) Potentially autoreactive naturally occurring transitional T3 B lymphocytes exhibit a unique signaling profile. J Autoimmun 38: 293–303.
33. Aletaha D, Smolen J (2005) The Simplified Disease Activity Index (SDAI) and the Clinical Disease Activity Index (CDAI): a review of their usefulness and validity in rheumatoid arthritis. Clin Exp Rheumatol 23: S100–108.
34. Aviszus K, Macleod MK, Kirchenbaum GA, Detanico TO, Heiser RA, et al. (2012) Antigen-specific suppression of humoral immunity by anergic ars/a1 B cells. J Immunol 189: 4275–4283.
35. Hughes-Austin JM, Deane KD, Derber LA, Kolfenbach JR, Zerbe GO, et al. (2012) Multiple cytokines and chemokines are associated with rheumatoid arthritis-related autoimmunity in first-degree relatives without rheumatoid arthritis: Studies of the Aetiology of Rheumatoid Arthritis (SERA). Ann Rheum Dis.
36. Scott DL, Wolfe F, Huizinga TW (2010) Rheumatoid arthritis. Lancet 376: 1094–1108.
37. Stastny P (1978) Association of the B-cell alloantigen DRw4 with rheumatoid arthritis. N Engl J Med 298: 869–871.
38. Perricone C, Ceccarelli F, Valesini G (2011) An overview on the genetic of rheumatoid arthritis: a never-ending story. Autoimmun Rev 10: 599–608.
39. Chatzikyriakidou A, Voulgari PV, Lambropoulos A, Drosos AA (2013) Genetics in rheumatoid arthritis beyond HLA genes: what meta-analyses have shown? Semin Arthritis Rheum 43: 29–38.
40. Ruyssen-Witrand A, Constantin A, Cambon-Thomsen A, Thomsen M (2012) New insights into the genetics of immune responses in rheumatoid arthritis. Tissue Antigens 80: 105–118.
41. de Almeida DE, Ling S, Holoshitz J (2011) New insights into the functional role of the rheumatoid arthritis shared epitope. FEBS Lett 585: 3619–3626.
42. de Vries RR, van der Woude D, Houwing JJ, Toes RE (2011) Genetics of ACPA-positive rheumatoid arthritis: the beginning of the end? Ann Rheum Dis 70 Suppl 1: i51–54.
43. Terrier B, Joly F, Vazquez T, Benech P, Rosenzwajg M, et al. (2011) Expansion of functionally anergic CD21-/low marginal zone-like B cell clones in hepatitis C virus infection-related autoimmunity. J Immunol 187: 6550–6563.

9

The Impact of DMARD and Anti-TNF Therapy on Functional Characterization of Short-Term T-Cell Activation in Patients with Rheumatoid Arthritis

Balázs Szalay[1], Áron Cseh[2], Gergő Mészáros[2], László Kovács[3], Attila Balog[3]*, Barna Vásárhelyi[1,4]

1 Department of Laboratory Medicine, Faculty of Medicine, Semmelweis University, Budapest, Hungary, **2** First Department of Pediatrics, Faculty of Medicine, Semmelweis University, Budapest, Hungary, **3** Department of Rheumatology, Faculty of Medicine, Albert Szent-Györgyi Health Center, University of Szeged, Szeged, Hungary, **4** MTA-SE, Pediatrics and Nephrology Research Group, Budapest, Hungary

Abstract

Rheumatoid arthritis (RA) is a chronic autoimmune disease characterized by a systemic dysfunction of T-cells. In this study we tested the impact of DMARD and anti-TNF agents on short-term activation characteristics of T-cells. We enrolled 12 patients with newly diagnosed RA (naïve RA) who were treated with methothrexate (MTX) and glucocorticsteroid (GCS) and 22 patients with established RA non responding to conventional DMARD therapy who were treated with different anti-TNF agents. Nine healthy volunteers served as controls. Blood samples were taken at baseline, then at 4th and 8th week of therapy. The characteristics of several intracellular activation processes during short-term activation of T-cells including cytoplasmic Ca^{2+} level, mitochondrial Ca^{2+} level, reactive oxygen species (ROS) and nitric oxide (NO) generation were determined by a novel flow-cytometry technique. At baseline, the tested processes were comparable to controls in naïve RA. During GCS therapy, cytoplasmic Ca^{2+} level and ROS generation decreased. After the addition of MTX to GCS cytoplasmic Ca^{2+} level became comparable to controls, while ROS generation decreased further. In DMARD non responders, cytoplasmic Ca^{2+} level was higher than controls at baseline. The cytoplasmic Ca^{2+} level became comparable to controls and ROS generation decreased during each of the three anti-TNF-α agent therapies. Mitochondrial Ca^{2+} level and NO generation were unaltered in all of the patient groups. These results indicate that intracellular machinery is affected in T-cells of RA patients. This may alter the behavior of T-cells during activation. Different therapeutic approaches may modulate the abnormal T-cell functions.

Editor: Jan P. Tuckermann, University of Ulm, Germany

Funding: The study was supported by Hungarian Scientific Research Fund (OTKA) (Grant no. 101661), Social Renewal Operational Programme (Grant no. TÁMOP-4.2.2.-08/1/KMR-2008-0004) and research grants from Abbott Laboratories and Pfizer. Attila Balog was supported by the Zoltán Magyary Scholarship (grant no. TÁMOP-4.2.4. A/2-11-1-2012-001). Abbott and Pfizer have provided an unrestricted research grant to facilitate the purchase of laboratory materials. The funders had no role in study design, data collection and analysis, decision to publish, or preparation of the manuscript.

Competing Interests: The authors confirm that their funding from commercial sources (Abbott Laboratories and Pfizer) does not alter their adherence to PLOS ONE policies on sharing data and materials. The drugs used for patients' treatment were prescribed by independent doctors, and were purchased and provided by assigned wholesalers in agreement with national contracts with the Hungarian National Health Fund, and reimbursed by the Hungarian National Health Fund. Participation in the study by the patients had no impact whatsoever on the therapeutic decisions made by the treating physicians.

* Email: balog.attila@med.u-szeged.hu

Introduction

Rheumatoid arthritis (RA) is the most common chronic autoimmune joint disease [1]. It has long been recognized that the immune phenotype (i.e. the prevalences of T-cell subsets) in RA is altered both in the synovium and in the peripheral blood [2,3]. Besides the alterations observed in the immune phenotype, there is increasing evidence in support of the notion that abnormal lymphocyte functions also contribute to the pathogenesis of RA. Specifically, an increased level of nitric oxide (NO) production [4], altered Ca^{2+} signaling [5] and the enhanced production of reactive oxygen species (ROS) [6] during activation are hallmarks of a T lymphocyte dysfunction in RA.

Several types of traditional disease-modifying anti-rheumatic drugs (DMARDs) and immunesuppressive agents have been demonstrated to influence the T-cell subset distribution and function, and it is increasingly acknowledged that this action may contribute to the therapeutic effects of such drugs [7]. Recently, we investigated in a follow-up study the changes in T-cell subsets in RA patients in response to conventional DMARD and biological therapies [8], but intracellular activation characteristics in response to these therapies are lacking at present. Moreover, no data are available as to whether the effects on T-cell function differ between individual types of anti-TNF-α agents. We have, therefore, performed a comprehensive follow-up investigation of a variety of T-cell functional parameters including cytoplasmic Ca^{2+} level, ROS generation, NO production and mitochondrial Ca^{2+} level in activated T-cells before and during the administration of synthetic DMARDs or three different anti-TNF-α agents [adalimumab (ADA), etanercept (ETA) and infliximab (IFX)].

Materials and Methods

Patients

Twelve patients with naiv RA and twenty two patients with established RA were enrolled in the study. The detailed clinical data and patient characteristics are presented in Table 1.

The naïve RA group (n = 12) had not received any treatment prior to our study. After the established RA diagnosis, DMARD therapy was initiated according to a fixed protocol, which was in agreement with current EULAR and Hungarian National treatment guidelines [9]. This included the administration of medium-dose oral glucocorticosteroid (GCS, methylprednisolone, 16 mg/day) alone for 4 weeks; then GCS was tapered to 8 mg/day and methotrexate (MTX) was started with a dose of 10 mg/week. Blood samples were taken before the initiation of DMARD therapy (baseline), then after 4 and 8 weeks of treatment (i.e. after 4 weeks on medium-dose GCS and after a further 4 weeks of combination therapy with tapered-dose GCS+MTX).

In the DMARD nonresponding group with established RA (n = 22) unresponding to standard DMARD combination therapy [i.e. MTX at 15 mg/week and leflunomide (LF) at 20 mg/day], anti-TNF-α therapy was initiated following the standard-of-care decision of the treating physician: ADA at 40 mg/2 weeks sc (n = 8); ETA at 50 mg/week sc (n = 7); or IFX on week 0, 2 and 6 at 3 mg/kg iv (n = 7). At this time, LF was discontinued, while MTX was given simultaneously. Blood samples were taken before the initiation of each anti-TNF-α agent (baseline), and then on Week 4 and 8 of therapy just before the administration of the actual dose of the drug. There were no differences in the baseline characteristics (age, disease duration, disease activity, rheumatoid factor etc.) of the patients in the different anti-TNF-α groups.

The nine age- and gender-matched healthy volunteers who served as controls had a negative history of rheumatic symptoms and a negative status upon detailed physical and laboratory examination. Written informed consent was obtained in advance from all participants. The project was approved by the Ethical Committee of the University of Szeged (ETT-TUKEB 905/PI/09). This study was conducted in full accordance with the Declaration of Helsinki (1964).

Cell preparation

Similarly to our previous study [10], 18 ml of lithium-heparin-anticoagulated blood was taken from all participants for the investigation of T-cells. Peripheral blood mononuclear cells (PBMCs) were separated by gradient centrifugation with Ficoll-Paque (GE Healthcare Life Sciences, Pittsburgh, PA, USA), washed twice with phosphate-buffered saline pH 7.4 (PBS; Central Pharmacy of Semmelweis University, Budapest, Hungary). The PBMCs were resuspended in modified RPMI medium (Sigma–Aldrich, St. Louis, MO, USA), the Ca^{2+} concentration of which was set to 2 mM. Samples were incubated with Fluo 3 AM, Rhod2 AM, dihydroethidium and DAF-FM diacetate (Molecular Probes, Carlsbad, CA, USA), which are sensitive to the cytoplasmic Ca^{2+} level, the mitochondrial Ca^{2+} level, the concentration of ROS and the level of nitric oxide, respectively. The staining conditions were identical to those reported previously [11]. Fluorescence signals were monitored for up to 10 min after the addition of phytohaemagglutinin (PHA) (Sigma–Aldrich, St. Louis, MO, USA), a non-specific activator of T-cells, in a final concentration of 20 μg/ml.

Cells were also stained with dyed antibodies against CD4 markers (Becton Dickinson, San Diego, CA, USA) allowing us to gate the cell populations to be monitored during activation.

Equipment and statistical analysis

All measurements were performed on a BD FACSAria flow cytometer (Becton Dickinson, San Jose, CA, USA). The kinetic parameters of intracellular processes were determined by using R (R Foundation for Statistical Computing, Vienna, Austria) as follows. The measurement time-frame was divided into 100 time intervals of equal length and the median values were calculated in each interval. The smoothing method of Lowess was applied to the median values and each value was referred to that measured at the beginning of the experiment, furnishing the relative parameter value, rpv. The following parameters were calculated from the rpv data: area under the curve (AUC), the maximum value (Max) and the time required to reach Max (tmax) (Figure 1). One unit (U) of the AUC is defined as a rpv of 1 in 1second. Detailed explanation of these parameters is published in a previous study [12].

Further statistical analysis based on the values of these parameters was performed with R and the Statistica 7 software package (Statsoft, Tulsa, OK, USA). The Mann-Whitney test was applied for the comparison of the data on the controls and the patients, while the paired data in each related patient group were compared by the Friedman test. When the Friedman test demonstrated significant differences, the post hoc Dunn test was used to identify which pairs were significantly different. Levels of $p<0.05$ were taken as statistically significant. The clinical data in Table 1 and the results in Table 2 are given as median [interquartile range].

Results

Naïve RA patients subjected to DMARD therapy

At baseline, the investigated intracellular parameters of the T-cells during short-term activation were similar to those of the controls (Table 2, Figure 2). At Week 4 of GCS therapy, the cytoplasmic Ca^{2+} response and the level of ROS production during T-cell activation had decreased significantly and become lower compared to the controls and the baseline values. At Week 8, cytoplasmic Ca^{2+} response had become comparable to the baseline and control levels, while the ROS production was further impaired.

DMARD nonresponder patients subjected to anti-TNF-α agents

At baseline, the cytoplasmic Ca^{2+} level was higher in this patient group than in the controls (Table 2, Figure 2). The other parameters investigated, including the mitochondrial Ca^{2+} levels, ROS and NO production were comparable to those observed in the controls with the exception of the subgroup treated later with ETA. (These patients exhibited an increased ROS generation capacity at baseline).

On Week 4 of anti-TNF-α therapy, the cytoplasmic Ca^{2+} level became comparable to controls, while ROS generation was decreased significantly to below the baseline, irrespective of the nature of the anti-TNF-α agent administered (including ETA). At this time point, the other parameters investigated were still comparable to those at the baseline in each patient group.

At Week 8, no significant alterations were detected relative to Week 4 in any of the parameters tested.

Discussion

This is the first study that provides a follow-up of T-cell activation characteristics in RA patients subjected to different therapeutic regimes. Our study involved two different RA groups: naïve RA and DMARD-non responding patients.

Table 1. Clinical data and patient characteristics.

	Age (years)	Gender (male/female)	Disease duration (years)	Rheumatoid factor (IU/ml)	Anti-MCV (IU/ml)	Timepoint	DAS-28 index	CRP (mg/l)	ESR (mm/h)
Naïve RA (n = 12)	56 [50–61]	5/7	0.3 [0.2–0.3]	104.7 [41.8–138.0]	65.1 [10.3–393.6]	**Baseline (without therapy)**	6.8 [6.1–7.1]	63.8 [26.4–96.6]	64 [35–91]
						Week 4, after medium-dose GCS therapy	4.0 [2.9–4.2]	2.8 [1.4–6.8]	14 [9–21]
						Week 8, after low-dose GCS and MTX therapy	2.4 [2.1–3.2]	3.4 [1.6–5.3]	19 [14–27]
Active RA with IFX therapy (n = 7)	54 [47–57]	4/3	10.0 [4.0–14.0]	110.0 [28.6–392.2]	17.4 [4.8–395.3]	**Baseline (on LF and MTX therapy)**	6.2 [5.7–6.8]	13.7 [11.8–19.7]	35 [30–48]
						Week 4 of IFX and MTX therapy	5.1 [4.5–5.6]	3.1 [2.1–6.9]	17 [13–29]
						Week 8 of IFX and MTX therapy	4.1 [3.2–4.5]	2.0 [1.6–2.4]	17 [11–20]
Active RA with ETA therapy (n = 7)	53 [51–61]	0/7	6.5 [3.8–11.3]	85.0 [22.9–236.7]	600.0 [39.7–1000]	**Baseline (on LF and MTX therapy)**	6.3 [6.2–6.8]	20.1 [12.7–54.4]	54 [44–62]
						Week 4 of ETA and MTX therapy	3.3 [2.6–4.4]	3.8 [2.0–5.7]	25 [14–29]
						Week 8 of ETA and MTX therapy	2.6 [2.4–2.8]	2.0 [2.0–5.9]	13 [11–36]
Active RA with ADA therapy (n = 8)	55 [52–59]	1/7	9.0 [7.3–10.0]	187.0 [102.3–377.3]	354.6 [71.0–857.9]	**Baseline (on LF and MTX therapy)**	6.1 [6.0–6.5]	29.7 [18.6–43.7]	46 [39–56]
						Week 4 of ADA and MTX therapy	3.4 [3.0–4.4]	9.4 [3.1–20.4]	28 [19–37]
						Week 8 of ADA and MTX therapy	3.4 [2.9–3.7]	5.2 [2.0–8.6]	26 [17–39]

GCS = glucocorticosteroid; MTX = methotrexate; LF = leflunomide; IFX = infliximab; ETA = etanercept; ADA = adalimumab; RA = rheumatoid arthritis; Anti-MCV = anti-mutated citrullinated vimentin; DAS-28 = disease activity score in 28 joints; CRP = c-reactive protein; ESR = erythrocyte sedimentation rate.
Data are expressed as median [interquartile range].

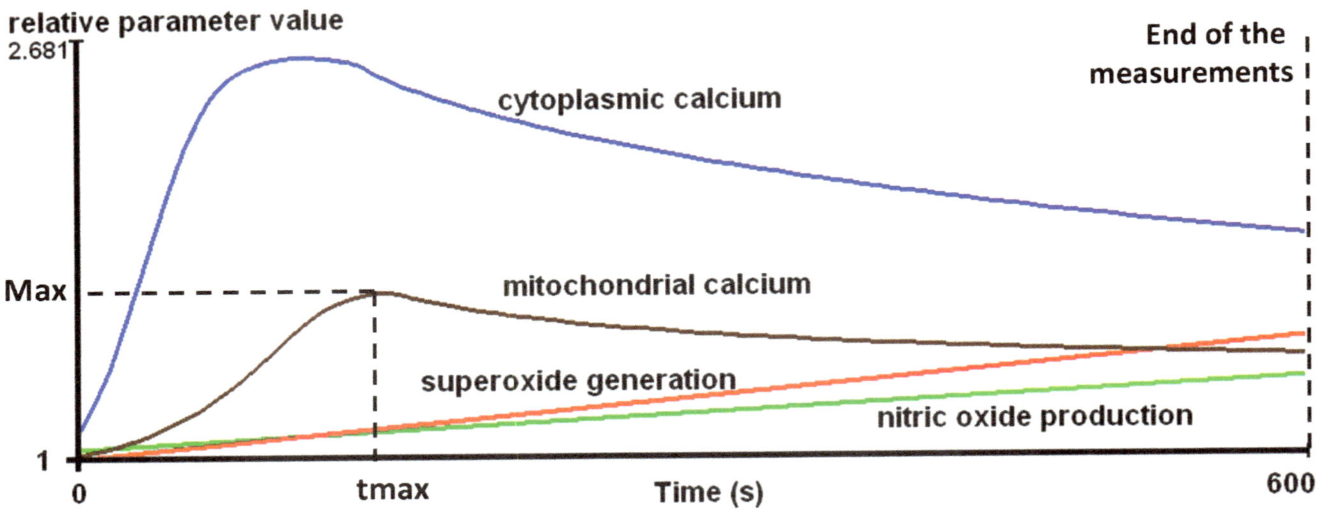

Figure 1. Schematic demonstration of kinetic parameters of the investigated intracellular processes during the activation of T-lymphocytes. Max = Maximum value, tmax = Time to reach maximum.

Naïve patients

There is a paucity of studies investigating T-cell activation characteristics in RA. The few data available suggest that increased levels of nitric oxide [13], intracellular Ca^{2+} [4] and ROS [6] are present in the T-cells of active RA patients and these abnormalities may contribute to the cellular dysfunction. However, in naïve RA patients we found that these parameters were comparable to those in the controls. The discrepancy between our results and previous studies could be due to the different populations tested as we enrolled newly diagnosed naïve RA subjects, while the published data involved a less specific RA population. Indeed, as we discovered in the case of patients who had suffered from RA for several years, these intracellular mechanisms may be affected in the later stage of the disease that does not respond to DMARD therapy.

The cytoplasmic Ca^{2+} response and ROS production during the short-term activation of T lymphocytes were suppressed relative to the baseline after 4 weeks of GCS therapy. In *in vitro* and *in vivo* animal studies GCS inhibited activated T-cell functions at several points of the intracellular signaling cascade [14]. GCS treatment limits PIP2 hydrolysis and IP3 production [15], down-regulates IP3 receptors [16] and also depletes internal Ca^{2+} stores [17]. Irrespective of the mechanism, the result at a cellular level is the reduction of the Ca^{2+} responses during short-term T-cell activation. GCS therapy also decreased intracellular ROS levels in human aortic smooth muscle cells [18]. These reported data are in accordance with our results indicating that GCS therapy has a major impact on the T-cell functionality in early RA.

After 1 month of MTX treatment, the cytoplasmic Ca^{2+} response during T-cell activation became comparable to controls. An in vitro animal study revealed evidence that MTX has IP3-like properties and mobilizes Ca^{2+} from the endoplasmic reticulum in a direct way without receptor activation [19]. The increase in the cytoplasmic Ca^{2+} level may reflect this effect (while it is still uncertain whether the normal appearance of the cytoplasmic Ca^{2+} level does indicate normal Ca^{2+} signaling in this situation).

In MTX-treated subjects, ROS generation was suppressed further. This phenomenon confirms previous results observed on RA synoviocytes, where MTX inhibited the production of ROS [20]. This finding may be of major clinical relevance, as excessive ROS production plays a critical role in the pathogenesis of RA [21]. Besides the role of extracellular ROS generation, it has also been demonstrated that increased intracellular ROS production amplifies the synovial inflammatory–proliferative response [22] and is characteristic of and augments the T-cell dysfunction in RA [23].

RA patients unresponding to DMARD therapy

In the second part of our study, we monitored T-cell functionality of RA patients on anti-TNF-α therapy. We also investigated whether different agents procure different effects on these parameters.

At baseline, (i.e. just before anti-TNF-α therapy) we found a higher cytoplasmic Ca^{2+} response to stimulation than in the controls. It was noteworthy that the increased Ca^{2+} signal became comparable to controls by Week 4 and remained unaltered at Week 8, irrespectively of the anti-TNF-α agent used. Although this occurred in almost all the patients, it is in contradiction with most of the published data that suggest hyporesponsiveness of the T-lymphocytes in RA [24,25].

The explanation of the discrepancy between the published and our own data is probably the different characteristics of the RA patients enrolled. The enrolled patients in the published studies were predominantly treated with NSAIDs (with no reported effect on the calcium metabolism in the T-cells). In contrast, we collected samples from patients who did not respond to DMARD therapy (that included MTX and LF). No effect of LF on T-cell Ca^{2+} signaling is known, while MTX has been documented to increase Ca^{2+} response. When LF was replaced by any of the anti-TNF-α agents, the cytoplasmic Ca^{2+} signal became comparable to controls. It is unclear whether this is due to the introduction of the anti-TNF-α agent and/or to the cessation of LF. Irrespective of the mechanism, our results should be regarded as characteristic of this specific RA subgroup. It is tempting to postulate that an increased cytoplasmic Ca^{2+} signal might possibly be used as a surrogate marker for the identification of RA patients in whom combination of MTX with leflunomide will not be sufficient and leflunomide is recommended to be replaced by an anti-TNF agent. This hypothesis should be evaluated further.

Table 2. Functional characteristics of intracellular processes in CD4+ cells following PHA activation in RA patients before and during therapy.

		Cytoplasmic Ca^{2+}			Reactive oxygen species generation			Nitric oxide production	Mitochondrial Ca^{2+}
		AUC (U)	Max (rpv)	t_{max} (s)	AUC (U)	Max (rpv)	t_{max} (s)	AUC (U)	AUC (U)
Control (n = 9)		89.06 [62.60–131.5]	1.211 [1.149–1.326]	444.8 [192.3–594.4]	75.43 [68.01–88.80]	1.239 [1.217–1.263]	594.5 [594.3–595.3]	5.501 [−6.919–35.98]	64.18 [42.85–97.89]
Naïve RA (n = 12)	**Baseline (without therapy)**	90.54 [73.45–206.5]	1.221 [1.166–1.581]	458.9 [172.6–594.5]	74.36 [50.26–90.26]	1.245 [1.178–1.308]	594.5 [594.0–595.2]	34.11 [−0.103–76.15]	63.03 [33.70–97.45]
	Week 4, after medium-dose GCS therapy	$44.55^{A,B}$ [21.11–74.37]	1.127^{A} [1.068–1.201]	234.2 [209.0–594.1]	$48.47^{A,B}$ [36.15–79.09]	1.172 [1.145–1.237]	594.7 [594.3–595.4]	−9.670 [−11.43–10.73]	40.11 [25.71–58.89]
	Week 8, after low-dose GCS and MTX therapy	60.67 [12.22–111.6]	1.232 [1.046–1.295]	306.5 [289.5–594.1]	49.75^{A} [45.87–54.55]	1.170^{A} [1.165–1.179]	594.6 [594.5–594.8]	3.180 [−12.39–11.74]	55.83 [19.47–72.22]
Active RA with IFX therapy (n = 7)	**Baseline (on LF and MTX therapy)**	145.1^{A} [126.8–207.4]	1.374^{A} [1.315–1.510]	594.1 [342.8–594.6]	65.04 [53.47–86.19]	1.223 [1.170–1.258]	594.6 [594.4–595.2]	24.62 [−7.701–95.59]	51.86 [44.98–81.62]
	Week 4 of IFX and MTX therapy	96.97 [4.403–162.7]	1.240 [1.032–1.352]	594.5 [276.2–594.6]	$39.92^{A,B}$ [33.42–67.93]	1.146^{A} [1.141–1.230]	594.4 [593.7–595.2]	19.82 [−14.59–30.06]	83.87 [51.44–166.5]
	Week 8 of IFX and MTX therapy	115.9 [59.33–141.1]	1.328 [1.242–1.347]	593.9 [288.0–594.9]	56.16^{A} [45.14–71.85]	1.186^{A} [1.167–1.220]	593.6 [593.1–595.5]	−2.549 [−16.00–25.92]	67.37 [42.57–118.9]
Active RA with ETA therapy (n = 7)	**Baseline (on LF and MTX therapy)**	141.2^{A} [109.1–235.6]	1.319^{A} [1.271–1.535]	372.0 [216.7–593.5]	94.55^{A} [81.39–111.0]	1.293 [1.242–1.372]	594.9 [594.2–595.6]	−0.087 [−12.70–22.17]	70.62 [59.08–128.8]
	Week 4 of ETA and MTX therapy	125.7 [64.09–159.1]	1.304 [1.147–1.396]	383.8 [246.1–594.1]	73.49^{B} [59.69–81.87]	1.235^{B} [1.188–1.275]	594.8 [594.1–595.3]	21.72 [−4.121–87.42]	50.93 [34.75–82.80]
	Week 8 of ETA and MTX therapy	92.11 [49.82–222.8]	1.231 [1.182–1.491]	312.5 [174.3–593.9]	72.37 [49.84–105.9]	1.226 [1.163–1.300]	593.9 [593.7–594.8]	8.466 [−8.267–62.04]	77.45 [26.15–94.89]
Active RA with ADA therapy (n = 8)	**Baseline (on LF and MTX therapy)**	144.4^{A} [128.0–199.8]	1.399^{A} [1.320–1.484]	557.9 [217.8–594.4]	81.89 [69.52–106.8]	1.258 [1.220–1.343]	594.5 [594.0–594.9]	15.86 [1.704–116.9]	77.94 [66.09–90.10]
	Week 4 of ADA and MTX therapy	93.91 [77.45–157.3]	1.227 [1.188–1.347]	497.4 [256.4–594.6]	63.21^{B} [34.48–77.15]	1.212 [1.155–1.240]	594.7 [594.2–595.5]	25.87 [−6.588–99.43]	66.84 [41.83–92.19]
	Week 8 of ADA and MTX therapy	107.6 [50.18–158.5]	1.262 [1.146–1.364]	432.4 [226.6–594.5]	73.95 [61.69–78.82]	1.230 [1.211–1.241]	594.2 [593.6–594.9]	60.43 [26.93–133.0]	71.77 [62.20–95.48]

Data are expressed as median [interquartile range].
[A]versus control $P<0.05$;
[B]versus baseline $P<0.05$.
AUC = area under the curve; Max = maximum value; t_{max} = time to reach maximum value; rpv = relative parameter value.
GCS = glucocorticosteroid; MTX = methotrexate; LF = leflunomide; IFX = infliximab; ETA = etanercept; ADA = adalimumab; RA = rheumatoid arthritis.

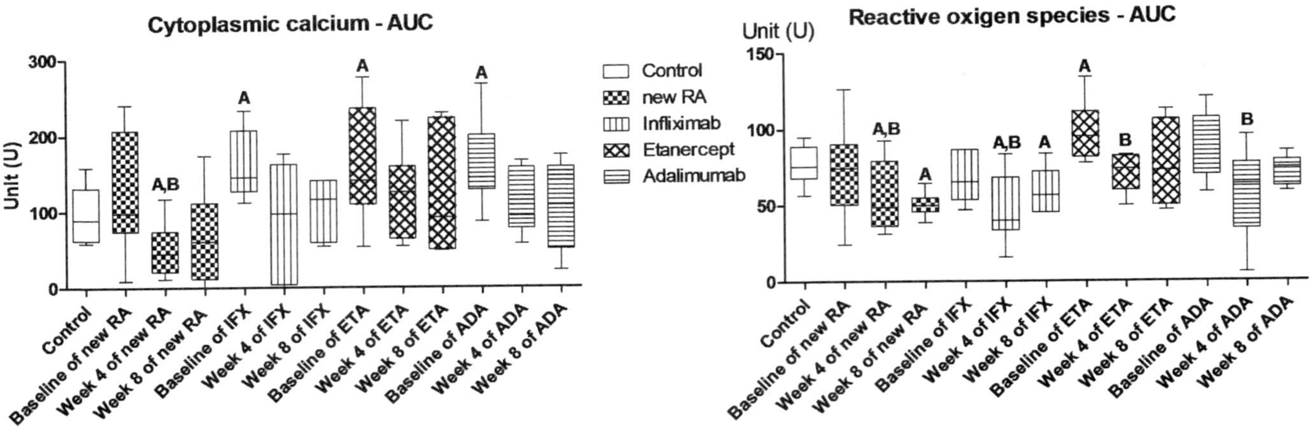

Figure 2. Area under the curve values of cytoplasmic calcium and reactive oxigen species in CD4+ cells. A-versus controls $P<0.05$; B-versus baseline $P<0.05$. AUC = area under the curve; RA = rheumatoid arthritis; IFX = infliximab; ETA = etanercept; ADA = adalimumab.

While our results also indicate that NO production and mitochondrial Ca^{2+} handling are not affected during short-term T-cell stimulation by anti-TNF agents in RA, we observed changes in intracellular ROS production during anti-TNF therapy. As discussed above, an increased intracellular ROS production may contribute to the prolonged inflammation observed in RA, and a reduction of ROS may therefore be a beneficial effect. We also found that the baseline ROS production was higher in the ETA-treated group and tended to be higher in the ADA group than in the controls. Although the overproduction of TNF-α is thought to be the main contributor to the increased ROS generation in RA, the effects of anti-TNF-α treatment have not been extensively studied in this RA patient subgroup.

The effect of anti-TNF agents on T-lymphocyte ROS production is not fully elucidated. Data are limited to neutrophils. Pay et al reported that IFX inhibited the production of ROS in neutrophils *in vitro* [26], while anti-TNF-α treatment has been stated to be ineffective on ROS production of the neutrophils in RA patients [27,28]. For T-lymphocytes, we demonstrated a significant decrease in all groups at Week 4 of anti-TNF-α therapy, irrespective of whether the baseline ROS production was higher than or comparable to the controls. This effect was most pronounced in the IFX-treated group and proved to be associated with significantly decreased ROS production. At Week 8, we found no changes in the production of ROS relative to that at Week 4; again, this type of anti-TNF action was comparable in the various treatment groups.

The limitations of our work

Evaluating these results one should note that because of the low number of patients enrolled, these observations are suitable for just hypothesis generation and the data can not be extrapolated to large patient cohorts.

In the DMARD nonresponding patients at initiation of anti-TNF-α therapy leflunomide was discontinued, but we could not investigate whether this effects the intracellular processes in any way.

Conclusions

This study on peripheral blood samples has provided comprehensive information regarding the functionality of T-cells in RA.

The intracellular T-cell activation processes (including cytoplasmic Ca^{2+}, ROS, NO generation and mitochondrial Ca^{2+}) during short-term T-cell activation were not altered in early RA. The therapeutic interventions exerted specific effects on the different parameters. GCS decreased cytoplasmic Ca^{2+} signal and the levels of ROS. Tapering the GCS dose and the introduction of MTX increased the cytoplasmic Ca^{2+} signal, but further decreased the levels of ROS. In DMARD non responding patients, the cytoplasmic Ca^{2+} level was higher than in the controls (possibly due to the treatment with MTX). After the introduction of TNF α inhibitors, the cytoplasmic Ca^{2+} signal became comparable to controls and the levels of ROS decreased. The extent of NO generation and the level of mitochondrial Ca^{2+} were not altered at any time during our study.

These results indicate that intracellular machinery is affected in T-cells of RA patients. This may alter the behavior of T-cells during activation. Different therapeutic approaches may modulate the abnormal T-cell functions.

Acknowledgments

We would like to thank Ambrus Kaposi for technical expertise.

Author Contributions

Conceived and designed the experiments: BS AB BV. Performed the experiments: BS LK AB. Analyzed the data: BS ÁC GM AB. Contributed reagents/materials/analysis tools: BS AB. Wrote the paper: BS AB BV. Designed the software and algorithm used in analysis: AC GM.

References

1. Scott DL, Wolfe F, Huizinga TW (2010) Rheumatoid arthritis. Lancet 376: 1094–1108.
2. McInnes IB, O'Dell JR (2010) State-of-the-art: rheumatoid arthritis. Ann Rheum Dis 69: 1898–1906.
3. Inman RD, El-Gabalawy HS (2009) The immunology of ankylosing spondylitis and rheumatoid arthritis: a tale of similarities and dissimilarities. Clin Exp Rheumatol 27: S26–32.
4. Nagy G, Clark JM, Buzas E, Gorman C, Pasztoi M, et al. (2008) Nitric oxide production of T lymphocytes is increased in rheumatoid arthritis. Immunol Lett 118: 55–58.
5. Nagy G, Clark JM, Buzás EI, Gorman CL, Cope AP (2007) Nitric oxide, chronic inflammation and autoimmunity. Immunol Lett 111: 1–5.
6. Phillips DC, Dias HK, Kitas GD, Griffiths HR (2010) Aberrant reactive oxygen and nitrogen species generation in rheumatoid arthritis (RA): causes and

consequences for immune function, cell survival, and therapeutic intervention. Antioxid Redox Signal 12: 743–785.
7. Vital EM, Emery P (2008) The development of targeted therapies in rheumatoid arthritis. J Autoimmun 31: 219–227.
8. Szalay B, Vasarhelyi B, Cseh A, Tulassay T, Deak M, et al. (2013) The impact of conventional DMARD and biological therapies on CD4+ cell subsets in rheumatoid arthritis: a follow-up study. Clin Rheumatol.
9. Smolen JS, Landewé R, Breedveld FC, Dougados M, Emery P, et al. (2010) EULAR recommendations for the management of rheumatoid arthritis with synthetic and biological disease-modifying antirheumatic drugs. Ann Rheum Dis 69: 964–975.
10. Szalay B, Mészáros G, Cseh Á, Ács L, Deák M, et al. (2012) Adaptive immunity in ankylosing spondylitis: phenotype and functional alterations of T-cells before and during infliximab therapy. Clin Dev Immunol 2012: 808724.
11. Mészáros G, Szalay B, Toldi G, Kaposi A, Vásárhelyi B, et al. (2012) Kinetic Measurements Using Flow Cytometry: New Methods for Monitoring Intracellular Processes. Assay Drug Dev Technol 10: 97–104.
12. Kaposi AS, Veress G, Vásárhelyi B, Macardle P, Bailey S, et al. (2008) Cytometry-acquired calcium-flux data analysis in activated lymphocytes. Cytometry A 73: 246–253.
13. Nagy G, Koncz A, Telarico T, Fernandez D, Ersek B, et al. (2010) Central role of nitric oxide in the pathogenesis of rheumatoid arthritis and systemic lupus erythematosus. Arthritis Res Ther 12: 210.
14. Van Laethem F, Baus E, Smyth LA, Andris F, Bex F, et al. (2001) Glucocorticoids attenuate T cell receptor signaling. J Exp Med 193: 803–814.
15. Baus E, Andris F, Dubois PM, Urbain J, Leo O (1996) Dexamethasone inhibits the early steps of antigen receptor signaling in activated T lymphocytes. J Immunol 156: 4555–4561.
16. Harr MW, Rong Y, Bootman MD, Roderick HL, Distelhorst CW (2009) Glucocorticoid-mediated inhibition of Lck modulates the pattern of T cell receptor-induced calcium signals by down-regulating inositol 1,4,5-trisphosphate receptors. J Biol Chem 284: 31860–31871.
17. Lam M, Dubyak G, Distelhorst CW (1993) Effect of glucocorticosteroid treatment on intracellular calcium homeostasis in mouse lymphoma cells. Mol Endocrinol 7: 686–693.
18. Marumo T, Schini-Kerth VB, Brandes RP, Busse R (1998) Glucocorticoids inhibit superoxide anion production and p22 phox mRNA expression in human aortic smooth muscle cells. Hypertension 32: 1083–1088.
19. Pagadigorria CL, Marcon F, Kelmer-Bracht AM, Bracht A, Ishii-Iwamoto EL (2006) Effects of methotrexate on calcium flux in rat liver mitochondria, microsomes and plasma membrane vesicles. Comp Biochem Physiol C Toxicol Pharmacol 143: 340–348.
20. Sung JY, Hong JH, Kang HS, Choi I, Lim SD, et al. (2000) Methotrexate suppresses the interleukin-6 induced generation of reactive oxygen species in the synoviocytes of rheumatoid arthritis. Immunopharmacology 47: 35–44.
21. Hassan SZ, Gheita TA, Kenawy SA, Fahim AT, El-Sorougy IM, et al. (2011) Oxidative stress in systemic lupus erythematosus and rheumatoid arthritis patients: relationship to disease manifestations and activity. Int J Rheum Dis 14: 325–331.
22. Hitchon CA, El-Gabalawy HS (2004) Oxidation in rheumatoid arthritis. Arthritis Res Ther 6: 265–278.
23. Griffiths HR, Dunston CR, Bennett SJ, Grant MM, Phillips DC, et al. (2011) Free radicals and redox signalling in T-cells during chronic inflammation and ageing. Biochem Soc Trans 39: 1273–1278.
24. Allen ME, Young SP, Michell RH, Bacon PA (1995) Altered T lymphocyte signaling in rheumatoid arthritis. Eur J Immunol 25: 1547–1554.
25. Carruthers DM, Naylor WG, Allen ME, Kitas GD, Bacon PA, et al. (1996) Characterization of altered calcium signalling in T lymphocytes from patients with rheumatoid arthritis (RA). Clin Exp Immunol 105: 291–296.
26. Pay S, Musabak U, Erdem H, Simsek I, Pekel A, et al. (2005) Chimerical anti-TNF-alpha, infliximab, inhibits neutrophil chemotaxis and production of reactive oxygen species by blocking the priming effect of mononuclear cells on neutrophils. Immunopharmacol Immunotoxicol 27: 187–198.
27. den Broeder AA, Wanten GJ, Oyen WJ, Naber T, van Riel PL, et al. (2003) Neutrophil migration and production of reactive oxygen species during treatment with a fully human anti-tumor necrosis factor-alpha monoclonal antibody in patients with rheumatoid arthritis. J Rheumatol 30: 232–237.
28. Capsoni F, Sarzi-Puttini P, Atzeni F, Minonzio F, Bonara P, et al. (2005) Effect of adalimumab on neutrophil function in patients with rheumatoid arthritis. Arthritis Res Ther 7: R250–255.

10

Bead Arrays for Antibody and Complement Profiling Reveal Joint Contribution of Antibody Isotypes to C3 Deposition

Burcu Ayoglu[1], Eszter Szarka[2], Krisztina Huber[2], Anita Orosz[2], Fruzsina Babos[3], Anna Magyar[3], Ferenc Hudecz[3,4], Bernadette Rojkovich[5], Tamás Gáti[5], György Nagy[5,6], Jochen M. Schwenk[1], Gabriella Sármay[2], József Prechl[7,8], Peter Nilsson[1]*, Krisztián Papp[1,7]*

1 Affinity Proteomics, SciLifeLab, School of Biotechnology, KTH Royal Institute of Technology, Stockholm, Sweden, 2 Department of Immunology, Eötvös Loránd University, Budapest, Hungary, 3 MTA-ELTE Research Group of Peptide Chemistry, Budapest, Hungary, 4 Department of Organic Chemistry, Eötvös Loránd University, Budapest, Hungary, 5 Department of Rheumatology, Polyclinic of the Hospitaller Brothers of St. John of God, Budapest, Hungary, 6 Department of Genetics, Cell and Immunobiology, Semmelweis University, Medical School, Budapest, Hungary, 7 MTA-ELTE Immunology Research Group, Budapest, Hungary, 8 Diagnosticum Ltd., Budapest, Hungary

Abstract

The development of antigen arrays has provided researchers with great tools to identify reactivities against self or foreign antigens from body fluids. Yet, these approaches mostly do not address antibody isotypes and their effector functions even though these are key points for a more detailed understanding of disease processes. Here, we present a bead array-based assay for a multiplexed determination of antigen-specific antibody levels in parallel with their properties for complement activation. We measured the deposition of C3 fragments from serum samples to reflect the degree of complement activation via all three complement activation pathways. We utilized the assay on a bead array containing native and citrullinated peptide antigens to investigate the levels of IgG, IgM and IgA autoantibodies along with their complement activating properties in serum samples of 41 rheumatoid arthritis patients and 40 controls. Our analysis revealed significantly higher IgG reactivity against the citrullinated fibrinogen β and filaggrin peptides as well as an IgA reactivity that was exclusive for citrullinated fibrinogen β peptide and C3 deposition in rheumatoid arthritis patients. In addition, we characterized the humoral immune response against the viral EBNA-1 antigen to demonstrate the applicability of this assay beyond autoimmune conditions. We observed that particular buffer compositions were demanded for separate measurement of antibody reactivity and complement activation, as detection of antigen-antibody complexes appeared to be masked due to C3 deposition. We also found that rheumatoid factors of IgM isotype altered C3 deposition and introduced false-positive reactivities against EBNA-1 antigen. In conclusion, the presented bead-based assay setup can be utilized to profile antibody reactivities and immune-complex induced complement activation in a high-throughput manner and could facilitate the understanding and diagnosis of several diseases where complement activation plays role in the pathomechanism.

Editor: Robert B. Sim, Oxford University, United Kingdom

Funding: This work was supported by the Hungarian Academy of Sciences, the Hungarian Scientific Research Fund (OTKA-PD 104779 and OTKA-NK 104846), ProNova VINN Excellence Centre for Protein Technology (VINNOVA, Swedish Governmental Agency for Innovation Systems), the János Bolyai Research Scholarship of the Hungarian Academy of Sciences, the Knut and Alice Wallenberg Foundation and SciLifeLab Stockholm. The funders had no role in study design, data collection and analysis, decision to publish, or preparation of the manuscript.

Competing Interests: J.P. is a paid employee of Diagnosticum Ltd. This does not alter the authors' adherence to PLOS ONE policies on sharing data and materials.

* E-mail: pkrisz5@gmail.com (KP); peter.nilsson@scilifelab.se (PN)

These authors contributed equally to this work.

Introduction

Antigen array-based methods allow screening for hundreds or thousands of potential targets of antibody reactivities and they are being increasingly utilized to identify novel antibody reactivities in the context of various pathological conditions such as autoimmune diseases [1–3]. The focus of such approaches is mostly limited only to determine the targets of antibodies, usually of IgG isotype. Yet, the information on targets of autoantibodies or antibodies towards infectious agents can be further enriched by screening for other antibody isotypes and by studying their effector functions.

Antigen-antibody immune complexes can induce various effector functions including activation of the complement system, yet the degree of antibody-induced complement activation is influenced by various factors such as antibody isotype composition, antibody affinity or glycosylation state [4]. Investigating the effector functions of antigen-antibody complexes can therefore potentially add another valuable dimension for categorizing antigens or classifying clinical samples in any given autoimmune or infectious disease.

The complement system is one of the first protection lines against pathogens. More than 30 proteins form an orchestrated enzyme cascade, which can be activated by classical, lectin or alternative pathways of the complement system. All these three pathways converge at the point of cleavage of the protein C3, the third complement component, followed by activation of the common terminal pathways [5]. Various molecular structures are able to initiate the activation of the complement system, *e.g.* immune complexes (classical pathway); certain carbohydrates (lectin pathway); or several microbes or aggregates of immunoglobulins (alternative pathway) [6]. The resulting complement cleavage products induce multiple immunological effects like opsonization of the antigen, induction of inflammation or lysis of certain pathogens; some of these effects are important not only for protection against invading microbes but also play a role in autoimmune diseases.

Rheumatoid arthritis (RA) is a systemic, inflammatory, autoimmune disease that affects 0.5–1% of the world population [7]. RA is characterized by formation of rheumatoid pannus in synovial membranes, which erode adjacent cartilage and bone, subsequently leading to joint destruction [8,9]. Rheumatoid factors (RF) – antibodies specific to the Fc part of IgG – can be detected in up to 70–80% of RA patients [10], but the specificity of RFs is not adequate as positive results occur in other autoimmune and infectious diseases and in up to 15% of healthy individuals, too [9,11]. Therefore, RF performs poorly as a screening test and should not be ordered in patients with minimal or no symptoms. Autoantibodies against citrullinated forms of peptides derived from various proteins are being suggested as promising disease markers for RA [12]. Citrullinated filaggrin was the first recognized protein, which proved to be a good candidate for detection of autoantibodies against anti-citrullinated peptides (ACPAs) [13]. But filaggrin is expressed in epithelial and not in RA-affected articular tissue, so citrullinated filaggrin is not the *in vivo* target but rather represents an *in vitro* cross-reactive antigen of ACPAs [14]. Masson-Bessière *et al.* showed that the main *in vivo* targets of citrullinated filaggrin-specific antibodies are deiminated forms of fibrinogen α and β chains, which are present in rheumatoid synovial membranes [8]. Other citrullinated protein targets in the joints like vimentin, collagen type II and α-enolase have also been previously investigated and some more are waiting for further characterization [12]. ACPA and RF define overlapping populations of RA patients. Joint destruction, comorbidities such as cardiovascular disease and other extra-articular manifestations are all prominent in the subset of patients positive for RF and ACPA [15].

The target of ACPA might be not only an autoantigen but also a viral antigen such as the citrullinated form of Epstein-Barr virus encoded nuclear antigen (EBNA-1), suggesting a possible role of Epstein-Barr virus (EBV) infection in the induction of disease-specific antibodies in RA [16]. EBV is a human γ-herpesvirus that infects more than 90% of the world population. EBV persists lifelong in the human host after the primary infection and is well controlled by the host's immune system, but it can cause a number of malignancies of lymphoid and epithelial origin in immunosuppressed individuals. EBNA-1 is expressed in all EBV infected cells and is the only viral protein regularly detected in all malignancies associated with EBV [17–19]. Antibodies against citrullinated peptides derived from EBNA-1 in contrast to the native form can differentiate between RA from non-diseased samples [16].

Assay setups based on suspension bead arrays currently offer a great sample throughput compared to planar array-based assay, allowing a highly multiplex analysis of up to 384 analytes in up to 384 samples per assay run [20]. Despite the presence of studies utilizing planar antigen arrays, there are no established protocols available to implement suspension bead-arrays for studying antigen-specific antibody reactivity and complement activation induced C3 deposition in a single assay. Here we describe development of an antigen bead-array based method for parallel detection of antibody isotypes and measurement of their complement activation properties. Our aim was to determine the optimal conditions and establish a workflow for parallel analysis of antibody reactivity and immune-complex induced complement activation on a suspension bead array platform. We demonstrated the utility of our method in the context of RA by screening serum samples for reactivity against citrullinated and non-citrullinated forms of various RA-related peptides. Furthermore, we tested the viral antigen EBNA-1 specific humoral responses in this serum sample cohort.

Materials and Methods

Ethics Statement

Serum samples were collected after written consent with ethical permission of the Scientific Research Ethics Committee of the Medical Scientific Board of Ministry of Human Resources (ETT TUKEB 5257-0/2010-1018EKU 376/PI/010).

Serum samples

Serum samples were collected from 41 RA patients with established disease and from 40 healthy volunteers. The diagnosis of the disease was established on the basis of the revised ACR/EULAR classification criteria [21]. Sample donor information for RA patients and non-diseased controls is summarized in Table 1. Serum samples were aliquoted within less than 2h after blood collection and were stored at –70°C without being exposed to any freeze-thaw cycle to preserve the complement activating property.

Peptide synthesis

The N-terminally biotinylated fibrinogen β chain (UniProt: P02675) derived peptides (Biotinyl-SGSG-^{60}RPAPPPISGG-GYRAR^{74} or Biotinyl-SGSG-^{60}**X**PAPPPISGGGY**X**A**X**^{74} where X stands for citrulline) [14] were purchased from Mimotopes Ltd. (Australia). The C-terminally biotinylated filaggrin (UniProt: P20930) related peptides (^{454}TRGRS^{458}-K-LCbiotin-Ttds or ^{454}T**X**GRS^{458}-K-LCbiotin-Ttds) were synthesized manually by solid phase peptide synthesis according to Fmoc/^{t}Bu strategy using biotinyl-6-aminohexanoic acid (LCbiotin) and 4,7,10-trioxa-1,13-tridecanediamino succinic acid linker (Ttds) and biotin [22,23]. Lysine was added to the C-terminus of the peptide for conjugation of the biotin derivatives to its ε-amino group of the side chain. The crude products were purified by HPLC. The amino acid sequence of the peptides was confirmed by ESI mass spectrometry.

Proteins and secondary antibodies

Properdin (Calbiochem); human IgG, IgM and IgA (Sigma); EBNA-1 protein (Tebu-Bio) and neutravidin (Thermo Scientific) were coupled to beads and utilized to determine the optimal assay conditions for measurement of complement activation. For detecting the various antibody isotypes, goat anti-human IgM (μ chain specific) $F(ab')_2$ –Cy3, goat anti-human IgG (γ chain specific) $F(ab')_2$ –PE or goat anti-human IgA (α chain specific) $F(ab')_2$ –DyL549 (Jackson ImmunoResearch Laboratories) antibodies were used. Goat anti-human complement C3 specific $F(ab')_2$ antibody (MyBioSource) was labeled with R-Phycoerythrin (Lightning-Link-R-Phycoerythrin Conjugation Kit, Innova Biosciences) according to manufacturer's protocol and was used to detect complement activation driven C3 deposition on beads.

Table 1. Demographics of the serum sample donors.

Atribute	RA Group	Control Group
Male/Female	10/31	13/27
Age (year)	56 (21–84)[a]	29 (19–65)
CCP2 Test +/−	38/3	
DAS index	4.2 (0.6–8.2)	
Disease duration (year)	4.5 (0–32)	

[a]Median and ranges in brackets are shown, where applicable. DAS - disease activity score.

Generation of suspension bead arrays

Proteins were coupled to carboxylated magnetic beads (MagPlex-C, Luminex Corp.) based on a previously published antigen coupling protocol [2] with minor changes. In brief, 10^6 beads per bead identity were distributed across 96-well plates (Greiner BioOne), washed and re-suspended in phosphate buffer (0.1 M NaH_2PO_4, pH 6.2) using a plate magnet and a plate washer (EL406, Biotek). The carboxyl groups on the surface of the beads were activated by 0.5 mg of 1-ethyl-3(3-dimethylamino-propyl) carbodiimide (Pierce) and 0.5 mg of N-hydroxysuccinimide (Pierce) in 100 µl phosphate buffer. After 20min incubation on a shaker (Grant Bio), beads were washed in MES buffer (0.05 M 2-(N-morpholino)ethanesulfonic acid, pH 5.0). For coupling of the following proteins to beads, 2-fold serial dilutions of the proteins with indicated starting concentrations were prepared in MES buffer: human IgG, IgM, IgA and properdin at 160 µg/ml; recombinant EBNA-1 protein at 80 µg/ml. Beads coupled in protein-free MES buffer were used as negative control. The coupling reaction was allowed to take place for 2h at RT, the beads were then washed 3x in PBS-T (0.05% Tween20 in PBS), re-suspended in 100 µl storage buffer (1% BSA, 0.05% Tween20, ProClin300 in PBS) and stored in plates at 4°C overnight. For efficient coupling of the peptides to the beads, the bead surface was first modified by covalent coupling of neutravidine (250 µg/ml) as described above. Then, 100 µl of each biotinylated peptide solution at 50 µM concentration was added to neutravidin-coated beads. Following an overnight incubation at 4°C, beads were washed 3x in PBS-T and re-suspended in 100 µl storage buffer. The final antigen suspension bead array was prepared by combining equal volumes of each bead identity and the mixture was re-suspended in storage buffer. After adjustment of the final volume to enable the transfer of 5 µl of bead solution per well, the beads were sonicated (Branson Ultrasonic Corp) and stored at 4°C until further use.

Assays on suspension bead arrays

Two types of assay buffers were utilized for the analysis of serum samples. An assay buffer supplemented with Ca^{2+} and Mg^{2+} (2.5 mM Ca^{2+}, 0.7 mM Mg^{2+}, 5% BSA, ProClin300 in PBS) was used for measurement of deposited C3 fragments, whereas an assay buffer supplemented with EDTA (25 mM EDTA, 5% BSA, ProClin300 in PBS) was used for detection of various antibody isotypes. Serum samples were diluted 1:10 (v/v) in assay buffer supplemented with 100 µg/ml neutravidin and incubated for 45 min on ice for pre-adsorption against neutravidin-specific antibodies. Using a liquid handler (CyBi-SELMA, CyBio), 50 µl of 1:10 diluted serum samples were transferred to 384 well plates containing 5 µl bead array per well. Following incubation at 37°C on a shaker (Grant Bio) for 1h, beads were washed 6x with 60 µl PBS-T on a plate washer (EL406, Biotek) and re-suspended in 50 µl of each secondary antibody solution. Anti-human C3–PE was used for detection of complement activation, whereas anti-human IgM–Cy3, anti-human IgG–PE or anti-human IgA–DyL549 antibodies were used for detection of bound antibody isotypes (**Figure 1**). All secondary antibodies were diluted 1:500 in a buffer consisting of 5% BSA, 0.05% Tween20 in PBS. After incubation with the secondary antibodies for 30 min, the beads were washed 3x with 60 µl PBS-T and re-suspended in 60 µl PBS-T for measurement by a FlexMap3D instrument (Luminex Corp.). At least 50 events per bead identity were counted and binding events were displayed as median fluorescence intensity (MFI) values.

Data Analysis

Data analysis and visualizations were performed using R [24] and various R packages or Prism 4 (GraphPad Software Inc.). Non-parametric Spearman's correlation and Mann-Whitney test were used, values were considered statistically significant if p-value < 0.05.

Results

Effect of serum sample dilution rate on complement activation

Complement activation is an enzyme cascade that requires relatively higher serum concentrations than usually applied for antibody detection methods. For identifying the optimal serum dilution rate, human IgG, IgA or properdin were coupled on beads with the aim of initiating the activation of classical, lectin & alternative or only alternative pathways, respectively. Beads were incubated with serially diluted normal human serum and the level of complement activation was determined by detection of deposited C3 fragments using an anti-human C3–PE antibody. Complement activation on beads coupled to classical pathway activator human IgG decreased with the increased serum dilution rate, yet a low level of C3 was detected in 1:160 diluted serum (***Figure 2B***). C3 detection for the beads coupled to human IgA, which is the lectin & alternative pathway activator, diminished when serum was diluted 1:20 or more (***Figure 2C***). Complement activation on beads coupled to properdin, which stabilizes the C3 convertase enzyme of the alternative pathway and induces an extreme activation of the alternative pathway, could be detected even in serum diluted 1:80 (***Figure 2D***). Very low MFI values for C3 detection on beads that were incubated in complement blocking EDTA supplemented buffer indicated that only the complement activation and not the passive binding of C3 molecules was measured by this method (***Figure 2B, 2C, 2D***).

Serum dilutions of 1:5 or less resulted in remarkably elevated background as revealed by the signal intensities for the "empty" beads, which were not coupled to any protein or peptide

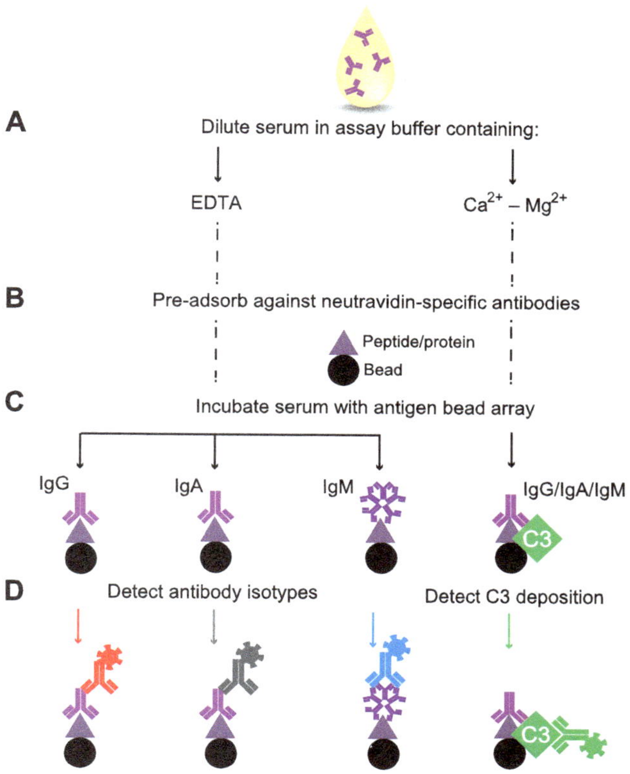

Figure 1. Schematic representation of assay workflow. A) Serum samples are diluted 1:10, either in a Ca^{2+}-Mg^{2+} containing assay buffer for detection of complement activation, or in an EDTA containing assay buffer for antibody detection. B) The samples are pre-adsorbed against neutravidin-specific antibodies. **C**) A mixture of beads coupled to various antigens is distributed into a 384-well plate and the pre-adsorbed samples are added to the bead array. **D**) Complement activation driven C3 deposition and different antibody isotypes are detected in parallel with fluorescently labeled secondary antibodies dispensed into individual wells of each quadrant of the 384-well plate.

(***Figure 2A***). Therefore, serum dilution rates of less than 1:10 were not suitable due to high background. On the other hand, the higher the serum dilution rate, the lower the C3 fragment deposition was on complement activator-coupled beads, highlighting the trade-off between low background and high MFI values for C3 detection. Serum diluted 1:10 in the Ca^{2+}- Mg^{2+} - buffer resulted in high C3 signal intensities on activator-coupled beads and yet gave low background on empty beads. Thus, a serum dilution rate of 1:10 was selected for use in further experiments.

Pronounced complement activation masks detectability of antibodies

Antibody-antigen immune complexes or directly bead-bound human antibodies can activate the complement system. Complement activation results in the deposition of complement fragments on bead surface and this phenomenon can potentially mask the detection of bead-bound antibodies. In order to evaluate the masking effect of complement components on antibody detection, human IgG or IgM coupled beads were incubated with 1:10 diluted normal human serum under assay conditions promoting (Ca^{2+}- Mg^{2+} - buffer) or blocking (EDTA - buffer) complement activation. Directly bead-bound antibodies were detected by anti-human IgG – PE and anti-human IgM - Cy3 secondary antibodies. As ***Figure 3A and 3B*** show, substantial complement deposition entirely diminished the signal intensities for the anti-human IgG antibody and decreased the signal intensities for the anti-human IgM antibody. A remarkable loss of signal intensity for the anti-human IgG antibody was also observed when the viral antigen EBNA-1 coupled beads were incubated with a seropositive serum sample ***(Figure 3C)***. Furthermore, the masking effect of complement activation diminished detectability of IgG-specific IgM rheumatoid factors as well ***(Figure 3D)***. Based on these results, EDTA containing assay buffer was used for detection of bead bound serum antibodies.

Detection of various rheumatoid factors and their complement activating properties

Sera of the majority of rheumatoid arthritis patients contain rheumatoid factors, namely autoantibodies against immunoglobulins [9]. Here, human IgG coupled beads were incubated with serum samples of RA patients and controls diluted 1:10 in EDTA-containing assay buffer and the bound human antibodies were detected by anti-human IgG, anti-human IgM or anti-human IgA secondary antibodies ***(Figure 4)***. Anti-human IgG antibody expectedly recognized the human IgG molecules coupled on beads; thus there was no significant difference between RA patients and controls. On the other hand, RA serum samples revealed significantly higher MFI values than control samples for the anti-human IgM and anti-human IgA antibodies, demonstrating the presence of IgG-specific IgM and IgA rheumatoid factors in RA patient sera ***(Figure 4A, Figure S1)***. The level of rheumatoid factors of IgM isotype in some serum samples reached 3000 AU, which can be considered as a high value, since the maximum anti-IgM signal intensities for beads coupled with highest concentration of IgM revealed 7000 AU. The level of rheumatoid factors of IgA isotype was relatively low even in RA patients, since it reached only 250 AU where the maximum anti-IgA signal intensity for beads coupled with highest concentration of IgA revealed 6000 AU.

Levels of IgG-specific IgM rheumatoid factors were measured also by ELISA, which revealed a strong positive correlation ($r = 0.927$) between the MFI values obtained on the bead array platform and the OD values in ELISA ***(Figure S2A)***. In parallel, human IgG coupled beads were also incubated with serum samples diluted 1:10 in Ca^{2+} and Mg^{2+}-containing buffer, providing assay conditions promoting activation of the complement system and the level of C3 deposition on beads was measured by the anti-human C3 antibody. Complement activation on human IgG coupled beads was significantly higher in sera of RA patients compared to controls ***(Figure 4A)***. As ***Figure 4B and 4C*** show, there was a very strong positive correlation ($r = 0.908$) between the MFI values for anti-C3 and anti-IgM antibodies. The correlations between MFI values for anti-IgA and anti-IgM antibodies ($r = 0.74$) and anti-IgA and anti-C3 ($r = 0.67$) antibodies were comparable.

Complement activating properties of autoantibodies against citrullinated peptides

Biotinylated citrulline or arginine-containing peptide pairs derived from filaggrin [36] and fibrinogen β [14] were coupled at their C- or N-terminal to neutravidin-coated beads through non-covalent but extremely strong and specific interaction, respectively. Serum samples needed first to be pre-adsorbed against neutravidin-specific antibodies before applying on bead arrays, since a number of serum samples were found to contain neutravidin-specific IgG and/or IgM antibodies, which would

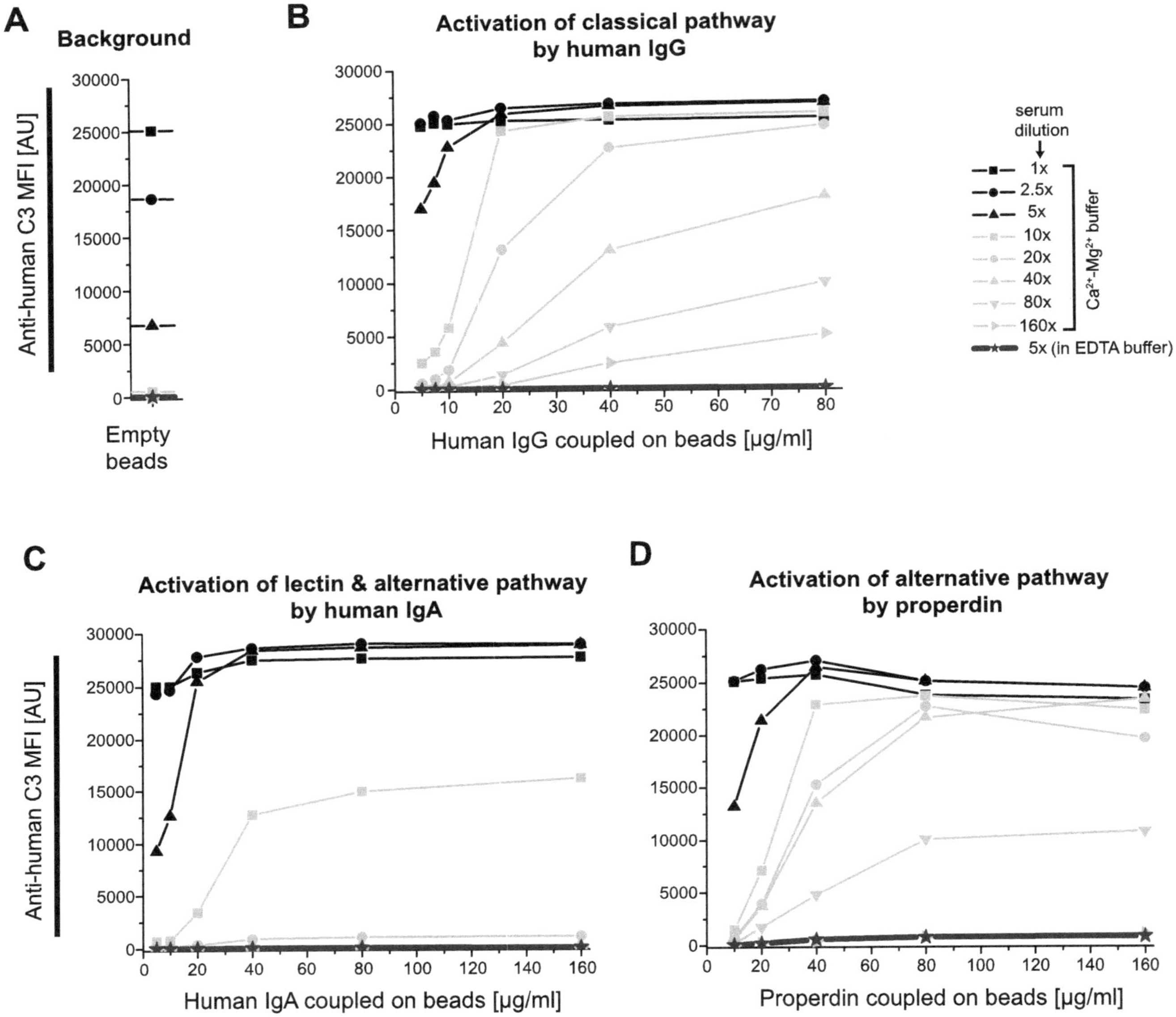

Figure 2. Dependence of complement activation on serum dilution rate. For measuring the background, classical, lectin & alternative and only alternative pathway activation, a serially diluted serum sample (1:1–1:160) was applied to empty, human IgG, human IgA and properdin-coupled beads, respectively. The assay buffer for serum dilution contained either Ca^{2+}-Mg^{2+}, which promotes complement activation, or EDTA, which blocks complement activation. Complement activation-driven C3 fragment deposition on beads was detected by PE-conjugated anti-human C3 antibody. Plots display for each serum dilution the respective median fluorescence intensity (MFI) value against varying concentrations of human IgG, human IgA and properdin coupled on beads. AU - arbitrary units

cause false positive signals ***(Figure S3A)***. Thus, both the Ca^{2+}-Mg^{2+} or EDTA-containing assay buffers were supplemented with 100 µg/ml neutravidin and the serum samples were diluted 1:10 in these buffers depending on whether C3 deposition or autoantibody level was measured.

As ***Figure 5A*** shows, in sera of RA patients there were only minimal amount of autoantibodies of IgG, IgA or IgM isotypes against the arginine-containing form of fibrinogen β chain peptide (^{60}RPAPPPISGGGYRAR^{74}) in sharp contrast to its citrullinated form (^{60}**X**PAPPPISGGGY**X**A**X**^{74}). The autoantibodies against the citrullinated form of fibrinogen β peptide also induced an increased complement activation in the RA patient group. The results were different regarding the filaggrin-derived peptides: complement activating autoantibodies of IgM isotype against the arginine-containing form of filaggrin (^{454}TRGRS^{458}) were detected in sera of both RA patients and controls. On the other hand, citrullinated filaggrin peptide (^{454}T**X**GRS^{458}) specific IgG antibodies were detected only in sera of RA patients and not of controls. Peptide-specific IgG autoantibody levels in RA patient sera were also confirmed by ELISA, where significant correlations were revealed between bead array and ELISA measurements for the citrullinated forms of peptides for fibrinogen β and filaggrin ***(Figure S2B)***.

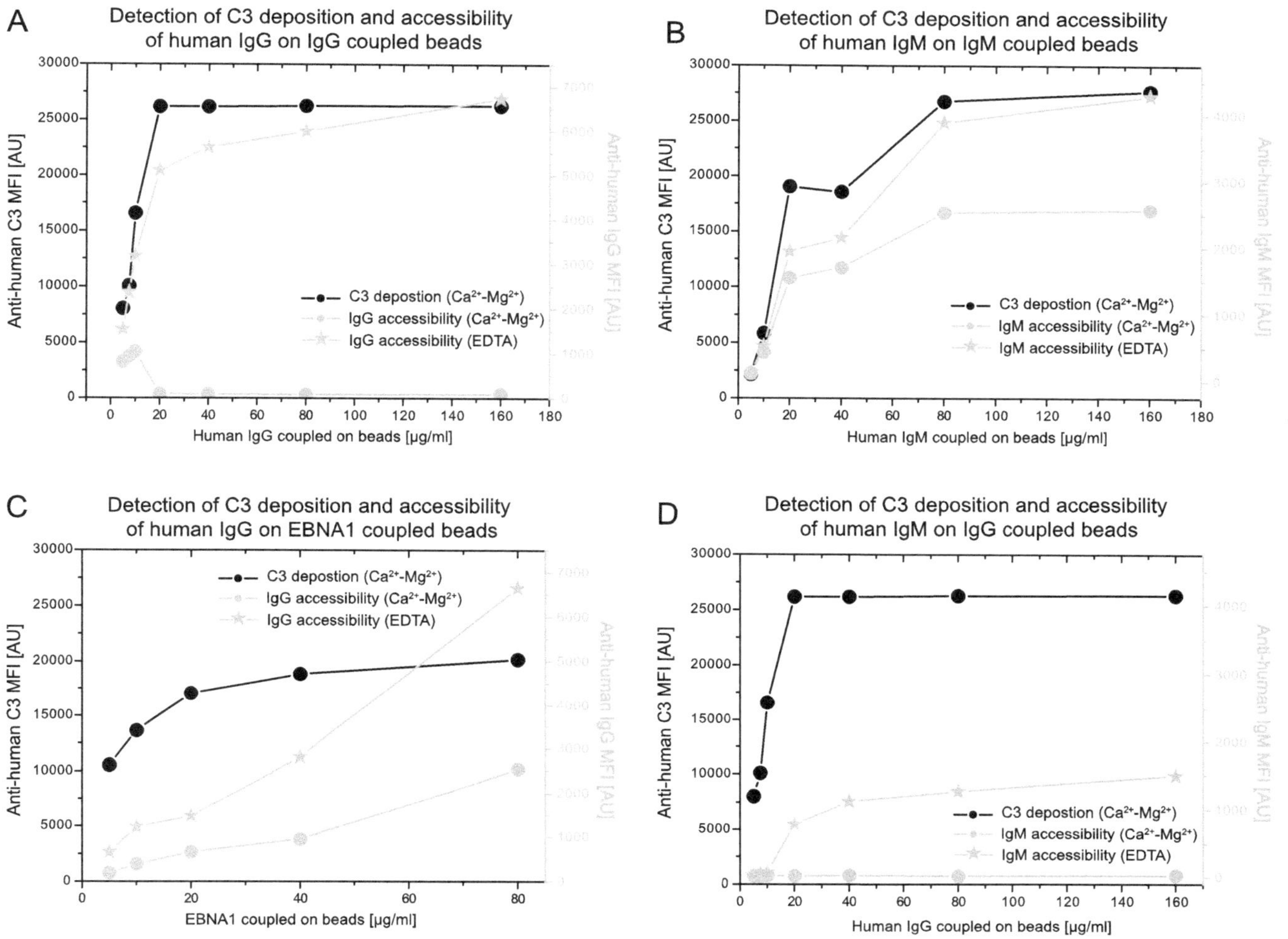

Figure 3. Complement activation masks detectability of antibodies. Human IgG *(A,D)*, human IgM *(B)* and EBNA-1 *(C)* coupled beads were incubated in 1:10 diluted serum. Ca^{2+}- Mg^{2+} (-●-) or EDTA (-*-) supplemented assay buffer was used for serum dilution. Anti-human C3-PE (black lines and axes), anti-human IgG-PE (gray lines and axes) or anti-human IgM-PE (gray lines and axes) secondary antibodies were used to measure the complement activation, IgG or IgM levels, respectively.

Antibodies against the viral antigen EBNA-1 and their complement activating properties

EBNA-1-specific IgG, IgM, IgA levels and their complement activating properties were measured in serum samples of RA patients and controls. Only the MFI values for the anti-IgM antibody on EBNA-1 coupled beads were significantly higher in sera of RA patients compared to controls ***(Figure 6A)***. There was also a significantly strong ($r = 0.714$) positive correlation between the levels of IgG-specific IgM rheumatoid factors and the anti-IgM signal intensities for EBNA-1 coupled beads ***(Figure S4.)*** Since most of the serum samples contain EBNA-1 specific IgG, the discriminating property of IgM signal intensities for EBNA-1 was supposedly derived from the rheumatoid factors that would bind to the EBNA-1 specific IgG antibody. Accordingly, there was a very high ($r = 0.898$) correlation between EBNA-1-specific C3 and IgG levels especially in control serum samples, which are not affected by the interference of rheumatoid factors ***(Figure 6B)***. The correlation between EBNA-1-specific IgA and C3 deposition was lower ($p = 0.539$) in control serum and non-significant in RA samples.

Discussion

We herein describe the development and application of a suspension-bead array based workflow for multiplex and parallel measurement of antigen-specific antibodies and complement activation in sera. To our current knowledge, this is the first study demonstrating the use of multiplex bead arrays for parallel measurement of antibody reactivity and complement activation towards various peptides and viral proteins in clinical samples within the same assay.

The complement system is an important part of the immune system and assessing the degree of complement activation can reveal important information about various pathophysiological processes. Human antibodies of different isotypes in complex with an antigen can induce complement activation to different extents. In general, the property of human antibody isotypes regarding activation of the classical pathway is as follows: IgM, IgG3> IgG1>>IgG2, while IgG4 and IgE do not activate the complement system and IgA activates only the alternative and lectin pathways [25]. Yet, different antibody clones of same isotype can initiate complement activation with very different efficacy [26], thus the direct measurement of antigen-specific complement

A

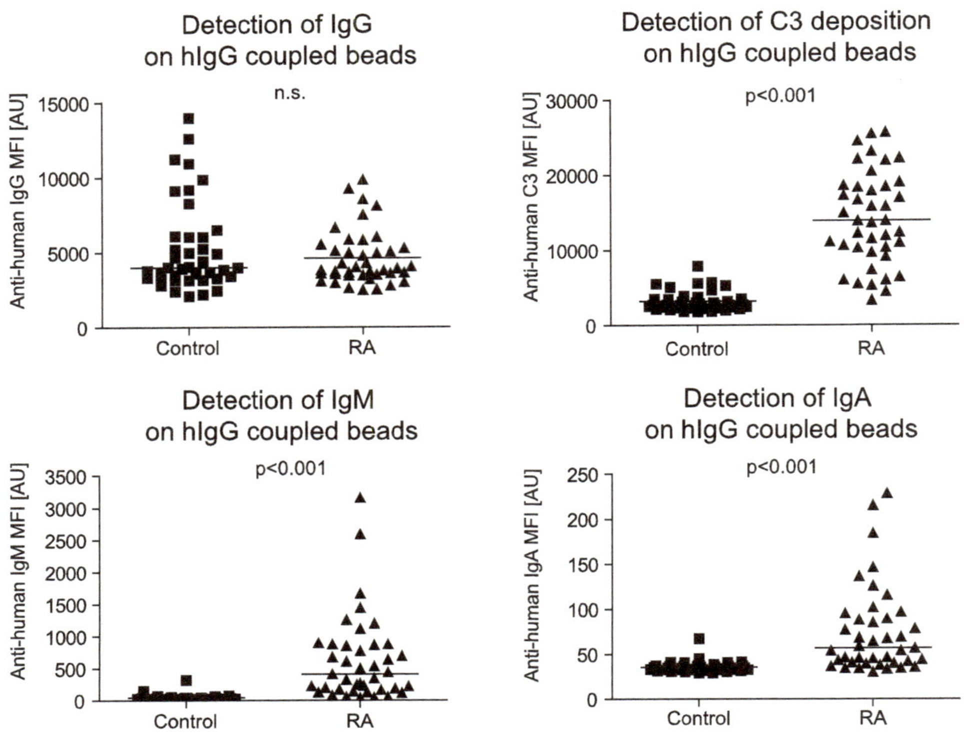

B

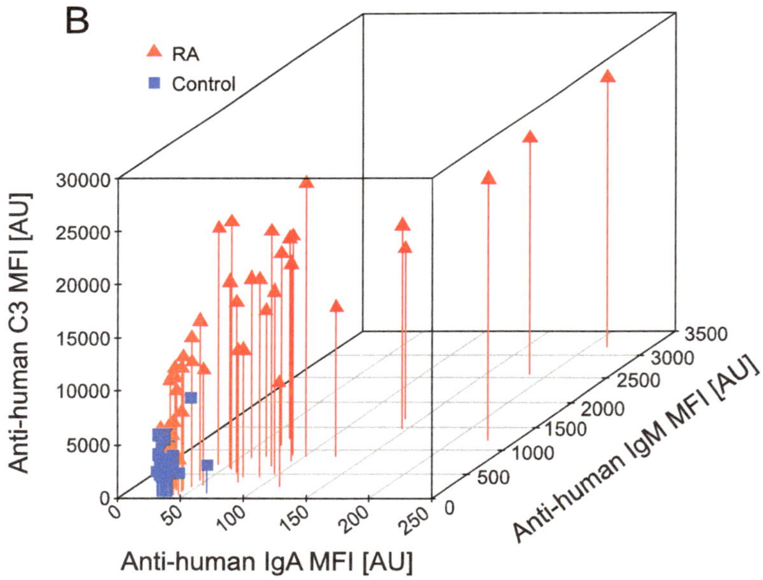

C

C3	–			
IgM	0.908	–		
IgG	n.s.	n.s.	–	
IgA	0.672	0.740	n.s.	–
	C3	**IgM**	**IgG**	**IgA**

Figure 4. Complement activation by rheumatoid factors. Following incubation of human-IgG coupled beads in sera of RA patients or non-diseased controls, bound IgG-specific rheumatoid factors and deposited C3 fragments were detected. ***A)*** Median fluorescence intensities (MFI) for anti-IgG, anti-IgM, anti-IgA and anti-C3 secondary antibodies are plotted separately for the RA patients and controls. Statistical differences between these two groups were calculated by Mann-Whitney non-parametric test. ***B)*** Anti-IgA, anti-IgM and anti-C3 MFI values for the human-IgG coupled bead within RA patient group (Δ) and controls (■) are plotted in a 3D graph for visualization of their correlation to each other. Anti-IgG MFI values are excluded from this plot since they not reveal a significant difference between the two groups. ***C)*** The table shows the Spearman's Rho correlation coefficients between anti-C3, anti-IgG, anti-IgM and anti-IgA MFI values in the entire sample cohort, where only statistically significant (p-value $<$ 0.05) correlation coefficients are shown and non-significant correlations are indicated by (n.s.).

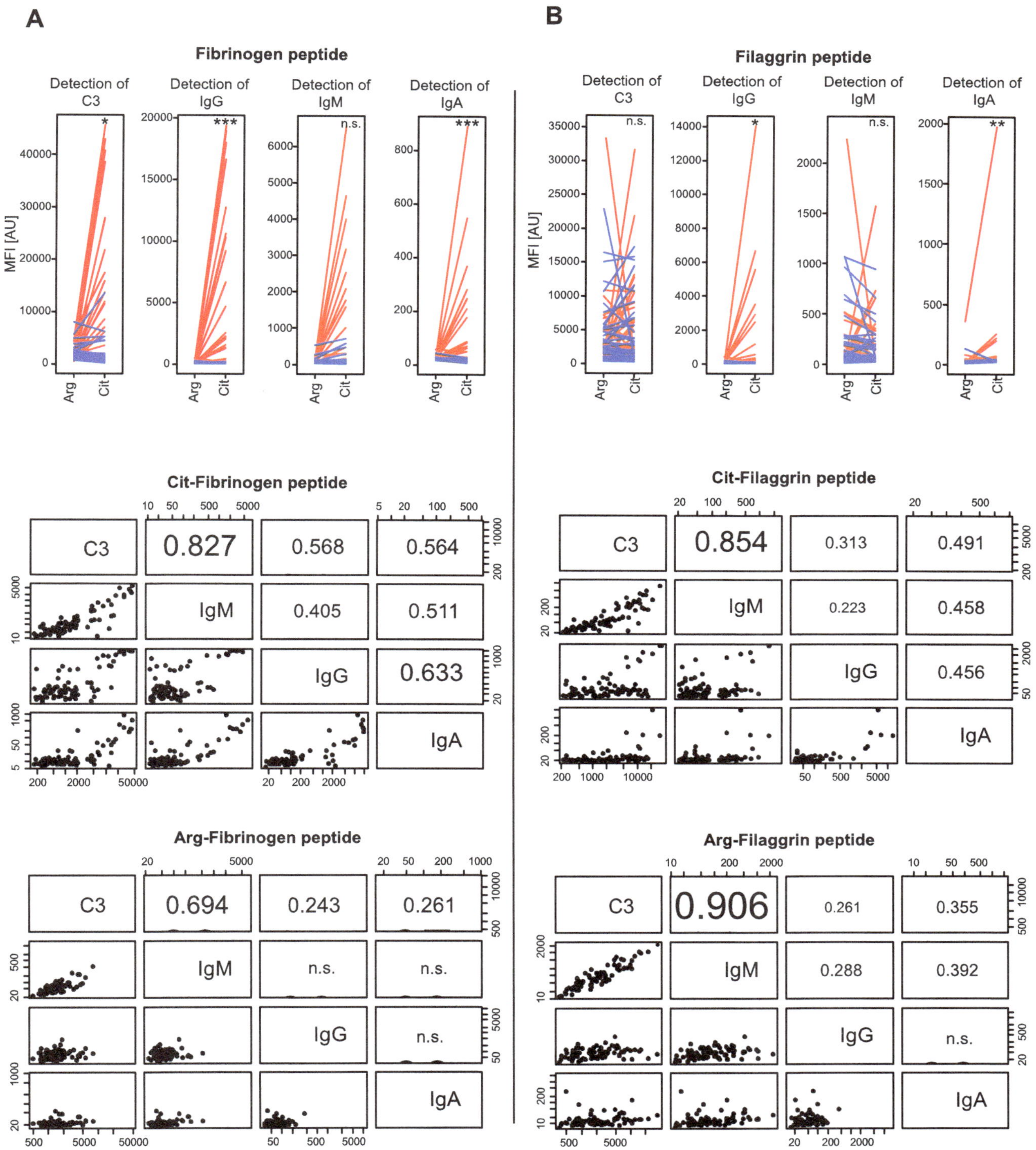

Figure 5. Detection of the level and the complement activating properties of autoantibodies against citrullinated peptides. The arginine or citrulline-containing form of fibrinogen β chain peptide (SGSG^{60}RPAPPPISGGGYRAR^{74} vs. SGSG^{60}XPAPPPISGGGYXAX^{74}) (A) and filaggrin peptides (^{454}TRGRS^{458}K vs. ^{454}TXGRS^{458}K) (B) were coupled on beads and incubated with serum samples to detect peptide-specific IgG, IgM, IgA autoantibody levels and their complement activating properties. Median fluorescent intensity (MFI) values for arginine or citrulline-containing forms of the peptides in RA patient group (red lines) or the control group (blue lines) are shown in the upper panel. Significance level of differences between controls and RA patients were calculated only for the citrullinated peptides by Mann-Whitney test and the p-values are indicated in the upper panel as follow: * p-value<0.05; ** p-value<0.01, ***p-value<0.001. Spearman's Rho correlation coefficients calculated between anti-C3, anti-IgG, anti-IgM and anti-IgA MFI values are shown for citrullined (middle panels) or native (lower panels) form of the peptides, where non-significant correlations are indicated by (n.s.).

A

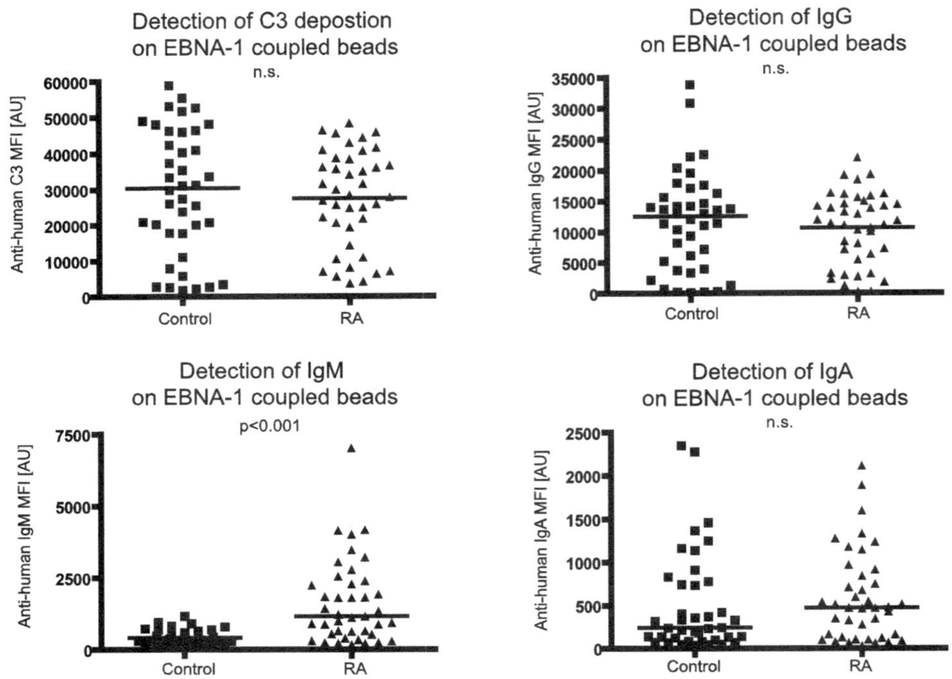

B

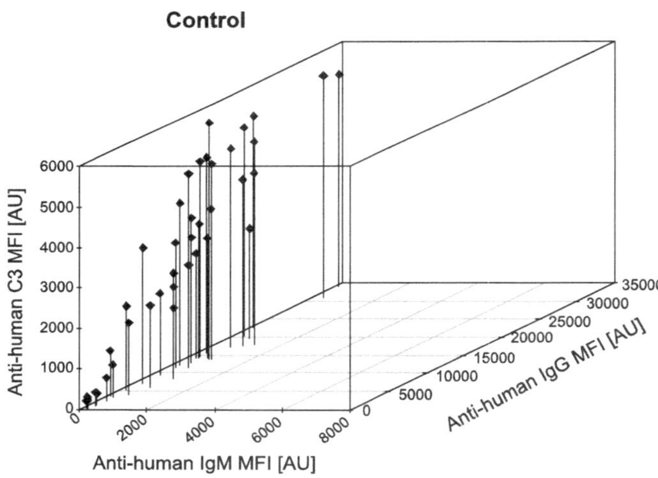

Control

C3	–			
IgM	n.s.	–		
IgG	0.898	n.s.	–	
IgA	0.539	n.s.	0.417	–
	C3	**IgM**	**IgG**	**IgA**

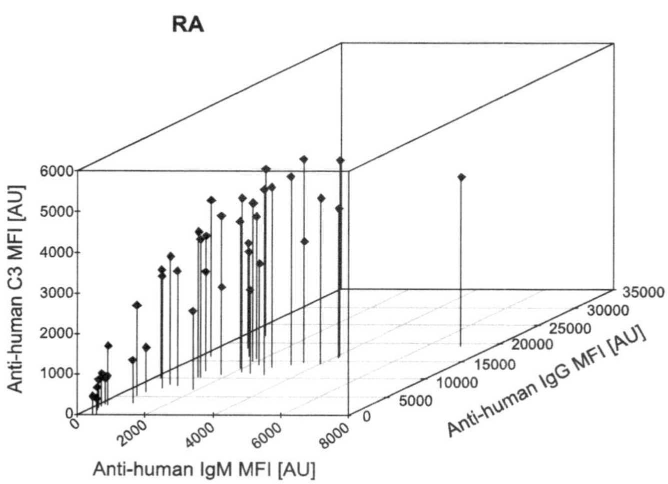

RA

C3	–			
IgM	0.700	–		
IgG	0.769	0.633	–	
IgA	n.s.	n.s.	n.s.	–
	C3	**IgM**	**IgG**	**IgA**

Figure 6. Level of EBNA-1 specific antibodies and their complement activation. EBNA-1 coupled beads were incubated with sera of RA patients and controls. ***A)*** Levels of bound human IgG, IgM and IgA antibodies along with the degree of complement activation are plotted for the two groups. Mann-Whitney non-parametric statistical test was used to calculate the statistical difference between the two groups. ***B)*** Signal intensities for anti-IgM, anti-IgA and anti-C3 for the controls (upper panel) and RA patients (lower panel) are plotted in a 3D graph. The tables show the Spearman's Rho correlation coefficients between anti-C3, anti-IgG, anti-IgM and anti-IgA signal intensities calculated separately for the control and RA patient groups. Only statistically significant (p-value<0.05) correlation coefficients are shown and non-significant correlations are indicated by (n.s.).

activation has many advantages. The clinical practice currently mainly focuses on measurement of overall complement activation and determines CH50 value or the level of C3 and C4 in the serum. ELISA tests allowing a separate analysis of the three complement activation pathways are also available [27,28]. However, when the assessment of antigen-specific complement activation is the goal, especially with the need to evaluate several candidate antigens in parallel, highly-multiplex systems such as planar [29] or suspension bead arrays offer a great advantage.

Wahrmann *et al.* previously showed a flow cytometry-based bead system to measure HLA alloantigen induced complement activation. They suggest detection of deposited C1q or C4 split products as an indication of complement activation and their data argues against the use of C3 fragment measurement, since it resulted in an alloantibody independent high background [30]. The authors applied undiluted serum that resulted in a very high background in our assay as well, but as ***Figure 2*** shows, if the bead array was incubated with a 1:10 diluted serum the background for the C3 detection disappeared and the antibody-dependent complement activation was measureable. In other published studies, C4 deposition was measured using an undiluted external complement source [31–34]; or bound externally added purified human C1q was detected after the antigen-coupled beads were treated with a mixture of heat-inactivated serum sample and C1q [35]. We measured C3 deposition as this reflects activation of any of the three pathways, which is particularly favorable since ACPAs can induce complement activation both through the classical and alternative pathways [36].

The own complement system of the tested serum sample itself was not utilized in any of these previous studies. Yet, utilizing the serum sample's own complement system can be favorable, since it reflects more precisely the individual-specific processes in the investigated serum sample as not only the presence of the complement activating antibody but also a responsive complement system is necessary for the complement activation. Avoiding the use of an external complement source can be especially attractive when highly multiplexed systems are used. External complement sources mostly consist of a mixture of normal human sera and the more ligand are tested the higher the possibility of getting false positive results due to using this serum mixture. On the other hand, inappropriate sample preparation, storage and transportation conditions or disease-related systemic complement consumption can decrease the complement activating capability of patient samples, which might lead to false negative results when the sample's own complement system is used as the complement source. Yet, in the presented assay setup, the intactness of the complement system in each sample can be easily inspected by including properdin-coupled beads in the assay. Properdin induces an extreme activation of the alternative pathway leading to C3 fragment deposition [37] and is more suitable as an internal control than the human IgG, as the RF would not alter the amount of bound C3 fragments. Very low amount of C3 deposition on properdin coupled beads indicates decreased complement level and necessitates sample exclusion or further normalization. By demonstrating that the complement system in the tested serum samples was intact and functioning with similar efficiency (***Figure S5***), we have used the own complement system of the serum samples which required a very strictly controlled storage of serum sample aliquots at $-70^{\circ}C$ by avoiding any repeated freeze-thaw cycles.

Here, an assay buffer containing physiologically equivalent concentrations of Ca^{2+} and Mg^{2+} ions was used for dilution of serum samples since these ions are essential for the activation of classical, lectin or alternative pathways, respectively. In addition, a relatively more concentrated serum condition is needed for measurement of complement activation than usually applied for detection of antibodies, where generally 1:100 or even more diluted serum can be utilized. Harboe *et al.* reported that hemolytic activity of the serum is lost at 1:16 dilution for assaying the alternative pathway and at 1:1024 dilution for assaying the classical pathway [38]. We have previously shown that 1:5–1:10 serum dilutions give the highest signal-to-noise ratios for complement measurement on nitrocellulose-coated protein microarray slides [39]. Trouw *et al.* also used a serum dilution of 1:10 in their ELISA based ACPA induced complement activation measurements [36]. Optimization of the serum dilution rate is though necessary for each assay platform, as the level of complement activation depends also on the type of the surface coating.. We observed a very high background on the empty beads when applying less than 1:5 times diluted serum, which is presumably the consequence of continuous alternative pathway tick-over that gives rise to reactive C3 fragments ***(Figure 2)***. Yet, serum diluted 1:10 in the presence of physiologically equivalent concentrations of Ca^{2+} and Mg^{2+} ions provided optimal conditions for complement measurement. But as ***Figure 3*** shows, this condition was not ideal for a parallel measurement of bound antibodies. Extensive complement fragment deposition on the site of activation masks the bound antibodies and prevents their detectability by the secondary antibodies. This effect was more pronounced regarding the detection of IgG than IgM ***(Figure 3)***. To circumvent this effect, either higher serum dilutions can be utilized [39] or the assay buffer can be supplemented with EDTA, which blocks the complement activation. Here we used the latter approach since our aim was to measure antibody levels under assay conditions as identical as possible to the conditions used for measurement of complement activation.

Here we have demonstrated the utility of multiplex antigen-specific complement activation measurement on the bead array platform both in the context of an autoimmune disease (rheumatoid arthritis) and for detection of a viral antigen (EBNA-1). There are evidences that complement activation contributes to the pathological processes of rheumatoid arthritis [40]. Rheumatoid factors are anti-human IgG Fc-specific autoantibodies of various isotypes (IgM, IgG, IgA, IgE) [41] and some of these autoantibodies can activate the complement system. There are discrepancies among the findings of previous studies concerning the prognostic value of rheumatoid factor isotypes [10,42]. We determined the levels of rheumatoid factors in sera of RA patients and non-diseased controls using human IgG coupled beads ***(Figure 4)***. The serum samples in the RA patient group revealed a significantly higher level of rheumatoid factors of IgM and IgA isotype than the control group, which is in agreement with the findings of previous studies [10]. Rheumatoid factors especially of IgM isotype induced very strong complement activation and C3 fragment deposition. The correlation between the abundance of rheumatoid factors of IgM isotype and C3 deposition was very strong (r = 0.908) ***(Figure 4C)*** and the classification power of IgM rheumatoid factors between RA patients and controls was high (AUC>0.97) ***(Figure S1)***. Samples collected from patients with a disease other than RA were not included in this study, as it would go beyond the scope of this study. Though in such a case, the classification power of rheumatoid factors might presumably be lower as high levels of rheumatoid factors are known to be present also in other diseases [11].

Measurement of anti-citrullinated peptide antibodies (ACPAs) in the context of RA shows higher specificity; in this study two peptide epitopes, one from fibrinogen β chain [14] and another one from filaggrin [9,22] protein were tested. These peptides represented the most dominant epitopes and were investigated in more detail ***(Figure 5)***. IgG reactivity against the citrullinated version of both fibrinogen β and filaggrin peptides were exclusively observed only in the sera of RA patients and not in controls. IgA reactivity against the citrullinated fibrinogen β peptide and C3 deposition also significantly discriminated RA patients from the controls. On the other hand, there were no significant differences between RA patients and controls regarding the IgM reactivity against both of the peptides. Especially in case of the filaggrin peptide, IgM autoantibodies recognizing even the native form of the peptide were present in sera of both RA patients and controls. These findings are in agreement with the results of our previous study, where the same filaggrin peptide pair was utilized in a planar protein microarray system [43]. As revealed by the strong correlation between anti-IgM and anti-C3 signal intensities (r> 0.8), the IgM autoantibodies against the filaggrin peptide present in sera of both sample cohorts could activate the complement system and did not result in a significant difference between RA patients and controls regarding the C3 levels.

Pratesi *et al.* suggested that also citrullinated forms of viral proteins such as the Epstein-Barr virus nuclear antigen 1 can be targets of ACPAs [16]. However, we utilized here only the native form of the EBNA-1 recombinant protein as a representative viral antigen and not because of any potential relevance to RA. Based on the fact that the majority of the population worldwide is seropositive for EBV, antibodies in sera against the immunodominant EBNA-1 protein are widespread [44] and we have confirmed this in our study as well ***(Figure 6A)***. Yet, we observed that EBNA-1 specific IgM reactivity significantly differed between RA patients and the controls. To elucidate this observation further, we investigated the correlation between the IgM reactivity against EBNA-1 and the level of rheumatoid factors of IgM isotype, which indeed revealed a strong correlation ***(Figure S4)***. Thus, the difference between RA patients and controls regarding the IgM reactivity against EBNA-1 is presumably caused as a pitfall by the presence of rheumatoid factors of IgM isotype in RA patient sera. Also Henle *et al.* previously found that rheumatoid factors can cause false-positive results in tests for EBNA-1 specific IgM antibodies [45]. The high level of complement-activating EBNA-1 specific IgG antibodies presumably overrode the complement activation of rheumatoid factors since the C3 signal intensities for EBNA-1 was high in sera of both the RA patients and controls. The interfering effect of rheumatoid factors regarding the EBNA-1 reactivity dictated to separately investigate the data derived from the RA patients and controls. In the control group, where the interfering effect of rheumatoid factors was not present, there was a very strong correlation (r = 0.898) between complement activation and IgG level ***(Figure 6B)***. IgA reactivity against EBNA-1 in a portion of the individuals was present in both sample groups. EBNA-1 protein contains a glycil-alanine (Gly-Ala) repeat region that was found as a dominant IgA antigen epitope for instance in patients with nasopharyngeal carcinoma but it was also shown that non-diseased serum samples might represent IgA reactivity against it, although with lower prevalence [46].

In conclusion, the findings we present here illustrate that antigen-specific immunoglobulin reactivity of various isotypes towards autoantigens or viral antigens and antigen-specific complement activation can be measured within the same assay and in a multiplex format using the suspension bead array platform. Measuring the C3 deposition allowed here to assess the joint effect of the three different possible complement pathways. Here we detected auto- and viral antigen-specific antibodies in the sera of RA patients and non-diseased controls, we investigated their complement activating properties and we also showed that rheumatoid factors have an interfering effect on complement activation measurement potentially causing false positive results. The suspension bead array-based workflow we developed and implemented here can be utilized to investigate any other autoimmune or infectious disease where the presence of complement activating antibodies has diagnostic value. Therefore, the presented approach is an important advancement for the analysis of autoantibody- or virus-associated immune pathologies.

Supporting Information

Figure S1 Classification power of rheumatoid factors and their complement activating properties. C3 fragment deposition and binding of IgM, IgG, IgA antibodies were measured on human-IgG coupled beads incubated with sera of 40 non-diseased controls and 41 RA patients. Receiver operating characteristic (ROC) curves and area under the curve (AUC) values are displayed on the figure.

Figure S2 Correlation between the bead array and ELISA measurements. ***A)*** Level of human IgG-specific IgM was determined in sera of RA patients by ELISA and on the bead array platform. Here, an ELISA plate was coated overnight with 5 µg/ml of human IgG in 0.05 M carbonate buffer, pH 9.5. Following washing with PBS-Tween, wells were blocked with blocking buffer (1% BSA, 0.05% Tween in PBS) at 37°C for 30 min. Wells were incubated in 200x diluted serum sample (diluted in blocking buffer) at 37°C for 1h. Following washing, bound human IgM was detected by rabbit anti-human IgM-HRP conjugate at 37°C for 1h. After TMB substrate development, OD was measured at 450 nm (reference 620 nm). ***B)*** Peptide-specific IgG levels in sera of RA patients and controls were also measured both by ELISA and on the bead array platform. For ELISA measurements, biotinylated peptides (1 µg/ml in PBS) were bound to neutravidin (5 µg/ml in PBS) pre-coated plates. Following washing with PBS-Tween, plates were blocked with blocking buffer (150 mM NaCl, 2% BSA in PBS) at 37°C for 30 min, then serum samples were added (1:100) in dilution buffer (2 M NaCl, 2% BSA in PBS). After an overnight incubation and washing the plate, rabbit anti-human IgG-HRP conjugate was added for 1h. Following TMB substrate development, OD was measured at 450 nm (reference 620 nm). The values derived from the ELISA and the bead array platform are plotted and Spearman' Rho correlation coefficients are indicated. OD - optical density; ELISA - enzyme-linked immunosorbent assay.

Figure S3 Presence of and pre-adsorption against neutravidin-specific antibodies in sera. ***A)*** Protein microarray technique was applied to determine the neutravidin-specific IgG and IgM levels in sera of each of the controls and RA patients. In short, 0.33 mg/ml neutravidin was printed in triplicates onto nitrocellulose covered glass slides by BioOdyssey Calligrapher miniarrayer (Bio-Rad). Following washing steps with PBS, slides were incubated with 1:20 diluted serum sample (25 mM EDTA, 5% BSA, 0.05% Tween 20 in PBS) at 37°C for 1h. Bound antibodies were detected by 1:2500 diluted DyLight 488-conjugated F(ab')$_2$ fragment of goat anti-human IgM (μ chain specific) and DyLight 649-conjugated F(ab')$_2$ fragment of goat anti-human IgG, (γ chain specific) (Jackson ImmunoResearch) antibodies. The neutravidin-specific IgG and IgM fluorescence intensity (FI) values of each serum sample are plotted. The arrow indicates the selected serum sample that was used in further experiments on the bead array platform. ***B)*** Neutravidin or EBNA-1 coupled beads were incubated in 1:10 diluted, untreated (black) or neutravidin pre-adsorbed (gray) serum. Here, serum was diluted in Ca^{2+}-Mg^{2+} - supplemented buffer for C3 detection and in EDTA-supplemented buffer for IgG and IgM detection. Neutravidin pre-adsorption diminished neutravidin-specific C3 and IgG levels, while it substantially decreased IgM levels. Neutravidin pre-adsorption had no effect on EBNA-1-specific signal intensities. ***C)*** Furthermore, neutravidin pre-adsorption had no effect on overall complement activation: classical pathway activator human IgG and alternative pathway activator properdin were coupled on beads at varying concentrations and incubated with 1:10 diluted, untreated (black square) or neutravidin pre-adsorbed (gray circle) serum. C3 fragment deposition was detected by the anti-human C3-PE antibody and the plots display the resulting MFI values.

Figure S4 Correlation between anti-IgM signal intensities for the viral antigen EBNA-1 and for human IgG-coupled beads. Anti-IgM MFI values for EBNA-1-coupled beads and for human IgG- coupled beads are plotted and Spearman's Rho correlation coefficient is indicated.

Figure S5 Distribution of anti-C3 signal intensities for properdin-coupled beads. Anti-C3 MFI values for all the tested serum samples on properdin-coupled beads are plotted. MFI values for all the samples were within 3 standard deviations (± 3SD) of the median.

Author Contributions

Conceived and designed the experiments: KP JP GS PN. Performed the experiments: KP BA ESZ KH AO FB AM FH. Analyzed the data: KP BA KH. Contributed reagents/materials/analysis tools: GYN BR TG. Wrote the paper: KP BA JMS PN JP.

References

1. Price JV, Haddon DJ, Kemmer D, Delepine G, Mandelbaum G, et al. (2013) Protein microarray analysis reveals BAFF-binding autoantibodies in systemic lupus erythematosus. J Clin Invest 123: 5135–5145.
2. Ayoglu B, Haggmark A, Khademi M, Olsson T, Uhlen M, et al. (2013) Autoantibody profiling in multiple sclerosis using arrays of human protein fragments. Mol Cell Proteomics 12: 2657–2672.
3. Miersch S, Bian X, Wallstrom G, Sibani S, Logvinenko T, et al. (2013) Serological autoantibody profiling of type 1 diabetes by protein arrays. J Proteomics 94: 486–496.
4. Prechl J, Papp K, Erdei A (2010) Antigen microarrays: descriptive chemistry or functional immunomics? Trends Immunol 31: 133–137.
5. Dunkelberger JR, Song WC (2010) Complement and its role in innate and adaptive immune responses. Cell Res 20: 34–50.
6. Walport MJ (2001) Complement. First of two parts. N Engl J Med 344: 1058–1066.
7. McInnes IB, Schett G (2007) Cytokines in the pathogenesis of rheumatoid arthritis. Nat Rev Immunol 7: 429–442.
8. Masson-Bessière C, Sebbag M, Girbal-Neuhauser E, Nogueira L, Vincent C, et al. (2001) The major synovial targets of the rheumatoid arthritis-specific antifilaggrin autoantibodies are deiminated forms of the alpha- and beta-chains of fibrin. Journal of immunology (Baltimore, Md: 1950) 166: 4177–4184.
9. Schellekens GA, de Jong BA, van den Hoogen FH, van de Putte LB, van Venrooij WJ (1998) Citrulline is an essential constituent of antigenic determinants recognized by rheumatoid arthritis-specific autoantibodies. The Journal of clinical investigation 101: 273–281.
10. Jónsson T, Valdimarsson H (1993) Is measurement of rheumatoid factor isotypes clinically useful? Annals of the rheumatic diseases 52: 161–164.
11. Shmerling RH, Delbanco TL (1991) The rheumatoid factor: an analysis of clinical utility. The American journal of medicine 91: 528–534.
12. Wegner N, Lundberg K, Kinloch A, Fisher B, Malmström V, et al. (2010) Autoimmunity to specific citrullinated proteins gives the first clues to the etiology of rheumatoid arthritis. Immunological reviews 233: 34–54.
13. Simon M, Girbal E, Sebbag M, Gomes-Daudrix V, Vincent C, et al. (1993) The cytokeratin filament-aggregating protein filaggrin is the target of the so-called "antikeratin antibodies," autoantibodies specific for rheumatoid arthritis. J Clin Invest 92: 1387–1393.
14. Sebbag M, Moinard N, Auger I, Clavel C, Arnaud J, et al. (2006) Epitopes of human fibrin recognized by the rheumatoid arthritis-specific autoantibodies to citrullinated proteins. European journal of immunology 36: 2250–2263.
15. Klareskog L, Catrina AI, Paget S (2009) Rheumatoid arthritis. Lancet 373: 659–672.
16. Pratesi F, Tommasi C, Anzilotti C, Chimenti D, Migliorini P (2006) Deiminated Epstein-Barr virus nuclear antigen 1 is a target of anti-citrullinated protein antibodies in rheumatoid arthritis. Arthritis and rheumatism 54: 733–741.
17. Levitskaya J, Coram M, Levitsky V, Imreh S, Steigerwald-Mullen PM, et al. (1995) Inhibition of antigen processing by the internal repeat region of the Epstein-Barr virus nuclear antigen-1. Nature 375: 685–688.
18. Paramita DK, Fatmawati C, Juwana H, Schaijk FGV, Fachiroh J, et al. (2011) Humoral Immune Responses to Epstein – Barr Virus Encoded Tumor Associated Proteins and Their Putative Extracellular Domains in Nasopharyngeal Carcinoma Patients and Regional Controls. 678: 665–678.
19. Young LS, Rickinson AB (2004) Epstein-Barr virus: 40 years on. Nat Rev Cancer 4: 757–768.
20. Drobin K, Nilsson P, Schwenk JM (2013) Highly multiplexed antibody suspension bead arrays for plasma protein profiling. Methods Mol Biol 1023: 137–145.
21. Aletaha D, Neogi T, Silman AJ, Funovits J, Felson DT, et al. (2010) 2010 rheumatoid arthritis classification criteria: an American College of Rheumatology/European League Against Rheumatism collaborative initiative. Ann Rheum Dis 69: 1580–1588.
22. Babos F, Szarka E, Nagy G, Majer Z, Sarmay G, et al. (2013) Role of N- or C-terminal biotinylation in autoantibody recognition of citrullin containing filaggrin epitope peptides in rheumatoid arthritis. Bioconjug Chem 24: 817–827.
23. Bartos A, Uray K, Hudecz F (2009) New biotin derivatives for labeling and solubilizing IgG peptides. Biopolymers 92: 110–115.
24. Team RDC (2011) R: A language and environment for statistical computing. R Foundation for Statistical Computing.
25. Roos A, Bouwman LH, van Gijlswijk-Janssen DJ, Faber-Krol MC, Stahl GL, et al. (2001) Human IgA activates the complement system via the mannan-binding lectin pathway. J Immunol 167: 2861–2868.
26. Seino J, Eveleigh P, Warnaar S, van Haarlem LJ, van Es LA, et al. (1993) Activation of human complement by mouse and mouse/human chimeric monoclonal antibodies. Clinical and experimental immunology 94: 291–296.
27. Seelen MA, Roos A, Wieslander J, Mollnes TE, Sjoholm AG, et al. (2005) Functional analysis of the classical, alternative, and MBL pathways of the complement system: standardization and validation of a simple ELISA. J Immunol Methods 296: 187–198.
28. Mollnes TE, Jokiranta TS, Truedsson L, Nilsson B, Rodriguez de Cordoba S, et al. (2007) Complement analysis in the 21st century. Mol Immunol 44: 3838–3849.
29. Papp K, Szekeres Z, Terenyi N, Isaak A, Erdei A, et al. (2007) On-chip complement activation adds an extra dimension to antigen microarrays. Mol Cell Proteomics 6: 133–140.
30. Wahrmann M, Exner M, Regele H, Derfler K, Körmöczi GF, et al. (2003) Flow cytometry based detection of HLA alloantibody mediated classical complement activation. Journal of Immunological Methods 275: 149–160.
31. Wahrmann M, Exner M, Haidbauer B, Schillinger M, Regele H, et al. (2005) [C4d]FlowPRA screening—a specific assay for selective detection of complement-activating anti-HLA alloantibodies. Human immunology 66: 526–534.

32. Wahrmann M, Exner M, Schillinger M, Haidbauer B, Regele H, et al. (2006) Pivotal role of complement-fixing HLA alloantibodies in presensitized kidney allograft recipients. American journal of transplantation: official journal of the American Society of Transplantation and the American Society of Transplant Surgeons 6: 1033–1041.
33. Wahrmann M, Bartel G, Exner M, Regele H, Körmöczi GF, et al. (2009) Clinical relevance of preformed C4d-fixing and non-C4d-fixing HLA single antigen reactivity in renal allograft recipients. Transplant international: official journal of the European Society for Organ Transplantation 22: 982–989.
34. Smith JD, Hamour IM, Banner NR, Rose ML (2007) C4d fixing, luminex binding antibodies - a new tool for prediction of graft failure after heart transplantation. American journal of transplantation: official journal of the American Society of Transplantation and the American Society of Transplant Surgeons 7: 2809–2815.
35. Chen G, Sequeira F, Tyan DB (2011) Novel C1q assay reveals a clinically relevant subset of human leukocyte antigen antibodies independent of immunoglobulin G strength on single antigen beads. Human immunology 72: 849–858.
36. Trouw LA, Haisma EM, Levarht EWN, van der Woude D, Ioan-Facsinay A, et al. (2009) Anti-cyclic citrullinated peptide antibodies from rheumatoid arthritis patients activate complement via both the classical and alternative pathways. Arthritis and rheumatism 60: 1923–1931.
37. Hourcade DE (2006) The role of properdin in the assembly of the alternative pathway C3 convertases of complement. J Biol Chem 281: 2128–2132.
38. Harboe M, Ulvund G, Vien L, Fung M, Mollnes TE (2004) The quantitative role of alternative pathway amplification in classical pathway induced terminal complement activation. Clinical and experimental immunology 138: 439–446.
39. Papp K, Vegh P, Hobor R, Erdei A, Prechl J (2012) Characterization of factors influencing on-chip complement activation to optimize parallel measurement of antibody and complement proteins on antigen microarrays. J Immunol Methods 375: 75–83.
40. Okroj M, Heinegård D, Holmdahl R, Blom AM (2007) Rheumatoid arthritis and the complement system. Annals of medicine 39: 517–530.
41. Gioud-Paquet M, Auvinet M, Raffin T, Girard P, Bouvier M, et al. (1987) IgM rheumatoid factor (RF), IgA RF, IgE RF, and IgG RF detected by ELISA in rheumatoid arthritis. Annals of the rheumatic diseases 46: 65–71.
42. Visser H, Gelinck LB, Kampfraath aH, Breedveld FC, Hazes JM (1996) Diagnostic and prognostic characteristics of the enzyme linked immunosorbent rheumatoid factor assays in rheumatoid arthritis. Annals of the Rheumatic Diseases 55: 157–161.
43. Szarka E, Babos F, Magyar A, Huber K, Szittner Z, et al. (2013) Recognition of new citrulline containing peptide epitopes by autoantibodies produced in vivo and in vitro by B cells of Rheumatoid arthritis patients. Immunology.
44. Fachiroh J, Schouten T, Hariwiyanto B, Paramita DK, Harijadi A, et al. (2004) Molecular diversity of Epstein-Barr virus IgG and IgA antibody responses in nasopharyngeal carcinoma: a comparison of Indonesian, Chinese, and European subjects. The Journal of infectious diseases 190: 53–62.
45. Henle G, Lennette ET, Alspaugh Ma, Henle W (1979) Rheumatoid factor as a cause of positive reactions in tests for Epstein-Barr virus-specific IgM antibodies. Clinical and experimental immunology 36: 415–422.
46. Mathew A, Cheng HM, Sam CK, Prasad U (1994) Serum IgA cross-reactivity between glycine-alanine repeat sequence of EBNA-1 and keratin or collagen in nasopharyngeal carcinoma. Clinical immunology and immunopathology 71: 164–168.

Clinical and Serological Features of Patients Referred through a Rheumatology Triage System because of Positive Antinuclear Antibodies

Christie Fitch-Rogalsky[1], Whitney Steber[1], Michael Mahler[2], Terri Lupton[1], Liam Martin[1], Susan G. Barr[1], Dianne P. Mosher[1], James Wick[1], Marvin J. Fritzler[1]*

1 Faculty of Medicine, University of Calgary, Calgary, Alberta, Canada, **2** INOVA Diagnostics Inc., San Diego, California, United States of America

Abstract

Background: The referral of patients with positive anti-nuclear antibody (ANA) tests has been criticized as an inappropriate use of medical resources. The utility of a positive ANA test in a central triage (CT) system was studied by determining the autoantibody profiles and clinical diagnoses of patients referred to rheumatologists through a CT system because of a positive ANA test.

Methods: Patients that met three criteria were included: (1) referred to Rheumatology CT over a three year interval; (2) reason for referral was a "positive ANA"; (3) were evaluated by a certified rheumatologist. The CT clinical database was used to obtain demographic and clinical information and a serological database was used to retrieve specific ANA and/or extractable nuclear antigen (ENA) test results. Clinical information was extracted from the consulting rheumatologist's report.

Results: 15,357 patients were referred through the CT system; 643 (4.1%) of these because of a positive ANA and of these 263 (40.9%) were evaluated by a certified rheumatologist. In 63/263 (24%) of ANA positive patients, the specialist provided a diagnosis of an ANA associated rheumatic disease (AARD) while 69 (26.2%) had no evidence of any disease; 102 (38.8%) had other rheumatologic diagnoses and 29 (11%) had conditions that did not meet AARD classification criteria. Of ANA positive archived sera, 15.1% were anti-DFS70 positive and 91.2% of these did not have an AARD.

Conclusions: This is the first study to evaluate the serological and clinical features of patients referred through a CT system because of a positive ANA. The spectrum of autoantibody specificities was wide with anti-Ro52/TRIM21 being the most common autoantibody detected. Approximately 15% of referrals had only antibodies to DFS70, the vast majority of which did not have clinical evidence for an AARD. These findings provide insight into the utility of autoantibody testing in a CT system.

Editor: Masataka Kuwana, Keio University School of Medicine, Japan

Funding: This project was funded and supported by resources from Mitogen Advanced Diagnostics Laboratory and as well as funds allocated to the Arthritis Society Research Chair by the University of Calgary, Division of Rheumatology, at the University of Calgary. The funders had no role in the study design, data collection and analysis, decision to publish, or preparation of the manuscript.

Competing Interests: This study was partly supported by the Mitogen Advanced Diagnostics Laboratory. M. Mahler is an employee of INOVA Diagnostics Inc. (San Diego), a manufacturer of autoantibody diagnostic kits. The HEp-2 slides were a kind gift from ImmunoConcepts Inc. (Sacramento, CA), and the anti-DFS70 assay kits were a gift of INOVA Diagnostics (San Diego, CA). M. Fritzler is a paid consultant, has received honoraria or has received gifts in kind from ImmunoConcepts Inc. (Sacramento, CA), Bio-Rad (Hercules, CA) and INOVA Diagnostics (San Diego, CA), Mikrogen GmbH (Neuried, Germany), Euroimmun GmbH (Lubeck, Germany) and Dr. Fooke Laboratorien GmbH (Neuss, Germany). There are no further patents, products in development or marketed products to declare. This does not alter adherence to all PLOS ONE policies on sharing data and materials, as detailed online in the guide for authors.

* E-mail: fritzler@ucalgary.ca

Introduction

The detection of anti-nuclear antibodies (ANA) has been established as an important adjunct to the diagnosis and classification of ANA-associated rheumatic diseases (AARD) such as systemic lupus erythematosus (SLE), systemic sclerosis (SSc), mixed connective tissue disease (MCTD), idiopathic inflammatory myopathies (IIM) and Sjögren's syndrome (SjS) [1]. Nevertheless, concerns have been raised about the ANA test as a screen for AARD [2,3] and that positive tests inappropriately prompt unwarranted referrals from primary and secondary care physicians to tertiary care specialists [4–6]. Some concerns about ANA tests as an approach to screening for AARD are based on studies of the frequency of ANA in the healthy individuals [7] and calculations of pre-test probabilities and the clinical challenge of interpreting a positive test when the patient has no apparent evidence for a definitive diagnosis of, nor meets the classification criteria for, an AARD [3–5,8].

The limitations of ANA and the related ENA tests have been offset by at least three key findings. First, for several decades it has been appreciated that some autoantibodies are highly specific for certain AARD [9,10]. Hence, when disease specific autoantibodies, such as anti-dsDNA antibodies in SLE, anti-centromere antibodies in SSc and anti-Jo-1 antibodies in IIM are detected in the absence of diagnostic or classification criteria for these conditions the clinician is often uncertain about the advice to give to the referring physician or the patient. This issue is linked to a second key finding wherein it now well established that ANA and disease-specific autoantibodies can pre-date the clinical diagnosis of AARD by as many as two decades [11–13]. Thus, in the context of a person with a positive ANA where the specific autoantibody is known, the physician should take care before advising the patient that they do not have an AARD. Third, there is growing evidence that autoantibodies directed against the dense fine speckled 70 (DFS70) antigen without accompanying disease specific antibodies are rare in AARD and may be useful biomarker to rule out these conditions [14–17]. All three of these issues are of particular importance when patients are referred to a rheumatology central triage system because of a positive ANA test. Key questions are: 1) are such referrals inappropriate and a waste of health care resources, and 2) can the specificities of ANA and related autoantibodies inform the triage process to define the urgency of a specific referral to a specialist? Accordingly, the goals of this study were firstly to examine the ANA/ENA profiles of patients referred through a rheumatology central triage system; secondly, to determine if ANA/ENA of a given specificity were attended by a specific diagnosis and, thirdly, to determine the frequency of autoantibodies directed to DFS70 in a ANA referral cohort and elucidate the possible association of these antibodies to a specific diagnosis.

Materials and Methods

Ethics Statement

This study was approved by the University of Calgary Conjoint Health Research Ethics Board (Ethics ID#: E-24353). Under the terms of this approval, all patient records and information was anonymized and de-identified prior to analysis, precluding the requirement of written informed consent. All clinical investigation was conducted according to the principles expressed in the Declaration of Helsinki.

Patients, Selection Criteria, Demographic and Clinical Information

We utilized an anonymous administrative database to evaluate the utility of autoantibody testing in the context of triage of referrals to the rheumatology service through a Central Referral and Triage (CReATe) service in the Calgary Health Region (Calgary, Alberta, Canada). This database includes the reason that the patient was referred for consultation, such as abnormal laboratory tests, signs or symptoms thought to suggest a rheumatic disease as well as baseline demographic data, working diagnoses and wait times. Of particular relevance to this study was the identification of patients referred to the rheumatology service because they had a positive ANA (ANA Referral Cohort: ARC). All individuals included in the ARC met the following criteria: (1) referred to Rheumatology Central Triage from in a sequential three year calendar time frame (n = 15,537); (2) reason for referral was a "positive ANA (n = 643); (3) were evaluated by certified rheumatology specialists at regional referral centres (n = 263) in Calgary, Alberta, Canada.

After the patient was seen by the consulting rheumatologist, a form was completed and information expressing the appropriateness of triage and final diagnosis was entered into the database. Final diagnoses were categorized as non-inflammatory disorders (e.g. fibromyalgia, osteoarthritis, tendonitis, and bursitis) or inflammatory diseases, including AARDs, rheumatoid arthritis (RA) and other systemic inflammatory arthritis. Accordingly, patients were grouped into three diagnostic categories (AARD, non-AARD and unresolved AARD). The AARD group included patients with a diagnosis of SLE, SSc, MCTD, IIM and SjS. The non-AARD included patients who had a definitive diagnosis but AARD was excluded. The third group (unresolved) consisted of patients without a final diagnosis or patients in which AARD insufficient classification criteria were not met and AARD could not be ruled out.

A second anonymous database that contained the serological data (see below) was extracted from the Mitogen Advanced Diagnostics Laboratory (MADL), Calgary, Alberta, Canada) master database. The two anonymous databases (CReATe and MADL) devoid of unique patient identifiers were merged using an anchored scrambled unique alphanumeric lifetime identifier (ULI) in order to maintain confidentiality.

A descriptive analysis of the combined dataset was performed, including the origin and number of referrals and autoantibody tests and results, triage categories, wait times and any delays in patient care resulting from requests for autoantibody tests. The number of patients referred because of a positive ANA test and their final diagnoses was tabulated. The primary analysis was the ability of an individual autoantibody to predict the diagnosis recorded by the consulting rheumatologist. This was gauged by determining the sensitivity, specificity, positive predictive value, negative predictive value and likelihood ratios for each test in relation to the final diagnosis, as well as the diagnostic categories described above. Secondary outcomes included the ability of individual or combined autoantibody results to predict the working diagnosis and triage category in order to assess how these results influence the triage process as it is currently designed. Agreement between the working diagnosis and the final diagnosis was assessed as a marker of referral quality.

Autoantibody Testing

The MADL performs ANA and ENA tests for the Calgary Health Region and surrounding catchment areas. ANA testing (including pattern and titer assessment) utilized HEp-2 cell substrates (HEp-2000, ImmunoConcepts Inc., Sacramento, CA) to screen for autoantibodies by indirect immunofluorescence (IIF) at a dilution of 1/160 [7] on the sera stored at MADL. All available samples were also tested for ANA specificities included in the ENA screening panel (chromatin, ribosomal P, Sm, U1RNP (ribonucleoprotein), SS-A/Ro60, Ro52/TRIM21, SS-B/La, Scl-70 (topoisomerase I), Jo-1 (histidyl tRNA synthetase) by addressable laser bead immunoassay (FIDIS, TheraDiag: Paris, France), anti-centromere by IIF pattern on HEp-2 cells and dsDNA by the *Crithidia lucilliae* IIF test (ImmunoConcepts, Sacramento, CA) [18]. Last, antibodies to DFS70/LEDGF were detected by a chemiluminescent immunoassay (QUANTA Flash DFS70, INOVA Diagnostics, San Diego, CA)[16,17].

Statistics

The data were evaluated using the Analyse-it software (Version 1.62; Analyse-it Software, Ltd., Leeds, UK). Positive and negative likelihood ratios (LR) were calculated for the individual autoantibodies. For statistical analysis, patients were grouped into AARD (SLE, SSc, SjS, IIM and MCTD) and non-AARD patients. Individuals in which diagnosis was not fully established and verified or in which AARD could not be ruled out were excluded from respective analyses.

Results

The clinical spectrum and referral diagnosis of all 15,357 patients referred to the Rheumatology service is represented in Figure 1. The majority of referrals were for evaluation of an inflammatory arthropathy (23.9%), arthralgia (26.6%) or a previously diagnosed AARD (12.1%), while smaller proportions were referred for consultation with respect to management of spondyloarthropathy (7.3%), osteoarthritis (6.7%), soft tissue rheumatism (3.1%) or vasculitis (1.4%). The ARC cohort of 263 patients from this referral group had an average age of 48.7 years (range 18–86, SD 83.53) and 92% were female. Approximately 68% of patients were referred from an urban center and 83.7% were referred by a family physician while the remainder were referred by subspecialist physicians: (in order of decreasing frequency) general internal medicine, neurology, respirology, otolaryngology, ophthalmology, dermatology, cardiology, hematology, obstetrics, general surgery, psychiatry. The mean interval from date of referral to when the patient was seen by the consultant was 165.4 days (range 25–551 days; SD 83.53).

Clinical information of the 263 ARC is summarized in Table 1. In total, 24% (n = 63) had a diagnosis of an AARD: SLE (9.1%; n = 24), SjS (9.1%; n = 24), SSc (2.3%; n = 6) and MCTD (1.9%; n = 5) followed by a spectrum of other AARDs or closely related conditions. Twenty-nine patients (11%) had equivocal evidence for an AARD and either did not meet sufficient criteria for classification or the consulting physician was unable to provide a definitive diagnosis (i.e. unresolved diagnosis): 13 (4.9%) undifferentiated connective tissue disease, 8 (3%) Raynaud's phenomenon, 5 (1.9%) inflammatory polyarthropathy and 3 (1.1%) discoid or cutaneous lupus. By comparison, 102 (38.8%) had a rheumatologic diagnosis but did not have an AARD, with osteoarthritis (9.9%), fibromyalgia (8.7%), arthralgia/myalgia (7.9%) and rheumatoid arthritis (RA) (2.3%) being the most common. Of note, 69 (26.2%) patients had no evidence for either an autoimmune or rheumatic disease. One hundred and sixteen patients (44.1%) of the ARC had a positive ENA test with the most common specificity being autoantibodies directed to Ro52/TRIM21 (n = 53; 45.7%), SS-A/Ro60 (n = 40; 34.5%), chromatin (n = 21; 18.5%), and SS-B/La (n = 19; 16.4%) (Table 2). The consultant's diagnosis linked to these anti-ENA autoantibodies is shown in Table S1 in File S1.

The IIF results of the ARC showed that the three most common primary ANA IIF patterns were speckled (n = 158; 60.1%),

Table 1. Consultant's Opinion of 263 Patients in the ARC.

Consultant's Diagnosis	N	%
AARD	**63**	**24**
Systemic lupus erythematosus	24	9.1
Sjögren's syndrome	24	9.1
Systemic sclerosis	6	2.3
Mixed connective tissue disease	5	1.9
Drug-induced lupus	2	0.8
Dermatomyositis	2	0.8
Unresolved AARD	**29**	**11**
Undifferentiated connective tissue disease	13	4.9
Raynaud's phenomenon	8	3.0
Inflammatory polyarthropathy	5	1.9
Discoid and cutaneous lupus	3	1.1
Other rheumatologic diagnoses	**102**	**38.8**
Osteoarthritis	26	9.9
Fibromyalgia	23	8.7
Arthralgia/myalgia	21	7.9
Rheumatoid arthritis	6	2.3
Neuromuscular/neuropathy	6	2.3
Mechanical back pain	5	1.9
Vasculitis/polymyalgia rheumatica	2	0.8
Other*	13	4.9
No findings for rheumatic or autoimmune disease	**69**	**26.2**

*Other includes gout, tendonitis, bursitis, patellofemoral syndrome, palindromic rheumatism, spondyloarthropathy, psoriatic arthritis, unspecified polyarthropathy.

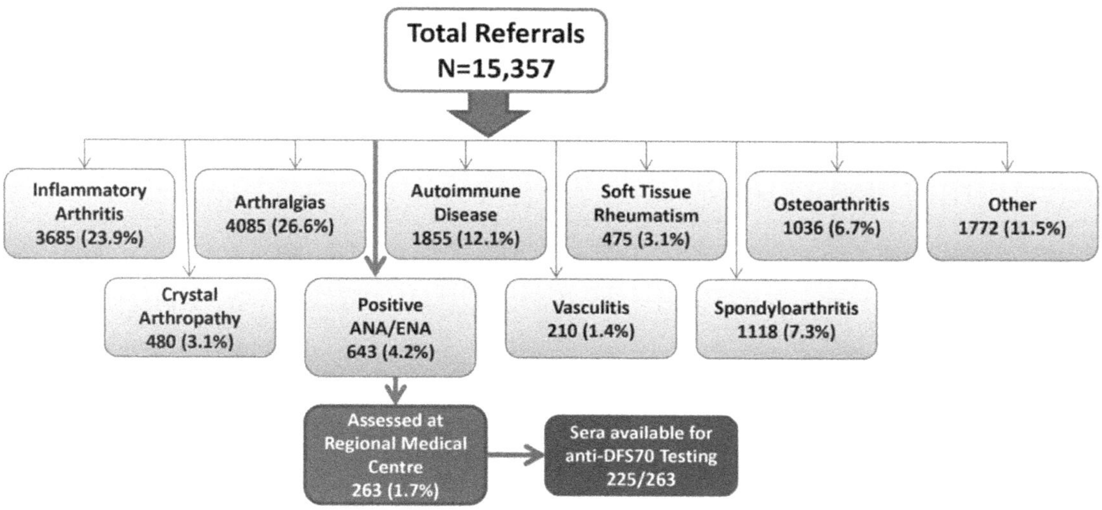

Figure 1. Derivation of the ARC via the diagnostic profile of 15,537 patients referred to rheumatology central triage over a three year audit period.

Table 2. Autoantibody Specificities of the 116 patients in the ARC with a positive anti-ENA*.

ENA Autoantibody**	N	%
Ro52/TRIM21	53	45.7
SS-A/Ro60	40	34.5
Chromatin	21	18.1
SS-B/La	19	16.4
Topoisomerase I (Scl-70)	17	14.7
U1 Ribonucleoprotein	17	14.7
Sm	14	12.1
Ribosomal P*	10	13.2
dsDNA*	10	13.2
Centromere	3	2.6
Jo-1	3	2.6
Unidentified	1	0.8

Note: 116/263 patients referred with a positive ANA had a detectable ENA autoantibody. Some patients had more than 1 autoantibody, hence % totals will not = 100.
*results available for 76 samples.
**Clinical diagnoses associated with specific autoantibodies see Table S1 in File S1.

nucleolar (n = 66; 25.1%), and homogeneous speckled (n = 55; 20.9%), with titers ranging from 1/160-1/5120 (Table S2 in File S1). Other IIF staining patterns included cytoplasmic (27.4%), multiple nuclear dots (26%), nuclear matrix and centromere (7.6%) and other less common patterns (Table S2 in File S1).

Anti-DFS70 antibodies

Thirty-four of the 225 (15.1%) archived sera tested positive for anti-DFS70 antibodies (Figure 2) and was the sole autoantibody detected in 24/34 (70.6%) of the sera. Among the anti-DFS70 antibody positive cohort, 33 had a definite diagnosis (one was unresolved) and of those 31/33 (93.9%) had no evidence of or fulfilled classification criteria for an AARD (Figure 3). The two patients with an AARD had SjS (one with coexistent anti-Ro52/TRIM21 antibodies). Sixteen (47.1%) anti-DFS70 positive patients had no evidence for any disease although three of these had autoantibodies typically associated with an AARD: one with anti-Scl-70/topo I and two with anti-chromatin antibodies. Other diagnoses in the anti-DFS70 antibody positive patients included Raynaud's phenomenon, osteoarthritis, RA, fibromyalgia and individual patients with polymyalgia rheumatica and psoriatic arthritis (Figure 2).

To analyze if autoantibodies might provide value in determining the urgency of referral we calculated the LRs for all anti-ENAs and for anti-DFS70 antibodies (Figure 3). The LR+ for AARD showed significant variations ranging from 0.0 (anti-Jo-1 antibodies) to 8.6 (anti-Ribo-P antibodies). The LR+ for non-AARD for anti-DFS70 antibodies was 5.4 and when considered in conjunction with other autoantibodies (no coexisting antibody/monospecific for anti-DFS70 antibodies) the LR+ increase to 10.9. Clarity on the usefulness of ANA, anti-ENA and anti-DFS70 antibody testing was illustrated by a supervised cluster analysis (Figure 4).

Discussion

Diagnosis of Patients with Positive ANA/anti-ENA antibodies

One of the time honored adjuncts to diagnosis of AARD or the broader spectrum of systemic autoimmune rheumatic diseases is autoantibody testing. In most of these conditions, autoantibodies are included as part of validated disease classification criteria [19–22]. Accordingly, on the backdrop of a wide range of protean clinical signs and symptoms, autoantibody tests, and the ANA test in particular, are often used as a screening tool for AARD by referring physicians [3,5,23–25]. The referral of patients with positive ANA and/or ENA to tertiary care specialists is a common practice that has met with some criticism [3,5,23,26,27], with one claim being that because pre-test probabilities of AARD is low, such referrals are unnecessary and a burden on the health care system resulting increased wait times for rheumatology consultations. This can be complicated when the referring physician has told the patient that they do or do not have an AARD. Such misdiagnoses (over-diagnosis or under-diagnosis) can have emotional and insurability consequences for the patient and a serious negative impact on health care resources, including inappropriate or delays in appropriate therapy culminating in poor clinical outcomes, such as irreversible organ damage or failure [5,28–30]. These issues also have ethical implications [31] and algorithms for how cost-effective and rational autoantibody testing could be harmonized and developed into a standardized schema is gaining international attention [23,24,32,32–37].

In 1989 Shiel and Jason [38] reported that patients referred to a community rheumatologist because of a positive ANA with a titer of 1/40 or greater (comprising 8.8% of all referrals compared to 4.1% in our study) received a specific diagnosis in 86.6% and of those, 51.4% had a connective tissue disease [38]. An interesting study by Narain et al [5] reported that of 263 patients referred with a presumptive diagnosis of SLE, 48% received a diagnosis of other conditions and 29% were seropositive for ANA but did not have autoimmune disease. Disconcertedly, 39 patients who were seropositive for ANA but had no autoimmune disease had been treated with corticosteroids at dosages as high as 60 mg/d. By comparison, a more recent study by Abeles and Ables [27] found that none of the patients referred to a specialist clinic with an ANA titer of <1/160 had an AARD, and like previous studies [39], the majority had soft tissue rheumatism and other pain syndromes. In our study, where the screening ANA test was performed at a serum dilution of 1/160, approximately 27% of patients referred because of a positive ANA/ant-ENA antibody test had an AARD, approximately 10% had equivocal evidence for AARD, and the remainder had a wide variety of rheumatic (i.e. rheumatoid arthritis) and non-rheumatic conditions. In another study of 50 ANA positive patients that did not fulfill sufficient criteria for classification of SLE, anti-Ro60/SS-A and anti- La/SS-B antibodies were the most common detectable anti-ENA antibodies (6%) using a limited diagnostic profile and while none of the patients with leukopenia, thrombocytopenia, fatigue and arthralgia did not evolve to a full diagnosis of SLE, the authors concluded that ANA positivity connoted a form of systemic autoimmunity [40]. By comparison, patients with arthritis, rash, Raynaud's phenomenon and anti- Ro60/SS-A autoantibodies did evolve to SLE. These observations are interesting in the context of our study since we have initiated a longitudinal study to determine which ACR patients with a positive ANA or anti-ENA antibody test that did not meet criteria for an AARD evolve into an AARD such as SLE.

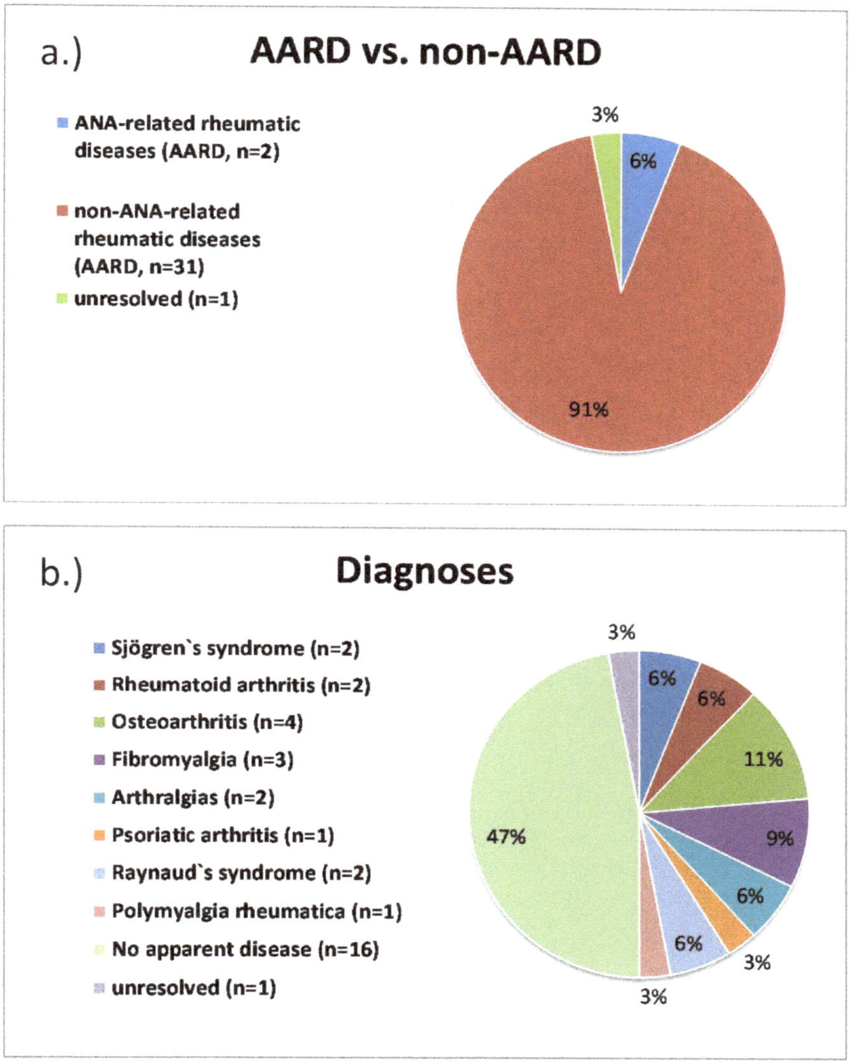

Figure 2. Clinical diagnoses of 34 patients with anti-DFS70 antibodies. Panel a.) frequency (%) of ANA-associated rheumatic diseases (AARD) and non-AARD. One patient with undifferentiated connective tissue disease did not match AARD or non-AARD and was classified as "unresolved". Panel b.) frequency of diagnoses of the patients with anti-DFS70 antibodies is shown.

The serum dilution at which screening ANA tests are performed lacks uniformity from laboratory to laboratory. A study by an international advisory committee comprised of representatives from fifteen participating laboratories concluded that the ANA screening dilution should be set at 1/160 to increase the specificity of the ANA test [7]. Nevertheless, as exemplified by the report of Abeles and Abeles [27] and others [38], many laboratories continue to test sera at lower screening dilutions. Based on our study it appears that even if the screening serum dilution is set at 1/160, more than one-half of patients do not have sufficient clinical evidence or classification criteria to make a diagnosis of an AARD at the time of evaluation by the consulting rheumatologist.

There is hope that a more thorough understanding of ANA and anti-ENA antibody specificities can help address some of the inherent shortcomings of ANA and anti-ENA antibody specificity and sensitivity. For example, mounting evidence indicates that the presence of anti-DFS70 antibodies is a useful biomarker found in ANA positive individuals the vast majority of whom did not have an AARD [14–17]. In the present study, approximately 15% of the ARC had antibodies directed to DFS70 and in the majority (73.5%) it was the only detectable autoantibody. Of these anti-DFS70 positive patients, only 2/33 (6.1%) had an AARD while approximately one-third had either no evidence for a disease or a variety of other non-AARD diagnoses such as osteoarthritis and fibromyalgia. In summation, our findings support previous studies indicating that anti-DFS70 antibodies tend to exclude the diagnosis of AARD [16,17,41] and the observation that the majority are "monospecific" for anti-DFS70 antibodies add further evidence to the potential value of routinely testing for these autoantibodies.

Use of Autoantibody Profiles to inform Patient Triage and Referral Systems

This is the first published study to evaluate the clinical diagnoses and serological parameters of patients referred to rheumatologists through a central triage system because of a positive ANA test. Access to rheumatologists is often inadequate to meet patient

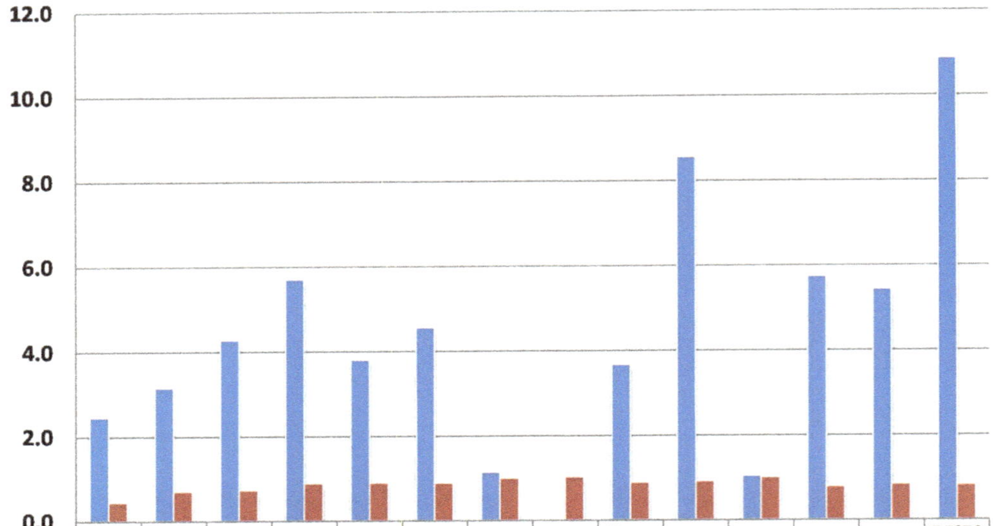

	ENA	Ro52	Ro60	SS-B	RNP	Sm	Scl-70	Jo-1	Chromatin	Rib	CENP	dsDNA	DFS70	DFS70 mono
Likelihood ratio (+)	2.5	3.2	4.3	5.7	3.8	4.6	1.1	0.0	3.7	8.6	1.0	5.7	5.4	10.9
Likelihood ratio (-)	0.4	0.7	0.7	0.9	0.9	0.9	1.0	1.0	0.9	0.9	1.0	0.8	0.8	0.8

Figure 3. Likelihood ratios differentiate AARD from non-AARD in ANA positive patients (n = 208, 55 excluded due to missing results; dsDNA based on 76 samples). NOTE: Anti-DFS70 positivity was indicative for non-AARD. 'DFS70 mono' represents patients that have anti-DFS70, but no other detectable autoantibody.

needs due to population growth, aging of the population, and a declining supply of specialists [42]. In our study, the average waiting time from referral to when the patient was seen by the consulting rheumatologist was 165 days (> five months). Although it is intuitive, there is evidence that an early and accurate diagnosis of patients with rheumatic diseases improves health outcomes while reducing health care costs [35,43–48]. In our study, the vast majority (~80%) of referrals for a positive ANA was from general practitioners (GPs) and at least one study has shown that the threshold used by GPs for referral to rheumatologists is low leading to lengthy wait times [49]. It was suggested that more frequent use of telephone consultations and improved diagnostic skills of GPs may alleviate the wait times. Another suggested approach was to use registered nurses and GPs themselves to do the triage [50], an approach that had a degree of diagnostic accuracy rivaling that of experienced rheumatologists. The limitation to this approach is that it seems an assumption that GPs are available for such activity because they are not as busy as rheumatologists. Using appropriately trained registered nurses and/or other allied health care personnel is the approach that we have taken to screen and adjudicate referrals as a "team" approach as recommended by others [51].

A key component to improving timely, efficient and appropriate access to specialist consultation and care is the ability of the triage team to assign a level of urgency to the referral. An effective and efficient triage system requires the formulation of a working diagnosis based on the information included in the referral letter [52]. This may be particularly difficult in rheumatology, as there are few diagnostic tests that can firmly establish a diagnosis. The diagnosis of AARD relies on a complete history, physical examination and investigations [34], and depends on the expertise of the care provider. In the context of rheumatology referrals

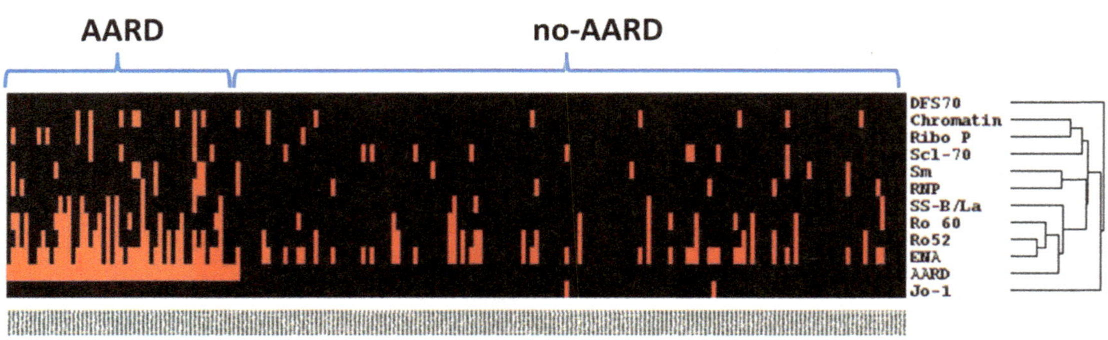

Figure 4. Supervised cluster analysis with patients sorted according to the presence or absence of ANA associated rheumatic disease (AARD) was performed with antibodies to extractable nuclear antigens (ENA), chromatin, ribosomal P and to DFS70. ENA, Ro52/TRIM21, SS-A/Ro60 and SS-B/La cluster most closely with AARD whereas DFS70 antibodies and Jo-1 demonstrate high distance clustering.

because of a positive ANA, our data suggest that patients with isolated anti-DFS70 autoantibodies do not require urgent referral to a specialist, whereas patients with anti-ENA antibodies and other AARD-specific autoantibodies, where early and accurate diagnosis is a goal, require rapid assessment for an AARD.

Limitations

This study was a cross-sectional study without patient follow-up to determine the longer term outcome of patients. The utility of ANA testing in a triage or referral setting or in diagnostic algorithms is complicated by a number of factors, most notably that autoantibodies often precede symptoms and overt evidence of disease by as much as two decades [53,54]. While this phenomenon is well established in medical literature, many physicians have yet to embrace the concept in their clinical evaluation of patients. To help understand the use of autoantibodies as predictors of diseases, the ARC in this study is being followed for long term clinical outcomes.

In addition, this study did not assess the economic impacts of the referral system. The cost effectiveness of autoantibody testing and its effective application to the clinical setting is clearly required [35], and if there were more effective ways to triage patients that will never develop an AARD, cost savings could be significant. To date, rather than a holistic cost-benefit analysis, cost analyses have tended to focus on the cost of the ANA test itself and related algorithms [3,23,36,37]. Of note, it has already been suggested that the detection of anti-DFS70 autoantibodies may result in meaningful cost savings [14,55] by the potential of reducing the additional testing in search of establishing the diagnosis of a systemic autoimmune rheumatic disease and in some cases the initiation of inappropriate therapy [5].

Future Considerations and Conclusions

With the emergence of novel biomarkers for AARD, it is thought that disease prevention and morbidity amelioration by establishing an early and accurate diagnosis will likely not rely on a single or any one class of biomarkers (i.e. autoantibody, genetic, metabolomic). Rather than a single autoantibody marker (i.e. anti-Scl-70/topo I, anti-dsDNA, anti-DFS70) it is likely that multiplexed autoantibody profiles will provide more important clinical information in the future. Our study suggests that the fine specificities of ANA and other autoantibodies are important to decide whether or not an urgent referral is needed. For example, based on other corroborating studies [15–17], our present study indicates that if the patient has isolated anti-DFS70 antibodies, then urgent referral is likely not required. However, if patients have certain anti-ENA, such as anti-dsDNA or anti-ribosomal P, then more urgent assessment is indicated.

Supporting Information

File S1 File contains Table S1 and Table S2. Table S1: Consultant Diagnosis of anti-ENA Antibody Positive Individuals. Table S2: Indirect Immunofluorescence Patterns of Sera from Patients in the Referral Cohort.

Acknowledgments

The authors acknowledge the technical support of Ms. Haiyan Hou, Jane Yang, Meifeng Zhang and the clinical input of the members of the Division of Rheumatology at the University of Calgary. The HEp-2 slides were a kind gift from ImmunoConcepts Inc. (Sacramento, CA) and the anti-DFS70 assay kits were a gift of INOVA Diagnostics (San Diego, CA).

Author Contributions

Conceived and designed the experiments: SB LM MJF. Performed the experiments: CR WS TL JW MJF. Analyzed the data: CR WS TL SB LM MM DM JW MJF. Contributed reagents/materials/analysis tools: MM MJF. Wrote the paper: CR WS MM MJF.

References

1. Mahler M, Fritzler MJ (2010) Epitope specificity and significance in systemic autoimmune diseases. Ann N Y Acad Sci 1183: 267–287.
2. Juby A, Johnston C, Davis P (1991) Specificity, sensitivity and diagnostic predictive value of selected laboratory generated autoantibody profiles in patients with connective tissue diseases. J Rheumatol 18: 354–358.
3. Man A, Shojania K, Phoon C, Pal J, de Badyn MH, et al. (2013) An evaluation of autoimmune antibody testing patterns in a Canadian health region and an evaluation of a laboratory algorithm aimed at reducing unnecessary testing. Clin Rheumatol 32: 601–608.
4. Esdaile JM, Joseph L, Abrahamowicz M, Li Y, Danoff D, et al. (1996) Routine immunologic tests in systemic lupus erythematosus: Is there a need for more studies? J Rheumatol 23: 1891–1896.
5. Narain S, Richards HB, Satoh M, Sarmiento M, Davidson R, et al. (2004) Diagnostic accuracy for lupus and other systemic autoimmune diseases in the community setting. Arch Intern Med 164: 2435–2441.
6. Yazdany J, Schmajuk G, Robbins M, Daikh D, Beall A, et al. (2013) Choosing wisely: the American College of Rheumatology's Top 5 list of things physicians and patients should question. Arthritis Care Res (Hoboken) 65: 329–339.
7. Tan EM, Feltkamp TEW, Smolen JS, Butcher B, Dawkins R, et al. (1997) Range of antinuclear antibodies in "healthy" individuals. Arthritis Rheum 40: 1601–1611.
8. Suarez-Almazor ME, Gonzalez-Lopez L, Gamez-Nava JI, Belseck E, Kendall CJ, et al. (1998) Utilization and predictive value of laboratory tests in patients referred to rheumatologists by primary care physicians. J Rheumatol 25: 1980–1985.
9. von Muhlen CA, Tan EM (1995) Autoantibodies in the diagnosis of systemic rheumatic disease. Semin Arthritis Rheum 24: 323–358.
10. Wiik AS (2005) Anti-nuclear autoantibodies: clinical utility for diagnosis, prognosis, monitoring, and planning of treatment strategy in systemic immunoinflammatory diseases. Scand J Rheumatol 34: 260–268.
11. Arbuckle MR, McClain MT, Rubertone MV, Scofield RH, Dennis GJ, et al. (2003) Development of autoantibodies before the clinical onset of systemic lupus erythematosus. N Engl J Med 349: 1526–1533.
12. Heinlen LD, McClain MT, Merrill J, Akbarali YW, Edgerton CC, et al. (2007) Clinical criteria for systemic lupus erythematosus precede diagnosis, and associated autoantibodies are present before clinical symptoms. Arthritis Rheum 56: 2344–2351.
13. Conrad K, Schlösser W, Fritzler MJ (2007) The predictive relevance of autoantibodies. In: Conrad K, Chan EKL, Fritzler MJ, Sack U, Shoenfeld Y, et al. editors. From Etiopathogenesis to the Prediction of Autoimmune Diseases: Relevance of Autoantibodies. Langerich, Germany: Pabst Scientific Publishers. pp. 16–31.
14. Muro Y, Sugiura K, Morita Y, Tomita Y (2008) High concomitance of disease marker autoantibodies in anti-DFS70/LEDGF autoantibody-positive patients with autoimmune rheumatic disease. Lupus 17: 171–176.
15. Mahler M, Hanly JG, Fritzler MJ (2012) Importance of the dense fine speckled pattern on HEp-2 cells and anti-DFS70 antibodies for the diagnosis of systemic autoimmune diseases. Autoimmun Rev 11: 642–645.
16. Mahler M, Parker T, Peebles CL, Andrade LE, Swart A, et al. (2012) Anti-DFS70/LEDGF Antibodies Are More Prevalent in Healthy Individuals Compared to Patients with Systemic Autoimmune Rheumatic Diseases. J Rheumatol 39: 2104–2110.
17. Miyara M, Albesa R, Charuel JL, El Amri M, Fritzler MJ, et al. (2013) Clinical phenotypes of patients with anti-DFS70/LEDGF antibodies in a routine ANA referral cohort. Clin Dev Immunol 2013: 703759.
18. Stinton LM, Barr SG, Tibbles LA, Yilmaz S, Sar A, et al. (2007) Autoantibodies in lupus nephritis patients requiring renal transplantation. Lupus 16: 394–400.
19. Petri M, Orbai AM, Alarcon GS, Gordon C, Merrill JT, et al. (2012) Derivation and validation of systemic lupus international collaborating clinics classification criteria for systemic lupus erythematosus. Arthritis Rheum 64: 2677–2686.
20. Funovits J, Aletaha D, Bykerk V, Combe B, Dougados M, et al. (2010) The 2010 American College of Rheumatology/European League Against Rheumatism classification criteria for rheumatoid arthritis: Methodological Report Phase I. Ann Rheum Dis 69: 1589–1595.
21. Johnson SR, Fransen J, Khanna D, Baron M, van den Hoogen F, et al. (2012) Validation of potential classification criteria for systemic sclerosis. Arthritis Care Res (Hoboken) 64: 358–367.

22. van den Hoogen F, Khanna D, Fransen J, Johnson S, Baron M, et al. (2013) Classification Criteria for Systemic Sclerosis: An ACR-EULAR Collaborative Initiative. Arthritis & Rheumatism 65: 2737–2747.
23. Tampoia M, Fontana A, Di Serio F, Maggiolini P, Pansini N (2003) Application of a diagnostic algorithm in autoantibody testing: assessment of clinical effectiveness and economic efficiency. Clin Chim Acta 333: 181–183.
24. Stinton LM, Fritzler MJ (2007) A clinical approach to autoantibody testing in systemic autoimmune rheumatic disorders. Autoimmun Rev 7: 77–84.
25. Lyons R, Narain S, Nichols C, Satoh M, Reeves WH (2005) Effective use of autoantibody tests in the diagnosis of systemic autoimmune disease. Ann N Y Acad Sci 1050: 217–228.
26. Fritzler MJ (2011) The antinuclear antibody (ANA) test: Last or lasting gasp? Arthritis Rheum 16: 19–22.
27. Abeles AM, Abeles M (2013) The clinical utility of a positive antinuclear antibody test result. Am J Med 126: 342–348.
28. Wiik AS, Gordon TP, Kavanaugh AF, Lahita RG, Reeves W, et al. (2004) Cutting edge diagnostics in rheumatology: on the role of patients, clinicians, and laboratory scientists in optimizing the use of autoimmune serology. Arthritis Care Res 51: 291–298.
29. Lateef A, Petri M (2012) Unmet medical needs in systemic lupus erythematosus. Arthritis Res Ther 14 Suppl: S4.
30. Bellando-Randone S, Guiducci S, Matucci-Cerinic M (2012) Very early diagnosis of systemic sclerosis. Pol Arch Med Wewn 122 Suppl 1:18–23: 18–23.
31. Bossuyt X, Louche C, Wiik A (2008) Standardisation in clinical laboratory medicine: an ethical reflection. Ann Rheum Dis 67: 1061–1063.
32. Kavanaugh AF, Solomon DH (2002) Guidelines for immunologic laboratory testing in the rheumatic diseases: Anti-DNA antibody tests. Arthritis Rheum 47: 546–555.
33. Solomon DH, Kavanaugh AJ, Schur PH (2002) Evidence-based guidelines for the use of immunologic tests: antinuclear antibody testing. Arthritis Rheum 47: 434–444.
34. Shojania K (2001) Rheumatology: 2. What laboratory tests are needed? Can Med Assoc J 162: 1157–1163.
35. Shoenfeld Y, Cervera R, Haass M, Kallenberg C, Khamashta M, et al. (2007) EASI - The European Autoimmunity Standardisation Initiative: a new initiative that can contribute to agreed diagnostic models of diagnosing autoimmune disorders throughout Europe. Ann N Y Acad Sci 1109: 138–144.
36. Bonaguri C, Melegari A, Dall'Aglio P, Ballabio A, Terenziani P, et al. (2009) An italian multicenter study for application of a diagnostic algorithm in autoantibody testing. Ann N Y Acad Sci 1173: 124–129.
37. Bonaguri C, Melegari A, Ballabio A, Parmeggiani M, Russo A, et al. (2011) Italian multicentre study for application of a diagnostic algorithm in autoantibody testing for autoimmune rheumatic disease: conclusive results. Autoimmun Rev 11: 1–5.
38. Shiel WC, Jason M (1989) The diagnostic associations of patients with antinuclear antibodies referred to a community rheumatologist. J Rheumatol 16: 782–785.
39. Gamez-Nava JI, Gonzalez-Lopez L, Davis P, Suarez-Almazor ME (1998) Referral and diagnosis of common rheumatic diseases by primary care physicians. Br J Rheumatol 37: 1215–1219.
40. Vlachoyiannopoulos PG, Tzavara V, Dafni U, Spanos E, Moutsopoulos HM (1998) Clinical features and evolution of antinuclear antibody positive individuals in a rheumatology outpatient clinic. J Rheumatol 25: 886–891.
41. Mariz HA, Sato EI, Barbosa SH, Rodrigues SH, Dellavance A, et al. (2011) ANA HEp-2 pattern is a critical parameter for discriminating ANA-positive healthy individuals and patietns with autoimmune rheumatic diseases. Arthritis Rheum 63: 191–200.
42. Qian J, Ehrmann FD, Bissonauth A, Menard HA, Panopalis P, et al. (2010) A retrospective review of rheumatology referral wait times within a health centre in Quebec, Canada. Rheumatol Int 30: 705–707.
43. Wiles NJ, Lunt M, Barrett EM, Bukhari M, Silman AJ, et al. (2001) Reduced disability at five years with early treatment of inflammatory polyarthritis: results from a large observational cohort, using propensity models to adjust for disease severity. Arthritis Rheum 44: 1033–1042.
44. Lard LR, Visser H, Speyer I, vander Horst-Bruinsma IE, Zwinderman AH, et al. (2001) Early versus delayed treatment in patients with recent-onset rheumatoid arthritis: comparison of two cohorts who received different treatment strategies. Am J Med 111: 446–451.
45. Emery P, Breedveld FC, Dougados M, Kalden JR, Schiff MH, et al. (2002) Early referral recommendation for newly diagnosed rheumatoid arthritis: evidence based development of a clinical guide. Ann Rheum Dis 61: 290–297.
46. Trouw LA, Mahler M (2012) Closing the serological gap: promising novel biomarkers for the early diagnosis of rheumatoid arthritis. Autoimmun Rev 12: 318–322.
47. Meacock R, Dale N, Harrison MJ (2013) The humanistic and economic burden of systemic lupus erythematosus: a systematic review. Pharmacoeconomics 31: 49–61.
48. Yang P, Kruh JN, Foster CS (2012) Antiphospholipid antibody syndrome. Curr Opin Ophthalmol 23: 528–532.
49. Lyons PA, Rayner TF, Trivedi S, Holle JU, Watts RA, et al. (2012) Genetically distinct subsets within ANCA-Associated Vasculitis. N Engl J Med 367: 214–223.
50. Gormley GJ, Steele WK, Gilliland A, Leggett P, Wright GD, et al. (2003) Can diagnostic triage by general practitioners or rheumatology nurses improve the positive predictive value of referrals to early arthritis clinics? Rheumatology (Oxford) 42: 763–768.
51. Wiik AS, Bizzaro N (2012) Missing links in high quality diagnostics of inflammatory systemicrheumatic diseases. It is all about the patient! Autoimmunity Highlights 3: 35–49.
52. Gran JT, Nordvag BY (2000) Referrals from general practice to an outpatient rheumatology clinic: disease spectrum and analysis of referral letters. Clin Rheumatol 19: 450–454.
53. Fritzler MJ (2011) Autoantibody Testing: Current Challenges and Future Opportunities. In: Conrad K, Chan EKL, Fritzler MJ, Humbel RL, Meroni PL, et al. editors. From Prediction to Prevention of Autoimmune Diseases. Berlin: Pabst Science Publishers.pp. 584–596.
54. Fritzler MJ (2012) Toward a new autoantibody diagnostic orthodoxy: understanding the bad, good and indifferent. Autoimmunity Highlights 3: 51–58.
55. Watanabe A, Kodera M, Sugiura K, Usuda T, Tan EA, et al. (2004) Anti-DFS70 antibodies in 597 healthy hospital workers. Arthritis Rheum 50: 892–900.

Accelerating Translational Research by Clinically Driven Development of an Informatics Platform

Imad Abugessaisa[1], Saedis Saevarsdottir[2], Giorgos Tsipras[1], Staffan Lindblad[3], Charlotta Sandin[2], Pernilla Nikamo[4], Mona Ståhle[4], Vivianne Malmström[2], Lars Klareskog[2], Jesper Tegnér[1]*

1 Unit of Computational Medicine, Department of Medicine, Center for Molecular Medicine, Karolinska Institutet, Stockholm, Sweden, **2** Rheumatology Unit, Department of Medicine, Center for Molecular Medicine, Karolinska Institutet, Stockholm, Sweden, **3** Medical Management Center, Department of Learning, Informatics, Management and Ethics, Karolinska Institutet, Stockholm, Sweden, **4** Dermatology and Venereology Unit, Department of Medicine, Karolinska Institutet, Karolinska University Hospital, Stockholm, Sweden

Abstract

Translational medicine is becoming increasingly dependent upon data generated from health care, clinical research, and molecular investigations. This increasing rate of production and diversity in data has brought about several challenges, including the need to integrate fragmented databases, enable secondary use of patient clinical data from health care in clinical research, and to create information systems that clinicians and biomedical researchers can readily use. Our case study effectively integrates requirements from the clinical and biomedical researcher perspectives in a translational medicine setting. Our three principal achievements are (a) a design of a user-friendly web-based system for management and integration of clinical and molecular databases, while adhering to proper de-identification and security measures; (b) providing a real-world test of the system functionalities using clinical cohorts; and (c) system integration with a clinical decision support system to demonstrate system interoperability. We engaged two active clinical cohorts, 747 psoriasis patients and 2001 rheumatoid arthritis patients, to demonstrate efficient query possibilities across the data sources, enable cohort stratification, extract variation in antibody patterns, study biomarker predictors of treatment response in RA patients, and to explore metabolic profiles of psoriasis patients. Finally, we demonstrated system interoperability by enabling integration with an established clinical decision support system in health care. To assure the usefulness and usability of the system, we followed two approaches. First, we created a graphical user interface supporting all user interactions. Secondly we carried out a system performance evaluation study where we measured the average response time in seconds for active users, http errors, and kilobits per second received and sent. The maximum response time was found to be 0.12 seconds; no server or client errors of any kind were detected. In conclusion, the system can readily be used by clinicians and biomedical researchers in a translational medicine setting.

Editor: Peter M.A. van Ooijen, University of Groningen, University Medical Center Groningen, Netherlands

Funding: This research is supported by Stockholm County Council (SLL), Swedish Research Council (Tegnér), Swedish Research Council, CERIC (Tegnér, Abugessaisa), Swedish Research Council, SerC (Tegnér, Abugessaisa), FP7 SYNERGY-COPD (Tegnér), IMI BTCure project (Klareskog, Abugessaisa), and Åke Wibergs Stiftelsen medicine research (Abugessaisa, Nikamo). The contribution of Nikamo was supported by Edvard Welande stiftelse Finsenstiftelse and Magn and Bergvalls Stiftelse. The funders had no role in study design, data collection and analysis, decision to publish, or preparation of the manuscript.

Competing Interests: The authors have declared that no competing interests exist.

* Email: jesper.tegner@ki.se

Introduction

Translational medicine, aimed at understanding etiology, molecular pathogenesis, clinical features, and prevention and treatment of diseases, depends on quantitative and high-quality data from patients during different stages of disease [1]. To this end, large amounts of clinical data are as a rule captured in electronic medical records (EMR), but increasingly also occasionally in dedicated registries on patients with specific diagnoses, thus capturing information on clinical characteristics of disease, laboratory data, response to therapies, and comorbidities. The success of translational medicine also relies on efficient utilization of data generated from emerging genomics technologies. Hence, to collect and manage large volumes of heterogeneous data has been recognized as a major enabler of translational informatics research [2]. However, unfortunately, these two pillars of translational medicine, clinical records and molecular data, along with their different parts, generally reside in disconnected informatics systems (figure 1). There is therefore an urgent need to reduce these barriers to accessing, sharing, reusing, and analyzing these different sources of data. A development mitigating this gap, thus enabling these data to be searchable across current data silos, would clearly spearhead the development and application of systems [3] and network-based [4,5] approaches supporting predictive precision medicine, as currently advocated by both the medical [6] and computational research communities [7].

These challenges and opportunities for systems-based translational research have been duly recognized recently. Several parallel efforts have consequently been undertaken to address this unmet need. Open-source initiatives include the i2b2 suite [8], a scalable software platform facilitating repurposing of clinical data into the research setting. This platform has been used to build a system for monitoring clinical trials by combining i2b2 with GenePattern, a suite of bioinformatics tools from Broad Institute

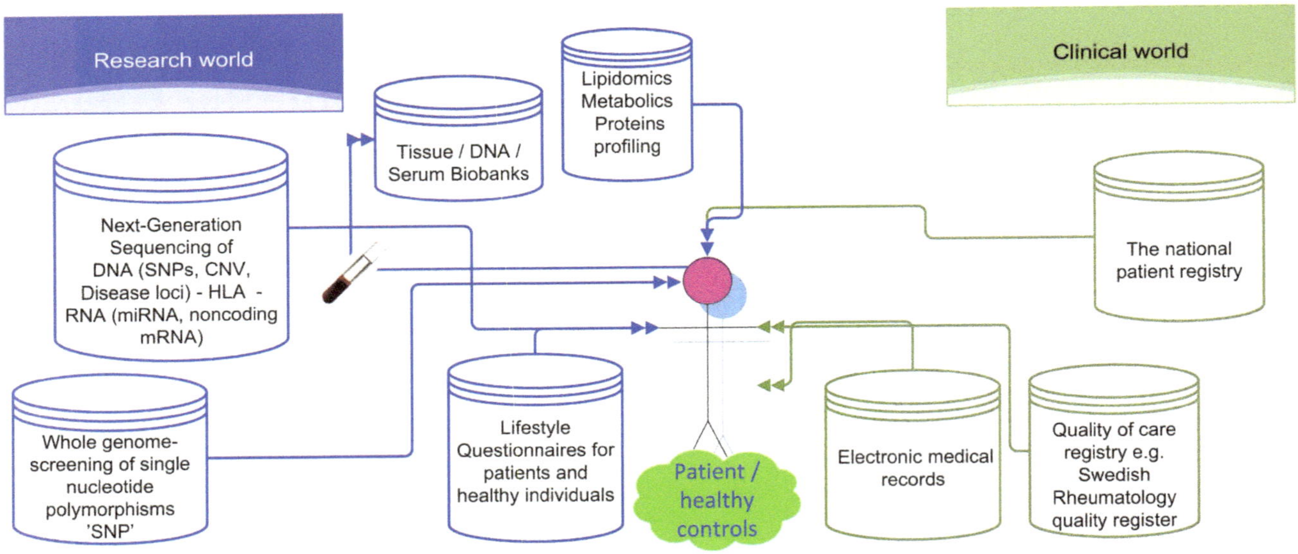

Figure 1. Schematic illustration of different types of database sources that need to be created for the analysis of cases (patients) versus healthy individuals (controls). Since these data are as a rule stored in different domains (clinical and research), a single case-control study needs to collect the data several times during a study, and this cycle must be repeated whenever a new case-control study is initiated.

[9]. This development has been orchestrated by the pharmaceutical company Johnson and Johnson and the Innovative Medicines Initiative (IMI) eTRIKS project (http://www.imi.europa.eu/content/etriks). However, the resulting system, referred to as tranSMART [10], requires professional software engineering support for the curation and import of data and applications, thus constituting a significant barrier for clinicians. To meet the requirements of clinicians, Stanford Medical Center has developed the STRIDE system [11], to support ongoing clinical research at Stanford University. For a review of these efforts including their pros and cons, and challenges in a broader context, see [12]. In contrast to these open-source or local efforts, a commercial vendor may first of all provide better support and usable graphical user interface (GUI) for clinicians and translational researchers, and secondly provide a secure platform capable of dealing with sensitive patient data in conjunction with molecular data. This possibility has recently been examined; one of the leading commercial platforms on the market, the Oracle Health Sciences Clinical Development Center suite developed by Oracle (http://www.oracle.com/us/corporate/press/350422), was evaluated in a translational research environment [13]. The study concluded that although the system performed well from a technical and usability point of view, there were still pending issues for a hospital or research group. In view of both open-source and commercial efforts, there is therefore ample room for new developments and further investigations of the real needs of clinical users. To this end, our requirements at Karolinska University Hospital, Karolinska Institutet and Stockholm County Council have guided and motivated us to initiate a research and development project aimed at building an informatics system for integrating healthcare and clinical research databases, hence bridging the clinical and research domains as illustrated in figure 1.

Here we show that our study design provides us with a firsthand view of real translational needs from clinical and biomedical users. Our case study describes and evaluates the first version of this system, T-MedFusion, which not only can integrate different kinds of data, thereby enabling translational research, but can also accelerate the research process by providing specific and detailed examples in the area of chronic inflammatory diseases such as psoriasis and rheumatoid arthritis (RA).

Materials and Methods

The RA study obtained approval from the ethical board at Karolinska Institute, Stockholm, Sweden.

Detailed and technical description of the assembly of methods and open-source software engineering tools used to develop T-MedFusion will be reported in a complementary manuscript. In brief, the T-MedFusion currently contains datasets from different ongoing clinical research studies at Karolinska University Hospital, such as the study of Venous thromboembolism, Non-Small Cell Lung Cancer and chronic inflammatory diseases.

Understanding translational researchers' data needs

In this section, we will illustrate our approach to acquire and collect end-user's needs and requirements mainly in two therapeutic areas; Psoriasis and Rheumatoid arthritis (RA).

We started by identifying the requirements and types of database sources, the data structure, type of queries and interfaces for clinical researchers, as well as ethical and organization rules and regulations. This initial step helped to define data sources, the storage method, use cases, and experimental platforms used to generate laboratory data. The identification of these components allowed us to create the required architecture for T-MedFusion. After defining the architecture layers of T-MedFusion, we used a prototype as a complementary method to simulate the behavior of the system, enabling end users to refine their ideas and requirements about the system. We developed multiple versions (prototypes) and asked the researchers to use the system to try different types of data extraction, retrieval, patient stratification, and so forth.

The users of T-MedFusion are biomedical and clinical researchers at the Center for Molecular Medicine (CMM), a translational medicine research environment hosting researchers and clinicians affiliated with different departments at the Karolinska Institute working with patient cohorts obtained from the clinical practice under the ruling of the Karolinska University Hospital and Stockholm County Council. To develop and test our method, we selected research groups conducting investigations targeting chronic inflammation diseases with an active cohort of patients at the clinic.

Clinical and metabolic profiles for psoriasis cases and controls

Psoriasis is a common disease affecting 2–3% of the human population including both men and women [14]. Psoriasis is said to be chronic, but the natural disease course is actually not known. Psoriatic arthritis (PsA) affects one-third of patients over time [15]. PsA is a clinical diagnosis based on clinical findings; at present there are no biomarkers available. Ample epidemiologic evidence supports a link between severe psoriasis and cardiovascular events [16,17]. Pathogenic mechanisms are incompletely known. Epidemiology also shows that psoriasis associates positively with metabolic dysfunction including obesity and vice versa, i.e., obesity increases the risk of developing psoriasis. However, putative mechanistic links between psoriasis and obesity are unclear. Hence, there is clear interest to perform future investigations across these diseases, thus defining the need for an integrative informatics platform supporting such queries across diseases.

The genetic contribution to psoriasis is overwhelming, and HLA-C is the main associated gene [18]. How HLA-C contributes to disease is still unknown, but it may involve altered presentation of a presumed autoantigen. Several recent genome-wide association studies have identified additional associated genes, the majority of which are involved in the immune system. These studies include unselected patient materials and reveal genes common to major subtypes, whereas genes associated with specific phenotypes may be missed. A striking example is the recent identification of the gene for pustular psoriasis, a rare and severe phenotype, where two independent groups reported mutations in the interleukin-36-receptor antagonist leading to deregulation of inflammation [19,20]. Psoriasis is immune-mediated and T cells play a prominent role. Depletion of T cells or interference with their activation are effective therapeutic strategies [21]. The hypothesis is that T cells under the influence of dendritic cells drive the disease. Novel treatments targeting such pathways provide powerful tools to understand psoriasis.

To address and investigate the above research questions, a data integration environment is required. The EMR (electronic medical record) of psoriasis patients and the clinical lab results of the cohort of 747 psoriasis patients stored at the dermatology clinic were used. All cases were included within 12 months of onset of skin disease and examined by the dermatologist in the group. All patients with joint irritations were examined by a specialist rheumatologist to ascertain the diagnosis of PsA. The metabolic profile, blood lipids, fasting blood sugar, and body mass index (BMI) of the cohort and the matched controls are stored in different systems at the clinic and CMM. The metabolic profile for each individual in the cohort consists of data collected at onset of disease (during 2000–2004) and 10 years after onset. The latter part of the study is ongoing; to date 225 individuals have been included for follow-up investigation.

Rheumatoid arthritis (RA)

RA is a chronic inflammatory joint disease. In addition to the synovial joints, RA may affect other organs. RA has a significant effect on the patient's life and employment. In Sweden, the incidence of RA is 0.5–1%; the cumulative prevalence was 0.77% [22].

T-MedFusion enables immunological studies of RA patients, aiming at increasing understanding of disease initiation and perpetuation. To perform such studies, researchers need to take into account and access both the genetic and serological profiles of the included patient material. The patient cohorts diagnosed with RA (defined by ACR 1987 or later ACR/Eular 2010) present three profiles: human leukocyte antigen-DR (HLA-DR) genotyping, genotype of 65 SNPs all predisposing for RA [23] (table 1), and detection of anti citrullinated peptide antibodies (ACPA:s) using the anti-CCP assays or antibodies IgG antibodies against citrullinated alpha-enclose peptide-1 (CEP-1) and citrullinated type-II collagen (citC1I) IgG antibodies against citrullinated vimentin [24,25].

Data sources and schemas in T-MedFusion

We started with the identification of data elements in the domain of knowledge (psoriasis and RA), identifying all entities (objects) composing the domain and the relationship among them. We used formal methods to define and model database sources. We used concept mapping [26] as a technique to define concepts and their attributes. Our starting point was therefore to identify and understand the data structure, regulations, and nature of each data source.

Patient clinical data

For each of the above diseases, the recruited patients have their clinical record stored within the hospital. A previously established system for exchange of structured data between the clinical records and a specific national registry for RA patients (named Swedish Rheumatology Quality of Care Registry (SRQ) was used for transfer of data from the clinical records to the Quality of Care Registry. However, a substantial part of the structured clinical data are also entered directly into the quality of care registry by the respective physicians (for information on the Swedish Rheumatology Quality of Care registry for RA; see [13,27]. In the present study, the clinical data from RA patients come from patients from Karolinska University Hospital registered in the Swedish Rheumatology Quality Registry. Researchers need to apply specifically for each study to the Register Steering Committee, after ethical approval of the study, to receive coded data from the register in order to perform research using the registry data.

In T-MedFusion we modeled and implemented attributes describing the disease duration (temporal), disease activity, and medication for RA patient (figure 2).

For the psoriasis patients, clinical phenotypes for the patients were collected at two time points, the first in 2002 and the 10-year follow-up starting in 2012. The basic clinical phenotype includes the development of the disease (healed, guttate, or plaque), psoriasis area severity index (PASI), BMI, low-density lipoprotein (LDL) levels, high-density lipoprotein (HDL) levels, triglyceride (TG) levels, HDL/LDL ratio, general skin examination, nails assessment, treatment, and so forth) (figure 3).

Biobank and cell register

The biobank and cell registry stores and manages biological specimens from patients and from relevant individuals in the population. Biological specimens are available mainly in the context of specific research into one or several diseases (RA and psoriasis). The biobank contains DNA, RNA, serum, plasma, information on different preparation methods and information on sample volume and of specific information on where the specimen is stored viable cells that are captured and stored from some patients, and the information on these cells is stored in the cell

Table 1. List of selected SNPs with their allele frequencies.

		Allele frequencies		
Rs number	**Locus**	**Major**	**Minor**	**Risk**
6314	HTR2A	C	T	C
1328674	HTR2A	C	T	T
548234	PRDM1	T	C	C
4781003	CIITA	C	T	T
4535211	PLCL2	G	A	A
10431908	CIITA	A	G	G
544167	C2	G	T	G
12746613	FCGR2A	C	T	T
4810485	CD40	G	T	G
10498441	NID2	A	G	A
10499194	OLIG3,TNFAIP3	C	T	C
2064476	HLA-DPB2	A	G	A
706778	IL2RA	C	T	T
2736340	BLK	A	G	G
26232	C5orf30	C	T	C
540386	TRAF6	C	T	C
231707	C4orf8	G	A	A
10402677	CEACAM1	G	A	A
42041	CDK6	C	G	G
2024301	CLEC4A;POU5F1P3	A	T	T
3807306	IRF5	A	C	A
10488631	IRF5;TNPO3	T	C	C
3761847	TRAF1/C5	A	G	G
7026551	C5	A	C	C
11586238	CD2,CD58	C	G	G
231735	CTLA4	G	T	G
13017599	REL	A	G	G
394581	TAGAP	T	C	T
2263484	C21orf74	A	C	C
6682654	CD244			
6859219	ANKRD55	C	A	C
13031237	REL	A	C	C
934734	SPRED2	A	G	G
11676922	AFF3	A	T	T
3087243	CTLA4	G	A	G
1678542	KIF5A	C	G	C
951500	CCL21	A	G	A
892188	GLP-1;FDX1L;ICAM5	C	T	T
1133104	CLEC4A;POU5F1P3	G	T	T
1980422	CD28	T	C	C
1859341	CEACAM8	A	G	G
3087456	CIITA	A	G	G
2271077	GALNTL2	A	G	A
2377422	CLEC4A;POU5F1P3	C	T	T
2476601	PTPN22	C	T	T
2812378	CCL21;C9orf144B	A	G	G
2240340	PADI4	C	T	T
6416647	CIITA	T	C	C

Table 1. Cont.

Rs number	Locus	Allele frequencies		
		Major	**Minor**	**Risk**
3890745	MMEL1	T	C	T
4272626	NHLH2	C	T	T
10258735	RPA3	A	G	G
3093023	CCR6	G	A	A
3218253	IL2RB	G	A	A
6822844	IL2,IL21	G	T	G
7234029	PTPN2	A	G	G
6457620	HLA-DRA	G	C	G
6920220	OLIG3,TNFAIP3	G	A	A
10413014	CEACAM8	A	G	G
7574865	STAT4	G	T	T
10468473	MAP2K4	G	A	A
10410147	CEACAM8	G	A	A
10919563	PTPRC	G	A	G
4750316	DKFZp667F0711/PRKCQ	G	C	G
2523451	MICA	A	G	G
6457617	HLA-DQ	C	T	C

registry database, which contains quantitative information about the number of cells available and other attributes.

Genotype variants, serology, and autoantibody

The genotype variants and serology data source contains information derived from the biobanked specimens, and these databases contain extensive information concerning the following: genotypes, both HLA-type and extensive SNP data; serology, covering titers of different RA-related autoantibodies (both IgG and IgA), such as CCP (Cyclic Citrullinated Peptide); and fine specificities [24,25]. For each patient a different measure from the synovial fluid and serum was stored. In addition, reference SNPs are stored and categorized according to gene risk level (Risk, major, minor). See table 1 for the list of selected SNPs with their allele frequencies.

System usability and interoperability

Through our research and implementation of T-MedFusion we used the iterative process development method, in which we allowed biomedical and clinical researchers to join in the process by testing the user interface and providing us with feedback for a new version.

To assure the usefulness of the system, we decided to consider and explore two complementary approaches. The first approach is

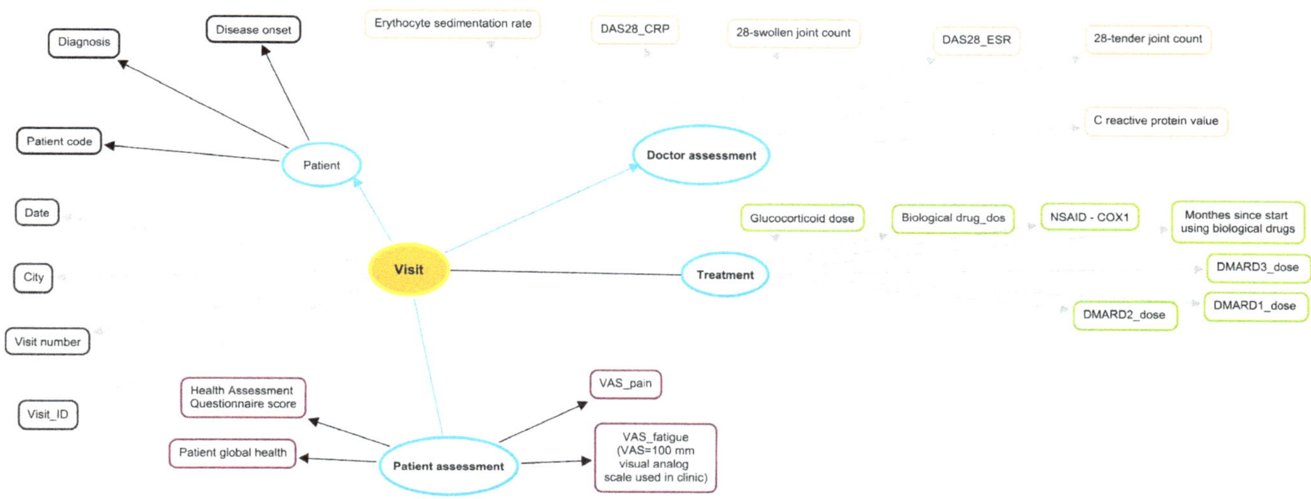

Figure 2. Basic data elements and associated attributes per patient visit to the clinic, as in the Swedish Rheumatology Quality Registry.

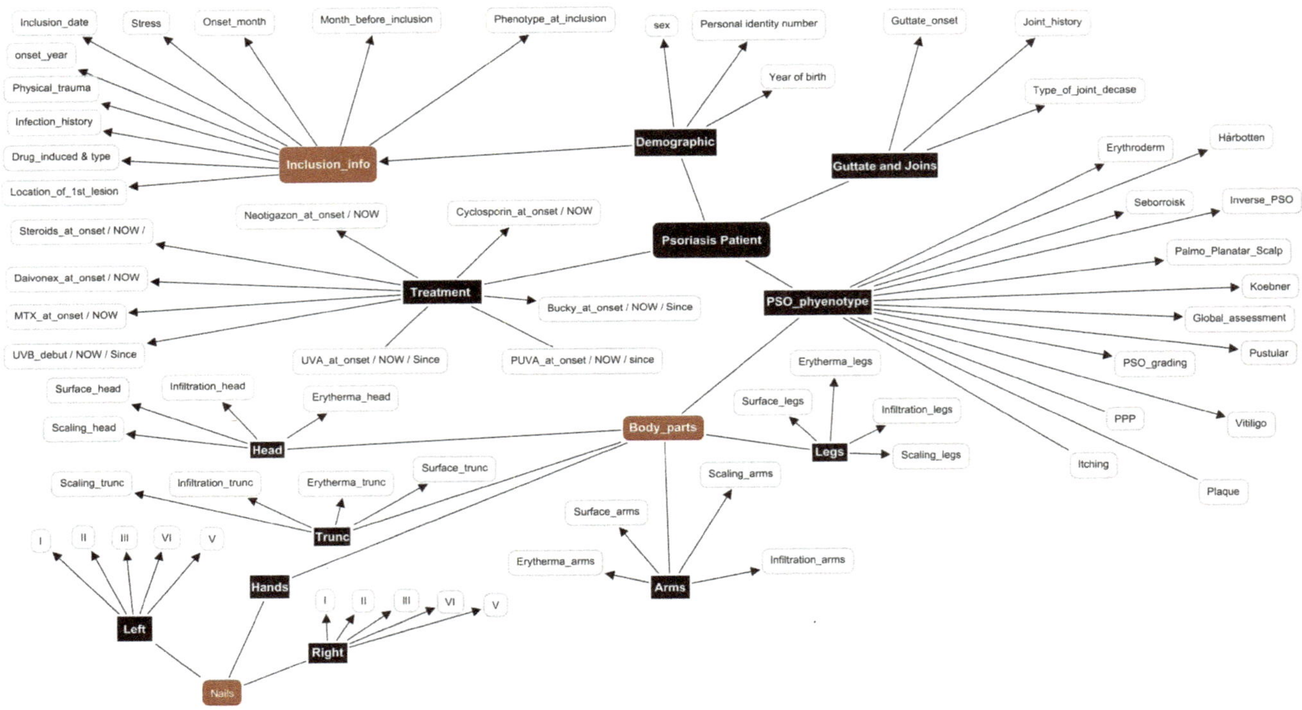

Figure 3. Clinical and metabolic profile of a psoriasis patient.

to make all user interaction based on a graphical user interface (GUI). The minimum requirements of the interface were to allow clinical and biomedical researchers to perform simple and complex queries on the fused databases. A simple query operates on a single source database, while a complex query retrieves data from fused database sources. In both cases, logical operations are supported. Such operations allow filtering the results according to specific expressions. The user interface enables the retrieval of a single record or group of records for a particular patient or sample. Also, it allows exporting output files into different file formats. The database is aggregated to the patient/sample level. The GUI for SNP data stored in T-MedFusion is illustrated in figure S1 serves as an example of the GUI layout in T-MedFusion.

The second approach is to perform a system performance evaluation study. Here we measure user satisfaction and acceptance of the system behavior based on the result of the performance evaluation. Through the performance evaluation and testing we obtained a quantitative measure to prove the effectiveness of the integration process and identify bottlenecks to overcome.

At the system level, we conducted a performance test to monitor the system's behavior under the following conditions:

- Increase the number of concurrent virtual users and monitor the reaction of the web service to the increased load.
- Operate the test for 120 hours (five days).
- Increase the number of virtual users from 1 to 20.
- Apply matrix and performance results.
- Response time: The elapsed time between the end of any inquiry or demand on a computer system and the beginning of a response (user query or sample selection).
- Average response time (during 120 hours). Maximum response time.
- Percentage of errors (during 120 hours), to identify any type of errors during the integration process.
- Test scenario: The investigator wants to select cells based on HLA type with preconditions of a cell count greater than 50,000,000 and SNP rs2064476 = AG and GG. This scenario involved integration of data from multiple sources available for the integration system. We obtained very good response time per virtual user, and we benchmarked the results with other systems.

The workflow and the implementation of the performance evaluation methods are illustrated in figure 4. The test was performed on a server running Redhat 5.5 Linux; the server configuration is Windows Intel 1.8 GHZ and 8 GB RAM. The server was running other applications during the test.

T-MedFusion supports interoperability with other systems as well. Through a friendly interface, the user can export the result of the query to many different formats. Importantly, we support integration via web services and provide the database in XML format and schema.

We implemented a web service (WS) in simple object access protocol (SOAP). The advantage of the WS implementation is that it allowed us to integrate T-MedFusion with the clinical decision support system (CDSS), as further elaborated in the Results section. Frequently in research and clinical environments we encounter different kinds of system for different functions. Such systems are developed by different vendors, each as a rule relying upon a different technology platform. A powerful best approach in integrating different software systems is to release WS based on well-defined service contracts in XML format.

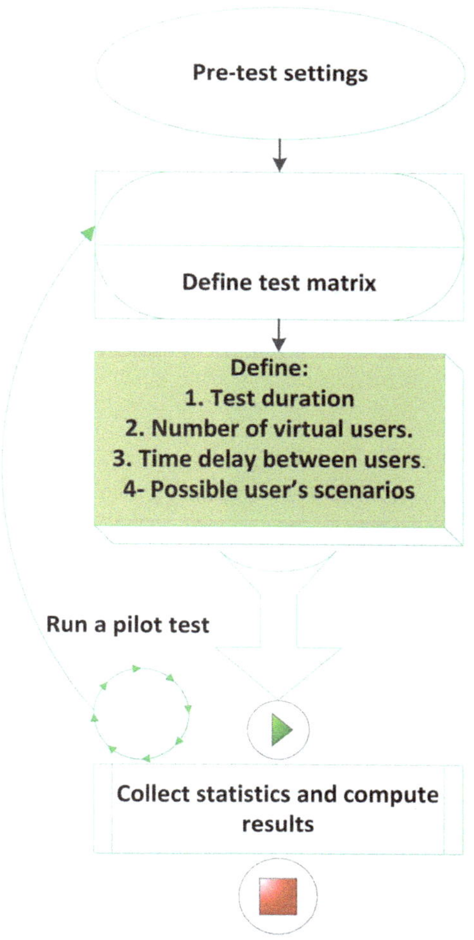

Figure 4. Flowchart depicting the performance evaluation method.

Results

As indicated within the introduction section, T-MedFusion has demonstrated the usefulness and capabilities to handle data from health care, clinical research and molecular data in different therapeutic areas and clinical specialties (Cardiovascular. Oncology, Dermatology and Rheumatology) within Karolinska institute and Karolinska University Hospital.

Here we first we explain the de-identification and security procedures implemented to protect patient and research data. These security requirements were the result of a dialogue between translational researchers and principal biomedical investigators, together with computational researchers. Secondly we report the results from a real-use case study of the system from investigators working on either psoriasis or rheumatoid arthritis, thus addressing the issue of the added practical value of an informatics system. Finally, we describe how to integrate T-MedFusion with the Clinical Decision Support System (CDSS) in the hospital clinic.

De-identification: Protecting patient privacy

The need for sharing and repurposing patient data in the translational research environment is constrained by several organizational and legal restrictions. One of the main barriers is the legitimate concern for protection of patient privacy [28]. It is therefore mandatory for any research institute to assure the protection of the patient information before making it accessible through any kind of platform. Coding processes approved by the local ethical committee were used for protection of identity of patients. Only a very limited group of named responsible clinicians/scientists have access to the coding keys, which allow identification of distinct individuals.

The de-identification process represents the first security layer in this system. This was complemented with additional layers to protect both privacy and the intellectual property rights and ownership of the database. In the next section we provide more details on the security protocol implemented in the system.

Multilayer security approach

In the present test cases, the users of the system were granted the necessary credentials to access the coded data either inside the firewall of the Center for Molecular Medicine (CMM) at Karolinska University Hospital or as a remote user outside CMM. Adhering to good practice, the database server was isolated from the application server. This solution has both advantages and disadvantages and has been debated with regard to server consolidation and multitier architecture [29].

The data stored in T-MedFusion were completely de-identified: all individually identifiable attributes were removed and replaced with virtual attributes for joining different schemas and helping in multiple table queries. The system was installed on a Linux web server and accessible through a web browser. The user requires a credential provided by the Principal Investigator (PI) to log in to the system through the browser. All tasks executed by the user were tracked. Saving documents and operations like deleting and uploading data required additional privileges and permission as determined by the PI See figure S2.

Our system has therefore been designed to be PI driven, thereby ensuring control of data and use in the hands of the PI instead of the local or central IT staff. This came through as a very clear requirement in the interaction with the users as a paramount requirement in the design of the system. The PI control of the system, in conjunction with a user-friendly interface, were key factors for success, since the need for daily support from software engineering to use the system was alleviated. It is clear that without this PI driven design we would not have been able to proceed further.

Improving cellular and immunological research in rheumatology

To assess the utility of the T-MedFusion platform for translational research, we asked whether the system could facilitate cellular and immunological research in the clinical rheumatology research unit. For example, it has hitherto been strenuous for researchers to systematically preselect cell samples based on clinical parameters.

At the rheumatology research laboratory, previous studies have been performed using donated patient material from Karolinska University Hospital. Patients donate several types of samples, primarily blood and synovial fluid, from which serum, DNA, and viable cells are retrieved and deposited in the RA biobank. The inclusion criteria for samples in a specific study, is typically based on serology and the availability of cells, while clinical information with regard to the samples is collected in the clinical setting and in the Swedish Rheumatology Quality of Care Registry; data from these sources are normally available to the cellular researcher only after specific search for information for each individual patients, something that has been a time-consuming and strenuous exercise.

Using our method, investigators are able to select research material based on the availability of the cell samples from the biobank, suitable genotype or serology status, and disease parameters from the clinical database (quality registry) in an efficient way. This facilitates and accelerates ongoing and future RA research at the clinical rheumatology research unit by enabling the identification of predictive markers such as immunological phenotypes.

For example, a common need is to be able to execute searches across several different data types using complex Boolean search criteria. As a rule, performing such queries requires each individual database to generate a list of hits. The next step is to combine these lists corresponding to the concatenated search criteria. This process is not only cumbersome but also prone to the introduction of errors. The simplified workflow supported by T-MedFusion, enabled by the introduction of methods instantiating data integration capabilities is as follows:

Pick a cell sample from the biobank based on the following criteria (Cx) using a Boolean search such that **C1** AND **C2** AND **C3** is true:

C1: Identify all samples where **HLA-DR** = ('*01/*04','*03/*04','*04','*04/*04','*04/*07','*04/*08','*04/*09','*04/*10','*04/*11','*04/*12','*04/*13','*04/*14','*04/*15','*04/*16').

C2: Only consider samples where the cell count is larger than 50×10^6 cells.

C3: SNP rs2064476 = Nucleobase: Adenine & Guanine (AG) and Guanine & Guanine (GG) from genotype data source.

The result of the Boolean query is shown in table 2.

Another example of workflow that also requires searches across different data sources is the challenge of determining how many patients are available with a certain human leukocyte antigen (HLA-DR) allele, antibody pattern, and disease severity from which cryopreserved cells, serum, and DNA samples are donated to the biobank.

A third example addresses the following question: Are there clinical differences (such as disease activity) between anti-CCP IgG versus anti-CCP single-positive and IgA/IgG double-positive RA patients? T-MedFusion provides the end users with a wide range of query capabilities to interact and retrieve the data from multiple data sources in a user-friendly and easy way. Tables 3-6 show example queries that are possible to perform.

As demonstrated above, the methods introduced by the T-MedFusion system make it feasible to perform complex queries across distinct data types without requiring manual concatenation of lists obtained from elaborate searches in distinct databases. Significantly reducing the barriers to performing these kind of queries facilitates translational research in that in-house data can be reused and investigated much more thoroughly.

Extract variation in antibody patterns

In addition to performing complex queries across distinct databases, investigators often want to extract time series patterns for longitudinal cohorts from either one or several data sources. Our system facilitates such analysis. For example, to explore the level of anti-citrullinated protein antibodies (ACPA) for an entire cohort and establish longitudinal cohort variation in antibody patterns, we can visually inspect the data in figure 5. For established longitudinal cohorts in RA or any other disease, the extraction and visualization of the time series will enable the investigator to study which fine specificities the anti-citrulline response displays (i.e., beyond the CCP-test). This method could be applied to any similar data for a cohort of patients.

Studying biomarker predictors of treatment response in RA patients

Recently, several effective immunologically designed treatments, commonly referred to as biological, have become available in the standard care of RA patients, improving their prognosis profoundly. However, the disease course varies widely among patients, and it is also clear that each of the new biological therapies is usually very effective in only a fraction of patients [30]. Non-responders to one specific therapy may, however, still respond to another drug, in part because it modifies another pathogenic pathway, which then may presumably be more prominent in the disease pathogenesis in that particular patient. Therefore, there is an urgent need in the clinic to identify (molecular) biomarkers that can predict the response to specific treatments at baseline. This may therefore support the accurate decision in selecting the correct treatment from the start, and the changes to biomarkers over time may also yield valuable information about the effects of such treatments. The T-MedFusion system is poised to be useful in the identification of such biomarkers, since the investigator can cross-link a response to therapy from the register-based follow-up data with molecular information collected in the research unit.

For example, with the availability of large numbers of biological samples collected at different time points for patients, an important issue for clinicians and investigators is to select samples according to predefined criteria within a defined time window for follow-up, in order to match those to clinical response data. One example is the selection of serum samples for RA patients at the baseline visit

Table 2. The output from a Boolean query from three sources of data.

Rs2064476	Number of cells (10^6)	Position	HLA-DR Type	cell source	CCP Serum
AG	13	01:F09	*04/*15	SFMC	438.9
AG	24	01:E10	*04/*15	SFMC	438.9
AG	17	01:H01	*04/*15	SFMC	238.9
AG	22	01:G02	*04/*15	SFMC	138.9
AG	53	01:B03	*04/*15	SFMC	538.9
AG	53	01:G04	*04/*15	SFMC	738.9
AG	31	01:H05	*04/*15	SFMC	738.9

Each row correspond to samples satisfying all three criteria (C1-C3). The position column pointed to the physical location of the cells in the freezer boxes. Cell source could be either synovial fluid mononuclear cells (SFMC) or peripheral blood mononuclear cells (PBMC), and the CCP-Serum column shows the serum levels of cyclic citrullinated peptide antibody.

Table 3. Retrieval of available peripheral blood mononuclear cell (PBMC) samples for each patient and the type of treatment the patient was undergoing at time of sampling.

Patient_ID								
Sample type	**Number of cells**	**Treatment**	**Treatment Dose**	**DMARD1**	**DMARD1 Dose**	**Cortisone**	**Cortisone Dose**	**NSAID**
PBMC	10	C	50 mg 7/d	Methotrexate	15 mg 0/			NSAID–COX1
PBMC	13,5	C	500 mg/d			Prednisolone	7.5 mg 1/d	
PBMC	10	C	500 mg/d			Prednisolone	5 mg 1/d	
SFMC	21,5	C	500 mg/d			Prednisolone	8.75 mg 1/d	
PBMC	13,5	C	50 mg 7/d	Methotrexate	15 mg 0/			

Table 4. Disease activity at different time points (visits to the clinic) for each patient in the cohort.

Patient_ID									
Pain scale	**Patients' Global**	**Health assessment questionnaire**	**Swollen Joints**	**Tender joints**	**ESR**	**C-reactive protein CRP**	**Disease activity score DAS28**	**DAS 28 CRP**	**Doctor assessment**
0	0	0	0	3	10	1	0	0	0
76	71	2	14	12	69	9,99	6,95	6,2	3
75	66	2	3	0	69	9,99	4,37	3,58	1
83	85	2,5	2	4	50	9,99	5,44	5,02	2
12	6	1,38	3	2	23	1	3,56	2,57	0

Table 5. Retrieval of cell samples according to HLA-DR type and sample date.

HLA, Dr04, cells per sample date				
Patient_ID				
RA Number	**HLA Type**	**Sample date**	**Sample type**	**Number of cells**
RA 1	*03/*08	Date A	SFMC	21,5
RA 2	*03/*08	Date B	PBMC	10
RA 3	*03/*08	Date C	PBMC	13,5

at treatment start and also at a follow-up visit, having available data on the outcome measure, e.g., disease activity scores (DAS) at these time points. To answer such a query, users need to extract the following information: treatment and DAS-related parameters from the clinical database, as well as sample and temporal information (sample donation date and time) from the biobank. The following algorithm describes the scenario of seeking serum samples in order to study the predictive value of biomarkers on patient response to treatment from the quality-of-care registry. From the RA biobank we have the following data:

- Total number of patients recruited in the study = 1622 active patients in the clinical database.
- Total number of serum samples in the biobank = 30,765. The samples are collected at the RA clinic and stored in the RA biobank at the CMM.

1. Identify and retrieve the clinical data for the cohort.
2. Extract treatment and DAS data for the selected cohort.
3. Identify and retrieve serum samples for the cohort in step 1.
4. Fuse the results from steps 1 and 3.
5. The result from step 4 is 22,279 (serum samples) out of 30,765 samples (according to predefined criteria on the serum sample volume and status in the freezer).
6. Extract all patients under treatment A = 1276 patients. Then extract two types of serum for this cohort according to:

   i. Initiation of DAS time window: Sample is selected if the sample has been collected at most 30 days before the DAS start date or up to 40 days after: 3204 serum samples satisfied this condition.

   ii. End DAS time window: Sample is selected if the sample has been collected at most 75 days before the DAS end date or up to 152 days after: 1952 serum samples satisfied the condition.

7. Repeat step 6 for treatment B, 95 patients: found 30 samples at Start DAS time window and 24 at End DAS time window.
8. Repeat step 6 for treatment C, 251 patients: found 215 samples at Start DAS time window and 221 at End DAS time window.

The system provides a summary of the above findings, as illustrated in table 7.

Without the integration capabilities of the T-MedFusion system, the above workflow would have been difficult and time-consuming to execute. Our methods readily thus enabled an integrative analysis of biomarkers corresponding to the following therapeutics: Infliximab, Adalimumab, Etanercept, Methotrexate (MTX).

Cohort stratification using waterfall filtering

In many cases an investigator needs to run a multi-criteria filtering process and stratify the research cohort. This type of filtering requires a complex query method. Through a waterfall filtering process, T-MedFusion supports patient stratification, as illustrated in figure 6. In this case the user wants to find all RA cases who are anti-CCP+ (having antibodies against cyclic citrullinated peptides), start with anti-TNF (anti-tumor necrosis factor) treatment, and have a baseline DAS28 with a follow-up visit in the two- to three-month time window. The system calculates the change in DAS28 and further filters the patients to a specific DAS28 value (X).

Exploration of metabolic profiles for psoriasis patients

Next we sought to evaluate the applicability of T-MedFusion methods in another disease area, namely translational research on psoriasis. We therefore created a database structure capable of storing the metabolic profiles of psoriasis cases and controls, with the aim being to explore whether a metabolic profile in a subset of psoriasis patients is associated with SNPs identified in other studies, such as SNPs of relevance for cardiometabolic disease and diabetes. Criteria that need to be fulfilled in the first round are the following:

Criteria of obesity and hyperlipidemia: BMI>29; LDL>4.3; Triglycerides>2.6, the total number of patients = 747 patients. The result is illustrated in table 8.

In the second round the criteria to be fulfilled are: BMI<25, Triglycerides<2 and LDL<4.

Total number of patients = 747 patients.

The results are illustrated in table 9.

For the entire cohort the system allows the researcher to visually explore the change in the psoriasis area severity index (PASI) at time 00 and after 10 years. PASI is a quantitative measurement of the severity of the skin disease, integrating involvement, redness, and thickness of lesions. In conclusion, our method permits a longitudinal analysis of a patient's metabolic profile.

Integration with clinical decision support system

At the RA clinic a clinical decision support system (CDSS) generated within the Swedish Rheumatology Quality of Care Register supports the doctors in their decisions about diagnosis, status of disease, and medication plan. The CDSS provides a simplified view of the patient's illness, treatment, and outcome. Currently the CDSS is based on data from the Quality of Care Registry, which also includes selected clinical laboratory test results. However, there is a need to integrate the clinical data and lab data with additional molecular data and findings from research.

Therefore, the current architecture of T-MedFusion was designed to provide a high level of interoperability with different

Table 6. Identification of the RA treatment type and dosage when the sample is collected from the patient.

Medication & sample							
Patient_ID							
Sample Type	**Treatment**	**Treatment Dose**	**Bio Basmand 1**	**Cortisone**	**Cortisone Dose**	**DMARD1**	**DMARD1 Dose**
Serum	C	50 mg 1/v	6	Prednisolone	2.5 mg 1/d	Methotrexate	20 mg 1/v
EDTA-plasma	C	50 mg 1/v	6	Prednisolone	2.5 mg 1/d	Methotrexate	20 mg 1/v
synovial	C	50 mg 1/v	6	Prednisolone	2.5 mg 1/d	Methotrexate	20 mg 1/v
DNA	C	50 mg 1/v	6	Prednisolone	2.5 mg 1/d	Methotrexate	20 mg 1/v
synovial	C	50 mg 1/v	6	Prednisolone	2.5 mg 1/d	Methotrexate	20 mg 1/v
DNA	C	50 mg 1/v	6	Prednisolone	2.5 mg 1/d	Methotrexate	20 mg 1/v

bioinformatics tools and workflows. This is possible through the so-called service-oriented architecture (SOA) [31]. The main feature of the SOA is enabling the reuse of information while maintaining a soft connection between the end users of the information platform (service consumer) versus the generators (systems). Using this architecture model the system can be interoperable with other infrastructures, thus making it possible to exchange different types of data stored in T-MedFusion with data stored in other systems. To illustrate this point we have performed a system-level integration between T-MedFusion and the RA CDSS (from the Quality of Care Registry) at Karolinska University Hospital.

The integration of T-MedFusion with the CDSS for RA at this stage will propagate the results of the ACPA tests from the research lab to the clinic. The knowledge about whether the patient is ACPA positive or negative is an important predictor for the need for result of treatment with some biologicals used in RA [32]. T-MedFusion can therefore enable the translation of the research results into clinical practice for predicting the eligibility of the patient for a specific treatment.

To introduce such information into the health-care system, the T-MedFusion transfers the research results about ACPA directly into the CDSS. The level of anti-citrullinated protein antibodies (ACPA) includes four parameters:

- CCP serum: Cyclic citrullinated peptide (CCP) - a diagnostic test for RA.
- Cit C1 IgG Serum: Cit C1 immunoglobulin G serum.
- Cit Eno IgG Serum: Cit enolase immunoglobulin G serum.
- Cit Fib IgG Serum: Cit fibrinogen immunoglobulin G serum.

The variant of RA (the ACPA-positive RA subset), is one of the genetically best characterized disease variants that exist, and a large number of studies have confirmed the effects of the genetic variants in RA diagnosis and treatment. Our entire approach is to firstly allow the clinicians to use the novel analyses of genetically complex diseases where different molecular phenotypes, here fine specificities of autoantibody re-activities, can be investigated. A second goal is to create a bridge between bench and bedside and translate research results to clinical care. Research wise, there has been very rapid development in this field recently (see [33,34,35]). All this combines to make the case of RA a very good example to demonstrate here.

The integration of T-MedFusion with the CDSS was achieved through the service integration platform hosted by Stockholm County Council as part of a specific project named 4D, where RA serves as a pilot project. The integration, using a web service based on requests and responses from the XML-based messaging protocol SOAP, was defined and agreed on in a service contract. The service contract (SC) is a technical agreement between the service provider (T-MedFusion) and consumer (CDSS). The exchange format and service communicate through service-oriented architecture and XML schemas. The SC consists of a web service description language (WSDL; figure 7) file with the associated XML schemas (XSD; figure 8), which is a document that describes all the rules, syntax and elements provided in the contract. The workflow and communication between the T-MedFusion and the CDSS is illustrated in figure 9.

A data-sharing model

T-MedFusion addresses researchers' challenges to maintain and manage research data in a long-term and persistent manner [36]. The system enables simplified procedures for uploading data from different formats. In addition to the database management, the implementation of T-MedFusion increases collaboration

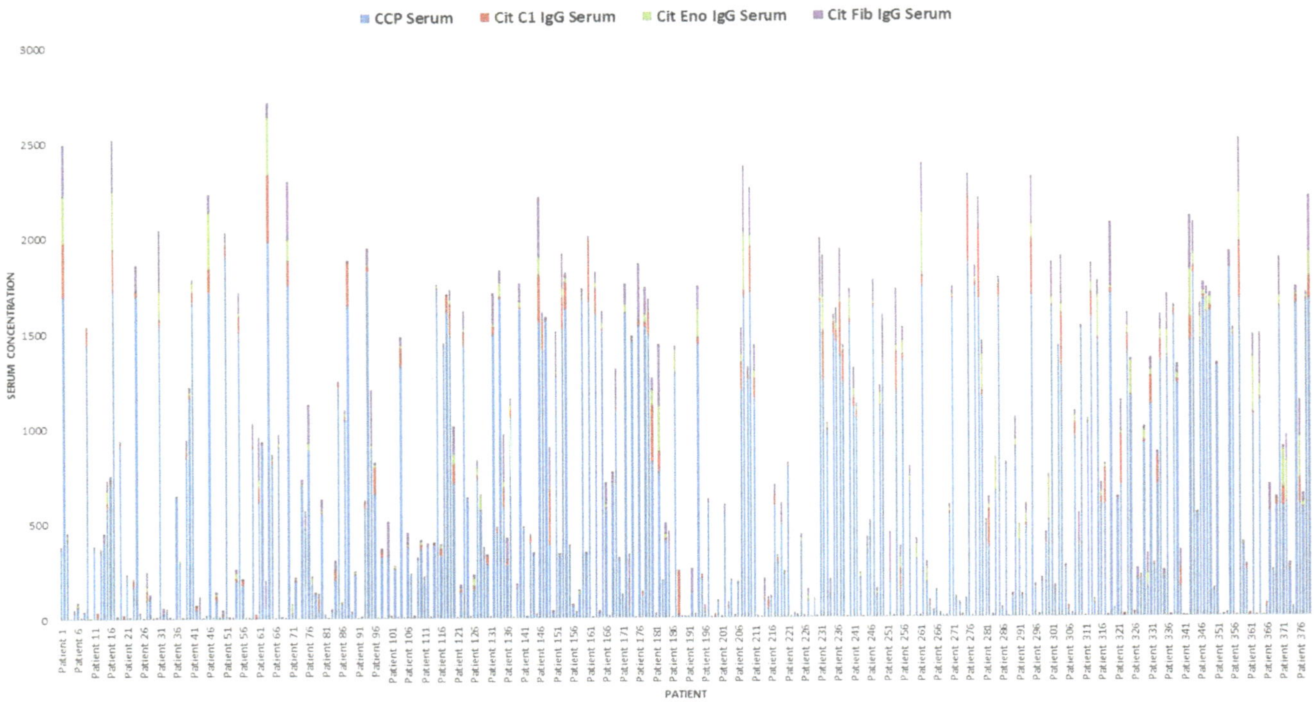

Figure 5. RA patient's profile for anti-citrullinated protein antibodies (ACPA). Each column in the x-axis represents one patient with four different serum concentrations. The y-axis represents concentration levels of the different serums (CCP, Cit C1 IgG, Cit Eno IgG and Cit Fib IgG).

possibilities and the sharing of research data and results across different research groups working in similar or different therapeutic areas. It also facilitates collaboration between biologists and bioinformaticians to further run advanced bioinformatics and computational modeling analysis. This since the process of accessing and mapping which data is available is significantly simplified, as this step is as a rule a major hurdle in numerous inter-disciplinary collaborative projects.

Outcome of the technical performance study

The results of the performance test are illustrated in data file (**SM: Data file S1. Performance evaluation results**) and table 10. We recorded the average response time in seconds for active users, http errors, and received and sent kbit per second. The maximum response time was found to be 0.12 second; no errors were detected. We observed some peaks during the second day of the test because heavy computation was run on the server, which took a lot of CPU time and memory.

The results show that the system response time is of sufficient quality and scales up with increasing workload (number of virtual users from single user up to twenty users at the same time).

Discussion

Our work as illustrated in this case study, effectively integrates requirements from the clinical and the software engineering perspectives in a translational medicine setting. The three principal achievements can be summarized as (a) a design of a user-friendly web-based investigator-driven system for data management and integration, while adhering to proper de-identification and security measures, using a modular three-layer architecture; (b) providing a real-world test of the system using clinical cohorts of rheumatoid arthritis and psoriasis; and (c) demonstrating interoperability, in that the system supports and integrates with a clinical decision support system for health care.

Below we elaborate on the challenges and opportunities in pursuing clinically driven informatics development, which includes developing appropriate tools facilitating data quality control and

Table 7. Summary of available serum samples in the RA biobank.

Treatment groups	Total number of patients	All serum samples	StartDAS		EndDAS	
			samples	patients	samples	patients
A	1276	22,279	3204	313	1952	288
B	95	22,279	30	9	24	5
C	251	22,279	215	53	221	36

Total number of patients and the classification of the samples according to the DAS time window (start and end).

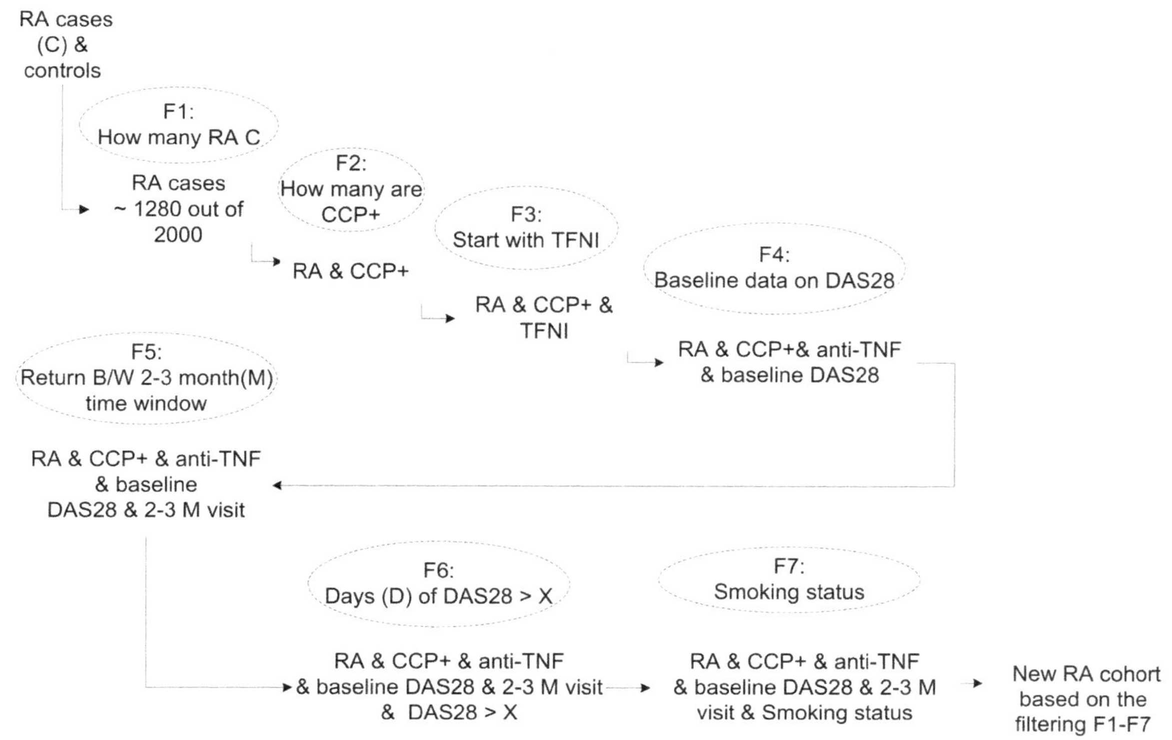

Figure 6. A waterfall query model to filter and stratify the patients according to specific criteria.

curation, data import, data integration, and possibilities for generalization to other disease areas while still having a modular and interoperable system. We close the discussion by some final remarks on future developments.

A clinically driven approach to integrate clinical and biomedical databases entails a number of challenges that might not have been readily apparent if a purely software engineering approach had been at work. For example, to have a system where the PI is in control of the environment is of uttermost importance, which should be considered together with the need for a user-friendly system enabling daily use by non-computer experts. To identify and meet those needs we therefore developed the methods and algorithms in close dialogue with clinical researchers in clinical settings. For example, we do not require the users to write query statements in scripting languages and thereby spend time dealing with syntax and computer commands. We augmented the query interface with information visualization methods to support cohort discovery through data visualization techniques. Moreover, we introduced a waterfall model to query and filter the cohorts using a wide range of inclusion and exclusion criteria. Finally, T-MedFusion reduces the required time to preselect biological samples based on clinical parameters such as disease activity and medication. The user interface allows the preparation of the research material according to the availability of the samples, suitable genotype or serology status, and various disease parameters.

Yet this work raised several challenges. It became clear that there is an urgent need for development of semi-automatic tools to facilitate the tasks such as quality control of data, import of data, identification of inconsistencies, and annotation. Such tools should

Table 8. Metabolic profile of psoriasis patients.

Question/condition	Number of patients	Criteria
BMI>29	92	BMI
BMI>29 & LDL>4.3	6	BMI & LDL
BMI>29 & LDL>4.3 and Triglycerides>2.6	0	BMI & LDL & Triglycerides
LDL>4.3	85	LDL
LDL>4.3 & Triglycerides>2.6	4	LDL & Triglycerides
Triglycerides>2.6	36	Triglycerides

Note: The criteria were BMI>29; LDL>4.3; Triglycerides>2.6 hyperlipidemia.

Table 9. Metabolic profile of psoriasis patients.

Question/condition	Number of patients	Criteria
BMI<25	379	BMI
BMI<25 & Triglycerides<2	359	BMI & Triglycerides
BMI<25 & LDL<4	335	BMI & LDL
BMI<25 & Triglycerides<2 & LDL<4	321	BMI & Triglycerides & LDL
Triglycerides<2	676	Triglycerides
Triglycerides<2 & LDL<4	556	Triglycerides & LDL
LDL<4	611	LDL

Note: The criteria were BMI<25, Triglycerides<2 and LDL<4.

be user-friendly in the hands of the clinical and biomedical scientist, while still being grounded in solid software engineering. Current systems targeting monitoring of clinical trials, [8] and [11], currently require sophistication in computer science beyond that of the translational scientist. Hence, extracting, importing, and loading data through the graphical user interface of the T-MedFusion system has been simplified by providing a wizard-based interface for importing data sets generated in the research lab (in several formats) into the system, thus enabling the biomedical scientist to perform data import without dealing with a command shell tool like Oracle SQL*Loader (sqlldr) [37], or an ETL tool like Pentaho (Kettle) data integration software package, in which the users need proper training in the design of metadata and taxonomy [38].

For a more extensive discussion of remaining challenges with respect to medical informatics systems, see [13] and [12]. An additional obstacle is that the quality and reusability of the data is also dependent upon proper annotation, which currently requires hands-on knowledge of the particular biomedical domain, generally beyond the abilities of the software architect. Hence, it is a challenge to develop methods that can mitigate this gap between the importance of annotation and the current more or less manual procedures for performing this work.

To support the practical demands from the users, we benefited from requirement engineering methods to determine their requirements. This guided our development and modification of techniques for data integration and system architecture. This is also important since we aim to design a system amenable to extension into other disease areas. Integration of several databases for large cohorts creates opportunities to query and understand relationships among the different data sets collected for the same patient. To achieve this feature, our methods provide a wide range of query capabilities with a usable interface. The main challenge met by the T-MedFusion system is the need for an underlying system architecture in which information can be stored, queried, accessed, annotated, and shared in numerous ways, while still

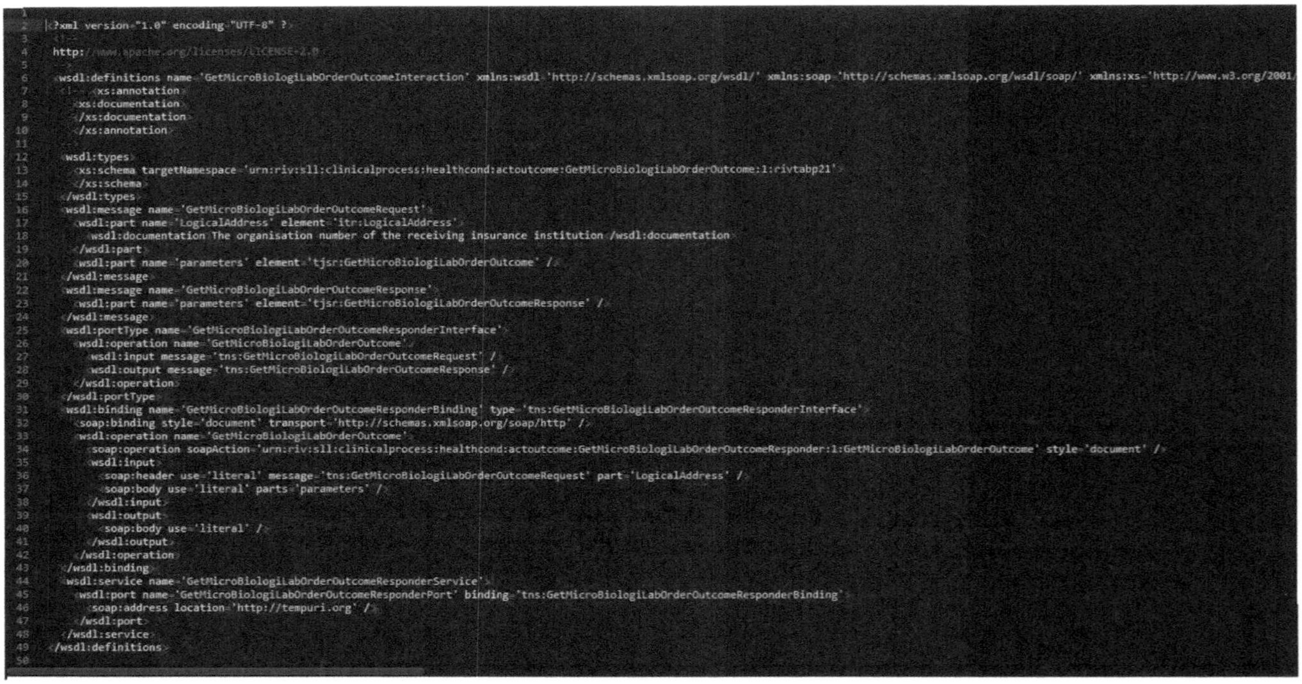

```
<?xml version="1.0" encoding="UTF-8" ?>
<!--
http://www.apache.org/licenses/LICENSE-2.0
-->
<wsdl:definitions name='GetMicroBiologiLabOrderOutcomeInteraction' xmlns:wsdl='http://schemas.xmlsoap.org/wsdl/' xmlns:soap='http://schemas.xmlsoap.org/wsdl/soap/' xmlns:xs='http://www.w3.org/2001/
  <!-- <xs:annotation>
    <xs:documentation>
    </xs:documentation>
    </xs:annotation>
  -->
  <wsdl:types>
    <xs:schema targetNamespace='urn:riv:sll:clinicalprocess:healthcond:actoutcome:GetMicroBiologiLabOrderOutcome:1:rivtabp21'>
    </xs:schema>
  </wsdl:types>
  <wsdl:message name='GetMicroBiologiLabOrderOutcomeRequest'>
    <wsdl:part name='LogicalAddress' element='itr:LogicalAddress'>
      <wsdl:documentation>The organisation number of the receiving insurance institution</wsdl:documentation>
    </wsdl:part>
    <wsdl:part name='parameters' element='tjsr:GetMicroBiologiLabOrderOutcome' />
  </wsdl:message>
  <wsdl:message name='GetMicroBiologiLabOrderOutcomeResponse'>
    <wsdl:part name='parameters' element='tjsr:GetMicroBiologiLabOrderOutcomeResponse' />
  </wsdl:message>
  <wsdl:portType name='GetMicroBiologiLabOrderOutcomeResponderInterface'>
    <wsdl:operation name='GetMicroBiologiLabOrderOutcome'>
      <wsdl:input message='tns:GetMicroBiologiLabOrderOutcomeRequest' />
      <wsdl:output message='tns:GetMicroBiologiLabOrderOutcomeResponse' />
    </wsdl:operation>
  </wsdl:portType>
  <wsdl:binding name='GetMicroBiologiLabOrderOutcomeResponderBinding' type='tns:GetMicroBiologiLabOrderOutcomeResponderInterface'>
    <soap:binding style='document' transport='http://schemas.xmlsoap.org/soap/http' />
    <wsdl:operation name='GetMicroBiologiLabOrderOutcome'>
      <soap:operation soapAction='urn:riv:sll:clinicalprocess:healthcond:actoutcome:GetMicroBiologiLabOrderOutcomeResponder:1:GetMicroBiologiLabOrderOutcome' style='document' />
      <wsdl:input>
        <soap:header use='literal' message='tns:GetMicroBiologiLabOrderOutcomeRequest' part='LogicalAddress' />
        <soap:body use='literal' parts='parameters' />
      </wsdl:input>
      <wsdl:output>
        <soap:body use='literal' />
      </wsdl:output>
    </wsdl:operation>
  </wsdl:binding>
  <wsdl:service name='GetMicroBiologiLabOrderOutcomeResponderService'>
    <wsdl:port name='GetMicroBiologiLabOrderOutcomeResponderPort' binding='tns:GetMicroBiologiLabOrderOutcomeResponderBinding'>
      <soap:address location='http://tempuri.org' />
    </wsdl:port>
  </wsdl:service>
</wsdl:definitions>
```

Figure 7. Segment of the WSDL file used to describe the SOAP service for integration T-MedFusion with CDSS.

```xml

<?xml version="1.0" encoding="UTF-8" ?>
<!--
  http://www.apache.org/licenses/LICENSE-2.0
  -->
<xs:schema xmlns:xs="http://www.w3.org/2001/XMLSchema"
    <xs:complexType name="GetMicroBiologiLabOrderOutcomeType">
     <xs:sequence>
       <xs:element name="patientId" type="core:PersonIdType"/>
       <xs:any namespace="##other" processContents="lax" minOccurs="0" maxOccurs="unbounded"/>
     </xs:sequence>
   </xs:complexType>
   <xs:complexType name="GetMicroBiologiLabOrderOutcomeResponseType">
     <xs:sequence>
       <xs:element name="ACPAResult" type="tns:ACPAResultType" minOccurs="0"/>
       <xs:any namespace="##other" processContents="lax" minOccurs="0" maxOccurs="unbounded"/>
     </xs:sequence>
   </xs:complexType>

   <xs:complexType name="ACPAResultType">
     <xs:sequence>
       <xs:element name="dateOfSample" type="core:DateType"/>
       <xs:element name="ACPA" type="xs:boolean"/>
       <xs:element name="ccp" type="xs:float"/>
       <xs:element name="cit_c1_igg" type="xs:float"/>
       <xs:element name="cit_eno_igg" type="xs:float"/>
       <xs:element name="cit_fib_igg" type="xs:float"/>
       <xs:any namespace="##other" processContents="lax" minOccurs="0" maxOccurs="unbounded"/>
     </xs:sequence>
   </xs:complexType>
</xs:schema>

```

Figure 8. The XML XSD file defining the basic element send from T-MedFusion to the CDSS via the SOAP services defined in the WSDL file.

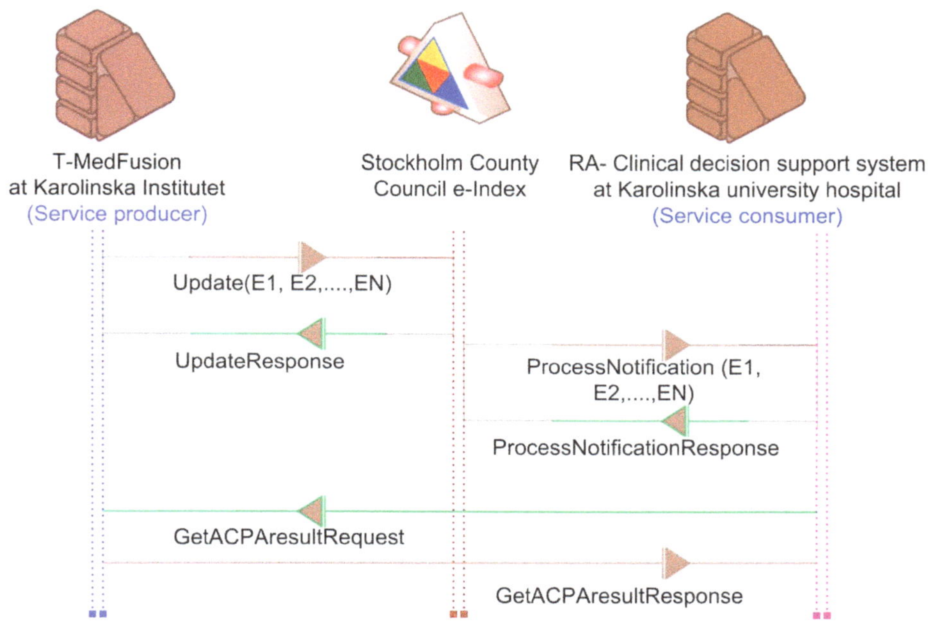

Figure 9. T-MedFusion (service provider) and the RA CDSS communicating through the Stockholm County Council exchange index (e-index). The e-index monitors the update service from T-MedFusion. Whenever a new ACPA result arrives, the e-index sends a notification to the CDSS. The CDSS sends a GetACPAresultRequest to T-MedFusion and as response obtains ACPA results for one or several patients. Streaming of the response and request services and communications between the systems are conducted through exchange of security certificates.

Table 10. Result of performance evaluation: Test execution parameters:Test status: finished, Test started at: 6/7/2012 8:04:55 PM, Test finished at: 6/12/2012 8:04:55 PM, Test duration: 120:00:00 hours (five days), Virtual users: 1–20.

System element	Total number of users	User think time in seconds	Response time, sec (with page elements)		HTTP errors (%)	Network errors (%)	Timeouts (%)
Response time in seconds for the user to load the login page	20	0	Minimum	Maximum	0	0,000034	0
			0.01	5.09	0	0,000034	0
Response time for the system user to log in to the system	20	0–8	0.03	5.13	0	0,000034	0
Response time to load the cell (from the biobank) and medication (from EMR)	20	0–5	0.76	38.3	0	0,000034	
Response time to search for patient's cell (from the biobank)	20	0–7	0.01	5.07	0	0,000034	0
Response time to get suggestions for search parameters from the biobank	20	0–9	0.11	27.6	0	0,000034	0
Response time to get suggestions for search parameters from the EMR	20	0–0	0.11	24.9	0	0,000034	0
Response time to get suggestions for search parameters and select one or more parameters	20	0–0	0.11	5.27	0	0,000034	0
Response time to get the final results of the query.	20	0–5	0.33	33.8	0	0,000034	0

respecting that different end users have different needs in terms of interface and research workflow.

We anticipate that the kind of system we have developed can readily be extended to cover other translational areas of research within the Karolinska University Hospital in a first wave of development. At a later stage T-MedFusion may serve as a mature platform that could be connected with transnational efforts at an international level. As a proof of principle we have presented the integration to the health care system and tools for clinical decision support, thus suggesting that the T-MedFusion platform can communicate readily with other national and transnational systems. This user-friendly design geared towards translational research has to a large degree approximated the components and functionalities of T-MedFusion, thereby serving as a "local" integrative and interoperable informatics platform.

There are several potential applications for the methods we introduced beyond the ones we have illustrated using RA and psoriasis. For example, in the cardiovascular disease area we have implemented the methods to study biomarkers for venous thromboembolism (VTE). In that project, clinical investigators are for example collecting lifestyle information for about 200 patients to be integrated with their EMRs, laboratory and screening tests, and VTE treatment. We are currently testing the same methods to integrate clinical data targeting approximately 150 patients diagnosed with lung cancer (non-small-cell lung carcinoma). Here our aim is to predict the outcome of stereotactic body radiation therapy (SBRT) [39], including induced side effects and toxicity. Furthermore, we are currently assessing whether it is feasible to apply the same architecture model to manage the breeding and associated genetics databases associated with experimental animal models.

Translation informatics systems should provide a technology-independent model of integration, which we illustrated in the last part of the Results section by describing how the service contract, defined as a set of rules governing the integration requirements between service consumers and service providers, facilitates interaction between researchers and clinicians and permits a secure flow of data between the bench and the clinic for an RA patient.

By providing interoperable and scalable systems as T-MedFusion, we aim to support researchers and clinicians in better understanding the capability of information system and software engineering to translate basic research results into clinical practice. Without appropriate understanding of the end users' needs at the clinic and in biomedical research, it is difficult to achieve progress. Likewise, nontechnical issues of ethics and security are highly important for gaining trust, facilitating the flow of information from bench to bedside, and providing the quantitative and high-quality data on patients and diseases that translation medicine critically depends on. Some sort of software infrastructure, such as T-MedFusion, is a prerequisite for repurposing clinical data into the research setting. In our continued work, we intend to improve the tool support for enabling and managing genomics and proteomics data from high throughput platforms. We expect that the fusion of different types of clinical information with rich omics data will improve the understanding of complex diseases and provide new insights into treatment methods and the efficacy and toxicity of drugs. Translational medicine is becoming increasingly dependent upon data captured in health care, clinical research, and molecular research. Yet there is an urgent need for integrative, interoperable informatics systems mitigating current barriers, thereby enabling systems analysis of diseases and therapeutic interventions. We conclude that the system can readily be used in a translational medicine setting in the hands of clinicians or biomedical researchers, while still being built according to robust and interoperable software engineering principles.

Supporting Information

Figure S1 User interface for SNP data stored in MedFusion.

Figure S2 Schematic description of the security layers of T-MedFusion.

File S1 Performance evaluation results.

Acknowledgments

The authors would like to thank Yvonne Kallberg for her valuable comments and feedback during prototype development of T-MedFusion and data curation.

Author Contributions

Conceived and designed the experiments: IA JT. Wrote the paper: IA JT MS VM SS. Usability evaluation: LK MS VM SS GT CS PN. Provided the link to the Swedish Rheumatology Quality Registry: LK SL. Read and proofed the final manuscript: All authors.

References

1. Armstrong AW, Reddy SB, Garg A (2012) Novel approach to utilizing electronic health records for dermatologic research: developing a multi-institutional federated data network for clinical and translational research in psoriasis and psoriatic arthritis. Dermatology online journal 18: 2.
2. Schadt EE, Linderman MD, Sorenson J, Lee L, Nolan GP (2010) Computational solutions to large-scale data management and analysis. Nature reviews Genetics 11: 647–657.
3. Clermont G, Auffray C, Moreau Y, Rocke DM, Dalevi D, et al. (2009) Bridging the gap between systems biology and medicine. Genome Med 1: 88.
4. Tan K, Tegner J, Ravasi T (2008) Integrated approaches to uncovering transcription regulatory networks in mammalian cells. Genomics 91: 219–231.
5. Vidal M, Cusick ME, Barabasi AL (2011) Interactome networks and human disease. Cell 144: 986–998.
6. Hood L, Flores M (2012) A personal view on systems medicine and the emergence of proactive P4 medicine: predictive, preventive, personalized and participatory. N Biotechnol 29: 613–624.
7. Hunter P, Coveney PV, de Bono B, Diaz V, Fenner J, et al. (2013) A vision and strategy for the virtual physiological human: 2012 update. Interface Focus 3: doi:10.1098/rsfs.2013.0004
8. Murphy SN, Weber G, Mendis M, Gainer V, Chueh HC, et al. (2010) Serving the enterprise and beyond with informatics for integrating biology and the bedside (i2b2). Journal of the American Medical Informatics Association: JAMIA 17: 124–130.
9. Reich M, Liefeld T, Gould J, Lerner J, Tamayo P, et al. (2006) GenePattern 2.0. Nature genetics 38: 500–501.
10. Szalma S, Koka V, Khasanova T, Perakslis ED (2010) Effective knowledge management in translational medicine. J Transl Med 8: 68.
11. Lowe HJ, Ferris TA, Hernandez PM, Weber SC (2009) STRIDE—An integrated standards-based translational research informatics platform. AMIA Annual Symposium proceedings/AMIA Symposium AMIA Symposium 2009: 391–395.
12. Tegner J, Abugessaisa I (2013) Pediatric systems medicine: evaluating needs and opportunities using congenital heart block as a case study. Pediatric research 73: 508–513.
13. Abugessaisa I, Gomez-Cabrero D, Snir O, Lindblad S, Klareskog L, et al. (2013) Implementation of the CDC translational informatics platform - from genetic variants to the national Swedish Rheumatology Quality Register. Journal of translational medicine 11: 85.
14. Nestle FO, Kaplan DH, Barker J (2009) Psoriasis. The New England journal of medicine 361: 496–509.
15. Gladman DD (2009) Psoriatic arthritis. Dermatologic therapy 22: 40–55.

16. Mallbris L, Akre O, Granath F, Yin L, Lindelof B, et al. (2004) Increased risk for cardiovascular mortality in psoriasis inpatients but not in outpatients. European journal of epidemiology 19: 225–230.
17. Gelfand JM, Neimann AL, Shin DB, Wang X, Margolis DJ, et al. (2006) Risk of myocardial infarction in patients with psoriasis. JAMA: the journal of the American Medical Association 296: 1735–1741.
18. Nair RP, Stuart P, Henseler T, Jenisch S, Chia NV, et al. (2000) Localization of psoriasis-susceptibility locus PSORS1 to a 60-kb interval telomeric to HLA-C. American journal of human genetics 66: 1833–1844.
19. Marrakchi S, Guigue P, Renshaw BR, Puel A, Pei XY, et al. (2011) Interleukin-36-receptor antagonist deficiency and generalized pustular psoriasis. The New England journal of medicine 365: 620–628.
20. Onoufriadis A, Simpson MA, Pink AE, Di Meglio P, Smith CH, et al. (2011) Mutations in IL36RN/IL1F5 are associated with the severe episodic inflammatory skin disease known as generalized pustular psoriasis. American journal of human genetics 89: 432–437.
21. Lowes MA, Bowcock AM, Krueger JG (2007) Pathogenesis and therapy of psoriasis. Nature 445: 866–873.
22. Neovius M, Simard JF, Askling J (2011) Nationwide prevalence of rheumatoid arthritis and penetration of disease-modifying drugs in Sweden. Annals of the rheumatic diseases 70: 624–629.
23. Stahl EA, Raychaudhuri S, Remmers EF, Xie G, Eyre S, et al. (2010) Genome-wide association study meta-analysis identifies seven new rheumatoid arthritis risk loci. Nature genetics 42: 508–514.
24. Hansson M, Mathsson L, Schlederer T, Israelsson L, Matsson P, et al. (2012) Validation of a multiplex chip-based assay for the detection of autoantibodies against citrullinated peptides. Arthritis research & therapy 14: R201.
25. Snir O, Widhe M, von Spee C, Lindberg J, Padyukov L, et al. (2009) Multiple antibody reactivities to citrullinated antigens in sera from patients with rheumatoid arthritis: association with HLA-DRB1 alleles. Annals of the rheumatic diseases 68: 736–743.
26. Wang WM, Cheung CF, Lee WB, Kwok SK (2008) Self-associated concept mapping for representation, elicitation and inference of knowledge. Know-Based Syst 21: 52–61.
27. Askling J, Fored CM, Geborek P, Jacobsson LT, van Vollenhoven R, et al. (2006) Swedish registers to examine drug safety and clinical issues in RA. Annals of the rheumatic diseases 65: 707–712.
28. O'Keefe CM, Connolly CJ (2010) Privacy and the use of health data for research. Medical Journal of Australia 193: 537–541.
29. Scourias J (1995) Aspects of Client/Server Database Systems.
30. van Vollenhoven RF (2009) Treatment of rheumatoid arthritis: state of the art 2009. Nature reviews Rheumatology 5: 531–541.
31. Joachim N, Beimborn D, Weitzel T (2013) The influence of SOA governance mechanisms on IT flexibility and service reuse. Journal of Strategic Information Systems 22: 86–101.
32. Tak PP (2012) A personalized medicine approach to biologic treatment of rheumatoid arthritis: a preliminary treatment algorithm. Rheumatology 51: 600–609.
33. Eyre S, Bowes J, Diogo D, Lee A, Barton A, et al. (2012) High-density genetic mapping identifies new susceptibility loci for rheumatoid arthritis. Nature genetics 44: 1336–1340.
34. Raychaudhuri S, Sandor C, Stahl EA, Freudenberg J, Lee HS, et al. (2012) Five amino acids in three HLA proteins explain most of the association between MHC and seropositive rheumatoid arthritis. Nature genetics 44: 291–296.
35. Klareskog L, Malmstrom V, Lundberg K, Padyukov L, Alfredsson L (2011) Smoking, citrullination and genetic variability in the immunopathogenesis of rheumatoid arthritis. Seminars in immunology 23: 92–98.
36. Ohno-Machado L (2012) To share or not to share: that is not the question. Science translational medicine 4: 165 cm115.
37. Blackwell B, Ravada S (2003) Oracle's technology for bioinformatics and future directions. Proceedings of the First Asia-Pacific bioinformatics conference on Bioinformatics 2003 - Volume 19. Adelaide, Australia: Australian Computer Society, Inc. pp. 35–42.
38. Casters M, Bouman R, Dongen Jv (2010) Pentaho Kettle Solutions: Building Open Source ETL Solutions with Pentaho Data Integration: Wiley Publishing. 720 p.
39. Okunieff P, Petersen AL, Philip A, Milano MT, Katz AW, et al. (2006) Stereotactic Body Radiation Therapy (SBRT) for lung metastases. Acta oncologica 45: 808–817.

13

Evolution of Direct Costs in the First Years of Rheumatoid Arthritis: Impact of Early versus Late Biologic Initiation - An Economic Analysis Based on the ESPOIR Cohort

Karine Chevreul[1,2,3]*, Georges Haour[1], Sandy Lucier[1], Stephanie Harvard[1,4], Marie-Laure Laroche[5,6], Xavier Mariette[7], Alain Saraux[8], Isabelle Durand-Zaleski[1,2,3,10], Francis Guillemin[9], Bruno Fautrel[4,11]

1 URC Eco Île-de-France (AP-HP), Hôtel Dieu, Paris, France, **2** Inserm, ECEVE, U1123, Paris, France, **3** Univ Paris Diderot, Sorbonne Paris Cité, ECEVE, UMRS 1123, Paris, France, **4** Pierre and Marie Curie University (UPMC) – Paris 6, UPMC GRC 08, Institut Pierre Louis d'Epidémiologie et Santé Publique, Paris, France, **5** Pharmacology and Toxicology Unit, Centre of Pharmacovigilance-Pharmacoepidemiology CHU, Limoges, France, **6** Limoges University, EA 6310 HAVAE, Faculty of Medicine, Limoges, France, **7** Paris XI University, Department of Rheumatology, Bicêtre University Hospital (AP-HP), Le Kremlin Bicêtre, France, **8** Brest University, Department of Rheumatology, La Cavale Blanche Hospital, Brest, France, **9** Lorraine University, EA 4360 APEMAC; INSERM CIC-EC CIE6, Nancy, France, **10** Department of Public Health, Henri Mondor-Albert Chenevilier Hospitals (AP-HP), Créteil, France, **11** AP-HP, Department of Rheumatology, La Pitié Salpêtrière University Hospital, Paris, France

Abstract

Objectives: To estimate annual direct costs of early RA by resource component in an inception cohort, with reference to four distinct treatment strategies: no disease modifying antirheumatic drugs (DMARDs), synthetic DMARDs only, biologic DMARDs in the first year ('first-year biologic', FYB), and biologic DMARDs from the second year after inclusion ('later-year biologic', LYB); to determine predictors of total and non-DMARD related costs.

Methods: The ESPOIR cohort is a French multicentric, prospective study of 813 patients with early arthritis. Data assessing RA-related resource utilisation and disease characteristics were collected at baseline, biannually during the first two years and annually thereafter. Costs predictors were determined by generalised linear mixed analyses.

Results: Over the 4-year follow-up, mean annual direct total costs per treatment strategy group were €3,612 for all patients and €998, €1,922, €14,791, €8,477 respectively for no DMARDs, synthetic DMARDs only, FYB and LYB users. The main predictors of higher costs were biologic use and higher Health Assessment Questionnaire (HAQ) scores at baseline. Being a biologic user led to a higher total cost (FYB Rate Ratio (RR) 7.22, [95% CI 5.59–9.31]; LYB RR 4.39, [95% CI 3.58–5.39]) compared to non-biologic users. Only LYB increased non-DMARD related costs compared to all other patients by 60%.

Conclusions: FYB users incurred the highest levels of total costs, while their non-DMARD related costs remained similar to non-biologic users, possibly reflecting better RA control.

Editor: Arvind Chopra, Center for Rheumatic Diseases, India

Funding: This study received funding from "la société francaise de rhumatologie", the french society for rhumatology. However, this funder had no role in study design, data collection and analysis, decision to publish, or preparation of the manuscript.

Competing Interests: The authors have declared that no competing interests exist.

* E-mail: karine.chevreul@urc-eco.fr

Introduction

Rheumatoid arthritis (RA) is an autoimmune disease causing chronic inflammation of the joints, often resulting in severe functional disability. The prevalence of RA in most world regions is under 1% of the population, [1] with an incidence of 0.2‰ to 0.5‰ [2].

In France, the mean annual direct cost of RA was estimated (costs are expressed in €2007 by applying the evolution of the consumption of care and medical goods price index in France. [3]) at €4,437 per patient in 2000 [4] and €9,345 in 2005. [5] Direct costs increased following the introduction of highly effective biologic disease modifying anti-rheumatic drugs (DMARDs), available since 2000 at more than ten times the cost of synthetic DMARDs. [6] With the expanded use of biologics, drugs are beginning to replace in-patient care as the greatest source of direct costs, [7–9] and differences in access to biologics will likely become the key variable in RA cost of illness across countries. [7] Used in patients with severe disease, biologics are currently not recommended as a first-line therapy due to safety and cost concerns. [10] While model results have demonstrated that early biologic initiation results in lower costs and improved quality-adjusted life expectancy, [11,12] real-life data are lacking on the mid- to long-term impact of biologics on the direct costs of RA, including the time of initiation of biologic therapy. Furthermore, cost of illness data from larger samples and among patients with early or mild

Table 1. Baseline patient characteristics.

	Whole pop.	Study pop.	Study population stratified on treatment strategy			
			No DMARDs	Synthetic DMARDs only	FYB	LYB
	(n = 813)	(n = 548)	(n = 51)	(n = 389)	(n = 42)	(n = 66)
Age in years	47.6 (12.6)	49.2 (11.6)	50.6 (11.1)	49.9 (11.5)	46.7 (12.2)	45.8 (11.9)
Female	624 (76.8%)	422 (77.0%)	36 (70.6%)	305 (78.4%)	33 (78.6%)	48 (72.7%)
Married	503 (61.9%)	358 (65.3%)	36 (70.6%)	258 (66.3%)	24 (57.1%)	40 (60.6%)
High school diploma	255 (31.4%)	171 (31. 2%)	19 (37.3%)	120 (30.9%)	11 (26.2%)	21 (31.8%)
Population of place of residence						
<5.000	274 (33.7%)	199 (36.3%)	24 (47.1%)	137 (35.2%)	12 (28.6%)	26 (39.4%)
>5.000 and <20.000	152 (18.7%)	100 (18.3%)	7 (13.7%)	76 (19.5%)	5 (11.9%)	12 (18.2%)
>20.000	366 (27.8%)	249 (45.4%)	20 (39.2%)	176 (45.2%)	25 (59.5%)	28 (42.4%)
Monthly household income (€)						
not reported	35 (4.2%)	20 (3.7%)	2 (3.9%)	11 (2.8%)	2 (4.8%)	5 (7.6%)
<1.220	154 (19.0%)	83 (15.2%)	9 (17.7%)	51 (13.1%)	5 (11.9%)	18 (27.3%)
>1.220 and <1.830	171 (21.1%)	114 (20.8%)	11 (21.6%)	83 (21.3%)	9 (21.4%)	11 (16.7%)
>1.830 and <2.440	156 (19.2%)	117 (21.4%)	12 (23.5%)	84 (21.6%)	9 (21.4%)	12 (18.2%)
>2.440 and <2.745	69 (8.5%)	53 (9.7%)	3 (5.9%)	43 (11.1%)	3 (7.1%)	4 (6.1%)
>2.745	228 (28.1%)	161 (29.4%)	14 (27.5%)	117 (30.1%)	14 (33.3%)	16 (24.2%)
Full health coverage	741 (91.1%)	510 (93. 1%)	46 (90.2%)	364 (93.6%)	38 (90.5%)	62 (93.9%)
Symptom duration (days)	214 (253)	102.1 (50.9)	103.2 (44.7)	98.5 (49.9)	109.8 (68.7)	117.8 (44.8)
Swollen joint count	7.19 (5.4)	7.5 (5.4)	5.8 (5.5)	7.5 (5.4)	9.8 (5.8)	7.8 (4.8)
Tender joint count	8.43 (7.0)	8.5 (7.0)	5.8 (5.9)	8.3 (7.1)	11.7 (6.8)	9.9 (6.7)
ESR (mm/1st hour)	29.43 (24.6)	29.3 (24.6)	19.9 (23.1)	29.0 (24.2)	40.6 (28.2)	30.9 (22.6)
CRP (mg/l)	22.15 (33.6)	21.6 (32.0)	14.5 (23.6)	21.2 (32.3)	28.2 (32.4)	25.2 (35.2)
IgM RF positive	372 (45.7%)	276 (50.3%)	8 (15.7%)	190 (48.8%)	31 (73.8%)	47 (71.2%)
ACPA positive	315 (39.0%)	250 (45.6%)	4 (7.8%)	168 (43.2%)	31 (73.8%)	47 (71.2%)
Typical damage on X-ray	110 (13.6%)	84 (15.3%)	2 (3.9%)	58 (14.9%)	11 (26.2%)	13 (19.7%)
DAS 28	5.11 (1.30)	5.12 (1.30)	4.27 (1.45)	5.08 (1.23)	5.95 (1.16)	5.49 (1.27)
HAQ	0.97 (0.68)	0.97 (0.68)	0.74 (0.65)	0.94 (0.67)	1.37 (0.76)	1.10 (0.65)
Satisfaction of ACR criteria (1987)	600 (73.8%)	417 (76.1%)	23 (45.1%)	305 (78.4%)	38 (90.5%)	51 (77.3%)
Satisfaction of ACR criteria (2010)	641/811 (79.0%)	456 (83.2)	25 (49.0%)	330 (84.8%)	42 (100%)	59 (89.4%)
Physician diagnostic certainty (0–100 VAS)	67.9 (24.5)	71.8 (23.8)	52.5 (23.9)	71.8 (23.6)	81.4 (16.8)	80.7 (19.2)
1st rheumatologist visit after RA onset[1]	74.9 (76.6)	76.9 (83.2)	63.1 (47.2)	75.9 (79.6)	110.8 (151.2)	70.7 (55.8)
DMARD initiation at 6-month visit	599/757 (79.1%)	452 (82.5%)	0 (0%)	353 (90.8%)	42 (100%)	57 (86.4%)
Hospitalization before baseline	193 (23.9%)	133 (24.4%)	11 (21.6%)	90 (23.1%)	15 (35.7%)	17 (25.8%)

Values are mean values (SD) or number of patients (%).
[1]Eular Guideline: 1st rheumatologist visit after RA onset <45 days; ESR = Erythrocyte sedimentation rate, CRP = C-Reactive Protein, DAS-28 = Disease Activity Score 28, HAQ = Health Assessment Questionnaire, ACR = American College of Rheumatology, VAS = Visual analogue scale, EULAR = European League Against Rheumatism, DMARD = Disease-modifying antirheumatic drug, ACPA = anti-citrullinated protein antibody.

disease is needed, as the majority of studies to-date have included only patients with established RA [13].

The *Etude et Suivi des Polyarthrites Indifférenciées Récentes* (ESPOIR) cohort is a multicentric, prospective study of French patients with early arthritis (EA). [14] Our objective was to estimate the annual direct costs of RA among patients in the ESPOIR cohort in their first four years of illness, to describe the distribution of costs by resource component and to identify factors associated with costs. In order to explore the economic and clinical impact of the time of biologic initiation, we sought to compare direct costs and disease activity between RA patients prescribed a biologic in their first year of disease treatment ('first-year biologic', FYB) and those prescribed a biologic later, after their first year of treatment ('later-year biologic', LYB).

Patients and Methods

Patients

The ESPOIR cohort recruited 813 patients in France between 2002 and 2005. [14] Patients were aged 18–70 years, had a rheumatologist's diagnosis of probable or certain RA or EA potentially becoming RA, with at least two swollen joints and symptom onset – first persistent arthritis according to the patient - between six months and six weeks before inclusion. History of DMARD use was limited to within two weeks before inclusion,

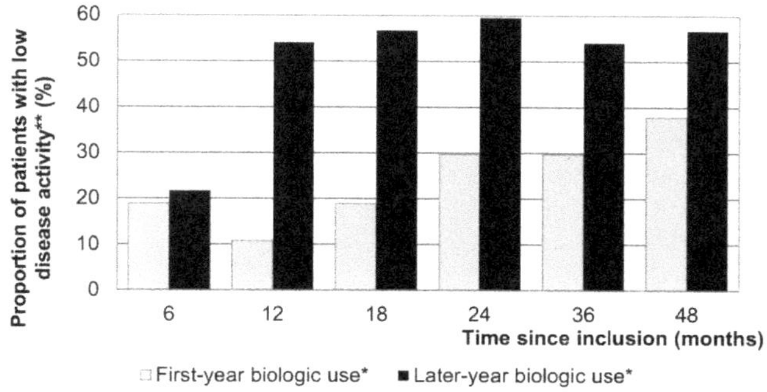

Figure 1. Disease activity per period among matched groups of FYB and LYB users.* 37 FYB users and 37 LYB users were matched for clinical and sociodemographic baseline characteristics using a logistic regression propensity score. ** Low disease activity is defined as DAS-28≤3.2.

while corticoid use was limited to a two-week prescription duration at a maximum mean dose of 20 mg/day of prednisone (four weeks for intra-articular injections). Due to the mode of recruitment, the cohort may be considered representative of the EA patient population in France and other similar countries. Patients were followed at one of 14 hospital centres every six months for a period of two years and every year thereafter. At each study visit after baseline, data were collected regarding health resource use since the previous visit, while data on patient sociodemographics, disease severity (health assessment questionnaire (HAQ) and Disease Activity Score on 28 joints (DAS-28) scores) and RA management were collected at every visit. The ethics committee of Montpellier approved the ESPOIR research programme in July 2002. All the patients signed an informed consent form before inclusion.

Costing Method: Definition and Sources of Costs

Our analysis included only direct RA costs from the French health system perspective, all three payers combined (i.e., statutory health insurance (SHI), complementary health insurance, and patients), divided between the cost of RA-specific drugs (either synthetic or biologic DMARDs) and costs of other healthcare resources. The cost of DMARDs was defined as the cost of the drugs themselves plus costs related to administration (e.g., day hospitalisations for intravenous biologics). Other healthcare costs included consultations with physicians and other health professionals, symptomatic treatments using non-DMARD drugs, imaging (X-rays, computerised tomography (CT scans), magnetic resonance imaging (MRI), gastric endoscopies, colonoscopies), transportation, hospitalisations (except for biologic administration -Infliximab, Rituximab, Abatacept – administered exclusively in a hospital setting) and clinical workups including blood tests. Because costs associated with the DRG coding version used were available only until 2007, costs were expressed using €2007 [3].

For both specialists and general practitioners, an average consultation fee was estimated using 2007 SHI tariffs and average extra billing. [15,16] Mean psychologist fees were derived from a survey. [17] Visits to physiotherapists were valued as the average tariff for patient education in inflammatory arthritis. [18] Nurse visits were valued as the tariff for 30 minutes of care by a skilled nurse plus a fixed average travel allowance [18].

Clinical workups were assigned their 2007 values based on expert opinion for inclusion, monthly and annual blood tests. [18] Transportation (ambulance and patient transport service) was

Table 2. Indicators comparing matched groups of FYB and LYB users per period.

	Time since inclusion (months)						
	0	6	12	18	24	36	48
Assistance needed in the last 6 months – (n (%))							
First-year biologic (n = 37)*	2 (5.41%)	4 (10.81%)	4 (10.81%)	3 (8.11%)	3 (8.11%)	5 (13.51%)	4 (10.81%)
Later-year biologic (n = 37)*	6 (16.22%)	5 (13.51%)	4 (10.81%)	3 (8.11%)	6 (16.22%)	7 (18.92%)	11 (29.73%)
RA caused disability - (n (%))							
First-year biologic	0 (0%)	1 (2.7%)	1 (2.7%)	2 (5.41%)	4 (10.81%)	7 (18.92%)	8 (21.62%)
Later-year biologic	0 (0%)	1 (2.7%)	2 (5.41%)	3 (8.11%)	4 (10.81%)	9 (24.32%)	11 (29.73%)
HAQ - (mean ± SD)							
First-year biologic	1.29±0.77	0.92±0.65	0.67±0.59	0.66±0.34	0.67±0.61	0.71±0.65	0.76±0.66
Later-year biologic	1.36±0.64	0.95±0.57	1.03±0.63	0.68±0.36	0.95±0.65	0.91±0.54	0.84±0.55
EQ-5D-5L utility - (mean ± SD)							
First-year biologic	0.31±0.35	0.43±0.36	0.54±0.36	0.53±0.31	0.54±0.34	0.57±0.3	0.49±0.37
Later-year biologic	0.23±0.33	0.38±0.29	0.39±0.3	0.39±0.33	0.42±0.34	0.44±0.31	0.48±0.34

*37 FYB users and 37 LYB users were matched for clinical and sociodemographic baseline characteristics using a logistic regression propensity score.

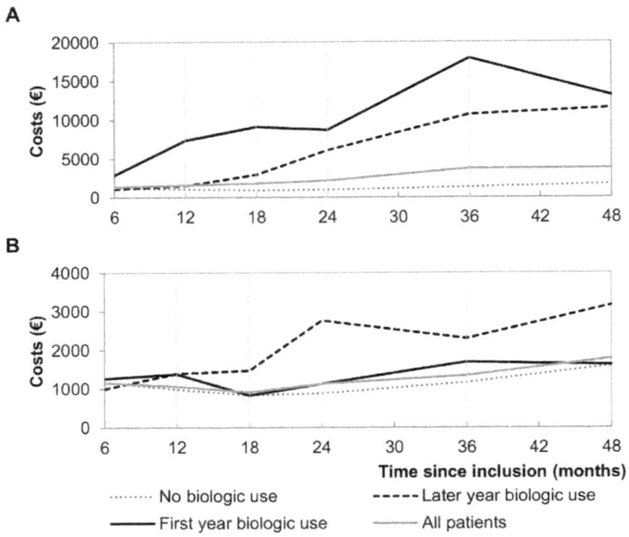

Figure 2. Mean costs per period according to treatment strategy. (A) Mean total costs according to treatment strategy; (B) Mean other health resource use costs according to treatment strategy.

valued by calculating an average cost per km and using a national average distance of 20 km to visit a rheumatologist [19].

Drugs were grouped according to their international nonproprietary names (INN), and their costs were calculated by estimating mean tariffs per milligram or per dose, weighted for the volumes sold in France in 2007 based on claims data. [18] The results were then multiplied by dosage and by prescription duration in days. Costs were estimated in each of the four treatment strategies, with patients divided into four mutually exclusive groups, the first two dividing non-biologic users into two groups and the last two dividing biologic users into two groups as well: 'no biologic use', synthetic DMARDs only, 'first-year biologic' (FYB) and 'later-year biologic' (LYB).

Hospitalisation costs were estimated according to diagnosis-related groups (DRG) using 2007 [20,21] cost estimations and were adjusted by the number of days. Costs were calculated for each six-month (or one-year) period and then summed in order to obtain the total cost over four years and the mean annual per-patient cost.

Statistical Analyses

Patient characteristics were described by the mean (SD) or number (%) and costs by the mean ± SD (median). Group comparisons were made using the Student t-test, the Wilcoxon Mann Whitney-test or the χ^2-test.

The clinical impact of the time of biologic initiation among biologic users was assessed by comparing the proportion of patients with low disease activity (DAS-28≤3.2), the proportion of patients needing assistance from other personnel, the proportion of patients with RA caused disability, mean HAQ and mean EuroQol Five Dimensional Questionnaire (EQ-5D-3L) throughout the study period in groups of FYB and LYB users matched on baseline characteristics using a logistic regression propensity score the variables of which were selected using the stepwise selection method.

A regression analysis was conducted to identify determinants of total direct costs in the first four years of illness for patients who had attended all follow-up visits. To assess the timeliness of biologic initiation, another regression analysis investigated determinants of other (non-DMARD) healthcare costs that reflect the patients' healthcare needs and level of disease activity. Because of the skewed distributions of both primary outcomes and the hierarchical structure of the data by center, we used generalised linear mixed models, which have been recommended for this type of cost data analysis. [22] Specifically, the fitted models were random intercept gamma regression models with log links. Coefficients were exponentiated to express effects as rate ratio (RR) estimates. For each model, the proportion of variance explained was calculated as the total variance from the fully unconditional model minus the total variance from the conditional model, divided by the total variance from the fully unconditional model. [23] The intraclass correlation coefficient (ICC), which is the proportion of the total variance that is accounted for by the center level, for each model was calculated as well. Variables were selected using the backward elimination method.

Variables used to investigate potential cost factors and to calculate propensity scores included patient sociodemographics, disease severity and RA management characteristics. Sociodemographic variables included age, sex, marital status, income and health insurance coverage. Disease severity indicators included hospitalisation at baseline or in the preceding six months (yes/no), functional ability at baseline expressed in four mutually exclusive groups (HAQ≤0.5; 0.5<HAQ≤1; 1<HAQ≤2; HAQ>2), [24] variation in HAQ in the first six months, presence of anti-cyclic citrullinated peptide (ACPA), presence of IgM rheumatoid factor at baseline and intensity of pain on a scale of 1 to 6. Effects of the DAS-28 score on costs were not investigated because it was highly correlated with the HAQ score (Pearson correlation coefficient = 0.60, $p<0.0001$), a fundamental outcome measure in RA. [24] Moreover, DAS-28 constitutes one of the main criteria for determining DMARD treatment strategies and thus would be a confounding factor. [25] RA management characteristics included physician certainty of RA diagnosis on a 0–100 visual analogue scale and treatment strategy.

Dropouts and missed study visits may be linked to patients' disease severity, and thus missing data may lead to bias in cost analyses. To address this issue and assess the robustness of the models, sensitivity analyses were conducted using a Markov chain Monte Carlo (MCMC) multiple imputation (24 cycles) method based on a multivariate normal distribution. Patients who missed all study visits and those who died during the study period remained excluded. Imputations concerned log-transformed costs per period (12.3% of missing data) as well as the variables FYB (4.5%) and LYB (22.5%), which were imputed without rounding. [26] The following variables were used in the imputation model: all variables tested for the complete case analyses as well as dummy variables to account for the multicentric structure of the data [27] and supplementary auxiliary variables correlated with the variables to be imputed as well as with their missingness. [28] Data were assumed to be missing at random. Imputed costs per period were back transformed and then summed. Regression analyses were performed on each imputed data set, and results were combined using Rubin's rules [29].

Statistical analyses were performed using SAS 9.3 (SAS Institute, Cary, North Carolina).

Results

Study Population

Two-thirds (n = 548) of the 813 patients in the ESPOIR cohort attended all follow-up visits and were included in the baseline analysis (Table 1). The majority (71.0%) were treated with

Table 3. Annual costs over the 4-year follow-up by resource component.

			Stratification on RA therapeutic strategy							
	Study population (n = 548)		No DMARD (n = 51)		Synthetic DMARD only (n = 389)		First-year biologic (n = 42)		Later-year biologic (n = 66)	
	Mean ± SD (median)	%	Mean ± SD (median)	%	Mean ± SD (median)	%	Mean ± SD (median)	%	Mean ± SD (median)	%
DMARDs/Biologics	1,767±4,141 (95)	49.0	0±0	0.0	180±231 (84)	9.4	12,816±5,760 (11,294)	86.6	5,462±3,582 (5,381)	64.4
Other healthcare use	1,844±3,251 (974)	51.0	998±1,147 (622)	100	1,742±3,478 (903)	90.6	1,974±1,639 (1,696)	13.4	3,016±3,490 (1,640)	35.6
All provider visits	318±406 (233)	8.8	174±147 (128)	17.4	308±432 (228)	16.0	382±336 (267)	2.6	446±382 (363)	5.2
Physicians[1]	200±14 (181)	5.5	127±100 (103)	12.8	195±107 (174)	10.1	224±118 (201)	1.5	269±125 (241)	3.2
Other health professionals[2]	118±354 (28)	3.2	46±94 (3)	4.6	113±385 (17)	5.9	158±289 (39)	1.1	177±324 (80)	2.1
Laboratory testing[3]	231±118 (218)	6.4	84±57 (72)	8.4	233±106 (223)	12.1	269±122 (243)	1.8	303±126 (288)	3.6
Imaging & other devices[4]	49±47 (35)	1.3	38±39 (30)	3.8	48±45 (34)	2.5	51±39 (36)	0.3	63±65 (42)	0.7
Transportation[5]	10±39 (0)	0.3	2±8 (0)	0.2	9±38 (0)	0.5	17±56 (0)	0.1	21±43 (0)	0.2
Inpatient care[6]	1,130±2,931 (176)	31.3	631±910 (95)	63.2	1,038±3,130 (95)	54.0	1,141±1,514 (552)	7.7	2,057±3,528 (796)	24.3
Non-DMARD medication	106±89 (88)	2.9	71±80 (37)	7.0	106±87 (89)	5.5	116±103 (105)	0.8	125±90 (103)	1.5
Total annual costs	3,612±5,407 (1423)	100	998±1,147 (62)	100	1,922±3,486 (1,146)	100	14,791±6,033 (13,726)	100	8,477±4,741 (8,121)	100

[1]Physician visit costs used were the following: 28.27€ for rheumatologists, 28.61€ for internists, 22.13€ for general practitioners and 30.56€ for orthopaedist surgeons.
[2]Health professional consultation costs used were the following: 11.30 € for nurses, 16.32 € for physiotherapists, 40.82 € for psychologists and 14.90 € for occupational therapists.
[3]Lab test costs used were the following: 173.80 € for inclusion biologic investigations, 28.86 € for monthly biologic tests and 42.63 € for annual biologic tests.
[4]Imaging and other devices costs included the following: 19.95 to 39.95 € for X-ray depending on the number of X-rays (19.95 € for the 1st X-ray, 39.95 € for the 2nd, 21.28 € for the 3rd, 20.00 € for the 4th), 69.00 € for MRI, 25.27 € for CT-scanner, 96.00 € for gastric endoscopy and 204.18 € for colonoscopy.
[5]Transportation costs were calculated on the basis of a reimbursement fee of 1.17 € per km.
[6]Inpatient costs were based on DRG tariffs.
DMARD = Disease-modifying antirheumatic drugs.

Table 4. Multivariate analysis of the effects of demographic and clinical variables and treatment strategy on total costs over 4 years.

	Complete case analysis (n = 548)		MCMC imputation model (n = 777)	
Variables	**Rate Ratio (95% CI)**	**P-value**	**Rate Ratio (95% CI)**	**P-value**
First year biologic use	7.22 (5.59–9.31)	<0.0001	7.74 (5.70–9.78)	<0.0001
Later year biologic use	4.39 (3.58–5.39)	<0.0001	4.54 (3.38–5.70)	<0.0001
HAQ score at baseline: >2	2.25 (1.76–2.88)	<0.0001	2.10 (1.52–2.67)	0.0002
HAQ score at baseline: 1 to ≤2	1.45 (1.23–1.69)	<0.0001	1.50 (1.22–1.78)	0.0006
Variation in HAQ score (per 0.25-point increase) between baseline and 6 month visit	1.07 (1.03–1.10)	<0.0001	1.06 (1.03–1.10)	0.0007
Doctor's evaluation of RA diagnostic <50% at baseline	0.73 (0.62–0.86)	0.0002	0.78 (0.65–0.91)	0.0014
Hospitalisation at baseline	1.32 (1.13–1.54)	0.0005	1.29 (1.07–1.50)	0.0083
Lives with a partner at baseline	0.67 (0.57–0.79)	<0.0001	0.69 (0.58–0.81)	<0.0001
Age (per 10-year increase) at baseline	–	–	1.11 (1.05–1.18)	0.0009
Full health coverage	–	–	0.67 (0.48–0.87)	0.0014
Family income>€1220	–	–	1.28 (1.03–1.52)	0.0264
Proportion of variance explained by model	53%		46% (44%–48%)[1]	
ICC	4.15%		5.97% (4.05%–8.53%)[1]	

The reported Rate Ratios describe the variations in costs expressed as a multiplicative factor for patients presenting the associated characteristic compared to those who did not, all other things being equal.
MCMC = Markov Chain Monte Carlo; CI = Confidence Intervalle; HAQ = Health Assessment Questionnaire; RA = Rheumatoid Arthritis; ICC = Intraclass Correlation Coefficient.
[1]Median and range for all 24 imputed datasets.

synthetic DMARDs only, while 9.3% received no DMARDs, 7.7% received a FYB and 12.0% received a LYB. LYB received biologics with a median duration of 2 years after inclusion (mean duration: 2.29 years, SD: 0.96).

Among the 265 excluded patients, baseline HAQ and DAS-28 scores were not different from the study population's ($p = 0.52$ and $p = 0.57$, respectively), nor was sex distribution ($p = 0.80$). However, excluded patients were slightly younger (45 vs. 49 years, $p = 0.002$), fewer were positive for ACPA (24.5% vs. 45.6%, $p < 0.0001$) and IgM rheumatoid factor (IgM RF) (36.2% vs. 50.4%, $p = 0.0001$) and fewer met the 1987 American College of Rheumatology (ACR) RA criteria (61.1% vs. 76.1%, $p < 0.0001$).

Table 5. Multivariate analysis of the effects of demographic and clinical variables and treatment strategy on other health resource use costs over 4 years.

	Complete case analysis (n = 548)		MCMC imputation model (n = 777)	
Variables	**Rate Ratio (95% CI)**	**P-value**	**Rate Ratio (95% CI)**	**P-value**
Later year biologic use	1.64 (1.32–2.05)	<0.0001	1.73 (1.28–2.18)	0.0016
HAQ score at baseline: >2	2.43 (1.87–3.17)	<0.0001	2.66 (1.87–3.45)	<0.0001
HAQ score at baseline: 1 to ≤2	1.48 (1.24–1.76)	<0.0001	1.51 (1.22–1.81)	0.0007
Variation in HAQ score (per 0.25-point increase) between baseline and 6 month visit	1.06 (1.03–1.10)	0.000	1.08 (1.04–1.11)	<0.0001
Doctor's evaluation of RA diagnostic <50% at baseline	0.76 (0.64–0.92)	0.004	0.82 (0.67–0.96)	0.0114
Hospitalisation at baseline	1.38 (1.16–1.64)	0.000	1.29 (1.06–1.51)	0.0113
Lives with a partner at baseline	0.65 (0.55–0.77)	<0.0001	0.72 (0.60–0.84)	<0.0001
Age (per 10-year increase) at baseline	–	–	1.10 (1.03–1.17)	0.0033
Proportion of variance explained by model	22%		17% (16%–19%)[1]	
ICC	4.85%		5.85% (4.21%–8.02%)[1]	

The reported Rate Ratios describe the variations in costs expressed as a multiplicative factor for patients presenting the associated characteristic compared to those who did not, all other things being equal.
MCMC = Markov Chain Monte Carlo; CI = Confidence Intervalle; HAQ = Health Assessment Questionnaire; RA = Rheumatoid Arthritis; ICC = Intraclass Correlation Coefficient.
[1]Median and range for all 24 imputed datasets.

The study population for the regression sensitivity analyses (n = 777) included the 813 cohort patients, less the seven who died during the study period and the 29 patients who attended no study visits following inclusion.

Impact of Time of Initiation of Biologics on Disease Activity

A comparison of groups of FYB and LYB users matched on baseline characteristics (baseline DAS-28 and HAQ scores not significantly different among two groups of equal sizes (n = 37) with p = 0.93 and p = 0.68 respectively after matching) shows that over the entire study period, FYB users compared to LYB users display lower proportions of patients with low disease activity (DAS-28≤3.2) (see Figure 1), lower proportions of patients needing assistance for daily activities, lower proportions of patients with RA caused disabilities, lower mean HAQ scores and higher mean EQ-5D-5L scores (see Table 2).

The variables retained in the propensity score model were: satisfaction of ACR criteria, HAQ level and home ownership status.

Descriptive Cost Analysis

The breakdown of costs by resource component is shown in Table 3. The mean annual total cost per patient over the four-year period was €3,612, with DMARD costs accounting for nearly half that amount. It can be seen in Figure 2 (A) that total costs increased year by year over the study period in all treatment strategy groups except for FYB users whose mean annual total costs decreased between year three and year four. Among other costs, hospitalisation was the largest component, constituting one-third of total costs with wide variation among groups. Hospitalisation costs for LYB users were more than three times higher than those of patients not treated with DMARDs.

For patients receiving biologics, DMARDs constituted the highest share of total costs. For FYB patients the mean annual cost per patient was more than five times higher than that of the rest of the population, nearly twice that of LYB users and nearly eight times that of patients receiving only synthetic DMARDs.

Other healthcare costs were one-third lower among FYB patients compared to LYB patients, representing an average annual offset of €1,042. Healthcare costs of FYB patients remained comparable to patients who received no biologic treatment (Figure 2 (B)), although FYB patients were likely to have a more active disease at inclusion (mean DAS-28:5.95 vs. 4.99, p<0.0001 and mean HAQ: 1.37 vs. 0.91, p<0.0001; see Table 1). This contrasted with LYB patient costs, which remained higher than those in all other groups and increased regularly over the four-year period with a peak increase 24 months after inclusion.

Grouping LYB patients by year of biologic initiation revealed that their total mean annual costs decreased with later initiation of biologics (total costs in order of year of biologic initiation: €10,661 (n = 32, 2nd year after inclusion), €7,592 (n = 16, 3rd year after inclusion) and €5,384 (n = 18, 4th year after inclusion) respectively), while their other mean annual costs remained comparable (healthcare costs by year of biologic initiation: €3,032, €2,941 and €3,053 respectively). Inferential statistics were not produced due to the small size of these groups.

Factors Associated with Costs

The results of the multivariate regression analyses of total costs and other healthcare costs are shown in Tables 4 and 5. The reported RR describe the variations in costs expressed as a multiplicative factor for patients presenting the associated characteristic compared to those who did not, all other things being equal.

The total and other healthcare costs models were similar in terms of significance and magnitude of effects. Higher HAQ scores at baseline, increase in HAQ score between baseline and the six-month study visit and hospitalisations at baseline or in the six months prior to inclusion were associated with higher costs, whereas living with a partner and having a doctor's certainty of RA diagnostic below 50% had the opposite effect. The strongest effects on costs were found for the use of biologic treatments and HAQ.

While the biologic treatment strategy induces the highest increase in total costs, with FYB showing a greater impact than LYB, only LYB shows a significant relation with other healthcare costs: plus 60% compared to all other patients.

Sensitivity analyses showed similar results but with additional significant effects. Higher age at baseline increased both types of cost, while high family income and full health coverage were only related to total costs with respectively increasing and decreasing effects.

The total costs model explained more than 50% of observed variations, while only 22% were explained by the other healthcare cost model. Furthermore, those variations were primarily driven by differences between patients rather than between medical centres' practices, with intraclass correlation coefficients lower than 5% when adjusted for patient-level variables.

Discussion

Our study reported the costs of a large sample of EA patients, more than 80% of whom satisfied the RA classification criteria. [30] With 71% of patients using only synthetic DMARDs and 19.7% using biologics, mean annual total costs in the cohort were €3,612 while mean other healthcare costs were €1,844.

High costs of RA in several countries have been described from both the societal and public payer perspectives, [7,13] with the latter most often estimating only direct costs of RA treatment. A recent overview in western countries estimated the average annual direct costs in €2007 at €4,208, [13] while another reported substantially higher costs in western European countries (€15,135) than in central or eastern European countries, (€3,532). [7] The ESPOIR cohort's direct costs were lower than those previously reported in the literature. [13,31,32] This could be partially explained by the fact that the present study explores the early stages of the disease, for which surgery and disability care are limited. Moreover, while previous studies found hospitalisations to be the largest cost share, [13,33] we found that it is currently attributable to RA-specific drug costs, particularly biologic therapies, which represent almost half of the direct four-year costs. The economic impact is significant for the French statutory health insurance, which bears almost the full cost of these drugs.

Our analysis revealed wide variations in direct medical costs among patients in the first four years of RA treatment depending on the treatment strategy. As expected, total costs over four years were over 70% higher for patients with FYB use compared to patients with LYB use. This difference was due to the increased cost of biologic DMARDs, as other costs were in fact lower among FYB patients compared to LYB users over the period. As shown in Figure 1 (B), FYB users' other healthcare costs remained at a lower level throughout the four-year study period than those of LYB users, indicating greater diminishment in disease progression among FYB users, which is supported by a higher proportion of patients with low disease activity (DAS-28≤3.2) (see Figure 2), lower rates of needed assistance and RA caused disability, higher HAQ levels and lower EQ-5D-3L utilities (see Table 2) among FYB users' after matching on baseline characteristics. Furthermore, FYB patients' other costs over four years did not differ significantly from those of patients who did not need biologic therapy, while they were more than 60% higher for LYB patients. This is consistent with previous findings according to which very early suppression of disease activity is likely to reduce patient costs [34].

As other authors have found [35,36] another significant cost driver was disease severity, as revealed by high HAQ values. In addition, when physicians were more confident in the RA diagnosis, they were more likely to use a step-up strategy [37,38] resulting in higher resource use.

We acknowledge some limitations regarding data quality, availability and follow-up and statistical analyses. Information related to blood tests and analgesic dosages was not recorded in a standardised manner, and thus we used standard packages defined by an expert. Transportation costs were also standardised, as covered distances were not reported. However, the impact of these limitations on the reported results should be small because they account for a minor proportion of total costs: blood tests (~5%), analgesics (<2%) and transportation (<1%). There was a substantial degree of missing values, with 33% of patients missing at least one follow-up visit. However, sensitivity analyses found the models to be robust. In addition, one may question the impact memory bias [39] may have on the quality of the data collected retrospectively given the length of time between study visits. Moreover, the overall study period may have been too short to reveal the longer term impact of biologic therapies on costs. Finally, we used 2007 prices and not more recent data. However the mean annual total costs in the cohort for 2011, obtained by applying the evolution of the consumption of care and medical goods price index in France was estimated at €3,616 which is quite similar to our 2007 results [3].

In our statistical analyses, the multiple imputation method we used to address the problem of missing data in the sensitivity analyses may have resulted in bias. We undertook log transformations of costs per period prior to implementing the multiple imputation in order to approach normality and obtain exclusively positive imputed costs following back transformation. Although some experts recommend such transformations, [40] more recent research has drawn attention to the limitations of this method, including degradation of the relationships between variables in the imputation model resulting in bias, and suggested approaches based on flexible non-normal distributions [41].

Our analysis suggests that early use of biologics may reduce other healthcare costs by slowing the evolution of the disease. We do not know the extent to which the high direct costs incurred from early use of biologics costs may be balanced in part by other health care cost offsets due to the reduction in the need for surgery or other interventions beyond the fourth year of the disease. Moreover, recent price reductions for biologics could make them more cost-effective, [42] thereby decreasing resistance to early use that may improve patients' lives.

Acknowledgments

The authors wish to thank Nathalie Rincheval, who did expert monitoring and data management, and all the investigators who recruited and followed the patients (F. BERENBAUM, Paris- Saint Antoine; M.C. BOISSIER, Paris-Bobigny; A. CANTAGREL, A. CONSTANTIN, Toulouse; B. COMBE, Montpellier; M. DOUGADOS, Paris-Cochin; P. FARDELONNE, P. BOUMIER, Amiens; B. FAUTREL, P. BOURGEOIS, Paris-La Pitié; R.M. FLIPO, Lille; P. GOUPILLE, Tours; F. LIOTE, Paris-Lariboisière; X. LE LOET Rouen; X. MARIETTE, Paris Bicêtre; O. MEYER, Paris Bichat; A.SARAUX, Brest; T. SCHAEVERBEKE, Bordeaux; J. SIBILIA, Strasbourg), as well as Karen Berg Brigham for her helpful review of the manuscript and Hassani Maoulida and Marie De Rosa for their participation in data management.

Author Contributions

Conceived and designed the experiments: KC BF IDZ. Performed the experiments: KC BF GH. Analyzed the data: GH SL SH. Contributed reagents/materials/analysis tools: SH MLL XM AS FG. Wrote the paper: KC GH SL SH FG BF.

References

1. Alamanos Y, Drosos AA (2005) Epidemiology of rheumatoid arthritis. Autoimmun Rev 4: 130–36.
2. Uhlig T, Kvien T (2005) Is rheumatoid arthritis disappearing? Ann Rheum Dis 64: 7–10.
3. Le Garrec M-A, Bouvet M, Koubi M (2012) Comptes nationaux de la santé – 2011. DREES (Direction de la recherche, des études, de l'évaluation et des statistiques). Available: http://www.drees.sante.gouv.fr/IMG/pdf/comptes_sante_2011.pdf. Accessed June 1st 2013.
4. Guillemin F, Durieux S, Daurès JP, Lafuma A, Saraux A et al. (2004) Costs of rheumatoid arthritis in France: a multicenter study of 1109 patients managed by hospital-based rheumatologists. J Rheumatol 31: 1297–304.
5. Kobelt G, Woronoff AS, Richard B, Peeters P, Sany J (2008) Disease status, costs and quality of life of patients with rheumatoid arthritis in France: the ECO-PR Study. Joint Bone Spine 75: 408–15.
6. Wolfe F, Michaud K (2010) The loss of health status in rheumatoid arthritis and the effect of biologic therapy: a longitudinal observational study. Arthritis Res Ther 12: R35.
7. Lundkvist J, Kastang F, Kobelt G (2008) The burden of rheumatoid arthritis and access to treatment: health burden and costs. Eur J Health Econ (Suppl 2): S49–60.
8. Fautrel B, Verstappen SM, Boonen A (2011) Economic consequences and potential benefits. Best Pract Res Clin Rheumatol 25: 607–24.
9. Rosery H, Bergemann R, Maxion-Bergemann S (2005) International variation in resource utilisation and treatment costs for rheumatoid arthritis: a systematic literature review. Pharmacoeconomics 23: 243–57.
10. Saag KG, Teng GG, Patkar NM, Anuntiyo J, Finney C et al. (2008) American College of Rheumatology 2008 recommendations for the use of nonbiologic and biologic disease-modifying antirheumatic drugs in rheumatoid arthritis. Arthritis Rheum 59: 762–84.
11. Finckh A, Bansback N, Marra CA, Anis AH, Michaud K et al. (2009) Treatment of very early rheumatoid arthritis with symptomatic therapy, disease-modifying antirheumatic drugs, or biologic agents: a cost-effectiveness analysis. Ann Intern Med 151: 612–21.
12. Benucci M, Saviola G, Manfredi M, Sarzi-Puttini P, Atzeni F (2011) Cost Effectiveness Analysis of Disease-Modifying Antirheumatic Drugs in Rheumatoid Arthritis. A Systematic Review Literature. Int J Rheumatol Doi:10.1155/2011/845496.
13. Franke LC, Ament AJ, van de Laar MA, Boonen A, Severens JL (2009) Cost-of-illness of rheumatoid arthritis and ankylosing spondylitis. Clin Exp Rheumatol 27: S118–23.
14. Combe B, Benessiano J, Brenbaum F, Cantagrel A, Daurès JP et al. (2007) The ESPOIR cohort: A ten-year follow-up of early arthritis in France: Methodology and baseline characteristics of the 813 included patients. Joint Bone Spline 74: 440–5.
15. Bories-Maskulova V (2008) Démographie et honoraires des médecins libéraux en 2006. Point de repère, Caisse nationale de l'Assurance Maladie 23. Available: http://www.ameli.fr/l-assurance-maladie/statistiques-et-publications/points-de-repere/n-23-demographie-honoraires-des-medecins-2006.php. Accessed June 1st 2013.
16. OECD Health Data (2007) ECOSANTE [database on the Internet]. Available: http://ecosante.fr/. Accessed June 1st 2013.
17. Chevreul K, Prigent A, Bourmaud A, Leboyer M, Durand-Zaleski I (2012) The cost of mental disorders in France. Eur Neuropsychopharmacol Doi: 10.1016/j.euroneuro.2012.08.012.
18. Caisse Nationale de l'Assurance Maladie des Travailleurs Salariés (CNAMTS) (2007) CCAMv10 2007: Common classification of medical procedures [database on the Internet]. Available: http://www.atih.sante.fr/index.php?id = 0003100028FF. Accessed June 1st 2013.
19. Coldefy M, Com-Ruelle L, Lucas-Gabrielli V, Marcoux L (2011) Les distances d'accès aux soins en France métropolitaine au 1er janvier 2007. IRDES (Institut de Recherche en Economie de la Santé). Available: http://www.irdes.fr/Publications/Rapports2011/rap1838.pdf. Accessed June 1st 2013.

20. Caisse Nationale de l'Assurance Maladie (CNAM) (2007) Medic'AM 2007 [database on the Internet] Available: http://www.ameli.fr/l-assurance-maladie/statistiques-et-publications/donnees-statistiques/medicament/medic-am-2002-2007.php.Accessed June 1st 2007.
21. Agence technique de l'information sur l'hospitalisation (ATIH) (2006) ENCC MCO 2006: National cost care for medecin surgery obstretics sector (acute care sector) [database on the Internet] Available: http://www.atih.sante.fr/index.php?id = 0000F00005FF.Accessed June 1st 2013.
22. Grieve R, Nixon R, Thompson SG, Normand C (2005) Using multilevel models for assessing the variability of multinational resource use and cost data. Health Econ 14: 185–96.
23. Raudenbush SW, Bryk AS (2001) Hierarchical Linear Models: Applications and Data Analysis Methods. Second Edition. Newbury Park, CA: SAGE. 79 p.
24. Fries JF, Spitz P, Kraines RG, Holman HR (1980) Measurement of patient outcome in arthritis. Arthritis Rheum 23: 137–45.
25. Smolen JS, Landewé R, Breedveld FC, Dougados M, Emery P et al. (2010) EULAR recommendations for the management of rheumatoid arthritis with synthetic and biological disease-modifying antirheumatic drugs. Ann Rheum Dis 69(6): 964–75.
26. Allison PD (2005) Imputation of Categorical Variables with PROC MI. Proceedings of the Thirtieth Annual SAS Users Group International (SUGI) Conference; 2005. Cary, North Carolina: SAS Institute Inc.
27. Graham JW (2009) Missing Data Analysis: Making It Work in the Real World. Annu Rev Psychol 60: 549–76.
28. Collins LM, Schafer JL, Kam C-M (2001) A comparison of inclusive and restrictive strategies in modern missing data procedures. Psychol Methods 6: 330–51.
29. Rubin DB (1987) Multiple Imputation for Nonresponse in Surveys. New York: John Wiley & Sons, Inc. 76 p.
30. Fautrel B, Combe B, Rincheval N, Dougados M, ESPOIR Scientific Commitee (2012) Level of agreement of the 1987 ACR and 2010 ACR/EULAR rheumatoid arthritis classification criteria: an analysis based on ESPOIR cohort data. Ann Rheum Dis 71: 386–89.
31. Adami S, Bernardi D, Rossi E, Rossini M, De Rosa M (2013) Drug use and Cost Evaluation In Rheumatoid Arthritis Patients. Value Health16: A221.
32. Kawatkar AA, Jacobsen SJ, Levy GD, Medhekar SS, Venkatasubramaniam KV et al. (2012) Direct medical expenditure associated with rheumatoid arthritis in a nationally representative sample from the medical expenditure survey. Arthritis Care Res (Hoboken) 64: 1649–56.
33. Fautrel B, Verstappen SMM, Boonen A (2011) Economic consequences and potential benefits. Best Pract Res Clin Rheumatol 25: 607–24.
34. Hallert E, Husberg M, Skogh T (2011) 28-joint count disease activity score at 3 months after diagnosis of early rheumatoid arthritis is strongly associated with direct and indirect costs over the following 4 years: the Swedish TIRA project. Rheumatology 50: 1259–67.
35. Michaud K, Messer J, Choi HK, Wolf F (2003) Direct medical costs and their predictors in patients with rheumatoid arthritis: a three-year study of 7,527 patients. Arthritis Rheum 48: 2750–62.
36. Zhu TY, Tam L-S, Li EK (2011) Societal costs of rheumatoid arthritis in Hong Kong: a prevalence-based cost-of-illness study. Rheumatology 50: 1293–1301.
37. Combe B, Landewe R, Lukas C, Bolosiu HD, Breedveld F et al. (2007) EULAR recommendations for the management of early arthritis: report of a task force of the European Standing Committee for International Clinical Studies Including Therapeutics (ESCISIT). Ann Rheum Dis 66: 34–45.
38. Knevel R, Schoels M, Huizinga TWJ, Aletaha D, Burmester GR et al. (2010) Current evidence for a strategic approach to the management of rheumatoid arthritis with disease-modifying antirheumatic drugs: a systematic literature review informing the EULAR recommendations for the management of rheumatoid arthritis. Ann Rheum Dis 69: 987–994.
39. Rubin DC, Baddeley AD (1989) Telescoping is not time compression: a model of the dating of autobiographical events. Mem Cognit 17: 653–61.
40. Schafer JL, Graham JW (2002) Missing data: our view of the state of the art. Psychol Methods 7: 147–77.
41. von Hippel PT (2013) Should a Normal Imputation Model be modified to Impute Skewed Variables? Sociol Methods Res 42: 105–38.
42. Finckh A, Bansback N, Liang MH, Boers M (2010) Cost-effectiveness of biologics in early rheumatoid arthritis. Ann Intern Med 152: 333–4.

14

Usual Interstitial Pneumonia Preceding Collagen Vascular Disease: A Retrospective Case Control Study of Patients Initially Diagnosed with Idiopathic Pulmonary Fibrosis

Masato Kono[1,2], Yutaro Nakamura[1]*, Noriyuki Enomoto[1], Dai Hashimoto[1], Tomoyuki Fujisawa[1], Naoki Inui[1], Masato Maekawa[2], Takafumi Suda[1], Thomas V. Colby[3], Kingo Chida[1]

1 Second Division, Department of Internal Medicine, Hamamatsu University School of Medicine, Hamamatsu, Japan, **2** Department of Laboratory Medicine, Hamamatsu University School of Medicine, Hamamatsu, Japan, **3** Department of Laboratory Medicine and Pathology, Mayo Clinic, Scottsdale, Arizona, United Sates of America

Abstract

Background: The aim of this study was to evaluate the cumulative incidence and the predictive factors for collagen vascular disease (CVD) in patients initially diagnosed with idiopathic pulmonary fibrosis (IPF), and to examine the features of patients who then developed CVD.

Methods: This was a retrospective review of 111 consecutive patients with IPF diagnosed at our institution. None of the patients fulfilled any of the CVD criteria from the American College of Rheumatology (ACR) within 6 months or more after the diagnosis of IPF.

Results: Ten patients (9.0%) developed CVD during the follow-up period: four had rheumatoid arthritis (RA); four had microscopic polyangiitis (MPA); one had systemic sclerosis (SSc); and one had SSc and Sjogren's syndrome (SjS). The mean time until CVD diagnosis was 3.9 years. The cumulative incidences of CVD at 1, 5, and 10 years were 0.91%, 9.85%, and 15.5%, respectively. Patients who developed CVD were significantly younger, more likely to be women and had a better prognosis than those with IPF. Cox proportional hazards regression analysis showed that female sex and the presence of lymphoid aggregates with germinal centers were significantly associated with the occurrence of CVD in patients initially diagnosed with IPF.

Conclusions: CVD is an important underlying condition in IPF, and shows better prognosis. The possibility of the development of CVD should remain a consideration in the follow-up of IPF.

Editor: Carol Feghali-Bostwick, Medical University of South Carolina, United States of America

Funding: This study was partly supported by a grant to the Diffuse Lung Diseases Research Group from the Ministry of Health, Labor and Welfare, Japan. The funders had no role in study design, data collection and analysis, decision to publish, or preparation of the manuscript.

Competing Interests: The authors have declared that no competing interests exist.

* E-mail: nakayuta@hama-med.ac.jp

Introduction

Interstitial pneumonia (IP) commonly complicates collagen vascular disease (CVD) [1–5], and it is well known that IP may be the first or only manifestation of CVD [6]. None of these patients with IP fulfill the diagnostic criteria for defined CVDs, and most may be diagnosed as idiopathic interstitial pneumonias (IIPs) [7,8]. It has been reported that patients with IIPs cannot be distinguished from those with IP associated with CVD (CVD-IP) before the systemic signs of CVD appear [6]. Although we sometimes encounter patients who fulfill the criteria for a CVD in the clinical course of IIP, the cumulative incidence and predictive factors associated with the occurrence of CVD remain unclear.

In patients with IIPs, non-specific interstitial pneumonia (NSIP) has been reported to be associated with autoimmune diseases including CVDs [9–11], and there are some reports of idiopathic NSIP preceding the diagnosis of CVD [11–14]. However, there are a few reports of patients who fulfill the criteria for a CVD after the diagnosis of idiopathic pulmonary fibrosis (IPF)/usual interstitial pneumonia (UIP) [4,15]. Recently, some patients with CVD-associated signs and symptoms who nonetheless failed to fulfill the criteria defined CVDs have been diagnosed using new criteria, such as those for undifferentiated connective tissue disease (UCTD) [16], lung-dominant connective tissue disease (LD-CTD) [17], and autoimmune-featured interstitial lung disease (AIF-ILD) [18]. However, these criteria are not always fulfilled in patients with IIPs preceding the diagnosis of CVD.

Here, we evaluated the cumulative incidence of CVD and the clinical features of patients who fulfilled the criteria for any CVD after an initial diagnosis of IPF. Furthermore, we examined the predictive factors associated with the development of CVD in patients initially diagnosed with IPF.

Patients and Methods

Patients and Diagnostic Criteria

We studied 155 consecutive patients with IPF who were diagnosed clinically or underwent surgical lung biopsy (SLB) at our institution from 1990 through 2007. The diagnosis of IPF was based on a history, physical examination, high-resolution computed tomography (HRCT) findings and/or histologic examination, and the appropriateness of the IPF diagnosis in each case was retrospectively reevaluated according to the current international diagnostic criteria [19]. Within at least 6 months of the initial diagnosis, none of the patients fulfilled the American College of Rheumatology (ACR) criteria defining CVDs, including rheumatoid arthritis (RA) [20], polymyositis/dermatomyositis (PM/DM) [21], systemic sclerosis (SSc) [22], systemic lupus erythematosus (SLE) [23] and Sjogren's syndrome (SjS) [24], or the Chapel Hill Consensus Conference criteria defining systemic vasculitis, including microscopic polyangiitis (MPA) [25]. The study protocol was approved by the Ethical Committee of Hamamatsu University School of Medicine. Patient approval and/or informed consent were waived because the study involved a retrospective review of patient records, images and pathologies. Our institutional review board determined that ethical approval was not necessary and did not require the patient's approval or informed consent.

Data Collection

Clinical data were obtained from patients' medical records. Laboratory findings, pulmonary function test results and bronchoalveolar lavage (BAL) data obtained at the time of the initial diagnosis were also recorded. For the patients who developed CVD, additional clinical data were obtained at the time of the CVD diagnosis. The duration of time until the CVD diagnosis and the cumulative incidence of CVD among patients with IPF were calculated.

High-resolution Computed Tomography (HRCT)

HRCT examinations of the lungs were performed on 1.0- or 1.5-mm-thick sections to evaluate radiographic abnormalities at the time of initial diagnosis. The HRCT images were based on previously published international criteria for IPF [19]. We reviewed the presence and the distribution of each of the following signs: consolidation, ground-glass opacity (GGO), reticulation, centrilobular nodules, honeycombing, traction bronchiectasis, lymph node enlargement, and cysts.

Pathological Review

Histological classification was based on the previously published criteria for IIPs and IPF [7,19]. A diagnosis of UIP was originally made histologically by a lung pathologist at our facility. Lung biopsy specimens were also reviewed by a second lung pathologist (T. V. C.) who was unaware of the clinical or physical findings. The degree of each of the following pathologic findings was scored semiquantitatively (absent, 0; mild, 1; moderate, 2; marked, 3): alveolar inflammation, fibrosis, intra-alveolar macrophages, organizing pneumonia, fibroblastic foci, and lymphoid aggregates with germinal centers. For lymphoid aggregates, the case was scored as 1 when there was one germinal center and as 3 when there were six or more in a low-power field (2×). The presence or absence of each of the following pathologic findings was also assessed: honeycombing, extensive pleuritis, prominent plasmacytic infiltration, and dense perivascular collagen including the histopathological features of the proposed provisional criteria for LD-CTD [17].

Statistical Methods

For two-group comparisons involving binary data, we used the chi-square test. Comparisons involving continuous data were made using the Mann-Whitney *U*-test. The cumulative survival probabilities and the cumulative incidence of CVD were estimated using the Kaplan-Meier method. The log-rank test was used to compare survival among the groups of patients. Cox proportional hazards regression analysis was used to identify significant variables predicting the development of CVD. Statistical analyses were performed using JMP Start Statistics (SAS Institute Inc., NC, USA). A P value <0.05 was considered significant.

Results

Patient Characteristics

Of the original 155 patients, 44 patients were excluded because of inadequate clinical information. The remaining 111 patients were included in this study. All of them were diagnosed with IPF (definite, n = 104; probable, n = 2; possible, n = 5) according to HRCT and/or the histopathological pattern [19] (**Figure 1**), and the clinical characteristics of these patients are shown in **Table 1**. During the observation periods (6.4±4.9 years), 10 patients (9%) developed CVD (all patients were initially diagnosed with definite IPF). We compared the clinical characteristics of patients who developed CVD and those with IPF at the initial diagnosis (**Table 1**). Compared to patients with IPF, those who developed CVD were younger and more often female. There were no statistically significant differences in smoking habits, observation period, or the rate of SLB between groups. Between-group comparisons revealed no significant difference in serum levels of lactate dehydrogenase (LDH), creatine phosphokinase (CPK), C-reactive protein (CRP), KL-6, surfactant protein-D (SP-D), PaO_2 in room air, or pulmonary function. BAL was performed in 83 patients (74.8%): in nine of 10 who developed CVD and in 74 of 101 who did not. The patients who developed CVD exhibited a reduced percentage of lymphocytes ($P = 0.04$) in comparison to those with IPF, but no other BAL findings were significantly different between the groups.

The clinical characteristics of the patients who developed CVD at the time of CVD diagnosis are shown in **Table 2**. These 10 patients included four patients with RA (40%), four patients with MPA (40%), one patient with SSc (10%), and one patient with overlap syndrome (SSc/SjS) (10%). This group included five women (50%). Age at the time of CVD diagnosis was 63.2±7.4 years. The average time from the initial diagnosis of IPF to the CVD diagnosis was 3.9±2.4 years. None of the patients had undergone treatment for IP with corticosteroids and/or immunosuppressive agents (ISA) prior to the development of CVD. Each had been diagnosed with CVD based on their symptoms and other findings associated with CVD. All four patients who developed RA showed polyarthralgia and positivity for rheumatoid factor (RF). In the four patients who developed MPA, two patients (Cases 7, 8) had alveolar hemorrhage, three patients (Cases 6, 7, 8) showed renal dysfunction with hematuria, two patients (Cases 5, 8) exhibited a purpuric rash with small-vessel vasculitis detected by skin biopsy, and all four patients showed positivity for myeloperoxidase antineutrophil cytoplasmic antibody (MPO-ANCA). Both patients who developed SSc showed Raynaud's phenomenon and scleroderma, and one patient (Case 10) also showed dry mouth with inflammation of the salivary glands associated with SjS. One patient died secondary to the acute exacerbation (AE) of IP (Case 6) and one patient died of unknown cause (Case 10). The deaths occurred at 5.8 and 3.8 years, respectively, from the initial diagnosis.

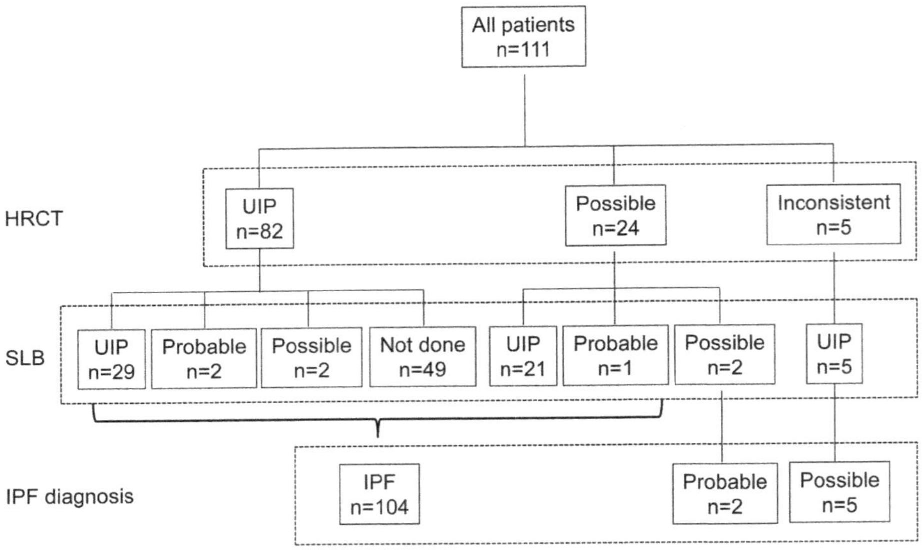

Figure 1. The algorithm for IPF diagnosis among enrolled patients. All 111 patients were diagnosed with IPF (definite, n = 104; probable, n = 2; possible, n = 5) according to the algorithm for IPF diagnosis. HRCT, high-resolution computed tomography; SLB, surgical lung biopsy; IPF, idiopathic pulmonary fibrosis; UIP, usual interstitial pneumonia.

Table 1. Patient characteristics.

Characteristics	All patients	CVD-IP	IPF	*P* value
No. of cases	111	10	101	
Age, yr	64.7±9.4	59.6±8.0	65.2±9.3	0.03
Gender, male/female	99/12	5/5	94/7	<0.001
Smoking habit, n Current/former/never	41/56/14	2/5/3	39/51/11	n. s.
Observation period, yr	6.4±4.4	8.7±5.9	6.1±4.2	n. s.
Surgical lung biopsy, n (%)	63 (56.8)	7 (70.0)	56 (55.4)	n. s.
Initial IPF diagnosis, n definite/probable/possible	104/2/5	10/0/0	94/2/5	n. s.
Laboratory data				
LDH, IU/L	253±85	280±89	251±84	n. s.
CPK, IU/L	90±48	101±62	89±46	n. s.
CRP, mg/dL	0.94±2.97	0.42±0.40	0.98±3.08	n. s.
KL-6, U/mL	1129±739	1707±1408	1096±694	n. s.
SP-D, ng/mL	273±195	357±179	269±196	n. s.
PaO_2 on room air, Torr	79.5±14.9	79.3±11.0	79.4±15.2	n. s.
Pulmonary function tests				
FVC, % predicted	84.2±20.9	83.7±21.7	84.2±20.9	n. s.
$FEV_{1.0}$, % predicted	81.9±9.2	84.0±4.3	81.7±9.6	n. s.
DLco, % predicted	84.5±25.1	86.4±30.6	84.2±24.7	n. s.
Bronchoalveolar lavage (BAL)*				
Macrophages, %	90.6±11.3	94.5±3.7	90.1±11.8	n. s.
Lymphocytes, %	6.2±8.0	3.0±3.5	6.6±8.3	0.04
Neutrophils, %	1.6±6.0	1.4±1.5	1.7±6.3	n. s.
Eosinophils, %	1.4±4.7	0.6±0.9	1.5±5.0	n. s.
CD4/CD8 ratio	2.8±2.4	3.4±2.6	2.7±2.5	n. s.

CVD, connective vascular disease; IPF, idiopathic pulmonary fibrosis; CVD-IP, interstitial pneumonia associated with collagen vascular disease; LDH, lactate dehydrogenase; CPK, creatine phosphokinase; CRP, C-reactive protein; SP-D, surfactant protein-D; FVC, forced vital capacity; $FEV_{1.0}$, forced vital capacity in 1 second; DLco; diffusion capacity for carbon monoxide; n. s., not significant.
*BAL was performed in 83 patients (74.8%): CVD-IP (n = 9), IPF (n = 74).

Table 2. Characteristics of the patients who had developed CVD at the time of CVD diagnosis.

Case	Age, yr	Sex, F/M	CVD	SLB	Duration until CVD diagnosis	Findings associated with CVD diagnosis	Treatment before CVD diagnosis	Outcome
1	63	F	RA	UIP	4yr4mo	Arthralgia	None	Alive
2	60	F	RA	UIP	2yr10mo	Arthralgia, Muscular pain	None	Alive
3	62	M	RA	UIP	1yr1mo	Arthralgia	None	Alive
4	66	F	RA	UIP*	4yr4mo	Arthralgia	None	Alive
5	64	M	MPA	UIP	3yr7mo	Rash (vasculitis)	Macrolide	Alive
6	76	M	MPA	None	6mo	Renal dysfunction	None	Dead
7	65	M	MPA	None	8yr	Alveolar hemorrhage, Renal dysfunction	None	Alive
8	66	F	MPA	None	4yr5mo	Alveolar hemorrhage, Rash (vasculitis), Renal dysfunction	None	Alive
9	64	M	SSc	UIP	7yr5mo	Raynaud, scleroderma	None	Alive
10	46	F	SSc/SjS	UIP	3yr	Raynaud, scleroderma, Dry mouth	None	Dead

CVD, connective vascular disease; yr, year; F, female; M, male; SLB, surgical lung biopsy; RA, rheumatoid arthritis; MPA, microscopic polyangiitis; SSc, systematic sclerosis; SjS, Sjogren's syndrome; UIP, usual interstitial pneumonia; mo, month.
*SLB was performed at the time of RA diagnosis.

Systemic Findings Associated with CVD and Autoantibodies

We compared the systemic findings associated with CVD and autoantibodies at the time of the initial diagnosis in patients who developed CVD and in those with a persistent diagnosis of IPF (**Table 3**). Anti-nuclear antibody (ANA) and RF test results were considered positive with a result ≥1+ or a titer of 1:40 and ≥15 IU/mL, respectively. No systemic findings associated with CVD or autoantibodies recorded at the time of the initial diagnosis differed between groups. About half of the patients with IPF had positive ANA results owing to the low cutoff level for ANA. In the patients who developed CVD, there were no positive findings of CVD-specific autoantibodies at the time of the initial diagnosis, except for ANA and RF. However, all patients who developed CVD had systemic findings associated with CVD and/or autoantibodies at the time of the CVD diagnosis. In particular, ANA was positive in 8/10 patients (80.0%) and RF was positive in 9/10 patients (90.0%) at the time of the CVD diagnosis.

HRCT and Pathological Findings

The HRCT and pathological findings in the patients who developed CVD and in those with IPF are shown in **Table 4**. The HRCT findings showed that there was no statistically significant difference between the groups with regard to the presence or distribution of each finding, including consolidation, GGO, reticulation, centrilobular nodules, honeycombing, traction bronchiectasis, lymph node enlargement, and cysts, at the initial diagnosis.

SLB was performed in 63 patients (56.8%): in seven of 10 who developed CVD and in 56 of 101 who did not. One patient who developed CVD (Case 4) was excluded from the statistical analysis because she had undergone SLB at the time of the RA diagnosis; this patient had fulfilled the clinical/radiologic criteria for IPF at the time of the initial diagnosis. The other six patients who developed CVD underwent SLB before the CVD diagnosis. Regarding each pathological finding listed in **Table 4**, the patients who developed CVD had significantly more lymphoid aggregates with germinal centers ($P<0.01$) than did patients with IPF. However, there were no statistically significant differences in the scores for alveolar inflammation, fibrosis, intra-alveolar macrophages, organizing pneumonia, fibroblastic foci, the presence of honeycombing, extensive pleuritis, prominent plasmacytic infiltration, or dense perivascular collagen between the groups. The pathological findings in the patients who developed CVD (Cases 1, 2, 5, 10) are shown in **Figure 2**. Interestingly, the pathological findings for one patient who underwent SLB at the time of the RA diagnosis (Case 4) showed a UIP pattern with prominent lymphoid follicles.

Treatment and Outcome

All of the patients who developed CVD were treated with corticosteroids alone or in combination with ISA therapy after the diagnosis of CVD. They were treated significantly more often than the patients with IPF ($P=0.01$) and also had a significantly higher rate of treatment with corticosteroids alone ($P=0.01$) (**Table 5**). Two of the patients who developed MPA (Cases 5, 7) were treated with corticosteroids and cyclophosphamide. Patients remaining in the IPF group had a higher rate of treatment with other agents, such as pirfenidone and N-acetylcysteine (NAC), than those who developed CVD. The patients who developed CVD had a higher rate of AE, although the difference was not statistically significant, and had significantly higher rates of overall death and death due to a respiratory cause ($P=0.04$, $P=0.02$, respectively).

Table 3. Systemic findings and autoantibodies in the patients who developed CVD and in those with IPF at the time of initial diagnosis.

Characteristics	CVD-IP	IPF	*P* value
Systemic findings			
Raynaud's phenomenon	1 (10.0)	3 (2.9)	n. s.
Arthralgias/joint swelling	0	3 (2.9)	n. s.
Photosensitivity	0	0	n. s.
Unintentional weight loss	1 (10.0)	2 (1.9)	n. s.
Morning stiffness	0	3 (2.9)	n. s.
Dry eye or dry mouth	0	3 (2.9)	n. s.
Dysphagia	0	0	n. s.
Recurrent unexpected fever	0	0	n. s.
Gastroesophageal reflex	0	1 (1.0)	n. s.
Skin change (rash)	0	3 (2.9)	n. s.
Oral ulceration	0	0	n. s.
Non-androgenic alopecia	0	0	n. s.
Autoantibodies, n (%)			
Anti-nuclear antibody	4/10 (40.0)	46/91 (50.5)	n. s.
Rheumatoid factor	3/9 (33.3)	19/85 (22.3)	n. s.
Anti-SCL 70 antibody	0/5 (0)	0/55 (0)	n. s.
Anti-SSA antibody	0/5 (0)	1/57 (1.7)	n. s.
Anti-SSB antibody	0/5 (0)	0/56 (0)	n. s.
Anti-Jo1 antibody	0/4 (0)	0/45 (0)	n. s.
Anti-centromere antibody	0/4 (0)	1/36 (2.7)	n. s.
Anti-RNP antibody	0/5 (0)	0/40 (0)	n. s.
Anti-DNA antibody	0/8 (0)	1/74 (1.3)	n. s.
MPO-ANCA	0/3 (0)	4/54 (7.4)	n. s.
PR3-ANCA	0/3 (0)	1/49 (1.9)	n. s.

CVD, connective vascular disease; IPF, idiopathic pulmonary fibrosis; CVD-IP, interstitial pneumonia associated with collagen vascular disease; MPO-ANCA, myeloperoxidase antineutrophil cytoplasmic antibody; PR3-ANCA, proteinase 3-antineutrophil cytoplasmic antibody; n. s., not significant.

A comparison of the survival curves from the time of initial diagnosis for patients who developed CVD and those who did not is shown in **Figure 3**. The former had a significantly better survival rate than the latter (log-rank test: $P<0.05$).

Cumulative Incidence of CVD and Predictive Factors for the Development of CVD in Patients with IPF

A Kaplan-Meier plot of the cumulative incidence of CVD is shown in **Figure 4**. The cumulative incidences of CVD at 1, 5, and 10 years were 0.91%, 9.85%, and 15.5%, respectively.

Factors predictive for the development of CVD at the initial diagnosis are shown in **Table 6**. Cox proportional hazards regression analysis showed that being female [hazard ratio 3.333, 95% confidence interval (CI) 0.732–6.441, $P<0.01$] and the score for lymphoid aggregates with germinal centers (hazard ratio 3.367, 95% CI 1.503–7.434, $P<0.01$) were significantly associated with the development of CVD in patients with IPF.

Discussion

In this retrospective study, we evaluated the cumulative incidence and the predictive factors for CVD in patients with IPF, and examined the features of patients who subsequently fulfilled the criteria for any CVD. The rate of development of CVD was 9% in consecutive patients initially diagnosed with IPF during the observation period, and the cumulative incidences of CVD at 1, 5, and 10 years were 0.91%, 9.85%, and 15.5%, respectively. It was difficult to predict the latency of CVD in patients with IPF based on systemic findings and the presence of autoantibodies, but Cox proportional hazards regression analysis showed that female sex and prominent lymphoid aggregates with germinal centers were significantly associated with the development of CVD in patients with IPF.

Pulmonary manifestation including IP commonly complicates CVD and increases the mortality and morbidity associated with CVD [26,27]. IP may be the first or only recognized manifestation of a CVD, and it is estimated to affect approximately 15–20% of patients with IIPs [6,9,10,26–28]. The development of CVD after an IIP diagnosis was documented best for SSc and PM/DM patients. It has been reported that IP precedes PM/DM in about 40% of patients [29]. It was also reported that SSc sine scleroderma (ssSSc)-associated IP might be present in IIP patients [30], developing in some cases into typical SSc [31].

In patients with IIPs, NSIP is reportedly associated with autoimmune disease, including CVD [9–11]. Previous studies have documented the development of CVD in patients with NSIP [11–14]. Sato *et al.* reported a small series of seven patients with histologically proven NSIP who later developed CVDs (PM/DM

Table 4. HRCT and pathological findings in the patients who developed CVD and in those with IPF at the time of initial diagnosis.

Characteristics	CVD-IP	IPF	*P* value
HRCT findings			
Subpleural, basal predominance, %	100	97.3	n.s.
Consolidation, %	20.0	11.7	n.s.
GGO, %	40.0	28.7	n.s.
Reticulation, %	100	98.9	n.s.
Centrilobular nodules, %	20.0	6.4	n.s.
Honeycombing, %	90.0	72.3	n.s.
Traction bronchiectasis, %	80.0	66.0	n.s.
Lymph node enlargement, %	10.0	5.3	n.s.
Cysts, %	40.0	26.6	n.s.
Pathological findings			
Alveolar inflammation*	1.41±0.58	1.30±0.51	n.s.
Fibrosis*	2.00±1.10	2.11±0.80	n.s.
Intra-alveolar macrophages*	0.83±0.75	1.21±0.73	n.s.
Organizing pneumonia*	0.33±0.81	0.13±0.33	n.s.
Fibroblastic foci*	0.75±0.52	1.08±0.60	n.s.
Honeycombing, %	83.3	62.5	n.s.
Lymphoid aggregates with germinal centers*	1.17±1.17	0.18±0.47	<0.01
Extensive pleuritis, %	16.7	10.7	n.s.
Prominent plasmacytic infiltration, %	16.7	12.5	n.s.
Dense perivascular collagen, %	0	1.8	n.s.

HRCT, high-resolution computed tomography; CVD, connective vascular disease; IPF, idiopathic pulmonary fibrosis; CVD-IP, interstitial pneumonia associated with collagen vascular disease; GGO, ground-glass opacity; n. s., not significant.
*scoring of the severity: absent 0, mild 1, moderate 2 and marked 3.

n = 4, SSc n = 1, RA n = 1, MPA n = 1) more than 6 months after the first presentation of NSIP [12]. Recently, in a large retrospective analysis, 3–10% of patients with idiopathic NSIP developed CVDs [13,14], with variable intervals between CVD occurrences (9 months to 8 years) [13].

However, there have been only a few reports of patients who developed CVD in presumed cases of IPF/UIP [4,15]. Lee *et al.* examined the histopathologic patterns and clinical features of 18 patients with RA-IP, and reported three patients in whom IP preceded the diagnosis of RA (1.6 years, 2.5 years, 7 years): two patients had UIP and one had NSIP [4]. Van der Kamp *et al.* reported three patients with IP as the first manifestation of SSc, and 1 of these three patients had biopsy-proven UIP 4 years prior to the SSc diagnosis [15]. The present study revealed that RA and MPA were the main CVDs that developed after the initial IP diagnosis. In the patients with IP-associated RA or MPA, the UIP pattern is seen more commonly than other pathological patterns [4,5,32]. CVD development after an IIP diagnosis might vary according to the histological pattern of the patient's IIP.

Although it was reported that younger patients with IPF, especially women, without clinical or serologic features at presentation may subsequently manifest clinical features of CVD [19], IIP patients could not be distinguished from CVD-IP patients before systemic signs of CVD appeared [6,12,13]. Our data showed similar results, but the pathological findings of lymphoid aggregates with germinal centers had clinical significance as a predictive factor of occult CVD in patients with IPF. Song *et al.* compared the pathological difference between CVD-UIP (most patients had RA and SSc) and IPF/UIP, and showed by multivariate analysis that germinal center score was the most discriminating factor for CVD-UIP [33]. Cipriani *et al.* also evaluated the difference between CVD-UIP and IPF/UIP by quantitative pathological assessment, and found that there was a trend toward more and larger lymphoid aggregates in the RA-UIP subset [34]. Our finding suggests that an UIP pattern with prominent germinal centers may be associated with subsequent CVD in IPF patients.

Some patients with IIPs have symptoms and/or autoantibodies suggestive of autoimmune disorders without fulfilling the criteria for defined CVDs [8]. Such patients can now be diagnosed based on new criteria, including those for UCTD [16], LD-CTD [17] and AIF-ILD [18]. We could speculate that patients exhibiting certain characteristics of CVD would subsequently fulfill the disease's official diagnostic criteria. However, in this study, there was no statistically significant difference between the patients who developed CVD and the remaining patients with IPF in the frequency with which patients fulfilled these criteria (UCTD, LD-CTD and AIF-ILD) at the time of the initial diagnosis (data not shown), suggesting that patients without symptoms of signs suggestive of CVD can develop CVD.

It has been reported that CVD-IP has a better prognosis than IIP [35,36]. The difference in outcome appears to be related to a better prognosis for CVD-UIP than IPF/UIP, rather than to the higher prevalence of NSIP [35,36]. In addition, the improved prognosis of CVD-IP could be attributable to the fact that subclinical or non-progressive IP is common. In contrast with IPF patients, those with CVD are more likely to be administered anti-inflammatory or immune-suppressive treatment, which might

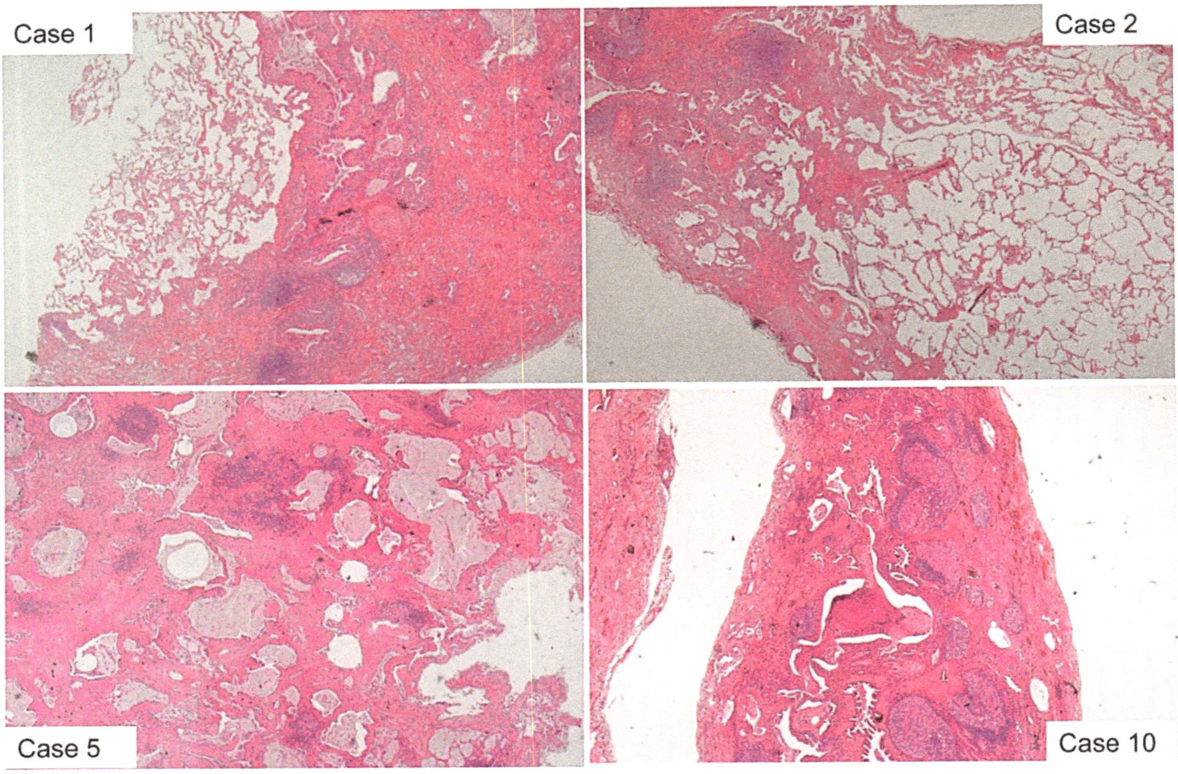

Figure 2. Pathological findings in the patients who developed CVD (Cases 1, 2, 5, 10). All patients showed a pathological UIP pattern at the time of the initial diagnosis. Lymphoid aggregates with germinal centers were prominent in the patients who developed CVD.

affect survival [27]. Our results also revealed that IPF patients who developed CVD (i.e., CVD-IP) had significantly better survival than those who did not, although some reports showed that there was no prognostic difference between IPF/UIP and IPF accompanied by the occult or probable form of CVD (i.e., antibody-positive IPF or LD-CTD) [33,37]. In terms of survival, IPF patients in our series survived longer (median survival time was 8.4 years; 5-year survival rate was 66.4%) than those in most other series [19]. The difference might be due to the fact that the patients included in our series had relatively early-stage disease. Further study including prospective research is needed in this regard.

Several recent reports showed that RA-UIP had a worse prognosis than the other histological patterns of RA-IP [36,38–40]. However, it is uncertain whether RA-UIP and IPF have equally poor prognoses. Indeed, in this study, the patients who developed CVD including RA-UIP had a better prognosis than did other patients with IPF. All the patients with RA-UIP were treated with corticosteroids and exhibited a slowly progressive course of disease without acute exacerbation during the observation period.

The present study has several limitations. First, this was a retrospective study from a single institution, and some patients were excluded because of inadequate information. In addition, the

Table 5. Treatment and outcome throughout the course of the patients who developed CVD and those with IPF.

	CVD-IP	IPF	*P* value
Treatment for IP, n (%)	10 (100)	61 (60.4)	0.01
Corticosteroids alone, n (%)	8 (80.0)	12 (11.8)	<0.01
Corticosteroids+ISA, n (%)	2 (20.0)	34 (33.6)	n. s.
Others, n (%)	0 (0)	23* (22.7)	0.09
Acute exacerbation, n (%)	1 (10.0)	30 (29.7)	n. s.
Death due to respiratory failure, n (%)	1 (10.0)	43 (42.5)	0.02
Overall death, n (%)	2 (20.0)	53 (52.4)	0.04

CVD, collagen vascular disease; IPF, idiopathic pulmonary fibrosis; CVD-IP, interstitial pneumonia associated with collagen vascular disease; ISA, immune suppressive agents; n. s., not significant.
*Pirfenidone (n = 14), N-acetylcysteine (NAC) (n = 5), intravenous immunoglobulin (IVIG) (n = 2), Pirfenidone+NAC (n = 1), Pirfenidone+IVIG (n = 1).

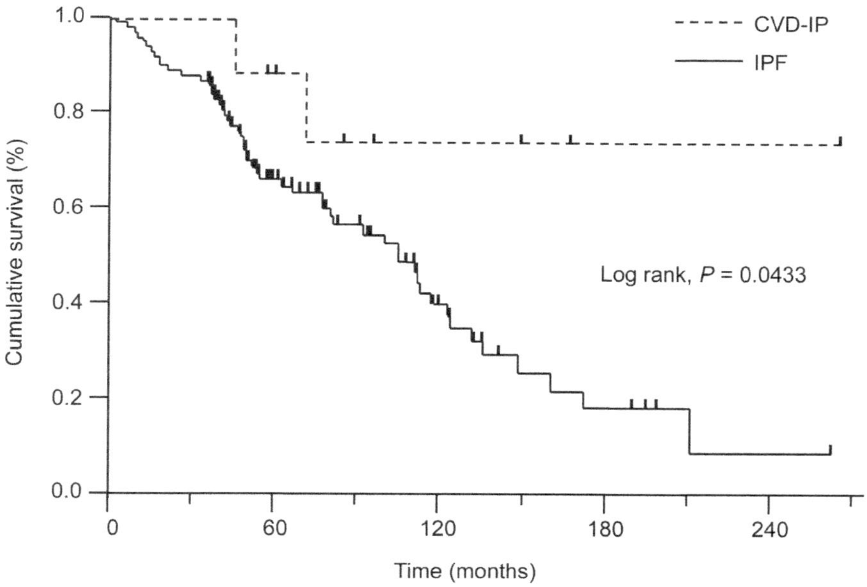

Figure 3. Survival curves for the patients who developed CVD and those with IPF. Patients who developed CVD had a significantly better survival rate than those with IPF (log-rank, $P = 0.0433$). IPF, idiopathic pulmonary fibrosis; CVD-IP, interstitial pneumonia associated with collagen vascular diseaseG.

IPF patients in our series were at a relatively early stage of disease and had longer survival than those in most other series. These were selection and recall biases. Second, although the present study included a relatively large number of patients with IPF, the sample size was too small to determine the precise cumulative incidence and clinical characteristics of those who developed CVD. Third, not all patients underwent SLB or were examined for all of the CVD-specific antibodies. Most patients could not be tested for new autoantibodies such as anti-cyclic citrullinated peptide (CCP) antibody and anti-aminoacyl-tRNA synthetase (ARS) antibody, and so on. In addition, the assays for identifying certain autoantibodies had changed during the study period. Fourth, it might be possible for the development of CVD to be suppressed by the use of immunomodulation drugs or an early observation period, including early death.

In conclusion, we suggest that some CVDs are an underlying condition in IPF and may have a better prognosis than IPF. Although it was unclear whether IP was actually the first

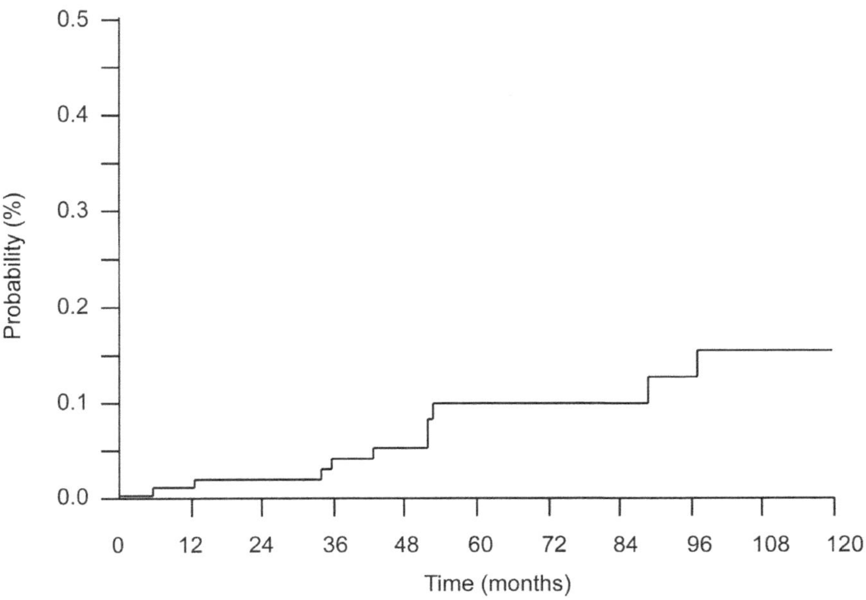

Figure 4. Cumulative incidence of CVD among patients with IPF. Cumulative incidences of CVD at 1, 5, and 10 years were 0.91%, 9.85%, and 15.5%, respectively.

Table 6. Predictive factors for the development of CVD in patients with IPF, according to univariate Cox proportional hazards analysis.

Variables	Hazard ratio	95% CI		*P* value
		Lower	Upper	
Age, year	0.955	0.891	1.023	0.189
Sex, female	3.333	1.732	6.441	<0.01
Symptoms associated with CVD*, positive	1.325	0.514	2.656	0.502
Autoantibodies, positive**	1.216	0.597	3.152	0.614
KL-6, U/mL	1.001	0.999	1.002	0.297
SP-D, ng/mL	1.001	0.996	1.004	0.566
FVC, % predicted	0.987	0.959	1.018	0.412
BAL lymphocytes, %	0.891	0.649	1.028	0.168
HRCT findings				
Consolidation, positive	1.196	0.278	2.801	0.747
GGO, positive	1.239	0.568	2.416	0.556
Centrilobular nodules, positive	1.360	0.315	3.196	0.593
Lymph node enlargement, positive	1.341	0.311	3.136	0.607
Pathological findings				
Alveolar wall inflammation, score	1.572	0.296	7.199	0.576
Fibroblastic foci, score	0.458	0.092	1.931	0.296
Honeycombing, positive	0.574	0.131	1.433	0.258
Lymphoid aggregates with germinal centers, score	3.367	1.503	7.434	<0.01

CVD, collagen vascular disease; IPF, idiopathic pulmonary fibrosis; CI, confidence interval; SP-D, surfactant protein-D; FVC, forced vital capacity; BAL, bronchoalveolar lavage; HRCT, high-resolution computed tomography; GGO, ground-glass opacity.
*one or more positive systemic symptoms in Table 2.
**one or more positive autoantibodies in Table 3.

manifestation of CVD or an incidentally coexisting disorder, it is very important to perform careful follow-up to watch for the development of CVD, especially RA, MPA, and SSc-associated diseases, in patients diagnosed with IPF.

Author Contributions

Conceived and designed the experiments: MK YN TS. Analyzed the data: MK YN NE DH TF NI MM TS TVC KC. Wrote the paper: MK YN TVC.

References

1. Douglas WW, Tazelaar HD, Hartman TE, Hartman RP, Decker PA, et al. (2001) Polymyositis-dermatomyositis-associated interstitial lung disease. Am J Respir Crit Care Med 164: 1182–1185.
2. Bouros D, Wells AU, Nicholson AG, Colby TV, Polychronopoulos V, et al. (2002) Histopathologic subsets of fibrosing alveolitis in patients with systemic sclerosis and their relationship to outcome. Am J Respir Crit Care Med 165: 1581–1586.
3. Ito I, Nagai S, Kitaichi M, Nicholson AG, Johkoh T, et al. (2005) Pulmonary manifestations of primary Sjogren's syndrome: a clinical, radiologic, and pathologic study. Am J Respir Crit Care Med 171: 632–638.
4. Lee HK, Kim DS, Yoo B, Seo JB, Rho JY, et al. (2005) Histopathologic pattern and clinical features of rheumatoid arthritis-associated interstitial lung disease. Chest 127: 2019–2027.
5. Kim EJ, Collard HR, King TE Jr (2009) Rheumatoid arthritis-associated interstitial lung disease: the relevance of histopathologic and radiographic pattern. Chest 136: 1397–1405.
6. Homma Y, Ohtsuka Y, Tanimura K, Kusaka H, Munakata M, et al. (1995) Can interstitial pneumonia as the sole presentation of collagen vascular diseases be differentiated from idiopathic interstitial pneumonia? Respiration 62: 248–51.
7. American Thoracic Society/European Respiratory Society International Multidisciplinary Consensus Classification of the Idiopathic Interstitial Pneumonias. This joint statement of the American Thoracic Society (ATS), and the European Respiratory Society (ERS) was adopted by the ATS board of directors, June 2001 and by the ERS Executive Committee, June 2001. (2002) Am J Respir Crit Care Med 165: 277–304.
8. Travis WD, Costabel U, Hansell DM, King TE Jr, Lynch DA, et al. (2013) An official American Thoracic Society/European Respiratory Society statement: Update of the international multidisciplinary classification of the idiopathic interstitial pneumonias. Am J Respir Crit Care Med 188: 733–748.
9. Cottin V (2006) Interstitial lung disease: are we missing formes frustes of connective tissue disease? Eur Respir J 28: 893–896.
10. Tzelepis GE, Toya SP, Moutsopoulos HM (2008) Occult connective tissue diseases mimicking idiopathic interstitial pneumonias. Eur Respir J 31: 11–20.
11. Romagnoli M, Nannini C, Piciucchi S, Girelli F, Gurioli C, et al. (2011) Idiopathic nonspecific interstitial pneumonia: an interstitial lung disease associated with autoimmune disorders? Eur Respir J 38: 384–391.
12. Sato T, Fujita J, Yamadori I, Ohtsuki Y, Yoshinouchi T, et al. (2006) Non-specific interstitial pneumonia; as the first clinical presentation of various collagen vascular disorders. Rheumatol Int 26: 551–555.
13. Park IN, Jegal Y, Kim DS, Do KH, Yoo B, et al. (2009) Clinical course and lung function change of idiopathic nonspecific interstitial pneumonia. Eur Respir J 33: 68–76.
14. Travis WD, Hunninghake G, King TE Jr, Lynch DA, Colby TV, et al. (2008) Idiopathic nonspecific interstitial pneumonia: report of an American Thoracic Society project. Am J Respir Crit Care Med 177: 1338–1347.
15. van der Kamp R, Tak PP, Jansen HM, Bresser P (2007) Interstitial lung disease as the first manifestation of systemic sclerosis. Neth J Med 65: 390–394.
16. Kinder BW, Collard HR, Koth L, Daikh DI, Wolters PJ, et al. (2007) Idiopathic nonspecific interstitial pneumonia: lung manifestation of undifferentiated connective tissue disease? Am J Respir Crit Care Med 176: 691–697.
17. Fischer A, West SG, Swigris JJ, Brown KK, du Bois RM (2010) Connective tissue disease-associated interstitial lung disease: a call for clarification. Chest 138: 251–256.
18. Vij R, Noth I, Strek ME (2011) Autoimmune-featured interstitial lung disease. A distinct entity. Chest 140: 1292–1299.
19. Raghu G, Collard HR, Egan JJ, Martinez FJ, Behr J, et al. (2011) ATS/ERS/JRS/ALAT Committee on Idiopathic Pulmonary Fibrosis. An official ATS/ERS/JRS/ALAT statement: idiopathic pulmonary fibrosis: evidence-based

guidelines for diagnosis and management. Am J Respir Crit Care Med 183: 788–824.
20. Arnett FC, Edworthy SM, Bloch DA, McShane DJ, Fries JF, et al. (1988) The American Rheumatism Association 1987 revised criteria for the classification of rheumatoid arthritis. Arthritis Rheum 31: 315–324.
21. Bohan A, Peter JB (1975) Polymyositis and dermatomyositis (first of two parts). N Engl J Med 292: 344–347.
22. (1980) Preliminary criteria for the classification of systemic sclerosis (scleroderma). Subcommittee for scleroderma criteria of the American Rheumatism Association Diagnostic and Therapeutic Criteria Committee. Arthritis Rheum 23: 581–590.
23. Tan EM, Cohen AS, Fries JF, Masi AT, McShane DJ, et al. (1982) The 1982 revised criteria for the classification of systemic lupus erythematosus. Arthritis Rheum 25: 1271–1277.
24. Vitali C, Bombardieri S, Moutsopoulos HM, Balestrieri G, Bencivelli W, et al. (1993) Preliminary criteria for the classification of Sjögren's syndrome. Results of a prospective concerted action supported by the European Community. Arthritis Rheum 36: 340–347.
25. Jennette JC, Falk RJ, Andrassy K, Bacon PA, Churg J, et al. (1994) Nomenclature of systemic vasculitides: the proposal of an international consensus conference. Arthritis Rheum 37: 187–192.
26. Antoniou KM, Margaritopoulos G, Economidou F, Siafakas NM (2009) Pivotal clinical dilemmas in collagen vascular diseases associated with interstitial lung involvement. Eur Respir J 33: 882–896.
27. Fischer A, du Bois R (2012) Interstitial lung disease in connective tissue disorders. Lancet 380: 689–698.
28. Mittoo S, Gelber AC, Christopher-Stine L, Horton MR, Lechtzin N, et al. (2009) Ascertainment of collagen vascular disease in patients presenting with interstitial lung disease. Respir Med 103: 1152–1158.
29. Yang Y, Fujita J, Tokuda M, Bandoh S, Ishida T (2002) Chronological evaluation of the onset of histologically confirmed interstitial pneumonia associated with polymyositis/dermatomyositis. Intern Med 41: 1135–1141.
30. Fischer A, Meehan RT, Feghali-Bostwick CA, West SG, Brown KK (2006) Unique characteristics of systemic sclerosis sine scleroderma-associated interstitial lung disease. Chest; 130: 976–981.
31. Lomeo RM, Cornella RJ, Schabel SI, Silver RM (1989) Progressive systemic sclerosis sine scleroderma presenting as pulmonary interstitial fibrosis. Am J Med 87: 525–527.
32. Homma S, Matsushita H, Nakata K (2004) Pulmonary fibrosis in myeloperoxidase antineutrophil cytoplasmic antibody-associated vasculitides. Respirology 9: 190–196.
33. Song JW, Do KH, Kim MY, Jang SJ, Colby TV, et al. (2009) Pathologic and radiologic differences between idiopathic and collagen vascular disease-related usual interstitial pneumonia. Chest 136: 23–30.
34. Cipriani NA, Strek M, Noth I, Gordon IO, Charbeneau J, et al. (2012) Pathologic quantification of connective tissue disease-associated versus idiopathic usual interstitial pneumonia. Arch Pathol Lab Med 136: 1253–1258.
35. Nakamura Y, Chida K, Suda T, Hayakawa H, Iwata M, et al. (2003) Nonspecific interstitial pneumonia in collagen vascular diseases: comparison of the clinical characteristics and prognostic significance with usual interstitial pneumonia. Sarcoidosis Vasc Diffuse Lung Dis 20: 235–241.
36. Park JH, Kim DS, Park IN, Jang SJ, Kitaichi M, et al. (2007) Prognosis of fibrotic interstitial pneumonia: idiopathic versus collagen vascular disease-related subtypes. Am J Respir Crit Care Med 175: 705–711.
37. Alhamad EH, Al-Kassimi FA, Alboukai AA, Raddaoui E, Al-Hajjaj MS, et al. (2012) Comparison of three groups of patients with usual interstitial pneumonia. Respir Med 106: 1575–1585.
38. Kim EJ, Elicker BM, Maldonado F, Webb WR, Ryu JH, et al. (2010) Usual interstitial pneumonia in rheumatoid arthritis-associated interstitial lung disease. Eur Respir J 35: 1322–1328.
39. Tsuchiya Y, Takayanagi N, Sugiura H, Miyahara Y, Tokunaga D, et al. (2011) Lung diseases directly associated with rheumatoid arthritis and their relationship to outcome. Eur Respir J 37: 1411–1417.
40. Nakamura Y, Suda T, Kaida Y, Kono M, Hozumi H, et al. (2012) Rheumatoid lung disease: prognostic analysis of 54 biopsy-proven cases. Respir Med 106: 1164–1169.

Decreased Circulating Visfatin Is Associated with Improved Disease Activity in Early Rheumatoid Arthritis: Data from the PERAC Cohort

Ondřej Sglunda[1], Heřman Mann[1,2], Hana Hulejová[1], Markéta Kuklová[1], Ondřej Pecha[3], Lenka Pleštilová[1], Mária Filková[1], Karel Pavelka[1,2], Jiří Vencovský[1,2], Ladislav Šenolt[1,2]*

1 Institute of Rheumatology, Prague, Czech Republic, **2** Department of Rheumatology, First Faculty of Medicine, Charles University in Prague, Prague, Czech Republic, **3** Technology Centre ASCR, Prague, Czech Republic

Abstract

Objective: To evaluate circulating visfatin and its relationship with disease activity and serum lipids in patients with early, treatment-naïve rheumatoid arthritis (RA).

Methods: Serum visfatin was measured in 40 patients with early RA before and after three months of treatment and in 30 age- and sex-matched healthy individuals. Disease activity was assessed using the Disease Activity Score for 28 joints (DAS28) at baseline and at three and 12 months. Multivariate linear regression analysis was performed to evaluate whether improved disease activity is related to serum visfatin or a change in visfatin level.

Results: Serum visfatin was significantly elevated in early RA patients compared to healthy controls (1.92 ± 1.17 vs. 1.36 ± 0.93 ng/ml; $p = 0.034$) and significantly decreased after three months of treatment (to 0.99 ± 0.67 ng/ml; $p < 0.001$). Circulating visfatin and a change in visfatin level correlated with disease activity and improved disease activity over time, respectively. A decrease in visfatin after three months predicted a DAS28 improvement after 12 months. In addition, decreased serum visfatin was not associated with an improved atherogenic index but was associated with an increase in total cholesterol level.

Conclusion: A short-term decrease in circulating visfatin may represent an independent predictor of long-term disease activity improvement in patients with early RA.

Editor: Oreste Gualillo, SERGAS, Santiago University Clinical Hospital, IDIS Research Laboratory 9, NEIRID Lab, Spain

Funding: This work was supported by a Ministry of Health of the Czech Republic (MHCR) grant (NT-13696-4), SVV project (264 511) and project of MHCR for conceptual development of a research organization (023728). The funders had no role in study design, data collection and analysis, decision to publish, or preparation of the manuscript.

Competing Interests: The authors have declared that no competing interests exist.

* Email: senolt@revma.cz

Introduction

Visfatin was originally discovered and named pre-B-colony enhancing factor [1] but was later renamed visfatin, reflecting its predominant secretion by visceral adipose tissue [2]. However, visfatin is also produced by several types of immune cells and synovial fibroblasts [3,4]. Recent studies have demonstrated the involvement of visfatin in innate immunity and inflammation [5], particularly in rheumatoid arthritis (RA). Visfatin is strongly up-regulated in the RA synovial lining layer and at sites of joint invasion, promoting synovial fibroblast motility and increasing the production of pro-inflammatory cytokines and matrix degrading enzymes by synovial fibroblasts and monocytes [3,6,7].

In RA, persistent synovial inflammation and invasive behaviour by activated synovial fibroblasts contribute to joint damage, leading to disability [8]. The discovery of novel molecules has contributed to a better understanding of RA pathogenesis and may lead to the identification of biomarkers that would allow for the monitoring of disease activity and individualising prognosis in RA patients [9]. Visfatin may represent a novel biomarker for disease severity. Some data indicate that visfatin is elevated in RA and may be associated with the degree of inflammation, clinical disease activity and radiographic joint damage [3,10,11]. However, these findings are not consistent throughout all studies [12–14].

The objective of the present study was to characterise 1) the association between serum visfatin level and disease activity in early RA, 2) the effect of treatment with conventional synthetic disease modifying drugs (csDMARDs) on the visfatin level and 3) the relationship between visfatin level and serum lipids.

Methods

Patients

A total of 40 patients (28 women) with early RA were included in the study. The inclusion criteria were as follows: 1) age >18 years, 2) fulfilment of the ACR/EULAR 2010 classification criteria for RA at baseline [15], 3) symptom duration of ≤6 months and 4) no or only symptomatic therapy with nonsteroidal antirheumatic drugs at baseline. Patients were prospectively followed in the Prague Early RA Clinic (PERAC) at the Institute of Rheumatology in the Czech Republic. The disease activity was assessed using the 28-joint count Disease Activity Score (DAS28-ESR). The control group consisted of 30 age- and sex-matched healthy individuals. Consent procedure was approved by the Ethics Committee of the Institute of Rheumatology. Each participant provided written informed consents prior to entering the study. Both original consents were given to the patients and documented in the patient's files.

Laboratory analysis

Fasting blood samples were collected from all patients at baseline and after three months. The samples were immediately centrifuged and stored at −20°C. The serum concentration of visfatin was measured using a commercially available enzyme-linked immunosorbent assay (ELISA) (Biovision, Milpitas, California, USA) as described previously [14]. The levels of serum anti-cyclic citrullinated peptide antibodies (anti-CCP) and IgM rheumatoid factor (IgM-RF) were measured using a standard ELISA assay (Test Line S.R.O., Czech Republic). CRP and total and HDL-cholesterol were determined using routine laboratory techniques.

Statistical analysis

Pearson's and Spearman's rank correlations were used in cases of normal and non-normal distributions. The T-test was used for normal variables, and the Mann-Whitney test was used for non-parametric variables. Multivariate linear regression analysis was performed to assess the influence of visfatin (its change) on disease activity and blood lipids. P values of less than 0.05 were considered to be statistically significant. Statistical analyses were performed using SPSS 17 (SPSS Inc., Chicago, IL, USA) and GraphPad Prism 5.0 (GraphPad Software, Inc., San Diego, CA, USA). The data are presented as the median [range] or mean and standard deviation (SD) in the case of abnormal or normal distribution.

Results

Patients and demographic data

Table 1 shows the baseline characteristics of patients and healthy controls included in the study. Twenty patients met the criteria for highly active disease (DAS28>5.1), 18 patients had moderate disease activity (3.2<DAS28≤5.1), and two patients had low disease activity (2.6<DAS28≤3.2) at baseline. Treatment with csDMARDS was initiated in 38 patients at baseline: 31 patients on methotrexate (mean weekly dose at month three was 15 mg; range, 10–20 mg), six on sulphasalazine and one on leflunomide. Additionally, 34 patients were receiving glucocorticoids (mean daily dose at month three was 5 mg; range, 1.25–15.0 mg of prednisone or equivalent per day). Two patients were initially only on glucocorticoids either due to planned pregnancy or elevated aminotransferases. After three months of treatment, a significant reduction in disease activity was observed (DAS28: from 5.3±1.5 to 2.8±1.3; CRP: from 7.7 [0.6–77.8] to 2.3 [0.2–14.3]; $p<0.001$ for all comparisons).

Visfatin is elevated in early RA and correlates with disease activity

The baseline visfatin level in early RA patients was significantly higher compared to that in healthy controls (1.92±1.17 vs. 1.36±0.93 ng/ml; $p=0.034$) (Fig. 1A). Using bivariate analysis, the visfatin level correlated positively with DAS28 ($r=0.383$, $p=0.015$) and CRP level ($r=0.456$, $p=0.003$) at baseline (Fig. 1B). The serum visfatin level was not related to age, gender or body mass index (BMI), but there was a negative association between visfatin and anti-CCP level ($r=-0.400$, $p=0.011$) albeit not with IgM-RF ($r=-0.045$, $p=0.787$).

A decreased visfatin level is associated with disease activity improvement

The serum visfatin level significantly decreased after three months compared to baseline (1.92±1.17 vs. 0.99±0.67 ng/ml; $p<0.0001$) (Fig. 1A). Similar to baseline, after three months of treatment, the visfatin level correlated with DAS28 ($r=0.338$, $p=0.035$) and CRP ($r=0.588$, $p=0.001$).

A decrease in visfatin level correlated with a decrease in DAS28 ($r=0.378$, $p=0.018$) and CRP ($r=0.386$, $p=0.015$) after three months (Fig. 2A). Furthermore, a decrease in visfatin level after three months correlated with a decrease in DAS28 ($r=0.354$, $p=0.027$) and CRP ($r=0.365$, $p=0.022$) after 12 months (Fig. 2B). Using multiple linear regression analysis, a visfatin decrease after three months predicted DAS28 improvement between baseline and month three ($p=0.021$, adjusted $R^2=11.9\%$) and between baseline and month 12 ($p=0.031$, adjusted $R^2=10.1\%$).

Visfatin level and lipid profile

The visfatin level did not correlate with serum lipids or atherogenic index at baseline in early RA patients (data not shown). While the mean total cholesterol (5.17±1.20 to 5.73±1.40 mmol/l; $p<0.001$) and HDL-cholesterol (1.07±0.25 to 1.32±0.29 mmol/l; $p<0.001$) significantly increased from baseline to month three, there was an improvement in the atherogenic index (4.02±1.35 to 3.50±1.29; $p<0.01$). Although a decrease in serum visfatin was not associated with an improved atherogenic index ($r=0.095$, $p=0.567$), the decrease was associated with an increase in total cholesterol ($r=-0.328$, $p=0.041$). A decrease in visfatin significantly and independently predicted an increase in total cholesterol in all RA patients ($p=0.015$). Another independent significant predictor in this model (adjusted $R^2=34.1\%$) was a decrease in CRP between baseline and month three ($p=0.007$).

Discussion

In this study, we have shown that an elevated visfatin level correlates with disease activity and that a decrease in visfatin level during the first three months of treatment independently predicts further disease activity improvement after 12 months in patients with treatment naïve early RA. The atherogenic index improved but was not related to visfatin reduction.

Consistent with previous studies demonstrating an increased visfatin level in patients with RA [3,10,14], we have shown that an elevated circulating visfatin in the early phase of the disease significantly decreased after three months of treatment. Because visfatin is up-regulated in several immune cells [3] and improvement in disease activity is associated with a decrease in macrophages in RA synovial tissue [16], a decrease in circulating visfatin may reflect a decrease in synovial immune cells following effective treatment. In addition, the visfatin level correlated with

Table 1. Baseline characteristics of patients with early rheumatoid arthritis (RA) and healthy controls.

Characteristics	Early RA (n = 40)	Healthy controls (n = 30)
Gender (F/M)	22/18	19/11
Age (years)	52±17	48±16
BMI	24±4.0	25±3.1
CRP (mg/l)	7.7 [0.6–77.8]	-
DAS28 score	5.25±1.50	-
RF positivity, n (%)	24 (60)	-
Anti-CCP positivity, n (%)	21 (53)	-
Drugs (csDMARDs/GC)	38/31	-

Anti-CCP, anti-cyclic citrullinated peptide antibody; RF, rheumatoid factor; CRP, C-reactive protein; DAS, disease activity score; csDMARDs, conventional synthetic disease modifying antirheumatic drugs; GC, glucocorticoids; RA, rheumatoid arthritis; F, female; M, male; MTX, methotrexate. The data are expressed as a mean (SD) or median [range].

clinical and laboratory measures of disease activity at baseline and during treatment, which has been reported in some [3,17], but not all, studies [12,14]. This inconsistency may be explained by differences in populations and treatments because in patients with long-term and active RA on biological therapy, an association between visfatin and disease activity was not observed [12,14].

Adipokines represent large group of highly bioactive substances secreted by adipocytes and immune cells that are involved in both metabolic and immunomodulatory functions. In addition to visfatin, Gonzalez-Gay et al demonstrated rapid reduction of serum resistin [18], but not adiponectin [19] levels in patients with long-term and active RA during anti-TNF-alpha therapy with infliximab. Resistin levels were positively associated with inflammatory markers of RA [18], whereas adiponectin levels were inversely associated with disease activity and low adiponectin levels clustered with metabolic syndrome features that reportedly contribute to atherogenesis in RA patients with severe disease [19].

We have found that a decrease in circulating visfatin correlates with disease activity improvement over the first three months of treatment. Furthermore, although baseline visfatin was not

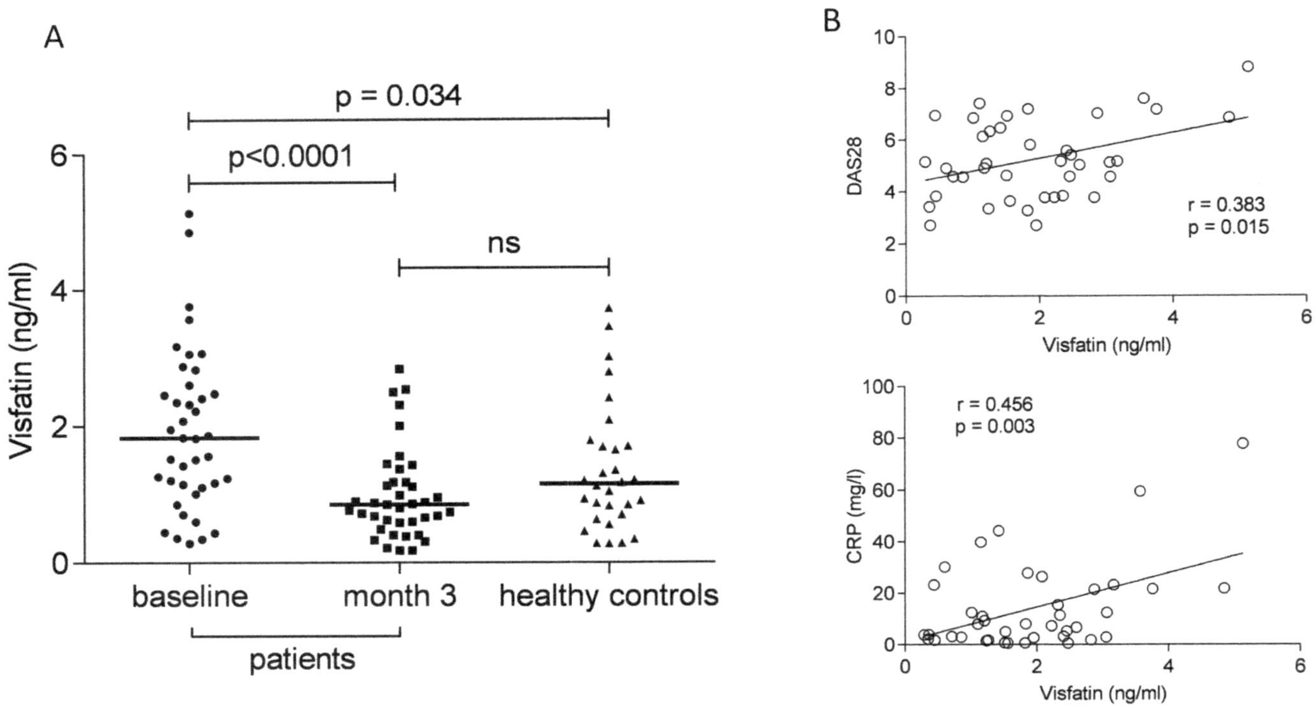

Figure 1. Comparison of serum visfatin levels between patients with early, treatment-naïve rheumatoid arthritis and healthy controls and change in serum visfatin after three months of treatment with conventional synthetic disease modifying antirheumatic drugs. (A). Association between baseline serum visfatin level and disease activity (B). CRP, C-reactive protein; DAS, disease activity score.

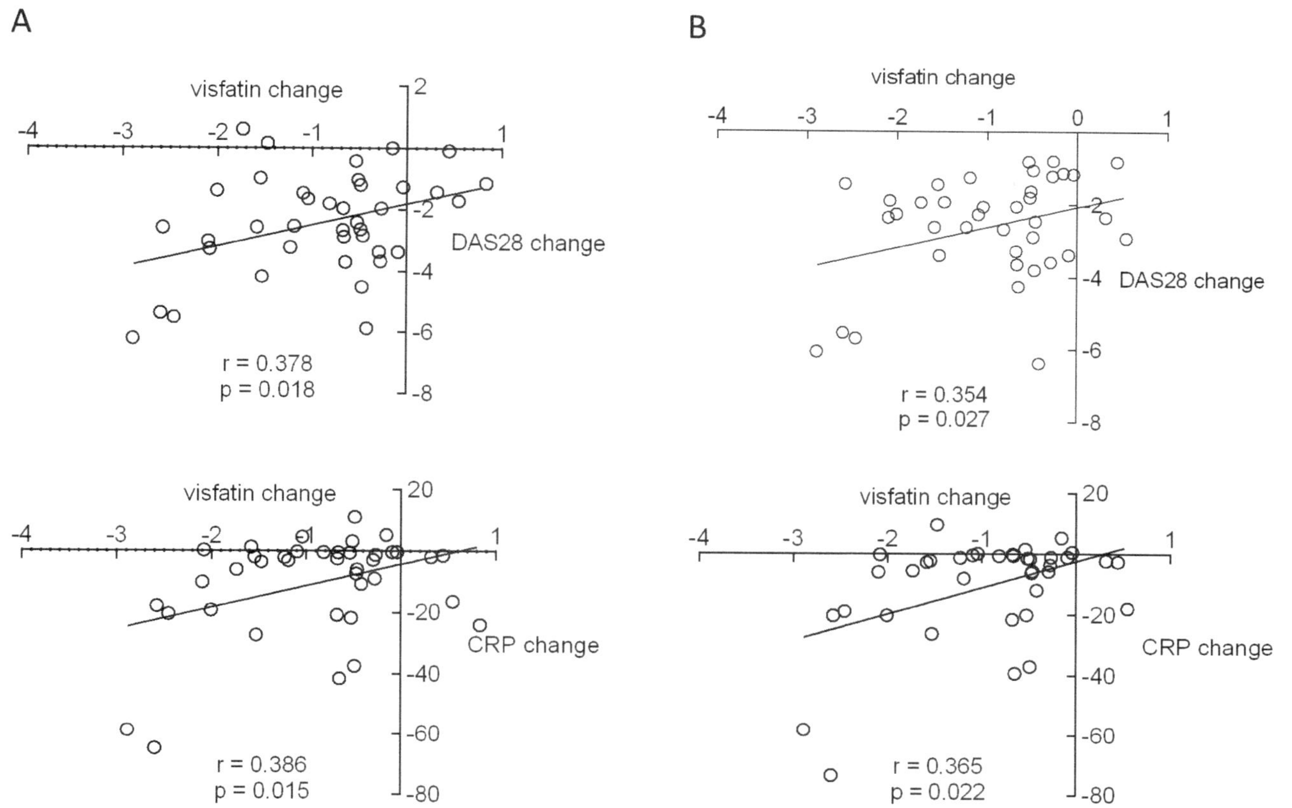

Figure 2. Correlations between visfatin reduction and disease activity improvement after three months (A) and between visfatin reduction after three months and disease activity improvement after 12 months (B). CRP, C-reactive protein; DAS, disease activity score.

predictive, the change of visfatin level over the first three months predicted disease activity improvement after 12 months of treatment. Thus, a higher visfatin level in treated RA patients may be associated with more severe disease and thus higher risk of structural progression as demonstrated previously [11,13]. These data further support a significant role for visfatin in the pathogenesis of RA.

There is evidence that a high visfatin level is associated with an increased risk of cardiovascular disease [20]. Klaasen et al. reported a relationship between a high visfatin level and an increased atherogenic index in adalimumab-treated RA patients and suggested that visfatin reduction can lead to decreased cardiovascular risk independent of disease activity [6]. However, in our study, the visfatin level correlated inversely with baseline total-cholesterol and its increase but not with atherogenic index. This finding may be explained by a different patient population and is consistent with a recent study by El-Hini et al. [20]. Because our patients had an improvement in atherogenic index during treatment [21], we suggest that the association between visfatin and total cholesterol level may be caused by dyslipidaemia, which occurs in early RA [21]. However, this hypothesis requires further investigation.

In conclusion, our study demonstrates an association between an elevated visfatin level and disease activity, and short-term reduction of visfatin is an independent predictor of long-term disease activity improvement in early, treatment-naïve RA patients. These results however need to be validated in larger and independent cohorts of patients with RA.

Acknowledgments

We thank all of the patients and healthy volunteers for blood donation.

Author Contributions

Conceived and designed the experiments: LS JV KP HM. Performed the experiments: HH MF. Analyzed the data: MK HH LP OP. Contributed reagents/materials/analysis tools: HH MF MK. Contributed to the writing of the manuscript: OS LS JV KP HM. Statistical analysis: OP. Enrolled patients to the study: LS HM.

References

1. Samal B, Sun Y, Stearns G, Xie C, Suggs S, et al. (1994) Cloning and characterization of the cDNA encoding a novel human pre-B cell colony-enhancing factor. Mol Cell Biol 14: 1431–7.
2. Fukuhara A, Matsuda M, Nishizawa M, Segawa K, Tanaka M, et al. (2005) Visfatin: a protein secreted by visceral fat that mimics the effects of insulin. Science 307: 426–30.
3. Brentano F, Schorr O, Ospelt C, Stanczyk J, Gay RE, et al. (2007) Pre-B cell colony-enhancing factor/visfatin, a new marker of inflammation in rheumatoid arthritis with proinflammatory and matrix-degrading activities. Arthritis Rheum 56: 2829–39.
4. Nowell MA, Richards PJ, Fielding CA, Ognjanovic S, Topley N, et al. (2006) Regulation of pre-B cell colony-enhancing factor by STAT-3-dependent interleukin-6 trans-signaling: implications in the pathogenesis of rheumatoid arthritis. Arthritis Rheum 54: 2084–95.
5. Luk T, Malam Z, Marshall JC (2008) Pre-B cell colony-enhancing factor (PBEF)/visfatin: a novel mediator of innate immunity. J Leukoc Biol 83: 804–16.

6. Klaasen R, Herenius MM, Wijbrandts CA, de Jager W, van Tuyl LH, et al. (2012) Treatment-specific changes in circulating adipocytokines: a comparison between tumour necrosis factor blockade and glucocorticoid treatment for rheumatoid arthritis. Ann Rheum Dis 71: 1510–6.
7. Présumey J, Courties G, Louis-Plence P, Escriou V, Scherman D, et al. (2013) Nicotinamide phosphoribosyltransferase/visfatin expression by inflammatory monocytes mediates arthritis pathogenesis. Ann Rheum Dis 72: 1717–24.
8. Ospelt C, Gay S (2008) The role of resident synovial cells in destructive arthritis. Best Pract Res Clin Rheumatol 22: 239–52.
9. Smolen JS, Aletaha D, Grisar J, Redlich K, Steiner G, et al. (2008) The need for prognosticators in rheumatoid arthritis. Biological and clinical markers: where are we now? Arthritis Res Ther 10: 208.
10. Otero M, Lago R, Gomez R, Lago F, Dieguez C, et al. (2006) Changes in plasma levels of fat-derived hormones adiponectin, leptin, resistin and visfatin in patients with rheumatoid arthritis. Ann Rheum Dis 65: 1198–201.
11. Rho YH, Solus J, Sokka T, Oeser A, Chung CP, et al. (2009) Adipocytokines are associated with radiographic joint damage in rheumatoid arthritis. Arthritis Rheum 60: 1906–14.
12. Gonzalez-Gay MA, Vazquez-Rodriguez TR, Garcia-Unzueta MT, Berja A, Miranda-Filloy JA, et al. (2010) Visfatin is not associated with inflammation or metabolic syndrome in patients with severe rheumatoid arthritis undergoing anti-TNF-alpha therapy. Clin Exp Rheumatol 28: 56–62.
13. Klein-Wieringa IR, van der Linden MP, Knevel R, Kwekkeboom JC, van Beelen E, et al. (2011) Baseline serum adipokine levels predict radiographic progression in early rheumatoid arthritis. Arthritis Rheum 63: 2567–74.
14. Senolt L, Krystufkova O, Hulejova H, Kuklova M, Filkova M, et al. (2011) The level of serum visfatin (PBEF) is associated with total number of B cells in patients with rheumatoid arthritis and decreases following B cell depletion therapy. Cytokine 55: 116–21.
15. Aletaha D, Neogi T, Silman AJ, Funovits J, Felson DT, et al. (2010) Rheumatoid arthritis classification criteria: an American College of Rheumatology/European League Against Rheumatism collaborative initiative. Ann Rheum Dis 69: 1580–8.
16. Haringman JJ, Gerlag DM, Zwinderman AH, Smeets TJ, Kraan MC, et al. (2005) Synovial tissue macrophages: a sensitive biomarker for response to treatment in patients with rheumatoid arthritis. Ann Rheum Dis 64: 834–8.
17. El-Hini SH, Mohamed FI, Hassan AA, Ali F, Mahmoud A, et al. (2013) Visfatin and adiponectin as novel markers for evaluation of metabolic disturbance in recently diagnosed rheumatoid arthritis patients. Rheumatol Int 33: 2283–9.
18. Gonzalez-Gay MA, Garcia-Unzueta MT, Gonzalez-Juanatey C, Miranda-Filloy JA, Vazquez-Rodriguez TR, et al. (2008) Anti-TNF-alpha therapy modulates resistin in patients with rheumatoid arthritis. Clin Exp Rheumatol 26: 311–6.
19. Gonzalez-Gay MA, Llorca J, Garcia-Unzueta MT, Gonzalez-Juanatey C, De Matias JM, et al. (2008) High-grade inflammation, circulating adiponectin concentrations and cardiovascular risk factors in severe rheumatoid arthritis. Clin Exp Rheumatol 26: 596–603.
20. Chang YH, Chang DM, Lin KC, Shin SJ, Lee YJ (2011) Visfatin in overweight/obesity, type 2 diabetes mellitus, insulin resistance, metabolic syndrome and cardiovascular diseases: a meta-analysis and systemic review. Diabetes Metab Res Rev 27: 515–27.
21. Boers M, Nurmohamed MT, Doelman CJ, Lard LR, Verhoeven AC, et al. (2003) Influence of glucocorticoids and disease activity on total and high density lipoprotein cholesterol in patients with rheumatoid arthritis. Ann Rheum Dis 62: 842–5.

Plasma Levels of IL-37 and Correlation with TNF-α, IL-17A, and Disease Activity during DMARD Treatment of Rheumatoid Arthritis

Ping-Wei Zhao[1]⁹, Wei-Guang Jiang[1]⁹, Li Wang[1], Zhen-Yu Jiang[2], Yu-Xing Shan[1], Yan-Fang Jiang[1]*

1 Key Laboratory of Zoonosis Research, Ministry of Education, The First Hospital, Jilin University, Changchun, China, **2** Department of Rheumatism, The First Hospital, Jilin University, Changchun, China

Abstract

The aim of this study was to assess the change of IL-37 concentrations in rheumatoid arthritis (RA) patients under Disease-modifying anti-rheumatic drug (DMARD) therapy, and to establish a correlation between Interleukin-37 and pro-inflammatory cytokines in plasma and disease activity. The plasma level of IL-37 was determined using ELISA in 50 newly diagnosed RA patients and 30 healthy controls (HC). Plasma levels of IL-17A, IL-6 and TNF-α were measured using flow a cytometric bead array assay. We found that the concentrations of IL-37, as well as IL-17A, IL-6 and TNF-α, were higher in plasma of RA patients compared to HCs. Compared to patients who did not respond to DMARD treatment, treatment of patients responsive to DMARDs resulted in down-regulation of IL-17A, IL-6 and TNF-α expression. The plasma level of the anti-inflammatory cytokine IL-37 was also decreased in drug responders after DMARD treatment. The plasma level of IL-37 in RA patients was positively correlated with pro-inflammatory cytokines (IL-17A, TNF-α) and disease activity (CRP, DAS28) in RA patients. IL-37 expression in RA and during DMARD treatment appears to be controlled by the level of pro-inflammatory cytokines. This results in a strong correlation between plasma levels of IL-37 and disease activity in RA patients.

Editor: Josep Bassaganya-Riera, Virginia Tech, United States of America

Funding: This study was supported by grants from the National Natural Science Foundation of China (No. 30972610 and 81273240), Jilin Province Science and Technology Agency (No. 20110716), the Health Department Research Projects in Jilin Province (2009Z054) and the Cutting-edge Science and Interdisciplinary Innovation Projects of Jilin University. The funders had no role in study design, data collection and analysis, decision to publish, or preparation of the manuscript.

Competing Interests: The authors have declared that no competing interests exist.

* E-mail: yanfangjiang@hotmail.com

⁹ These authors contributed equally to this work.

Introduction

Rheumatoid arthritis (RA) is a chronic inflammatory disorder with autoimmune etiology characterized by joint inflammation, T cell infiltration of the synovium, synovial hyperplasia, neoangiogenesis, involvement of many catabolic cytokines, and progressive destruction of articular cartilage and bone [1]. Multiple pro-inflammatory cytokines involved in RA contribute to the proliferation of synovial tissue and joint erosion [2]. We hypothesize that an imbalance between pro-inflammatory cytokines and anti-inflammatory cytokines may be a primary factor in disease progression.

TNF-α is a pivotal pro-inflammatory cytokine in the pathogenesis of RA that is known to induce adhesion molecule and proteinase gene expression, and play a major role in the progression of joint destruction and proliferation of synoviocytes [3]. IL-6 is another pro-inflammatory cytokine with multiple functions, and is believed to play a pivotal role in the inflammatory process, in osteoclast-mediated bone resorption, and in synovitis. In autoimmunity, IL-6 may induce pro-inflammatory T-helper 17 (Th17) cell differentiation and B-cell antibody production [4–6]. IL-17A is one of the most important mediators involved in T cell-mediated synovial inflammation and contributes to bone destruction through increase of migration, chemokine gene expression, and invasiveness of synoviocytes in RA [7,8]. Therefore, therapies targeting these cytokines or their receptors are recognized as effective treatments for patients with RA [9].

IL-37 is a newly defined member of the IL-1 cytokine family, and it is a key cytokine in regulating inflammation [10]. Expression of IL-37 in macrophages or epithelial cells almost completely inhibits the synthesis of pro-inflammatory cytokines [11,12]. In addition, IL-37 protein can be up-regulated by pro-inflammatory cytokines and inflammatory stimuli [12,13]. IL-37 acts as an essential inhibitor of inflammation and innate immunity in various diseases [14]. Marcel F Nold. *et al.* have reported that immunohistochemical staining of synovial lining from RA patients revealed greater amounts of IL-37 compared to that of HCs [13]. In this study, we assessed the plasma levels of IL-37 in RA patients, and analyzed the relationship between IL-37 and pro-inflammatory cytokines or disease activity.

Disease-modifying anti-rheumatic drugs (DMARDs) help to ease symptoms and to slow progression of RA. Methotrexate is often the first drug given for rheumatoid arthritis [15]. In this study we combined methotrexate with Leflunomide, another DMARD, and determined the expressions of both pro- and anti-inflammatory cytokines in RA patients during DMARD therapy.

Table 1. Demographic and clinical characteristics of subjects.

Group	HCs	Drug responder (n = 34)		Drug-nonresponder (n = 16)	
		Before	After	Before	After
ESR (mm/hour)	13(4–19)	53(28–120)*	21(7–65)*#	69(15–105)*	60(30–95)*
CRP (mg/dl)	4.2(0.3–6.2)	31.6(0.61–141)*	7.6(1.66–40.9)*#	18.9(3.8–104)*	16.4(0.8–93.7)*
RF (IU/ml)	14(0.4–27)	319.4(0.11–1270)*	58 (3.37–501)*#	265.7(25.8–1440)*	163(2.57–1020)*
RF (+/−)	NA	31/3	9/25	15/1	14/2
Anti-CCP (IU/ml)	4.32(0.24–6.29)	547(0.67–2476)*	51.3(5.4–798)*#	652(35.6–2778)*	359(21.9–2250)*
Anti-CCP (+/−)	NA	33/1	7/24	16/0	15/1
DAS28	NA	6.39(3.76–9.85)*	3.38(1.65–5.07)*#	7.15(3.9–10.12)*	5.27(3.74–9.96)*

Data shown are median (range) of each group of subjects. RF: rheumatoid factor; ESR: erythrocyte sedimentation rate; CRP: C-reactive Protein; CCP: cyclic citrullinated peptide; DAS28: Disease Activity Score in 28 joints; NA: not applicable;
*$P<0.05$ vs. HCs;
#$P<0.05$ vs. baseline values.

Materials and Methods

Patients

Fifty newly diagnosed (<12 months of disease duration) RA patients were recruited sequentially at the inpatient service of the First Hospital of Jilin University from March 2011 to October 2012 and were orally treated weekly with 10 mg methotrexate (MTX, Shanghai Xinyi Pharmacy, Shanghai, China), and daily with 20 mg Leflunomide (Fujian Huitian Pharmacy, Fujian, China) for 90 consecutive days. Thirty age- and sex-matched healthy volunteers were included in this study. Individual patients with RA were diagnosed, according to the diagnosis criteria established by the American College of Rheumatology [16], and the disease severity of individual patients was evaluated using the disease activity score 28 (DAS28) [17]. According to disease severity classification of RA patients, serious disease activity is defined as DAS28>5.1; medium disease activity is defined as 3.2< DAS28<5.1; a fundamentally alleviated pathologic condition is defined as 2.6<DAS28<3.2; and complete improvement is defined as DAS28<2.6. According to the European League Against Rheumatism (EULAR) response criteria, a decrease in the DAS28 score of 0.6 or less is considered a poor response, while a decrease of greater than 1.2 indicates a moderate or good response, dependent on whether an individual's DAS28 score at the end point is above or below 3.2, respectively. All RA patients included in this study had initial DAS 28 scores of >3.2 during the activity phase of the disease. The first blood sample was collected from patients before the initiation of treatment with DMARDs. Following DMARD therapy, we defined drug-responders as patients whose DAS28 score decreased by more than 1.2 points, while non-responders were defined by a decrease of the DAS28 score by 0.6 points or less. None of the patients had been treated with DMARDs, immunosuppressive, or other drugs, or had other chronic inflammatory or autoimmune diseases prior to the first sampling. None of the patients were treated with NSAIDs or glucocorticoids except for MTX plus leflunomide during RA therapy. Sera of RA patients and healthy controls were stored at −80°C prior to evaluation of cytokines. All subjects signed an informed consent form prior to the initiation of the study, which was approved by the Ethics Committee of the First Hospital of Jilin University.

Laboratory Tests

Full blood counts and erythrocyte sedimentation rates (ESR) of individual subjects were determined. Levels of serum C-reactive protein (CRP), rheumatoid factor (RF), and anti-cyclic citrullinated peptide (anti-CCP) were determined by scatter turbidimetry using a Siemens special protein analyzer (Siemens Healthcare Diagnostics Products, GmbH, Germany).

Measurement of IL-37 by ELISA

Plasma level of IL-37 in HCs and RA patients were assayed using a commercially available enzyme-linked immunosorbent assay (ELISA) kit (human IL-37 ELISA, AdipoGen, Switzerland). A polyclonal antibody specific for IL-37 was used for coating of 96-well microtiter plates. Briefly, individual sera were diluted in Diluent 1X at 1:2. 100 μl of the different standards were added into the appropriate wells in duplicate. 100 μl of diluted plasma were added in duplicate into additional wells. The plate was covered and incubated overnight at 4°C. After extensive washing to remove unbound compounds, IL-37 was recognized by the addition of 100 μl of polyclonal antibody specific for IL-37 (detection antibody). After removal of excess polyclonal antibody, 100 μl HRP-conjugated anti-rabbit IgG (secondary antibody conjugate) was added. Following a final wash, the bound peroxidase activity was quantified using 100 μl of the substrate 3,3′,5,5′-tetramethylbenzidine (TMB). The color reaction was developed at ambient temperature in the dark for 10 minutes. The intensity of the color reaction was measured at 450 nm after acidification and was directly proportional to the concentration of IL-37 in the standards. According to a standard curve established using recombinant IL-37, the concentration of serum IL-37 in individual samples were calculated. The detection range of the IL-37 ELISA kit was 0.016–1 ng/mL.

Cytometric Bead Arrays of Serum Cytokines

The plasma levels of TNF-α, IL-6, and IL-17A in HCs and RA patients were determined by cytometric bead array (CBA) [18], according to the manufacturer's protocol (BD Biosciences, San Joes, USA). Briefly, 25 μl of individual sera were used in duplicate for analysis, as described previously [19]. The serum concentrations of cytokines were quantified using the CellQuestPro and CBA software (Becton Dickinson) on a FACSCalibur cytometer (BD Biosciences).

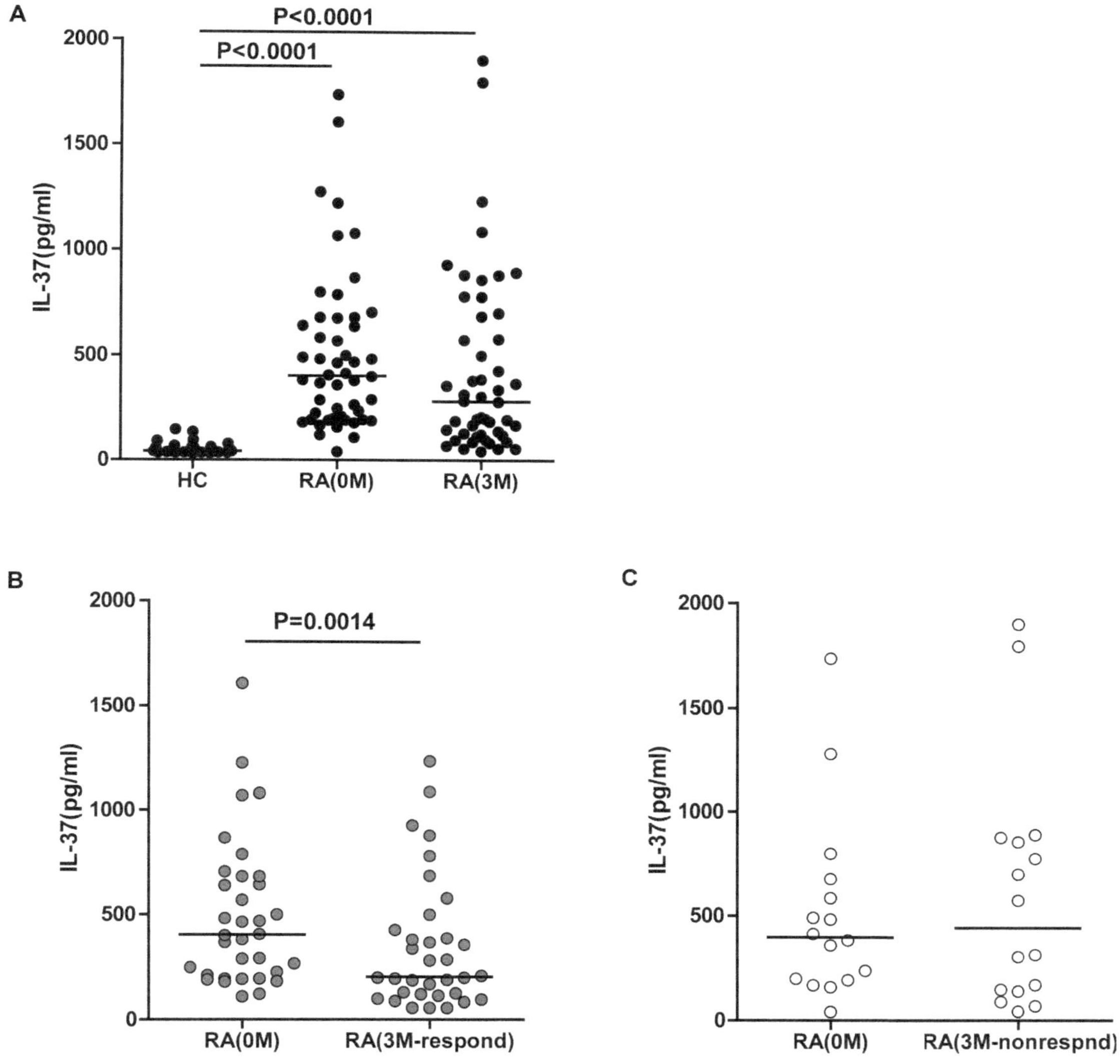

Figure 1. Plasma levels of IL-37 in RA patients. (**A**) Plasma levels of IL-37 in HCs and the total RA patient cohort at baseline, and after three months of DMARD treatment. (**B**) Plasma levels of IL-37 in drug responders compared to the same patients at baseline (grey dots). (**C**) Plasma levels of IL-37 in drug non-responders compared to the same patients at baseline (white dots). The horizontal lines indicate the median values of the different groups. The difference between the groups was analyzed by Mann-Whitney test and Wilcoxon signed rank tests for unpaired and paired comparisons, respectively.

Statistical Analysis

All data are expressed as median and range unless specified. The difference between the groups was analyzed by Mann-Whitney test and paired Wilcoxon signed rank tests using SPSS 18.0 software for unpaired and paired comparisons, respectively. The relationship between variables was evaluated using the Spearman rank correlation test. A two-side P value <0.05 was considered statistically significant.

Results

Demographic and Clinical Characteristics of Study Subjects

Fifty plasma samples from RA patients (41 female and 9 male) (range 32–63 years of age) and 30 samples from age- and sex-matched healthy volunteers were analyzed in this study. ESR, CRP, RF, anti-CCP and DAS28 were higher in patients with RA than in HCs (in all cases $P<0.05$). Following DMARD therapy for three months, these clinical parameters decreased in patients responding to treatment, compared to the same parameters at base line; however, there was no statistically significant difference between the same parameters in non-responders before and after DMARD treatment (Table 1).

Plasma Levels of IL-37 in RA Patients during DMARD Treatment

It has been reported that IL-37 plays an anti-inflammatory role in various diseases [14]. However, the effect of DMARD treatment on IL-37 in RA patients has not yet been established. Therefore, this study assessed the levels of plasma IL-37 in RA patients before and after DMARD treatment, and in comparison to HCs. The plasma levels of IL-37 in the full cohort of RA patients before treatment were significantly higher compared to levels in HCs (Fig. 1A, $P<0.0001$). However, there was no

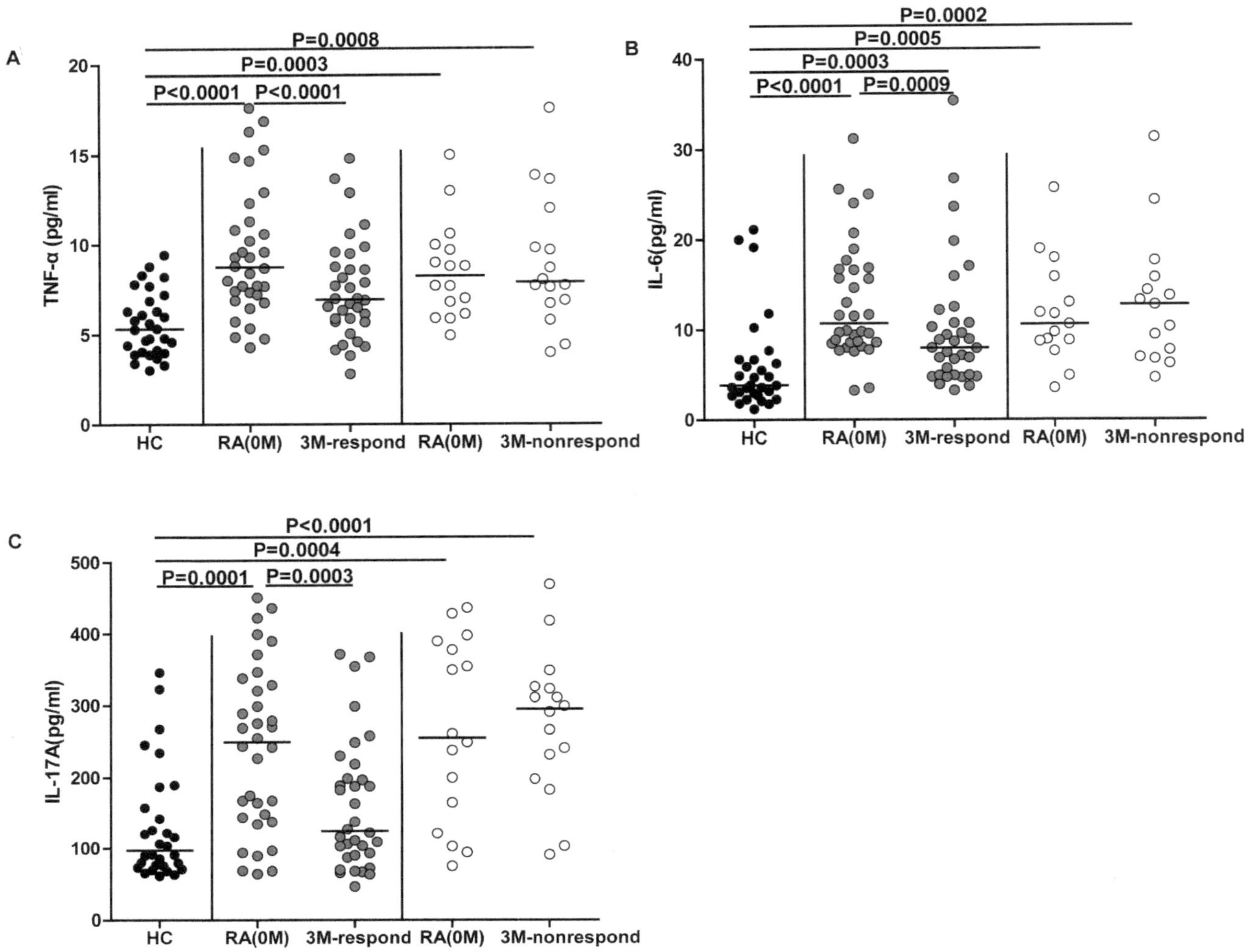

Figure 2. Plasma levels of TNF-α, IL-6 and IL-17A in RA patients. (**A**) Plasma levels of TNF-α in HCs, drug responders, and drug non-responders at baseline and after three months of treatment. (**B**) Plasma levels of IL-6 in HCs, drug responders (grey dots), and drug non-responders at baseline and after three months of treatment (white dots). (**C**) Plasma levels of IL-17A in HCs, drug responders (grey dots), and drug non-responders at baseline and after three months of treatment (white dots). The horizontal lines indicate the median values of the different groups. The difference between the groups was analyzed by Mann-Whitney test and Wilcoxon signed rank tests for unpaired and paired comparisons, respectively.

statistically significant difference between IL-37 levels before and after three months of DMARD treatment for the full patient cohort. Based on the effect of DMARD treatment on the DAS28 score, the 50 RA patients were divided into two groups: 34 patients were determined as being responsive to DMARD treatment, while the other 16 patients were determined to be unresponsive to DMARD treatment. As shown in Fig. 1B, plasma levels of IL-37 decreased in drug-responsive RA patients compared to the same patients at baseline (Fig. 2B, $P = 0.0014$). However, there was no statistically significant difference between IL-37 levels in RA patients not responding to treatment compared to the same patients at baseline (Fig. 2C).

Plasma Levels of TNF-α, IL-6 and IL-17A in RA Patients during DMARD Treatment

TNF-α, IL-6 and IL-17A play a crucial role in the progression of RA [3,4,7]. In this study, we determined plasma levels of these cytokines in RA patients following DMARD treatment. Consistent with previous studies, plasma levels of TNF-α were significantly higher in both groups of RA patients at base line compared to TNF-α levels in HCs (Fig. 2A, $P<0.0001$ and $P = 0.0003$, respectively). The plasma levels of IL-6 were also higher in both groups of RA patients at baseline compared to HCs (Fig. 2B, $P< 0.0001$ and $P = 0.0003$, respectively). Furthermore, the plasma levels of IL-17A in both groups of RA patients at baseline were also elevated compared to IL-17A levels in HCs (Fig. 2C, $P = 0.0001$ and $P = 0.0004$, respectively). Following DMARD treatment for three months, drug responders among the RA patients had lower levels of plasma TNF-α, IL-6 and IL-17A than before treatment (Fig. 2A, $P<0.0001$; 2B, $P = 0.0009$ and 2C, $P = 0.0003$, respectively). In contrast, there was no statistically significant difference between the plasma levels of these cytokines in drug non-responders before and after treatment.

Correlation of IL-37 with Other Cytokines in RA Patients

The relationship between IL-37 and pro-inflammatory cytokines in the plasma of RA patients has not yet been investigated. We found that the plasma levels of IL-37 in RA patients were

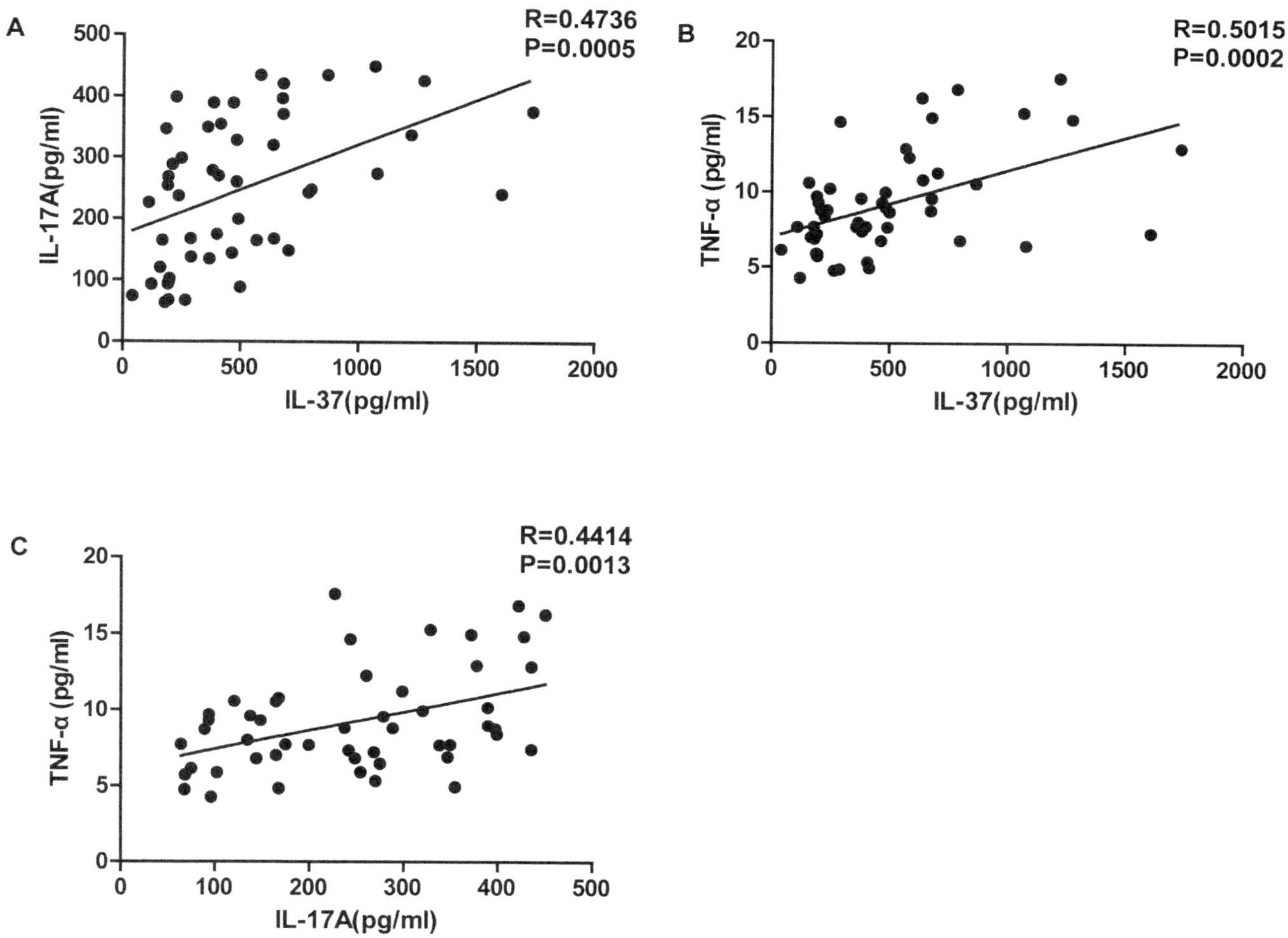

Figure 3. Correlation between IL-37 and other cytokines in RA patients. (**A**) Correlation between IL-37 and IL-17A in plasma of RA patients. (**B**) Correlation between IL-37 and TNF-α in plasma of RA patients. (**C**) Correlation between IL-17A and TNF-α in plasma of RA patients. The relationship between variables was evaluated using the Spearman rank correlation test.

positively correlated with IL-17A (Fig. 3A, R = 0.4736, P = 0.0005) and TNF-α (Fig. 3B, R = 0.5015, P = 0.0002) levels. Additionally, the plasma levels of IL-17A were positively correlated with TNF-α (Fig. 3C, R = 0.4414, P = 0.0013).

Correlation of IL-37 with Disease Activity in RA Patients

We analyzed the relationship between IL-37 and disease activity in RA patients, and found that plasma IL-37 was positively correlated with CRP (Fig. 4A, R = 0.4738, P = 0.0005) and the DAS28 score (Fig. 4B, R = 0.5454, P<0.0001) in RA patients. In addition, plasma TNF-α was positively correlated with CRP (Fig. 4C, R = 0.5184, P = 0.0001) and ESR (Fig. 4D, R = 0.3649, P = 0.0092) in RA patients.

Discussion

RA is a chronic, systemic inflammatory disease that is characterized by inflammatory cell infiltration, synovial cell proliferation, destruction of cartilage and aberrant post-translational modifications of self-proteins [20]. Numerous cytokines, both pro- and anti-inflammatory, have been detected in inflammatory diseases, and the balance between these opposing cytokine activities has been shown to regulate disease severity [21]. RA is closely associated with increased expression of TNF-α, IL-6, and IL-17A [22]. Therefore, inhibition of TNF-α, IL-6, and IL-17A expression is a promising strategy for the development of novel anti-RA therapies.

The anti-inflammatory mechanism of IL-37 is still not clear. There are currently two hypotheses: either IL-37 is secreted into the extracellular space to inhibit the actions of pro-inflammatory cytokines or their receptors [23], or IL-37 translocates to the nucleus where it interacts with Smad3 to interrupt transcription of pro-inflammatory cytokine genes [10,12,13]. IL-37 has been shown to significantly suppress IL-1β-induced expression of IL-1α, IL-8, IL-6, chemokines MIP-2/CXCL-2, MCP-5/CCL-12, and BCA-1/CXCL13, IL-23, IL-1RA, IL-17, IL-18, IFN-γ and TNF-α in several cell types [24]. In contrast, pro-inflammatory cytokines IL-18, IFN-γ, IL-1β and TNF-α can increase synthesis of IL-37 in human peripheral blood mononuclear cells [12,24]. It has been reported that immunohistochemical staining of the synovial lining in active RA revealed larger amounts of IL-37 compared to HCs [13]. The IL- 37 protein was also detected in plasma of patients with severe Systemic Lupus Erythematosus [25] and in lamina propria macrophages of patients with Crohn's disease [12]. However, plasma concentrations of IL-37 in RA patients have not yet been reported. Our data show that plasma

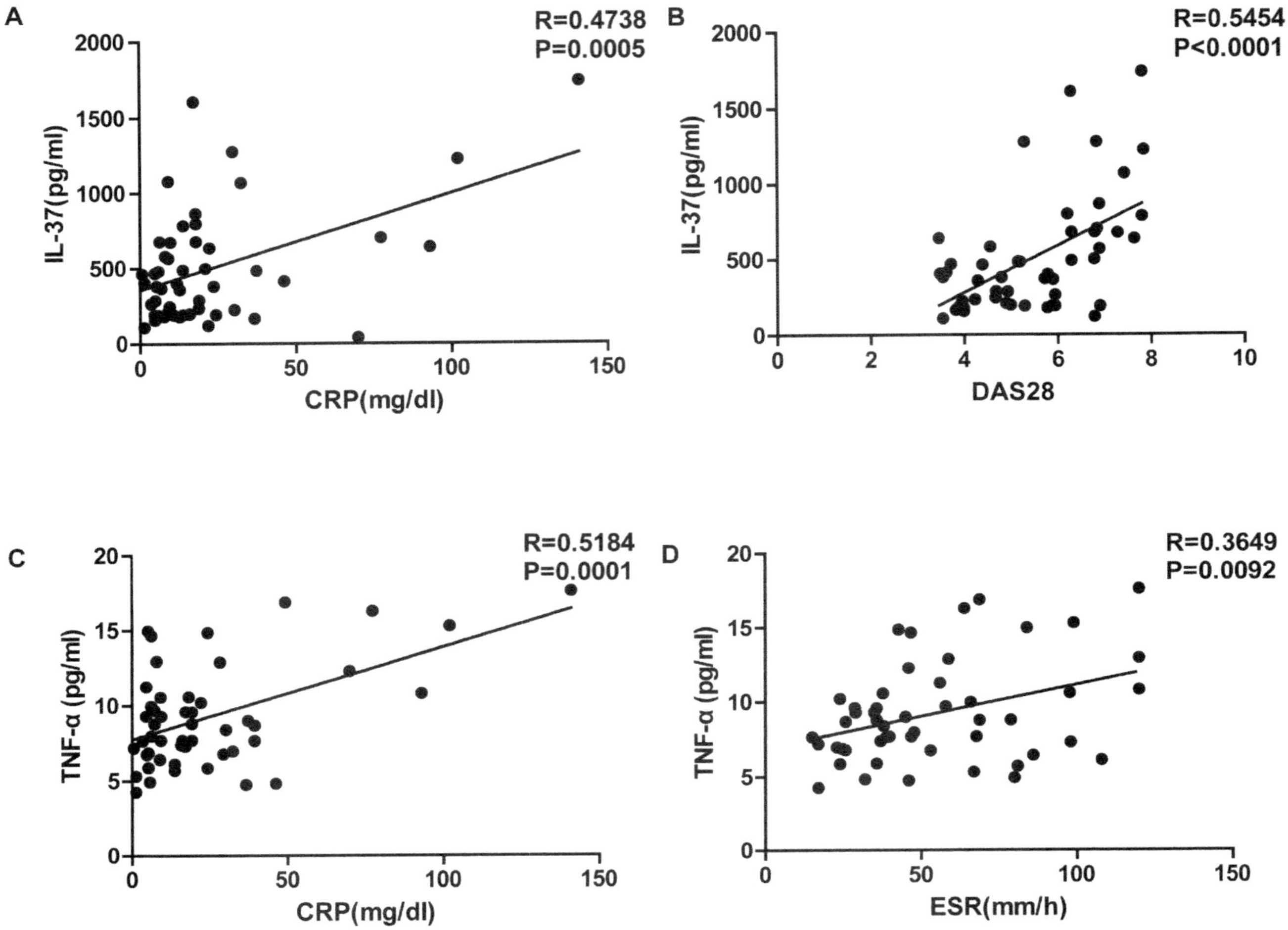

Figure 4. Correlation between plasma levels of IL-37 and disease activity in RA patients. (**A**) Correlation between plasma levels of IL-37 and CRP in RA patients. (**B**) Correlation between plasma levels of IL-37 and the DAS28 score in RA patients. The relationship between variables was evaluated using the Spearman rank correlation test.

levels of IL-37 were significantly higher in active RA patients compared to HCs. This suggests that IL-37 may be activated by pro-inflammatory cytokines or other unknown factors in the acute phase of RA.

TNF-α, IL-6 and IL-17A have been considered to be the pivotal cytokines in the pathogenesis of RA, as they are present at biologically significant levels in RA synovial tissue and in synovial fluid [26,27]. In good agreement, we found that the plasma levels of TNF-α, IL-17A and IL-6 were significantly higher in RA patients than in HCs. Following DMARD treatment, the plasma levels of TNF-α, IL-6 and IL-17A significantly decreased in drug responders. However, there was no significant decrease in cytokine levels in patients who did not respond to DMARD treatment. These data suggest that DMARD treatment in responders resulted in alleviation of the severity of arthritis by down-regulation of pro-inflammatory TNF-α, IL-6 and IL-17A cytokine expression. The plasma levels of IL-37 in drug-responding RA patients also decreased significantly, compared to IL-37 levels before treatment, suggesting that the expression of IL-37 was mostly controlled by pro-inflammatory cytokine levels.

In this study, we found that the plasma level of IL-37 was positively correlated with TNF-α in RA patients. Consistent with our results, a previous study reported that TNF-α could effectively increase the synthesis of IL-37 in PBMCs, using immunoblot analysis of cell lysates [13]. It has been reported that IL-17A is strongly dependent on TNF-α in the early stages of experimental arthritis, and could induce the production of TNF-α at later stages of experimental arthritis [28,29]. Consistent with these studies, our results indicated that the plasma levels of IL-17A were positively correlated with TNF-α in RA patients with active disease. In addition, the plasma levels of IL-37 were also positively correlated with IL-17A in RA patients. The lack of correlation between IL-6 levels and other cytokines, or the severity of the disease may be attributed to the relatively small sample size.

IL-37 has been reported to be protective against septic shock [12,13], DSS-induced colitis [30], concanavalin A-induced hepatitis [31], and in an experimental model of ischemia/reperfusion (I/R)-induced hepatitis [32]. These effects are related to the ability of IL-37 to reduce the production of pro-inflammatory cytokines and chemokines [31]. However, the correlation between IL-37 and disease activity in RA patients has not yet been investigated. We found that the plasma level of IL-37 was positively correlated with both CRP and DAS28. This is consistent with the notion that both the levels of IL-37 and the disease activity are determined by the same underlying factors, most likely the levels of pro-inflammatory cytokines.

In conclusion, the plasma levels of IL-37, as well as TNF-α, IL-6 and IL-17A, were found to be significantly increased in RA patients compared to HCs, and decreased in drug responders following DMARD treatment. In addition, plasma levels of IL-37 were positively correlated with the levels of pro-inflammatory cytokines TNF-α and IL-17A, and also with the disease activity in RA patients. Our data are consistent with the notion that the expression of IL-37 is mostly controlled by pro-inflammatory cytokines during the acute phase and the recovery phase of RA. This suggests that IL-37 may be part of a feed-back loop to control inflammation. However, this mechanism does not work effectively to control inflammation during active RA, either because the expression of IL-37 is inadequate, or because the effect of IL-37 is neutralized by unknown factors. These novel findings may provide new insights into understanding the pathogenesis of RA. More detailed studies are warranted to better understand the role of IL-37 in regulating the pathogenesis of RA. Our future studies will determine the role and mechanisms of IL-37 in regulating the pathogenic process of RA.

Author Contributions

Conceived and designed the experiments: YJ. Performed the experiments: PZ WJ. Analyzed the data: ZJ. Contributed reagents/materials/analysis tools: LW. Wrote the paper: PZ YJ. Designed the software used in analysis: YS.

References

1. Scott DL, Wolfe F, Huizinga TW (2010) Rheumatoid arthritis. Lancet 376: 1094–1108.
2. Corvaisier M, Delneste Y, Jeanvoine H, Preisser L, Blanchard S, et al. (2012) IL-26 is overexpressed in rheumatoid arthritis and induces proinflammatory cytokine production and Th17 cell generation. PLoS Biol 10: e1001395.
3. Chu K, Zheng H, Li H, Zhang Y, Zhang X, et al. (2013) Shuangtengbitong tincture treatment of collagen-induced arthritis via downregulation of the expression of IL-6, IL-8, TNF-alpha and NF-kappaB. Exp Ther Med 5: 423–428.
4. Hashizume M, Mihara M (2011) The roles of interleukin-6 in the pathogenesis of rheumatoid arthritis. Arthritis 2011: 765624.
5. Zhou L, Ivanov, II, Spolski R, Min R, Shenderov K, et al. (2007) IL-6 programs T(H)-17 cell differentiation by promoting sequential engagement of the IL-21 and IL-23 pathways. Nat Immunol 8: 967–974.
6. Park JY, Pillinger MH (2007) Interleukin-6 in the pathogenesis of rheumatoid arthritis. Bull NYU Hosp Jt Dis 65 Suppl 1: S4–10.
7. Kurebayashi Y, Nagai S, Ikejiri A, Koyasu S (2013) Recent advances in understanding the molecular mechanisms of the development and function of Th17 cells. Genes Cells 18: 247–265.
8. van Hamburg JP, Corneth OB, Paulissen SM, Davelaar N, Asmawidjaja PS, et al. (2013) IL-17/Th17 mediated synovial inflammation is IL-22 independent. Ann Rheum Dis.
9. Lubberts E, van den Berg WB (2003) Cytokines in the pathogenesis of rheumatoid arthritis and collagen-induced arthritis. Adv Exp Med Biol 520: 194–202.
10. Sharma S, Kulk N, Nold MF, Graf R, Kim SH, et al. (2008) The IL-1 family member 7b translocates to the nucleus and down-regulates proinflammatory cytokines. J Immunol 180: 5477–5482.
11. Dunn E, Sims JE, Nicklin MJ, O'Neill LA (2001) Annotating genes with potential roles in the immune system: six new members of the IL-1 family. Trends Immunol 22: 533–536.
12. Boraschi D, Lucchesi D, Hainzl S, Leitner M, Maier E, et al. (2011) IL-37: a new anti-inflammatory cytokine of the IL-1 family. Eur Cytokine Netw 22: 127–147.
13. Nold MF, Nold-Petry CA, Zepp JA, Palmer BE, Bufler P, et al. (2010) IL-37 is a fundamental inhibitor of innate immunity. Nat Immunol 11: 1014–1022.
14. Akdis M, Burgler S, Crameri R, Eiwegger T, Fujita H, et al. (2011) Interleukins, from 1 to 37, and interferon-gamma: receptors, functions, and roles in diseases. J Allergy Clin Immunol 127: 701–721 e701–770.
15. Simon LS (2000) DMARDs in the treatment of rheumatoid arthritis: current agents and future developments. Int J Clin Pract 54: 243–249.
16. Arnett FC, Edworthy SM, Bloch DA, McShane DJ, Fries JF, et al. (1988) The American Rheumatism Association 1987 revised criteria for the classification of rheumatoid arthritis. Arthritis Rheum 31: 315–324.
17. Prevoo ML, van't Hof MA, Kuper HH, van Leeuwen MA, van de Putte LB, et al. (1995) Modified disease activity scores that include twenty-eight-joint counts. Development and validation in a prospective longitudinal study of patients with rheumatoid arthritis. Arthritis Rheum 38: 44–48.
18. Morgan E, Varro R, Sepulveda H, Ember JA, Apgar J, et al. (2004) Cytometric bead array: a multiplexed assay platform with applications in various areas of biology. Clin Immunol 110: 252–266.
19. Tarnok A, Hambsch J, Chen R, Varro R (2003) Cytometric bead array to measure six cytokines in twenty-five microliters of serum. Clin Chem 49: 1000–1002.
20. Biswas S, Sharma S, Saroha A, Bhakuni DS, Malhotra R, et al. (2013) Identification of novel autoantigen in the synovial fluid of rheumatoid arthritis patients using an immunoproteomics approach. PLoS One 8: e56246.
21. Feldmann M, Brennan FM, Maini RN (1996) Role of cytokines in rheumatoid arthritis. Annu Rev Immunol 14: 397–440.
22. McInnes IB, Schett G (2007) Cytokines in the pathogenesis of rheumatoid arthritis. Nat Rev Immunol 7: 429–442.
23. Bufler P, Azam T, Gamboni-Robertson F, Reznikov LL, Kumar S, et al. (2002) A complex of the IL-1 homologue IL-1F7b and IL-18-binding protein reduces IL-18 activity. Proc Natl Acad Sci U S A 99: 13723–13728.
24. Tete S, Tripodi D, Rosati M, Conti F, Maccauro G, et al. (2012) IL-37 (IL-1F7) the newest anti-inflammatory cytokine which suppresses immune responses and inflammation. Int J Immunopathol Pharmacol 25: 31–38.
25. Song L, Qiu F, Fan Y, Ding F, Liu H, et al. (2013) Glucocorticoid regulates interleukin-37 in systemic lupus erythematosus. J Clin Immunol 33: 111–117.
26. Matsuno H, Yudoh K, Katayama R, Nakazawa F, Uzuki M, et al. (2002) The role of TNF-alpha in the pathogenesis of inflammation and joint destruction in rheumatoid arthritis (RA): a study using a human RA/SCID mouse chimera. Rheumatology (Oxford) 41: 329–337.
27. Md Yusof MY, Emery P (2013) Targeting interleukin-6 in rheumatoid arthritis. Drugs 73: 341–356.
28. Moran EM, Mullan R, McCormick J, Connolly M, Sullivan O, et al. (2009) Human rheumatoid arthritis tissue production of IL-17A drives matrix and cartilage degradation: synergy with tumour necrosis factor-alpha, Oncostatin M and response to biologic therapies. Arthritis Res Ther 11: R113.
29. Kramer JM, Gaffen SL (2007) Interleukin-17: a new paradigm in inflammation, autoimmunity, and therapy. J Periodontol 78: 1083–1093.
30. McNamee EN, Masterson JC, Jedlicka P, McManus M, Grenz A, et al. (2011) Interleukin 37 expression protects mice from colitis. Proc Natl Acad Sci U S A 108: 16711–16716.
31. Sakai N, Van Sweringen HL, Belizaire RM, Quillin RC, Schuster R, et al. (2012) Interleukin-37 reduces liver inflammatory injury via effects on hepatocytes and non-parenchymal cells. J Gastroenterol Hepatol 27: 1609–1616.
32. Bulau AM, Fink M, Maucksch C, Kappler R, Mayr D, et al. (2011) In vivo expression of interleukin-37 reduces local and systemic inflammation in concanavalin A-induced hepatitis. ScientificWorldJournal 11: 2480–2490.

An Osteoprotegerin Gene Polymorphism Is Associated with an Increased Risk of Hip Fracture in Japanese Patients with Rheumatoid Arthritis: Results from the IORRA Observational Cohort Study

Shinji Yoshida[1,2], Katsunori Ikari[1*], Takefumi Furuya[1], Yoshiaki Toyama[2], Atsuo Taniguchi[1], Hisashi Yamanaka[1], Shigeki Momohara[1]

1 Institute of Rheumatology, Tokyo Women's Medical University, Tokyo, Japan, **2** Department of Orthopaedic Surgery, Keio University School of Medicine, Tokyo, Japan

Abstract

Introduction: Patients with rheumatoid arthritis (RA) have a higher prevalence of osteoporosis and hip fracture than healthy individuals. Multiple genetic loci for osteoporotic fracture were identified in recent genome-wide association studies. The purpose of this study was to identify genetic variants associated with the occurrence of hip fracture in Japanese patients with RA.

Methods: DNA samples from 2,282 Japanese patients with RA were obtained from the DNA collection of the Institute of Rheumatology Rheumatoid Arthritis cohort (IORRA) study. Six single nucleotide polymorphisms (SNPs) that have been reported to be associated with fractures in recent studies were selected and genotyped. Forty hip fractures were identified with a maximum follow-up of 10 years. The genetic risk for hip fracture was examined using a multivariate Cox proportional hazards regression model.

Results: The risk analyses revealed that patients who are homozygous for the major allele of SNP rs6993813, in the *OPG* locus, have a higher risk for hip fracture (hazard ratio [95% CI] = 2.53 [1.29–4.95], $P = 0.0067$). No association was found for the other SNPs.

Conclusions: Our results indicate that an *OPG* allele is associated with increased risk for hip fracture in Japanese patients with RA.

Editor: Rui Medeiros, IPO, Inst Port Oncology, Portugal

Funding: This work was supported by grants provided by the Japanese Ministry of Education, Culture, Sports, Science and Technology Grant-in-Aid for Scientific Research (KI, SM), the Japanese Ministry of Health, Labour and Welfare (SM, HY). The funders had no role in study design, data collection and analysis, decision to publish, or preparation of the manuscript.

Competing Interests: No conflict of interest has been declared by the authors.

* Email: kikari@ior.twmu.ac.jp

These authors contributed equally to this work.

Introduction

Rheumatoid arthritis (RA) is a complex polygenic disorder of unknown etiology characterized by chronic inflammation and joint destruction, resulting in deteriorated physical function and increased risk of falling. [1–3] Patients with RA have a higher prevalence of osteoporosis and hip fracture than healthy individuals. [4–6] Several clinical risk factors for osteoporotic fracture in RA patients have been reported thus far. [7] Bone mineral density (BMD) is the major predictor of osteoporotic fracture, [5] and the fracture risk assessment tool was developed based on the use of clinical risk factors, including the presence of RA. [8] Recently, multiple genetic risk loci for BMD and osteoporotic fracture were identified in a meta-analysis of genome-wide association studies in people of European descent. [9] However, it is unknown if these genetic risk loci may contribute to fracture risk in non-white populations or in patients with RA. The purpose of the present study was to validate the association and to identify genetic variants associated with the occurrence of hip fracture in Japanese patients with RA. We hope that results from this study will increase our understanding of the genetic basis of hip fracture.

Materials and Methods

Study population

Tokyo Women's Medical University Genome Ethics Committee approved the present study (217C) and each individual signed an informed consent form after receiving a verbal explanation of

Table 1. Demographic, clinical and therapeutic data at the time of an enrollment in IORRA.

Factor	median (interquartile range) or n (%)	
Age, years	57.0	(48.5–64.2)
Sex, female	1949	(85.4)
Duration of disease, years	7.0	(2.0–13.0)
BMI, kg/m^2	21.1	(19.3–23.2)
DAS28	4.2	(3.4–5.1)
J-HAQ	0.8	(0.3–1.4)
RF, positive*	1801	(82.2)
ACPA, positive†	1908	(86.8)
History of smoking, ever	755	(34.5)
History of TKR, ever	99	(4.3)
DMARDs use, ever	1949	(85.4)
Methotrexate use, ever	980	(43.2)
Biologic use, ever	45	(2.0)
Corticosteroid use, ever	1119	(49.0)
Bisphosphonate use, ever	93	(4.1)
Active vitamin D use, ever	82	(3.6)

*Maximum value of RF measured in the cohort project during 2000–2010 for each individual was used.
†Cut-off = 4.5 IU/ml.
IORRA, Institute of Rheumatology Rheumatoid Arthritis cohort study; BMI, body mass index; DAS28, disease activity score in 28 joints; J-HAQ, the Japanese version of Health Assessment Questionnaire; RF, rheumatoid factor; ACPA, anti-citrullinated peptide antibody; TKR, total knee replacement; DMARDs, disease modifying antirheumatic drugs.

the study; the Genome Ethics Committee also approved consent procedure. This study was a part of the Institute of Rheumatology, Rheumatoid Arthritis cohort (IORRA) study, a single-institution–based, large-scale, prospective observational cohort study with an enrollment of over 5,000 Japanese patients with RA, which began in 2000. [7,10,11] DNA samples from 2,282 Japanese patients with RA were obtained from the IORRA DNA collection. All of the patients satisfied the American College of Rheumatology 1987 revised criteria for the classification of RA.

SNP selection and genotyping

Six single nucleotide polymorphisms (SNPs) reported to be associated with fractures in the recent European study [9] were selected and genotyped: rs6993813, in the osteoprotegerin (*OPG*) locus; rs6696981, in the zinc finger and BTB domain containing 40 (*ZBTB40*) locus; rs3130340, in the major histocompatibility complex (*MHC*) locus; rs3018362, in the receptor activator of the nuclear factor-κB (*RANK*) locus; rs11189505, in the spectrin β nonerythrocytic 1 (*SPTBN1*) locus; and rs2306033, in the low-density lipoprotein receptor-related protein 4 (*LRP4*) locus. Genotyping was performed using the TaqMan fluorogenic 5′ nuclease assay according to the manufacturer's instructions (Applied Biosystems, Tokyo, Japan). [11] Duplicate samples and negative controls were included to ensure accuracy of SNP genotyping. All polymerase chain reactions were performed using the GeneAmp PCR System 9700 (Applied Biosystems), and endpoint fluorescent readings for TaqMan assays were done on an

Table 2. Multivariate Cox proportional hazards model of each SNP associated with the occurrence of hip fracture.

Locus	SNP	MAF*	Risk allele	HR (95%CI)	*P*
OPG	rs6993813	0.423 (C/T)	C	2.53 (1.29–4.95)	0.0067
ZBTB40	rs6696981	0.218 (G/T)	G	1.42 (0.70–2.87)	0.33
MHC	rs3130340	0.140 (T/C)	T	0.78 (0.38–1.58)	0.48
RANK	rs3018362	0.312 (A/G)	A	1.12 (0.59–2.14)	0.73
SPTBN1	rs11898505	0.216 (G/A)	G	1.28 (0.64–2.55)	0.48
LRP4	rs2306033	0.363 (A/G)	G	1.05 (0.41–2.69)	0.094

All analyses were adjusted for independent non-genetic factors: age, body mass index, Japanese version of Health Assessment Questionnaire disability score, and history of total knee replacement. [7].
*Alleles are listed as major allele/minor allele.
SNP, single nucleotide polymorphism; MAF, minor allele frequency; HR, hazard ratio; CI, confidence interval; *OPG*, osteoprotegerin; *ZBTB40*, zinc finger and BTB domain containing 40; *MHC*, major histocompatibility complex; *RANK*, receptor activator of the nuclear factor-κB; *SPTBN1*, spectrin β nonerythrocytic 1; *LRP4*, low-density lipoprotein receptor-related protein 4.

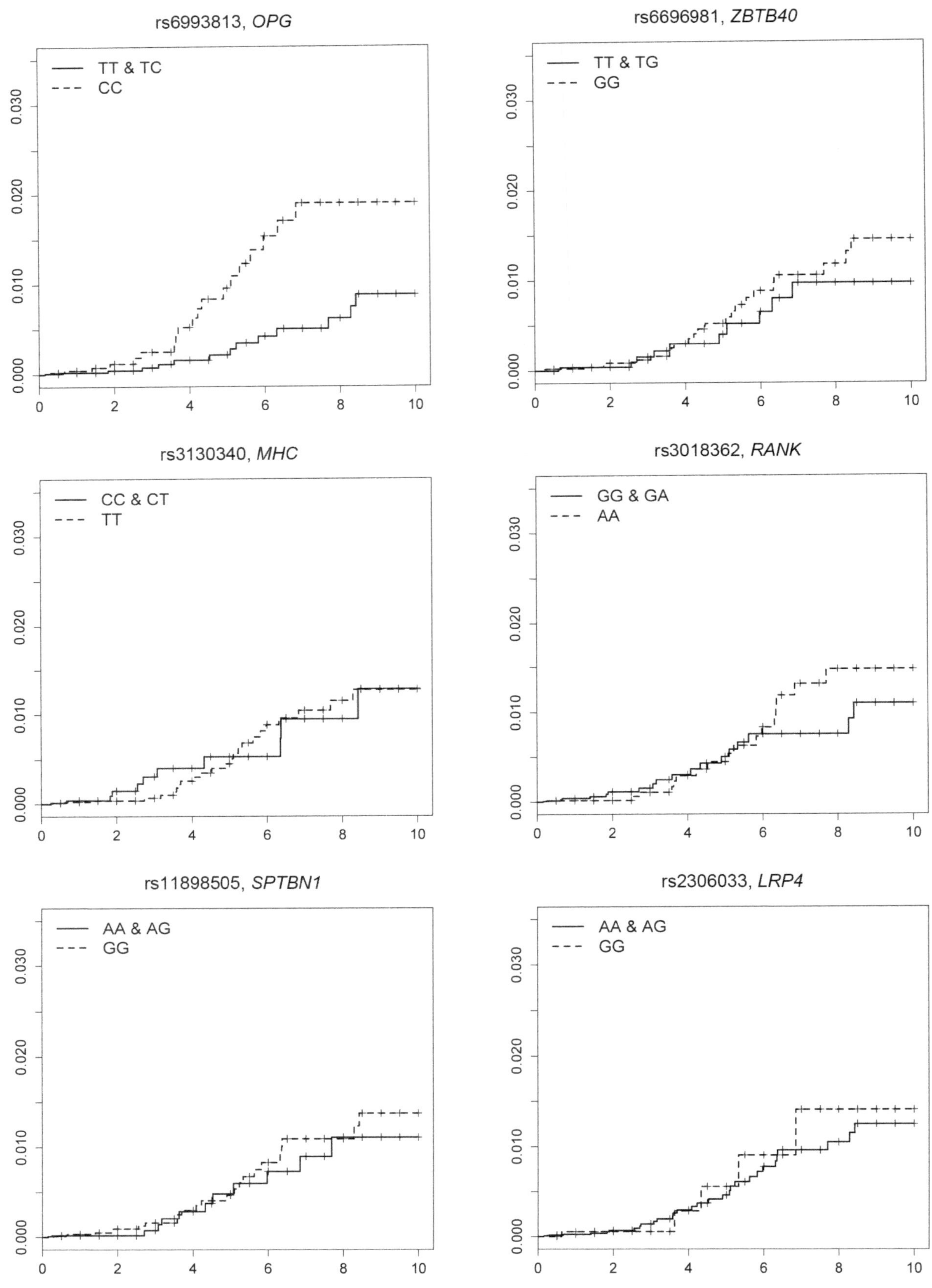
rs6993813, *OPG*
TT & TC
CC
rs6696981, *ZBTB40*
TT & TG
GG
rs3130340, *MHC*
CC & CT
TT
rs3018362, *RANK*
GG & GA
AA
rs11898505, *SPTBN1*
AA & AG
GG
rs2306033, *LRP4*
AA & AG
GG
0.000
0.010
0.020
0.030
0
2
4
6
8
10

Figure 1. Cumulative incidence of hip fracture for patients who were homo- or heterozygous for the non-risk allele and patients homozygous for the risk allele of each single nucleotide polymorphism (by the Kaplan-Meier method). Homozygous for the risk allele of rs6993813 (C) in the *OPG* locus was significantly associated with the occurrence of hip fracture ($P = 0.0067$).

ABI PRISM 7900 HT Sequence Detection System (Applied Biosystems), as described elsewhere. [11]

Assessment of hip fracture

The occurrence of hip fractures after enrollment in IORRA was determined from the responses to a patient questionnaire every 6 months from October 2000 to October 2010, with a maximum follow-up period of 10 years (median, 7.5 years). The data were confirmed by review of medical records and radiographs, as described elsewhere. [7,12] Only the occurrence of the first hip fracture reported by patients was included in this study. Hip fractures caused by major trauma such as car accidents were excluded. A total of 40 hip fractures in 40 patients were identified and included in this study.

Statistical analyses

This study used longitudinal data analyses to define whether the reported risk allele of each SNP was associated with the occurrence of hip fracture in Japanese RA patients. [9] The length of time from the date of enrollment in IORRA to the date of occurrence of hip fracture was calculated. A multivariate Cox proportional hazards model was used to examine the association of risk alleles of each SNP with the occurrence of hip fracture in 2,282 patients. Adjustments were made for the following independent non-genetic risk factors: age, body mass index, the Japanese version of the Health Assessment Questionnaire disability score, and history of total knee replacement, which we have previously shown to be clinical risk factors for the occurrence of hip fracture. [7] The proportional hazards assumption for the Cox model was assessed using log-minus-log plots for survival analysis. All statistical analyses were performed using the R software package (http://www.r-project.org/).

Results

Demographic, clinical, and therapeutic data of 2,282 patients at the time of enrollment in IORRA are shown in Table 1. The overall genotyping success rate was 97.5% and the genotyping concordance rate was 100% as assessed by duplicate samples. After the application of quality control criteria for genotyping (removal of samples that consistently failed for >16.7% [1/6] SNPs and removal of SNPs with a call rate <95% after removing samples that consistently failed), 2,210 of the 2,282 samples and all SNPs were accepted for the analyses. The studied SNPs were found to be in Hardy-Weinberg equilibrium.

A multivariate Cox proportional hazards model revealed that patients who are homozygous for the major allele of SNP rs6993813, in the *OPG* locus, had a higher risk for hip fracture compared to other patients (HR [95% CI] = 2.53 [1.29 to 4.95], $P = 0.0067$ [$\alpha = 0.0083$ after Bonferroni correction], Table 2, Figure 1). No associations were found for the other SNPs (Table 2).

Discussion

This study demonstrated that a polymorphism of rs6993813 in *OPG* was significantly associated with the occurrence of hip fracture in Japanese patients with RA. To date, many genome-wide association studies have identified multiple genetic risk loci for osteoporosis and osteoporotic fracture. [9,13] We recently identified that a *GC* polymorphism related to serum vitamin D concentration was significantly associated with the occurrence of hip fracture. [12] However, the genetics of fracture remain poorly understood in the Asian population, and genetic constitution may differ among populations. [14,15] Therefore, it is important to validate whether the previous findings are relevant to other ethnic groups.

The *OPG* gene encodes known regulators of bone remodeling and maintains a fine balance between bone formation and resorption involving osteoblasts and osteoclasts, potentially contributing to pathophysiological mechanisms of osteoporosis and osteoporotic fracture. [16] OPG is a member of the RANK-RANKL-OPG signaling pathway and is important to BMD genetics, and appears to have an influence on fracture risk. [17] Indeed, therapeutic targeting of the RANK-RANKL-OPG signaling pathway clearly influences fracture risk. [18]

The strength of this study is that the samples were relatively large and followed up for comparatively long periods. The data were based on a single-institution cohort study of Japanese patients with RA. Therefore, the differences between regions, races, and treatment strategies are expected to have had minimal influence on the results.

The possible limitation of this study is that we could not evaluate the influence of BMD because the data were not available for most patients. A bigger sample size could increase the statistical power to detect minor effects on events. It is likely that we were not able to validate associations of other genes and fracture risk due to the insufficient statistical power of this study. Further studies are required to confirm these associations and dissect the fracture risk, independently of BMD.

In conclusion, our data demonstrated that rs6993813 in *OPG* was significantly associated with increased risk of hip fracture in Japanese patients with RA. These results should contribute to a better understanding of bone metabolism and establishment of models for prediction of fracture risk in RA patients.

Acknowledgments

We thank all DNA donors for making this study possible. We appreciate the members of Institute of Rheumatology, Tokyo Women's Medical University for their effort on the IORRA cohort. We are also grateful to Ms Erika Abe, Ms Kaori Arai and Ms Akiko Sato for their technical assistance and to Dr Eisuke Inoue for his guidance and suggestions in statistical analyses.

Author Contributions

Conceived and designed the experiments: KI SY. Performed the experiments: SY KI. Analyzed the data: SY KI. Contributed reagents/materials/analysis tools: KI TF YT AT HY SM. Contributed to the writing of the manuscript: SY KI.

References

1. Armstrong C, Swarbrick CM, Pye SR, O'Neill TW (2005) Occurrence and risk factors for falls in rheumatoid arthritis. Ann Rheum Dis 64: 1602–1604.
2. Smulders E, Schreven C, Weerdesteyn V, van den Hoogen FH, Laan R, et al. (2009) Fall incidence and fall risk factors in people with rheumatoid arthritis. Ann Rheum Dis 68: 1795–1796.

3. Hayashibara M, Hagino H, Katagiri H, Okano T, Okada J, et al. (2010) Incidence and risk factors of falling in ambulatory patients with rheumatoid arthritis: a prospective 1-year study. Osteoporos Int 21: 1825–1833.
4. Kim SY, Schneeweiss S, Liu J, Daniel GW, Chang CL, et al. (2010) Risk of osteoporotic fracture in a large population-based cohort of patients with rheumatoid arthritis. Arthritis Res Ther 12: R154.
5. Orstavik RE, Haugeberg G, Uhlig T, Mowinckel P, Falch JA, et al. (2004) Self reported non-vertebral fractures in rheumatoid arthritis and population based controls: incidence and relationship with bone mineral density and clinical variables. Ann Rheum Dis 63: 177–182.
6. Huusko TM, Korpela M, Karppi P, Avikainen V, Kautiainen H, et al. (2001) Threefold increased risk of hip fractures with rheumatoid arthritis in Central Finland. Ann Rheum Dis 60: 521–522.
7. Furuya T, Inoue E, Hosoi T, Taniguchi A, Momohara S, et al. (2013) Risk factors associated with the occurrence of hip fracture in Japanese patients with rheumatoid arthritis: a prospective observational cohort study. Osteoporos Int 24: 1257–1265.
8. Kanis JA, Johnell O, Oden A, Johansson H, McCloskey E (2008) FRAX and the assessment of fracture probability in men and women from the UK. Osteoporos Int 19: 385–397.
9. Styrkarsdottir U, Halldorsson BV, Gretarsdottir S, Gudbjartsson DF, Walters GB, et al. (2008) Multiple genetic loci for bone mineral density and fractures. N Engl J Med 358: 2355–2365.
10. Yamanaka H, Seto Y, Tanaka E, Furuya T, Nakajima A, et al. Management of rheumatoid arthritis: the 2012 perspective. Mod Rheumatol 23: 1–7.
11. Kobayashi S, Ikari K, Kaneko H, Kochi Y, Yamamoto K, et al. (2008) Association of STAT4 with susceptibility to rheumatoid arthritis and systemic lupus erythematosus in the Japanese population. Arthritis Rheum 58: 1940–1946.
12. Yoshida S, Ikari K, Furuya T, Toyama Y, Taniguchi A, et al. A GC polymorphism associated with serum 25-hydroxyvitamin D level is a risk factor for hip fracture in Japanese patients with rheumatoid arthritis: 10-year follow-up of the Institute of Rheumatology, Rheumatoid Arthritis cohort study. Arthritis Res Ther 16: R75.
13. Estrada K, Styrkarsdottir U, Evangelou E, Hsu YH, Duncan EL, et al. (2012) Genome-wide meta-analysis identifies 56 bone mineral density loci and reveals 14 loci associated with risk of fracture. Nat Genet 44: 491–501.
14. Okada Y, Wu D, Trynka G, Raj T, Terao C, et al. (2014) Genetics of rheumatoid arthritis contributes to biology and drug discovery. Nature 506: 376–381.
15. Okada Y, Terao C, Ikari K, Kochi Y, Ohmura K, et al. (2012) Meta-analysis identifies nine new loci associated with rheumatoid arthritis in the Japanese population. Nat Genet 44: 511–516.
16. Simonet WS, Lacey DL, Dunstan CR, Kelley M, Chang MS, et al. (1997) Osteoprotegerin: a novel secreted protein involved in the regulation of bone density. Cell 89: 309–319.
17. Boyce BF, Xing L (2007) Biology of RANK, RANKL, and osteoprotegerin. Arthritis Res Ther 9 Suppl 1: S1.
18. Cummings SR, San Martin J, McClung MR, Siris ES, Eastell R, et al. (2009) Denosumab for prevention of fractures in postmenopausal women with osteoporosis. N Engl J Med 361: 756–765.

18

From Synovial Tissue to Peripheral Blood: Myeloid Related Protein 8/14 Is a Sensitive Biomarker for Effective Treatment in Early Drug Development in Patients with Rheumatoid Arthritis

Ivy Y. Choi[1], Danielle M. Gerlag[1¤a], Dirk Holzinger[2,3], Johannes Roth[3], Paul P. Tak[1*¤b¤c]

1 Division of Clinical Immunology and Rheumatology, Academic Medical Center/University of Amsterdam, Amsterdam, the Netherlands, 2 Department of Paediatric Rheumatology and Immunology, University Children's Hospital Muenster, Muenster, Germany, 3 Institute of Immunology, University Hospital Muenster, Muenster, Germany

Abstract

Objective: The change in number of CD68-positive sublining macrophages in serial synovial biopsies has been successfully used to discriminate on the group level between effective and ineffective treatment during early drug development in rheumatoid arthritis (RA) patients. Measurement of a soluble biomarker would clearly have practical advantages. Therefore, we investigated the sensitivity to change of myeloid related protein (MRP)8/14 in serum.

Methods: 139 RA patients who received known effective biologics (infliximab, adalimumab and rituximab) and 28 RA patients who received placebo/ineffective therapies were included. MRP8/14 levels were analyzed in baseline and follow-up serum samples and the standardized response mean (SRM) was calculated to determine the sensitivity to change of MRP8/14 in comparison to C-reactive protein (CRP) levels and the disease activity score evaluated in 28 joints (DAS28).

Results: In patients treated with effective treatment, the SRM for MRP8/14 was moderate (0.56), but in patients treated with placebo/ineffective treatment the SRM was 0.06, suggesting that this biomarker is perhaps not susceptible to placebo effects in proof-of-concept studies of relatively short duration. In contrast, the SRM for DAS28 was high for effective treatment (1.07), but also moderate for ineffective treatment (0.58), representing the placebo effect. The SRM for CRP was low in the effective (0.33) and ineffective (0.23) treatment groups.

Conclusion: These data support the notion that quantification of changes in MRP8/14 serum levels could be used to predict potential efficacy of novel antirheumatic drugs in an early stage of drug development. A positive result would support the rationale for larger, conventional clinical trials to determine whether the effects are clinically relevant.

Editor: Oliver Frey, University Hospital Jena, Germany

Funding: This research was supported by the Center for Translational Molecular Medicine (project TRACER, grant 04I-202) and the Innovative Medicines Initiative project BTCure (grant agreement number 115142-1). The funders had no role in study design, data collection and analysis, decision to publish, or preparation of the manuscript.

Competing Interests: The authors have declared that no competing interests exist.

* Email: paul-peter.x.tak@gsk.com

¤a Current address: GlaxoSmithKline Research & Development, Cambridge, United Kingdom
¤b Current address: University of Cambridge, Cambridge, United Kingdom
¤c Current address: GlaxoSmithKline Research & Development, Stevenage, United Kingdom

Introduction

Rheumatoid arthritis (RA) is a chronic systematic inflammatory disease affecting the synovial tissue in multiple joints. In spite of significant improvement in treatment, there is still a significant subset of patients that does not respond sufficiently to currently available medicines. Thus, there is still a need for treatments with a novel mechanism of action, and several of these are currently in development. The conventional approach towards clinical trials during early drug development is however not sustainable due to the high costs involved in testing large numbers of patients to provide proof of mechanism; slow recruitment rates due to improved standard of care as well as the large number of competing clinical trials; and ethical considerations: why would one unnecessarily expose large numbers of patients to placebo or experimental drugs that are likely to be ineffective in light of the high attrition rates during early drug development?

Therefore, we have previously proposed a fundamentally different approach towards phase Ib/IIa clinical trials: small, high density-of-data clinical trials evaluating biomarkers associated with common final pathogenetic pathways known to be relevant for the disease, biomarkers associated with the proposed specific mechanism of action, and trends towards clinical improvement. [1] We have previously identified and validated the expression of CD68+ cells in the synovial tissue of RA patients as a biomarker that is related to changes in clinical signs and symptoms independent of the primary mechanism of action. [2–4] We have recommended a rethinking of the decision to move ahead to large clinical trials when there is no trend towards clinical improvement, no specific effect related to the mechanism of action, and no change in CD68+ macrophage numbers in the synovium after treatment. [1] If this is the case, the drug might not hit the target effectively or the target may not be the right one. However, when there is a signal in at least one of these three variables, the next step would be to test the drug in conventional studies to determine whether the biological effect translates into clinically meaningful improvement. This screening approach, where the change in the number of CD68-positive sublining macrophages in serial arthroscopic synovial biopsy specimens is used to discriminate on the group level between effective treatment and ineffective during early drug development, has been successfully used to test a wide variety of experimental medicines, [1,5] allowing early go/no go decisions related to further clinical development. Such proof of mechanism studies may not only help to screen for potential efficacy, but may also help to optimize the range of dosages to be tested in the phase II/III trials.

While synovial biopsy is a safe and generally well-tolerated procedure in experienced hands [6], a limitation of this approach is that it is only used in a limited number of centers. Moreover, serial synovial biopsy is mainly restricted to the knee, ankle and wrist joints, affecting recruitment as not all patients with active RA have clinical involvement of these joints. Thus, there is a clear need for a biomarker reflecting the changes in monocyte/macrophage infiltration and activation in the synovial compartment in response to treatment, but which can be measured in the peripheral blood to screen for potential efficacy on the group level during early drug development.

Myeloid-related protein (MRP)-8 and MRP-14 are calcium-modulated proteins that regulate myeloid cell function and control inflammation. The heterodimer MRP8/14 is released during the interaction of monocytes with activated endothelium, probably at sites of local inflammation. [7] Therefore, we investigated the sensitivity to change of this soluble biomarker in RA patients in small clinical trials of short duration, similar to how this would be used in early phase Ib/IIa proof of mechanism clinical trials.

Materials and Methods

We investigated the changes after treatment with three known effective biologics: infliximab, adalimumab and rituximab; these open label prospective clinical trials have been described before. [8] Briefly, in the first cohort, 34 patients were treated with infliximab 3 mg/kg intravenously at baseline, week 2, week 6 and subsequently every 8 weeks. [9] In the second cohort (ISRCTN68762628), 85 patients received adalimumab 40 mg subcutaneously at baseline and every other week, [10] and in the third cohort (ISRCTN05568900), 20 patients were treated with intravenous infusions of 1000 mg rituximab at day 1 and 15 after premedication with 2 mg clemastine fumarate and 1000 mg acetaminophen but without methylprednisolone [11].

We also analyzed data obtained in 3 randomized, controlled clinical trials of treatment strategies that were shown to be ineffective in RA: C5a receptor-antagonist (C5aR; n = 6), [12] a human C-C chemokine receptor type 2 blocking antibody (CCR2; n = 8), [13] C-C chemokine receptor type 5 inhibitor (CCR5, n = 13), [5] and one patient treated with placebo in a randomized, double-blind, placebo-controlled study with abatacept (Clinicaltrials.gov NCT00420199) in patients with RA. [14] Targeting C5aR, CCR2 and CCR5 has been shown ineffective in RA in these placebo-controlled, phase Ib/IIa trials. [5,12,13] The studies were performed in the Academic Medical Centre/University of Amsterdam and approved by the Medical Ethics Review Board of the Faculty of Medicine (AMC-UvA). All patients gave written informed consent.

We collected serum samples at baseline and at a follow up visit after initiation of effective treatment or placebo/ineffective treatment. The follow up samples were the samples taken after baseline. For trials with effective treatment as well as C5aR antagonists and anti-CCR5 antibodies, the follow up samples were obtained 4 weeks after baseline. For the trial with anti-CCR2 antibodies, the follow up sample was taken at day 43. In the trial with placebo versus abatacept, the follow up sample was taken at day 113. Serum levels of MRP8/14 complexes were determined by double-sandwich enzyme-linked immunosorbent assay (ELISA) system, performed in the laboratory of the University of Münster, as described previously. [8,15] For comparison with earlier studies, internal control sera were used as a reference in all ELISA studies. The readers of the laboratory assay were blinded for the clinical details and samples were analyzed in a random order. In addition, we measured serum C-reactive protein (CRP) serum levels at these

Table 1. Baseline characteristics of patients enrolled in the effective and placebo/ineffective treatment groups.

	Effective treatment (n = 139)	Placebo/ineffective treatment (n = 28)	p-value
Female, n (%)	106 (76.3)	18 (64.3)	0.186
Age (years)	55 (47–63)	51 (36–59)	0.097
EULAR responder, n (%)	110 (79.1)	10 (35.7)	<0.0001
TJC68	10 (6–17)	10 (4–12)	0.093
SJC68	7 (4–12)	8 (6–11)	0.633
ESR	22 (12–37)	28 (18–56)	0.122
CRP	9 (3.5–22)	13 (6–47)	0.029
DAS28-CRP	4.72 (4.05–5.87)	4.77 (4.41–5.46)	0.662

Median and interquartile range or percentages are shown. EULAR responder = good or moderate responder according to the European League Against Rheumatism Response, TJC68 = tender joint count of 68 joints, SJC68 = swollen joint count of 68 joints, ESR = erythrocyte sedimentation rate, CRP = C-reactive protein, DAS28-CRP = disease activity score based on CRP. P-value <0.05 was considered statistically significant. Significance of the comparison is determined by the chi-square test or the Mann-Whitney test.

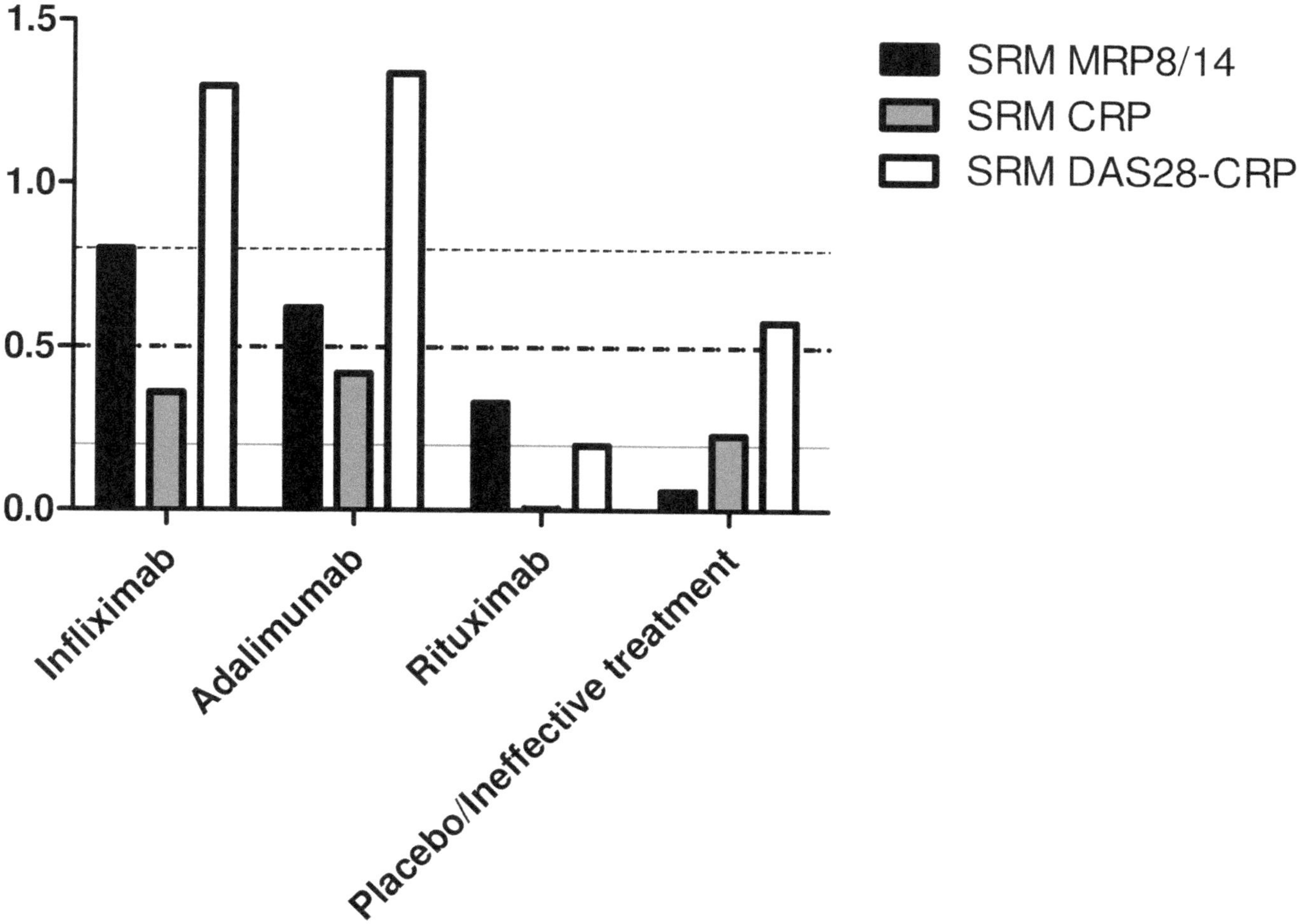

Figure 1. Sensitivity to change of MRP8/14 serum levels compared to DAS28 and CRP serum level. Standardized response mean (SRM) of the change in myeloid related protein 8/14 (MRP8/14), C-reactive protein (CRP) and disease activity score evaluated in 28 joints (DAS28-CRP) 4 weeks after treatment with infliximab (n = 34), adalimumab (n = 85), rituximab (n = 20) and treatment with placebo or ineffective therapy (n = 28). The solid line indicates the 0.2 SRM cut off point (low), the thick dotted line indicates the 0.5 SRM cut off point (moderate) and the thin dotted line indicates the 0.8 SRM cut off point (high).

time points and determined the disease activity score evaluated in 28 joints (DAS28-CRP).

Statistical analysis

Continuous data were described as median and interquartile range (IQR) if not normally distributed. The chi-square test was used to compare categorical characteristics. Mann-Whitney U test was used to compare continuous variables. All statistical analyses were performed with SPSS 20.0 software (IBM Corp., Armonk, NY). A p-value <0.05 was considered statistically significant. The standardized response mean (SRM), a measure of sensitivity to change, was calculated by dividing the mean change over time by the standard deviation of that change. The SRM of the clinical scores (CRP and DAS28-CRP) and MRP8/14 were calculated to evaluate the ability of these measurements to detect changes over time in the effective treatment groups (infliximab, adaliumab and rituximab treatment) and in the ineffective/placebo group (patients who received placebo or treatment with C5aR antagonist, anti- CCR2 or anti-CCR5 antibodies). An SRM>0.8 is considered high, representing a change of at least four fifths of a standard deviation of the change in the score. An SRM of 0.5 is defined as having moderate potential to detect changes, and an SRM of 0.2 as having low potential.

Results

One hundred thirty-nine patients treated with a known effective treatment and 28 patients treated with a placebo or ineffective treatment were included and analyzed in this study. Baseline characteristics of the patients treated with effective treatment or placebo/ineffective treatment are shown in Table 1. Age and gender were representative of typical RA cohorts. The response rate, as determined by the EULAR response, is as expected significantly higher in the group of patients treated with known effective treatment ($p<0.0001$). Tender and swollen joint counts of 68 joints (TJC68 and SJC68) at baseline were comparable between these groups. There were also no significant differences in baseline levels of erythrocyte sedimentation rate (ESR) and DAS28-CRP between the groups. Baseline CRP serum levels were significantly higher in the placebo/ineffective treatment group compared to the effective treatment groups ($p = 0.029$).

Sensitivity to change of MRP8/14 serum levels compared to DAS28 and CRP serum levels

In the first cohort (infliximab treatment), the SRM for MRP8/14 was 0.80 and the SRM for DAS28-CRP was 1.42 (Figure 1). Similarly, in the second cohort (adalimumab treatment), the SRM for MRP8/14 was 0.62 and the SRM for DAS28-CRP was 1.34 (Figure 1). The MRP8/14 biomarker exhibited consistently higher sensitivity to change than CRP in these anti-TNF cohorts, which was 0.36 and 0.42, respectively (Figure 1). In the third cohort (rituximab treatment), the SRM for MRP8/14 was 0.33 and the SRM for DAS28-CRP was 0.18 (Figure 1). In this cohort, the SRM for CRP was 0.00 (Figure 1). The SRM for MRP8/14 for the pooled effective treatment groups was 0.56, the SRM for DAS28-CRP was 1.07 and the SRM for CRP was 0.33.

In the studies with placebo/ineffective treatment, the SRM for MRP8/14 was 0.06, while the SRM for DAS28-CRP was 0.58 (Figure 1). The SRM for CRP in this group was 0.23 (Figure 1).

Sensitivity to change of CRP remains low if only patients with higher CRP levels at baseline are included in the analysis

To test whether CRP may have higher sensitivity to change if only patients with higher CRP levels at baseline are included, we calculated the SRM for CRP if CRP at baseline >5 mg/L. The SRM for CRP in the infliximab, adalimumab and rituximab was 0.46, 0.54 and 0.00, respectively. The SRM for CRP for the pooled effective treatment groups remained low (SRM of 0.40) and also remained low for the ineffective/placebo group (SRM of 0.26).

Sensitivity to change of MRP8/14 remains low in responders after ineffective/placebo treatment

As described in table 1, there was a 35.7% clinical response rate in the ineffective/placebo treatment group. When we calculated the SRM for MRP8/14 in EULAR good/moderate responders after known ineffective or placebo treatment, the sensitivity to change for MRP8/14 remained low (SRM of 0.12). In this group, the SRM for DAS28-CRP was 1.62 and the SRM for CRP was 0.35.

Discussion

We investigated the potential of soluble MRP8/14 as a biomarker to screen for initial evidence of efficacy on the group level during early drug development in small proof-of-mechanism trials in RA patients. The SRM for MRP8/14 in the two anti-TNF cohorts indicates a moderate to high potential to detect change. We also confirmed high sensitivity to change for DAS28 in this study, in line with our previous observations. [3] The relatively high values for DAS28 in the two anti-TNF cohorts compared to the rituximab cohort, might perhaps be explained in part by the early effects of TNF inhibitors on the central nervous system, [16] affecting the patient reported outcomes. Changes in MRP8/14 levels and DAS28 do suggest an effect of rituximab 4 weeks after the first infusion, but the values are relatively low due to the time point that is early for this specific mechanism of action and due to the fact that no methylprednisolone pre-treatment was given.

The sensitivity to change for serum levels of MRP8/14 resembles that for expression of CD68 positive macrophages in synovial tissue samples in patients treated with effective treatments across different mechanisms of action. [2,3] Of importance, this soluble biomarker does not appear to be susceptible to placebo effects, expectation bias or regression to the mean in proof of mechanism studies of relatively short duration in contrast to DAS28, with an SRM of 0.58 (moderate sensitivity to change) in the placebo/ineffective treatment studies. The SRM of MRP8/14 was low in EULAR responders after ineffective/placebo treatment, which supports the notion that this biomarker is not susceptible to placebo effects in studies of short duration.

The test characteristics of CRP were also clearly not as good as those for MRP8/14 in discriminating between effective and ineffective treatment. To exclude the possibility that this results could be explained by a relatively low CRP level at baseline in some of the patients, we calculated the SRM for CRP excluding all the cases with relatively low levels with a similar result.

Taken together, the results suggest that serial measurement of MRP8/14 levels in peripheral blood could be used as a biomarker to screen for initial evidence of efficacy on the group level during early drug development. This study provides the rationale for future validation studies using known effective drugs with a distinct mechanism of action such as tocilizumab, abatacept and tofacitinib compared to placebo and ineffective experimental treatments.

Author Contributions

Conceived and designed the experiments: PPT. Performed the experiments: DH JR. Analyzed the data: IYC. Contributed reagents/materials/analysis tools: DH JR. Contributed to the writing of the manuscript: IYC DMG PPT.

References

1. Gerlag DM, Tak PP (2008) Novel approaches for the treatment of rheumatoid arthritis: lessons from the evaluation of synovial biomarkers in clinical trials. Best Pract Res Clin Rheumatol 22: 311–323. S1521-6942(08)00014-4 [pii];10.1016/j.berh.2008.02.002 [doi].
2. Haringman JJ, Gerlag DM, Zwinderman AH, Smeets TJ, Kraan MC, et al. (2005) Synovial tissue macrophages: a sensitive biomarker for response to treatment in patients with rheumatoid arthritis. Ann Rheum Dis 64: 834–838. ard.2004.029751 [pii];10.1136/ard.2004.029751 [doi].
3. Wijbrandts CA, Vergunst CE, Haringman JJ, Gerlag DM, Smeets TJ, et al. (2007) Absence of changes in the number of synovial sublining macrophages after ineffective treatment for rheumatoid arthritis: Implications for use of synovial sublining macrophages as a biomarker. Arthritis Rheum 56: 3869–3871. 10.1002/art.22964 [doi].
4. Bresnihan B, Pontifex E, Thurlings RM, Vinkenoog M, El-Gabalawy H, et al. (2009) Synovial tissue sublining CD68 expression is a biomarker of therapeutic response in rheumatoid arthritis clinical trials: consistency across centers. J Rheumatol 36: 1800–1802. 36/8/1800 [pii];10.3899/jrheum.090348 [doi].
5. van Kuijk AW, Vergunst CE, Gerlag DM, Bresnihan B, Gomez-Reino JJ, et al. (2010) CCR5 blockade in rheumatoid arthritis: a randomised, double-blind, placebo-controlled clinical trial. Ann Rheum Dis 69: 2013–2016. ard.2010.131235 [pii];10.1136/ard.2010.131235 [doi].
6. Gerlag D, Tak PP (2005) Synovial biopsy. Best Pract Res Clin Rheumatol 19: 387–400. S1521-6942(05)00006-9 [pii];10.1016/j.berh.2005.01.005 [doi].
7. Frosch M, Strey A, Vogl T, Wulffraat NM, Kuis W, et al. (2000) Myeloid-related proteins 8 and 14 are specifically secreted during interaction of phagocytes and activated endothelium and are useful markers for monitoring disease activity in pauciarticular-onset juvenile rheumatoid arthritis. Arthritis Rheum 43: 628–637. 10.1002/1529-0131(200003)43:3<628::AID-ANR20>3.0.CO;2-X [doi].
8. Choi I, Gerlag DM, Herenius M, Thurlings R, Wijbrandts C, et al. (2013) MRP8/14 serum levels as a strong predictor of response to biological treatments in patients with rheumatoid arthritis. Ann Rheum Dis.
9. Wijbrandts CA, Dijkgraaf MG, Kraan MC, Vinkenoog M, Smeets TJ, et al. (2008) The clinical response to infliximab in rheumatoid arthritis is in part dependent on pretreatment tumour necrosis factor alpha expression in the synovium. Ann Rheum Dis 67: 1139–1144. ard.2007.080440 [pii];10.1136/ard.2007.080440 [doi].
10. Wijbrandts CA, van Leuven SI, Boom HD, Gerlag DM, Stroes EG, et al. (2009) Sustained changes in lipid profile and macrophage migration inhibitory factor levels after anti-tumour necrosis factor therapy in rheumatoid arthritis. Ann Rheum Dis 68: 1316–1321. ard.2007.086728 [pii];10.1136/ard.2007.086728 [doi].

11. Thurlings RM, Vos K, Wijbrandts CA, Zwinderman AH, Gerlag DM, et al. (2008) Synovial tissue response to rituximab: mechanism of action and identification of biomarkers of response. Ann Rheum Dis 67: 917–925. ard.2007.080960 [pii];10.1136/ard.2007.080960 [doi].
12. Vergunst CE, Gerlag DM, Dinant H, Schulz L, Vinkenoog M, et al. (2007) Blocking the receptor for C5a in patients with rheumatoid arthritis does not reduce synovial inflammation. Rheumatology (Oxford) 46: 1773–1778. kem222 [pii];10.1093/rheumatology/kem222 [doi].
13. Vergunst CE, Gerlag DM, Lopatinskaya L, Klareskog L, Smith MD, et al. (2008) Modulation of CCR2 in rheumatoid arthritis: a double-blind, randomized, placebo-controlled clinical trial. Arthritis Rheum 58: 1931–1939. 10.1002/art.23591 [doi].
14. Conaghan PG, Durez P, Alten RE, Burmester GR, Tak PP, et al. (2013) Impact of intravenous abatacept on synovitis, osteitis and structural damage in patients with rheumatoid arthritis and an inadequate response to methotrexate: the ASSET randomised controlled trial. Ann Rheum Dis 72: 1287–1294. annrheumdis-2012-201611 [pii];10.1136/annrheumdis-2012-201611 [doi].
15. Holzinger D, Frosch M, Kastrup A, Prince FH, Otten MH, et al. (2012) The Toll-like receptor 4 agonist MRP8/14 protein complex is a sensitive indicator for disease activity and predicts relapses in systemic-onset juvenile idiopathic arthritis. Ann Rheum Dis 71: 974–980. annrheumdis-2011-200598 [pii];10.1136/annrheumdis-2011-200598 [doi].
16. Hess A, Axmann R, Rech J, Finzel S, Heindl C, et al. (2011) Blockade of TNF-alpha rapidly inhibits pain responses in the central nervous system. Proc Natl Acad Sci U S A 108: 3731–3736. 1011774108 [pii];10.1073/pnas.1011774108 [doi].

Inhibition of HMGB1-Induced Angiogenesis by Cilostazol via SIRT1 Activation in Synovial Fibroblasts from Rheumatoid Arthritis

Hye Young Kim[1,§], So Youn Park[1,§], Sung Won Lee[3], Hye Rin Lee[1], Won Suk Lee[1,2], Byung Yong Rhim[2], Ki Whan Hong[1], Chi Dae Kim[1,2]*

1 Medical Research Center for Ischemic Tissue Regeneration, Pusan National University, Yangsan, Gyeongnam, Republic of Korea, **2** Department of Pharmacology, School of Medicine, Pusan National University, Yangsan, Gyeongnam, Republic of Korea, **3** Department of Internal Medicine, College of Medicine, Dong-A University, Busan, Republic of Korea

Abstract

High mobility group box chromosomal protein 1 (HMGB-1) released from injured cells plays an important role in the development of arthritis. This study investigated the anti-angiogenic effects of cilostazol in collagen-induced arthritis (CIA) of mice, and the underlying mechanisms involved. The expressions of HIF-1α, VEGF, NF-κB p65 and SIRT1 in synovial fibroblasts obtained from rheumatoid arthritis (RA) patients were assessed by Western blotting, and *in vitro* and *in vivo* angiogenesis were analyzed. Tube formations by human microvascular endothelial cells (HMVECs) were significantly increased by direct exposure to HMGB1 or to conditioned medium derived from HMGB1-stimulated RA fibroblasts, and these increases were attenuated by cilostazol, the latter of which was blocked by sirtinol. HMGB1 increased the expression of HIF-1α and VEGF and concomitantly increased nuclear NF-κB p65 and DNA binding activity, but these effects of HMGB1 were inhibited by cilostazol. SIRT1 protein expression was time-dependently decreased (3–24 hr) by HMGB1, which was recovered by pretreatment with cilostazol (1–30 μM) or resveratrol, accompanying with increased SIRT1 deacetylase activity. In the tibiotarsal joint tissues of CIA mice treated with vehicle, HIF-1α- and VEGF-positive spots and CD31 staining were markedly exaggerated, whereas SIRT1 immunofluorescence was diminished. These variables were wholly reversed in cilostazol (30 mg/kg/day)-treated mice. Furthermore, number of blood vessels stained by von Willebrand factor antibody was significantly lower in cilostazol-treated CIA mice. Summarizing, cilostazol activated SIRT1 and inhibited NF-κB-mediated transcription, thereby suppressing the expression of HIF-1α and VEGF. In addition, cilostazol caused HIF-1α deacetylation by enhancing SIRT1 activity and reduced VEGF production, thereby had an anti-angiogenic effect *in vitro* studies and in CIA murine model.

Editor: Christina Bursill, Heart Research Institute, Australia

Funding: This work was supported partly by the programs of the National Research Foundation of Korea (NRF) funded by the Ministry of Education, Science and Technology (NRF-2013R1A2A2A01067921 and NRF-2011-0009020). The funders had no role in study design, data collection and analysis, decision to publish, or preparation of the manuscript.

Competing Interests: The authors have declared that no competing interests exist.

* Email: chidkim@pusan.ac.kr

§ These authors contributed equally to this work.

Introduction

Rheumatoid arthritis (RA) is characterized by uncontrolled hyperplastic synovium and inflammatory synovitis associated with the chronic production of proinflammatory cytokines and low oxygen tension. Hypoxia is a characteristic feature of RA synovitis, because limited vascular capacity makes it difficult to meet the greater oxygen demands of hyperplastic synovium present in active RA. Consequently, a state of chronic hypoxia is produced, which induces new vessel formation via the induction of pro-angiogenic mediators [1,2]. Cellular response to hypoxia is driven by the hypoxia-inducible factor (HIF), which induces the expressions of large numbers of genes by interacting with specific promoter elements termed hypoxia-responsive elements [3]. Furthermore, the cytokines, IL-1β and TNF-α are known to increase HIF-1 protein accumulation in synovial fibroblasts (SF) by increasing its mRNA expression [4,5]. High mobility group box chromosomal protein 1 (HMGB 1) levels are largely elevated in the synovial fluid samples of RA patients and potently trigger arthritis, and HMGB1 is reported to be actively secreted by macrophages or passively released by necrotic cells [6,7]. Moreover, HMGB1 promotes the release of proinflammatory cytokines (TNF-α, IL-1β, and IL-6) from macrophages in synovial fluid [8,9]. Hamada et al. [10] showed hypoxia increases extracellular HMGB-1, which localizes preferentially to regions of tissue hypoxia in arthritis lesions. In addition, these workers observed the attenuation of inflammatory pathology in a collagen-induced arthritis (CIA) mouse model after HMGB-1 neutralization, which suggests that tissue hypoxia and resultant extracellular

HMGB-1 upregulation play important roles in the development of arthritis.

Several studies have shown that HMGB1 signals through RAGE or the toll-like receptors TLR2 and TLR4, and the activation of these receptors result in the activation of NF-κB, and thus, enhance the productions of proinflammatory cytokines and angiogenic factors in hematopoietic and endothelial cells, promoting inflammation [11]. Forsythe et al. [12] demonstrated the involvement of HIF-1 in the activation of VEGF transcription in hypoxic cells, and it was separately reported that HIF-1 binds to hypoxia-responsive element in the promoter region of the VEGF gene, and thus, upregulates VEGF expression [13].

Cilostazol is a phosphodiesterase type III inhibitor, and has been reported to exert potent anti-inflammatory effects. The anti-inflammatory actions of cilostazol suppress NAD(P)H oxidase-dependent superoxide formation, cytokine production (TNF-α, IL-1β etc.), and release of chemokines associated with reduced monocyte adhesion to HUVECs [14,15]. As the underlying mechanisms involved, the anti-inflammatory actions of cilostazol were attributed to the cAMP-dependent protein kinase activation and to the suppression of NF-κB gene transcription [16,17]. On the other hand, Lim et al. [18] proposed SIRT1 modulates cellular adaptation to hypoxia by targeting HIF-1α, and that SIRT1 directly deacetylates and inactivates HIF-1α. Furthermore, they revealed that SIRT1 prevents the secretion of VEGF in hypoxia, indicating SIRT1-induced deacetylation is responsible for inhibiting HIF-1 signaling.

Given that HIF-1α and VEGF signaling pathways play important roles in the regulation of angiogenesis, we hypothesized that cilostazol might regulate the HIF-1α and VEGF levels induced by HMGB1 in the SFs of RA. Thus, we investigated the signal pathways responsible for the inhibitory effect of cilostazol on synovial angiogenesis, and in particular, we attempted the following questions: (1) Does cilostazol suppress the expressions of HIF-1α and VEGF by inhibiting NF-κB activation? (2) Does cilostazol attenuate HIF-1α activity by enhancing SIRT1 expression and deacetylase activity? In addition, we sought to confirm that cilostazol inhibits HMVEC tube formation using an *in vitro* technique and by examining blood vessel formation *in vivo* in the arthritic synovia of CIA mice.

Results

Suppression by cilostazol of HMGB1-induced tube formation *in vitro*

We investigated whether the observed *in vitro* effect of HMGB1 on angiogenic processes is directly interfered with by cilostazol. When human microvascular endothelial cells (HMVECs) were directly exposed to HMGB1 (100 ng/ml) for 7 hr, tube formation significantly increased from 20.4±2.9 tubes/well (control) to 43.6±6.4 tubes/well ($P<0.01$), and pretreatment with 10 μM cilostazol reduced this HMGB1-stimulated tube formation to 18.5±3.5 tubes/well ($P<0.05$) (Fig. 1A and B).

Based on the expectation that HMGB1-treated RA fibroblasts produce high levels of angiogenic factors, we compared HMVEC tube formation after treating them with conditioned medium (CM) derived from HMGB1 (100 ng/ml, for 48 hr)-stimulated RA fibroblasts or CM from vehicle-treated fibroblasts. CM was diluted 1:5 in assay medium. Upon exposure of HMVECs to CM, the numbers of tubes formed increased significantly [(12.3±3.9 (vehicle group) to 34.5±4.0 tubes/well (HMGB1-treated), $P<0.001$)] (Fig. 1 Cb, c and Db, c). However, after pretreatment with 10 μM cilostazol, the number of tubes per well formed by these CM-treated HMVECs were significantly decreased ($P<0.001$) (Fig. 1Cd and Dd), and this decrease was prevented by pretreatment with sirtinol (20 μM, an inhibitor of SIRT1) (Fig. 1Ce and De). Additionally, pretreatment with YC-1 (30 μM, HIF-1α inhibitor) [19] inhibited HMGB1-induced tube formation, indicating that HIF-1α is involved in HMGB1-induced tube formation.

Cilostazol suppressed the elevations of HIF-1α mRNA and protein expressions induced by HMGB1 in RA SFs

We also examined the effect of exogenous HMGB1 on HIF-1α mRNA and protein levels in RA SFs. As shown in Fig. 2A and B, the expressions of HIF-1α mRNA ($F_{3,12}=31.94$, $P<0.0001$) and protein ($F_{3,12}=15.15$, $P<0.0002$) were significantly elevated by treating SFs with 100–500 ng/ml of HMGB1 ($P<0.001$). Correspondingly, HIF-1α protein expression was time (3–24 hr)-dependently increased ($F_{4,15}=54.01$, $P<0.0001$) by HMGB1 (100 ng/ml) (Fig. 2C).

To determine whether cilostazol suppresses HMGB1-induced upregulations of HIF-1α mRNA and protein, we pretreated RA SFs with cilostazol (1, 10 and 30 μM) for 4 hr prior to culturing them with 100 ng/ml HMGB1 for 12 hr. Increased HIF-1α protein expression by HMGB1was significantly reduced by cilostazol in a concentration-dependent manner [from 1.74±0.39 (100 ng/ml HMGB1) to 0.83±0.15 fold by cilostazol at 30 μM; $P<0.001$)]. Resveratrol (20 μM) had an effect similar to cilostazol on HIF-1α protein levels (Fig. 2D). Increased expression of HIF-1α mRNA by HMGB1 was also significantly inhibited by cilostazol (10 or 30 μM), and this was prevented by 1 μM of KT5720 (cAMP-dependent protein kinase inhibitor). Additionally, HIF-1α mRNA was significantly suppressed by pretreatment with chetomin (10 nM, $P<0.001$; an inhibitor of hypoxia-inducible transcription [20] as well as by Bay11–7082 [1 μM, $P<0.001$; an inhibitor of IκBα phosphorylation [21], pretreated for 30 min] (Fig. 2E). These results strongly suggest the involvement of NF-κB in the expression of HIF-1α mRNA and protein by HMGB1. Accordingly, HIF-1α protein level changes paralleled those of HIF-1α mRNA in response to HMGB1 and cilostazol (Fig. 2F). However, HIF-1β protein expression was not affected by HMGB1 (data not shown).

Suppression by cilostazol of elevated VEGF mRNA and protein expression by HMGB1

HIF-1 was reported to bind to hypoxia-responsive element in the promoter region of the VEGF gene and to upregulate VEGF expression [12]. Thus, we first checked that VEGF mRNA and protein levels are increased in SF of RA in response to HMGB1. VEGF mRNA levels increased time (3–24 h)-dependently by over 2 fold at 12–24 hr ($F_{4,20}=13.73$, $P<0.0001$) (Fig. 3A) and concentration-dependently to 1.90±0.26 fold ($F_{3,12}=16.24$, $P<0.0002$) by 100 ng/ml HMGB1 ($P<0.001$) (Fig. 3B). Similarly, VEGF protein expression was also time- and concentration-dependently elevated by HMGB1 (Fig. 3C and D).

It was determined whether the HMGB1-induced VEGF mRNA expression and protein release were suppressed by cilostazol. When cilostazol (1–100 μM) was co-treated with HMGB1 (100 ng/ml), HMGB1 (100 ng/ml)-induced increased VEGF mRNA expression was concentration-dependently reduced by cilostazol (1–100 μM) ($F_{5,18}=21.38$, $P<0.0001$) (Fig. 3E). Furthermore, HMGB1-induced increased VEGF release (control, 159±12 ng/ml to 285±11 ng/ml by 100 ng/ml HMGB1) was significantly attenuated by 10 μM cilostazol (to 195±11 ng/ml, $P<0.001$), and this attenuation was wholly prevented by pretreatment with KT5720 (1 μM, $P<0.001$). In addition,

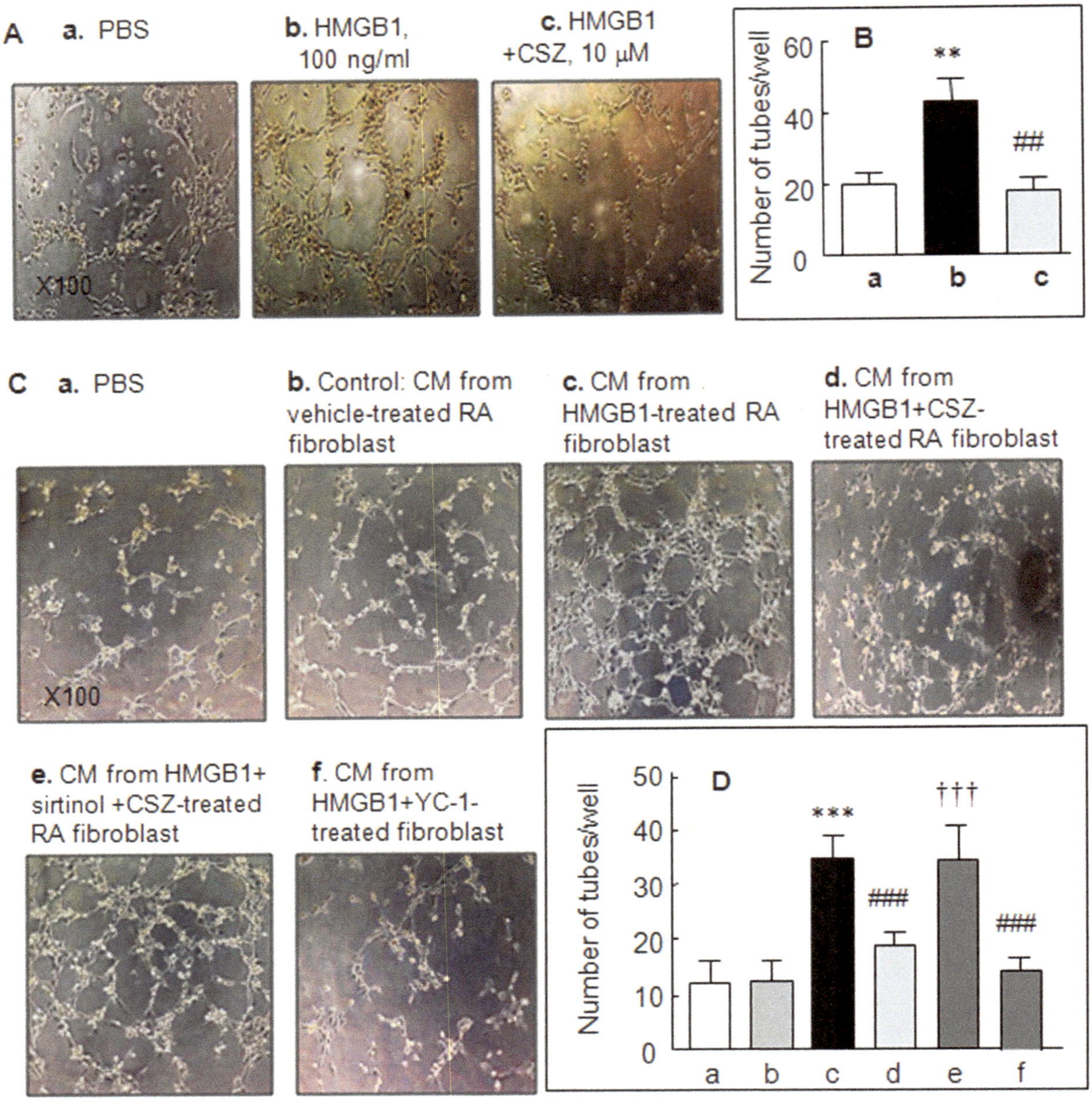

Figure 1. Suppression of endothelial cell tube formation by cilostazol (CSZ). Photographs of tube formation induced by HMGB1 (100 ng/ml), which was applied directly to the HMVECs in the absence and the presence of 10 μM of cilostazol (A) and by conditioned medium (CM) derived from cultures of HMGB1 (100 ng/ml for 48 hr)-treated RA synovial fibroblasts (C). Diluted CM was added to the culture medium after adding HMVECs to Matrigel. Cultures were photographed after 9 hr (×100). (B and D) Quantitative analyses: Results are mean numbers ±SEM of tubes per well for 4–5 experiments. $^{**}P<0.01$, $^{***}P<0.001$ vs. PBS (phosphate-buffered saline); $^{\#\#}P<0.01$, $^{\#\#\#}P<0.001$ vs. HMGB1 alone; $^{\dagger\dagger\dagger}P<0.001$ vs. 10 μM cilostazol.

pretreatment with either YC-1 (30 μM, a HIF-1α inhibitor) or chetomin (10 nM, an inhibitor of hypoxia-inducible transcription) significantly suppressed HMGB1-induced VEGF release, which strongly suggest involvement of HIF-1α in VEGF production (Fig. 3F).

These findings were further confirmed by an immunofluorescence study. When RA SFs were stained after being exposed to HMGB1 (100 ng/ml) for 24 hr, VEGF was largely expressed in the perinuclear region, but after pretreatment with cilostazol (10 μM) in the presence of HMGB1, this VEGF expression was greatly diminished (Fig. 3G). These results also suggest that HMGB1-induced increased VEGF release is reduced by cilostazol.

Inhibition of NF-κB p65 activation by cilostazol

It has been previously demonstrated that NF-κB is a direct modulator of HIF-1α expression, and that HIF-1α promoter is responsive to selective NF-κB subunits [22]. Accordingly, we assessed the suppressive effect of cilostazol on NF-κB p65 activation in HMGB1-stimulated RA SFs. Stimulation of SFs with HMGB1 (10–500 ng/ml, for 30 min) caused concentration-dependent increase in expression of phosphorylated IκB, and nuclear NF-κB p65 expression was significantly increased [1.69±0.17 fold ($P<0.001$) by 100 ng/ml HMGB1] (Fig. 4A and B). Furthermore, the DNA binding activity of NF-κB p65 was

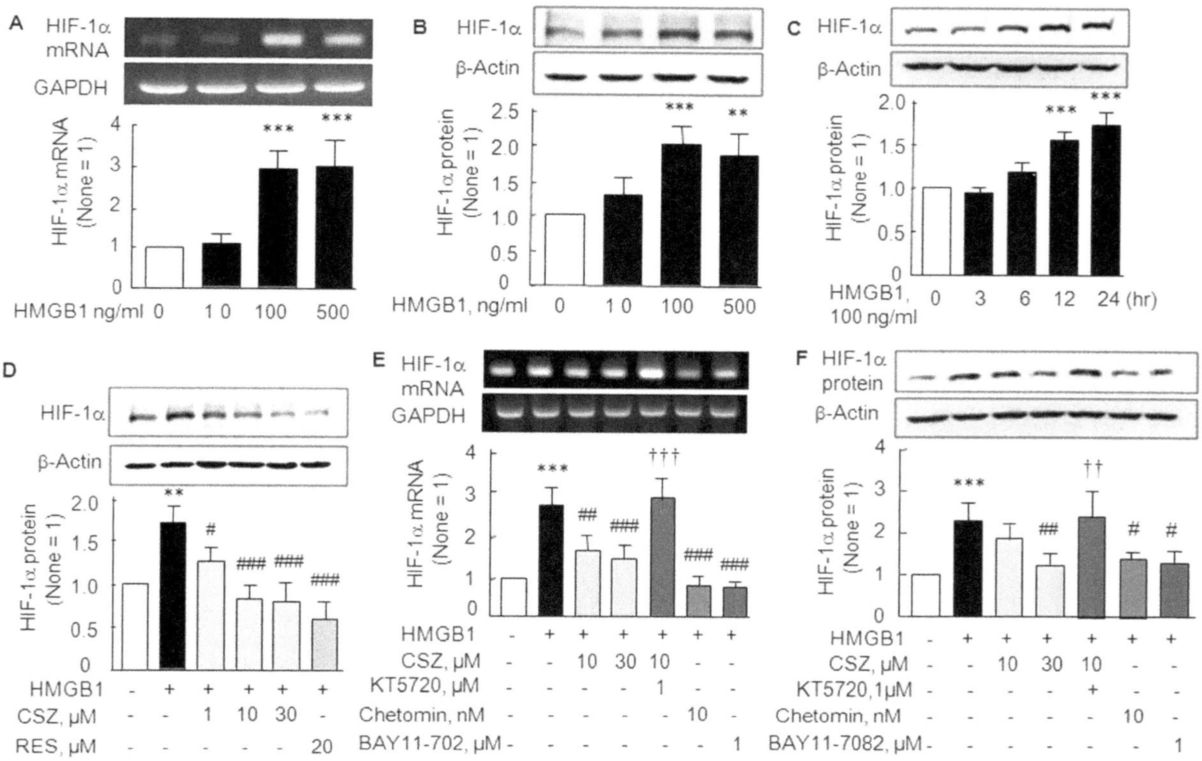

Figure 2. Elevations of HIF-1α mRNA and protein expressions by HMGB1 and their inhibition by cilostazol. (A and B) Concentration-dependent HMGB1 (10–500 ng/ml)-induced increases in the mRNA and protein expressions of HIF-1α. (C) Time (3, 6, 12, and 24 hr)-dependent increases in HIF-1α protein levels in the presence of 100 ng/ml of HMGB1. (D) Concentration-dependent decrease of HMGB1 (100 ng/ml)-induced HIF-1α protein by cilostazol (CSZ; 1, 10 and 30 μM) and resveratrol (RES, 20 μM). (E and F) Reverse of cilostazol-induced decrease in HIF-1α mRNA (E) and protein (F) by KT5720 (1 μM; a cAMP-dependent protein kinase inhibitor), and significant suppression of HMGB1-induced HIF-1α mRNA by chetomin (10 nM, an inhibitor of hypoxia-inducible transcription) and by Bay11–7082 (1 μM, an inhibitor of IκBα phosphorylation). Results are the means ±SEM of 4–5 experiments. **$P<0.01$, ***$P<0.001$ vs. no treatment; #$P<0.05$, ##$P<0.01$, ###$P<0.001$ vs. HMGB1 alone; †††$P<0.001$ vs. 10 μM cilostazol.

concentration-dependently increased by HMGB1 (10–500 ng/ml), which was attenuated by pretreatment with glycyrrhizin (50 μM; an inhibitor of HMGB1 to DNA binding in cells) [23] and with Bay11–7082 (1 μM; an inhibitor of IκBα phosphorylation and NF-κB activation [21]) (Fig. 4C). Correspondingly, HMGB1 (100 ng/ml)-induced increase in expression of phosphorylated IκB [1.50±0.07 fold ($P<0.001$, N = 4)], nuclear translocation of NF-κB p65 and its DNA binding activity were all concentration-dependently repressed by cilostazol, respectively (Fig. 4D, E and F). Interestingly, the HMGB1-induced increase in phosphorylated IκBα, NF-κB nuclear translocation and DNA binding activity were significantly reduced by 20 μM of resveratrol, a known SIRT1 activator.

In line with these results, we verified the functional correlation between HMGB1 and proinflammatory cytokine productions in the absence or the presence of cilostazol by ELISA. As shown in Fig. 4 G and H, stimulation of RA SFs with HMGB1 (10–500 ng/ml) for 48 hr significantly increased the productions of IL-6 and MCP-1 (by 100 ng/ml HMGB1: IL-6 to 12.00±1.76 pg/ml, $P<0.05$ and MCP-1 to 28.03±3.52 pg/ml, $P<0.05$) in culture medium, and these increases were significantly suppressed by cilostazol pretreatment (10 μM). Furthermore, these suppressions by cilostazol were reversed by subsequent treatment with KT5720 (1 μM).

Cilostazol increased SIRT1 expression and deacetylase activity

The effect of HMGB1 on the SIRT1 expression was explored in SFs. SIRT1 protein expression significantly decreased in a time (3–24 hr)-dependent manner after exposing RT SFs to HMGB1 (100 ng/ml) ($F_{4,15} = 39.06$, $P<0.0001$). When pretreated with cilostazol (1–30 μM) or resveratrol (20 μM) for 2 h prior to HMGB1 and cultured for 12 hr, HMGB1-induced decreases in SIRT1 protein expression were significantly restored by cilostazol (1.77±0.19 fold by 10 μM cilostazol, $P<0.001$) and by 20 μM resveratrol (1.66±0.27 fold, $P<0.01$) (Fig. 5A and B).

It has been previously reported by Lim et al. (18) that upregulation of SIRT1 leads to the deacetylation and inactivation of HIF-1α in hypoxia. We assessed SIRT1 activities in SFs by Western blots using an antibody specific for acetylated histone 4 lysine 16 residues (H4 Ac-k16). HMGB1significantly stimulated H4 Ac-k16 immunoreactivity (2.02±0.13 fold, $P<0.001$), which was significantly decreased by cilostazol (10 μM; to 1.29±0.22 fold, $P<0.01$ and 30 μM; to 1.08±0.22 fold, $P<0.001$) and by resveratrol (20 μM), and the effect of cilostazol was strongly blocked by sirtinol (20 μM, a SIRT1 inhibitor) (Fig. 5C). These results suggest that increased cilostazol-coupled SIRT1-mediated deacetylase activity prevented the HMGB1-induced acetylation of HIF-1α in SFs.

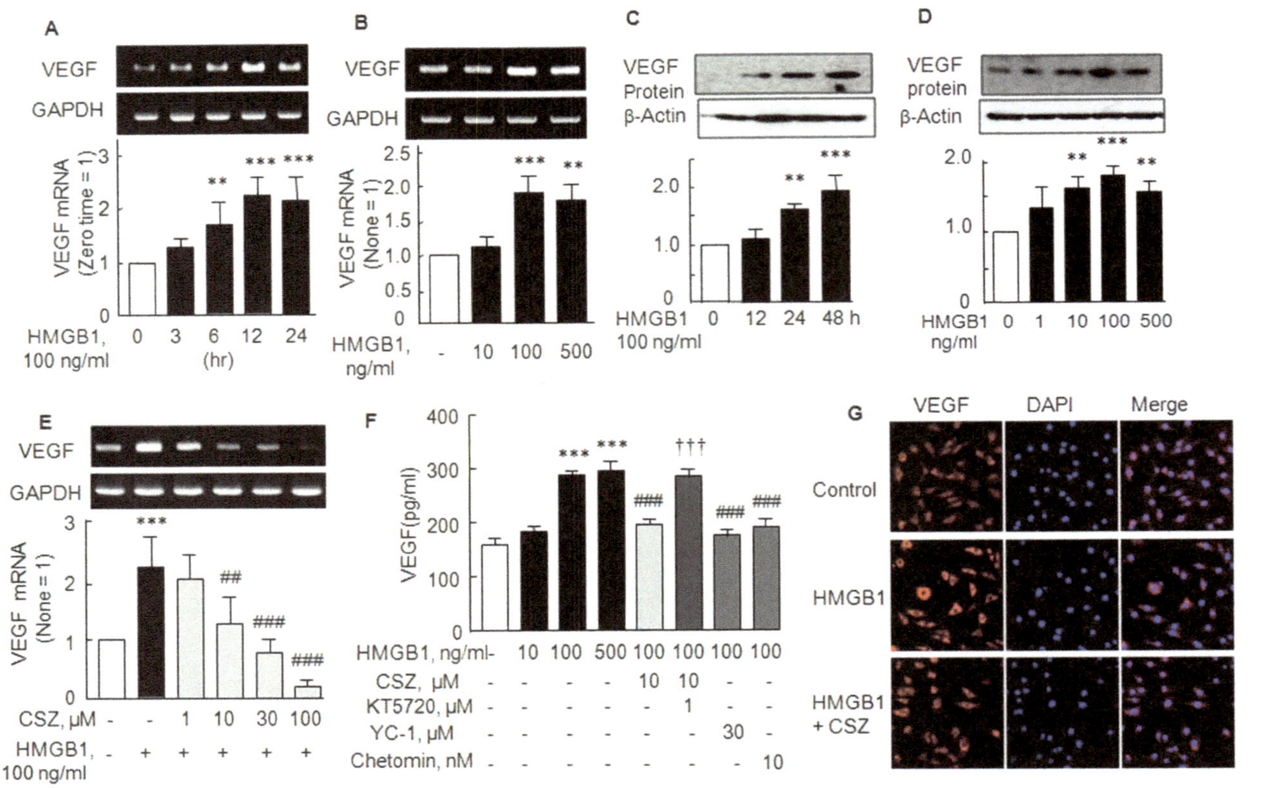

Figure 3. Suppression of HMGB1-induced elevations of VEGF mRNA and protein expressions by cilostazol. (A, B, C and D) Time- and concentration-dependent increases in VEGF mRNA and protein expressions stimulated by HMGB1. (E) Concentration-dependent suppression of HMGB1-stimulated VEGF mRNA expression by cilostazol (1–100 μM). (F) HMGB1-induced increase in VEGF releases and the attenuation of VEGF release by 10 μM cilostazol, by 30 μM YC-1 (HIF-1α inhibitor), and by 10 nM chetomin. The effect of cilostazol was blocked by KT5720 (KT, 1 μM) pretreatment. (G) Representative immunofluorescence photographs showing greater VEGF (+)-staining in HMGB1-treated synovial fibroblasts (24 hr), compared with control synovial fibroblasts. After treatment with cilostazol (10 μM), VEGF (+)-staining was obviously reduced. Results are expressed as means ±SEM of 4–5 experiments. $^{**}P<0.01$, $^{***}P<0.001$ vs. no treatment; $^{\#\#}P<0.01$, $^{\#\#\#}P<0.001$ vs. 100 ng/ml HMGB1 alone; $^{\dagger\dagger\dagger}P<0.001$ vs. 10 μM cilostazol.

Since HMGB1-stimulated NF-κB activation was inhibited by cilostazol, we examined whether HMGB1-induced NF-κB p65 and acetyl-p65 expression were affected by cilostazol in the SIRT1 gene silenced RA SFs. With silencing of the SIRT1 gene (~50% reduction in SIRT1 protein expression; Fig. 5D), cilostazol failed to reduce expression of NF-κB p65 and acetyl-p65 expression, whereas expression of NF-κB p65 and acetyl-p65 were decreased by cilostazol in cells transfected with scrambled siRNA duplex (negative control) (Fig. 5E, F), indicating the involvement of SIRT1 in the action mechanism of cilostazol.

Immunohistochemistry and immunofluorescence studies in CIA mice

Histological study (H & E staining) revealed attenuated synovial tissue inflammation and reduced inflammatory cell infiltration in the tibiotarsal joints of mice treated with cilostazol (30 mg/kg/day). We adopted an immunofluorescence approach to determine whether cilostazol stimulates SIRT1 expression and suppresses the expressions of HIF-1α and VEGF in knee joints. In the vehicle-treated CIA mice, SIRT1 was expressed at low levels, whereas HIF-1α and VEGF were highly expressed. Interestingly, in mice treated with cilostazol (30 mg/kg/day), HIF-1α- and VEGF-positive spots were markedly attenuated, whereas SIRT1 immunofluorescence was markedly increased (Fig. 6A).

Additionally, CD31 expression, a marker of blood vessels, was high in vehicle-treated knee joints of CIA mice, and this was markedly attenuated in cilostazol-treated CIA mice as shown in control mice. To quantitatively analyze synovial angiogenesis, tibiotarsal joint tissue sections were stained with polyclonal rabbit anti-human von Willebrand factor (vWF, a marker of endothelial cells), and numbers of blood vessels were counted in joint sections. As shown in Fig. 6B, pronounced vWF staining area and vessel numbers were increased in the inflammatory synovial pannus areas of the paws of CIA mice treated with vehicle, and these were significantly diminished in cilostazol-treated CIA mice, indicating that cilostazol strongly attenuated angiogenesis in the synovium of the knee joints of CIA mice.

Discussion

The major findings of the present study are that cilostazol inhibits *in vitro* tube formation by HMVECs and *in vivo* blood vessel formation with increased inflammatory severity in the arthritic synovium of CIA mice. The study confirms that the signaling pathways involved in HMGB1-induced HIF-1α expression and VEGF release involve NF-κB activation in RA SFs. Additionally, the study shows that cilostazol has two inhibitory effects, that is, (1) it inhibits HMGB1-induced increases in phosphorylated IκBα and the nuclear translocation of NF-κB,

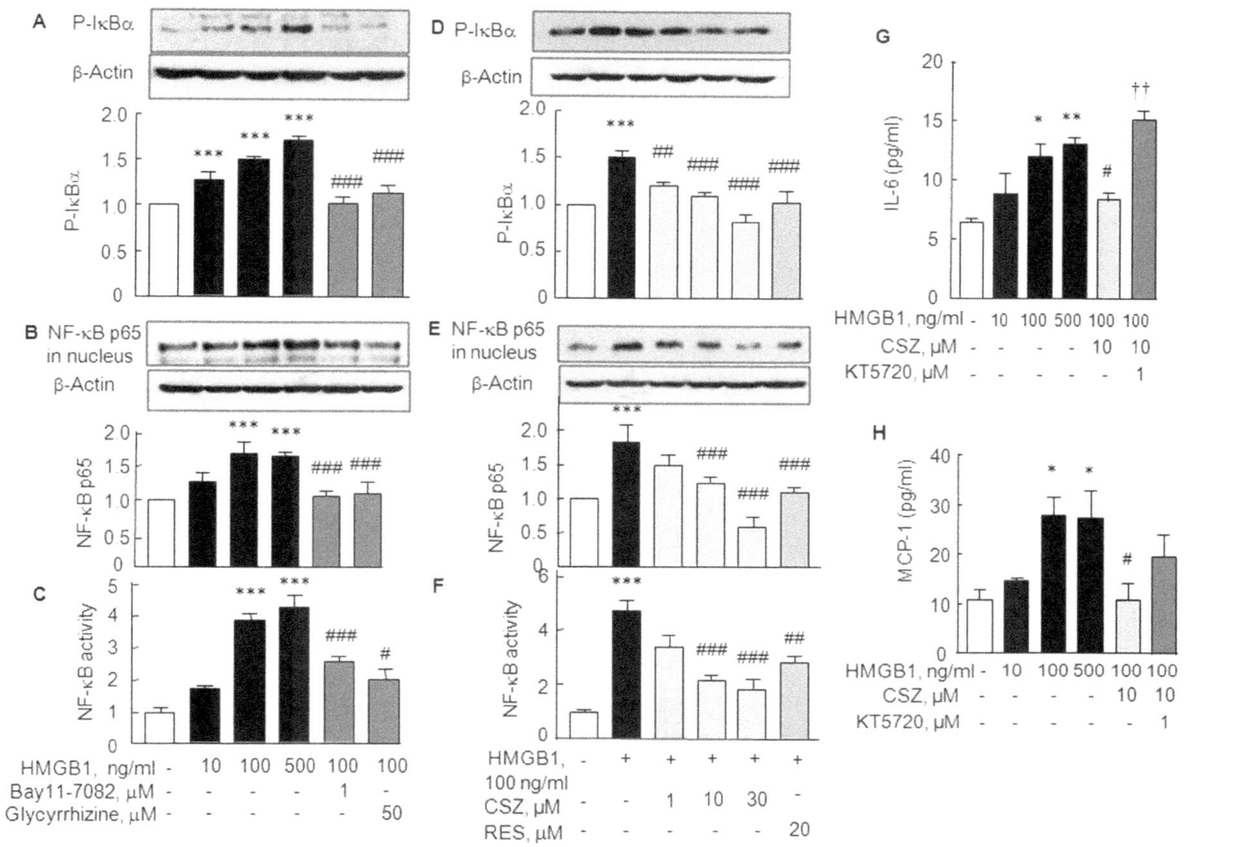

Figure 4. Inhibition of NF-κB p65 expression and activity by cilostazol. (A, B and C) HMGB1-induced increase in phosphorylated IκBα (A) and increase in the nuclear translocation of NF-κB (B) and DNA binding activity of NF-κB in synovial fibroblasts (C). These effects were inhibited by glycyrrhizin (50 μM, an inhibitor of HMGB1 binding to DNA) and by Bay11–7082 (1 μM). (D, E and F) Cilostazol (CSZ; 1, 10 and 30 μM) and resveratrol (RES; 20 μM) decreased phosphorylated IκBα (D), nuclear NF-κB (E) levels and DNA binding activity of NF-κB (F). (G, H) Suppression of HMGB1-stimulated production of proinflammatory cytokines, IL-6 and MCP-1, by cilostazol (10 μM) and the reversal of this suppression by KT5720 (1 μM) in cultured medium. Results are the means ±SEM of 3–4 experiments. *$P<0.05$, **$P<0.01$, ***$P<0.001$ vs. no treatment; $^{\#}P<0.05$, $^{\#\#}P<0.01$, $^{\#\#\#}P<0.001$ vs. HMGB1 alone; $^{\dagger\dagger}P<0.01$ vs. 10 μM cilostazol.

and thus suppresses HIF-1α expression, and (2) it inactivates HIF-1α by enhancing SIRT1 deacetylase activity, thereby suppressing VEGF expression at the mRNA and protein levels, and consequently inhibiting synovial angiogenesis (Fig. 7). Furthermore, our results provide first evidence that HMGB1 requires the upregulation of HIF-1α/VEGF for endothelial tube formation.

It has been established synovial inflammation is accompanied by fibroblast proliferation and neutrophil infiltration and by angiogenesis in RA patients. The uncontrolled proliferation of the synovial lining layer leads to microenvironmental changes resulting in hypoxic conditions [5,16]. HMGB1 is either actively secreted by macrophages or passively released from necrotic cells [6,7]. Furthermore, extracellular HMGB1 has been abundantly demonstrated in synovitis, that is, in the intra-articular fluids of RA patients and in animal models of arthritis [24]. In line with these results, Hamada et al. [10] have emphasized that concentration of HMGB1 significantly correlate with tissue hypoxia, indicating that extracellular HMGB1 plays a role as a coupling factor between hypoxia and inflammation in arthritis.

The cellular response to hypoxia is mainly driven by the transcription factor HIF [25]. Thus, in this study, measurement of HIF-1α protein in the presence of HMGB1 was considered as a marker of hypoxia. HIF-1 is a heterodimeric transcription factor and is composed of HIF-1α, which is oxygen regulated, and HIF-1β, which is expressed constitutively in the nucleus [26]. Our results show that exogenously applied HMGB1 markedly upregulated HIF-1α mRNA and protein levels, but not HIF-1β in RA SFs. Furthermore, these upregulations were significantly suppressed by cilostazol pretreatment, and these suppressions were reversed by KT5720, which concurs with the findings of Torii et al. [27]. In addition, VEGF mRNA and protein releases, which were increased time- and concentration-dependently by over 2 fold by HMGB1, were significantly attenuated by cilostazol. It was documented by Chun et al. [19] that YC-1 as a HIF-1α inhibitor blocked the induction of VEGF mRNAs. Considering that HMGB1-induced VEGF release and tube formation were inhibited by YC-1 and chetomin, an inhibitor of hypoxia-inducible transcription [20], it is likely considered that cilostazol-induced suppression of HMGB1-stimulated tube formation is ascribed to down-regulation of HIF-1α-linked VEGF release.

Recently, it was revealed NF-κB is a direct modulator of HIF-1α expression, and HIF-1α promoter is responsive to selective NF-κB subunits [22]. Furthermore, the classic hypoxia-responsive gene VEGF is present at high levels in the serum and synovial fluid of RA patients [28,29]. In an experiment on IKK-2-deficient mice, NF-κB was proved to be required for HIF-1α protein

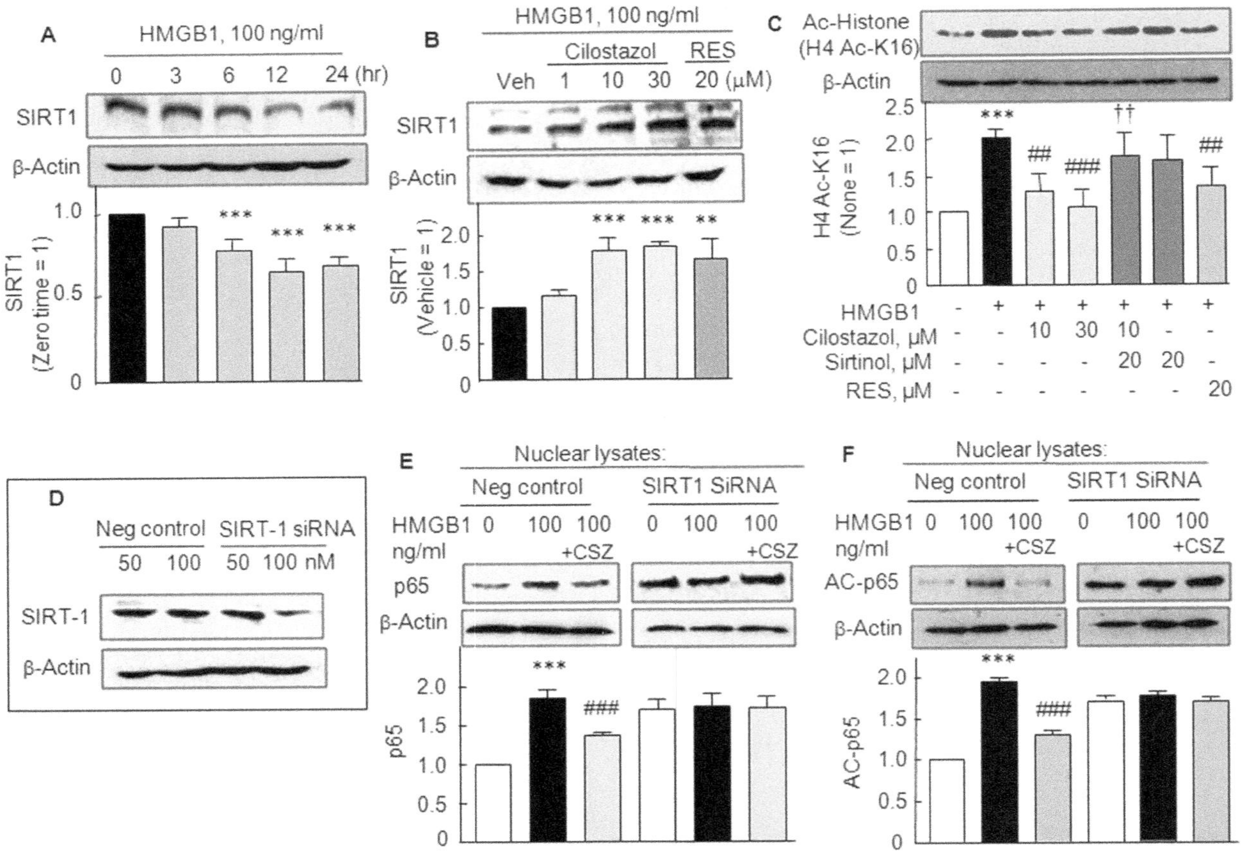

Figure 5. Increased SIRT1 expression and deacetylase activity by cilostazol. (A) Time (3–24 hr)-dependent decrease in SIRT1 protein expression after exposure to HMGB1 (100 ng/ml), and (B) recovery of reduced SIRT1 expression by cilostazol (1–30 μM) and by resveratrol (RES, 20 μM). (C) HMGB1-induced increase in H4 acetyl-k16 (H4 Ac-K16) immunoreactivity was decreased by cilostazol (10 and 30 μM) and resveratrol (RES, 20 μM). Cilostazol-induced decrease in H4 Ac-K16 was prevented by sirtinol (20 μM). (D) Analyses of SIRT1 knockout RA SFs compared with negative control cells. Cilostazol (10 μM) failed to induce expression of SIRT1 in RA SF cells transfected with SIRT1 siRNA oligonucleotide (100 nM) as contrasted to negative control. (E and F) Loss of the effect of cilostazol on the elevated expressions of p65 and acetyl (AC)-p65 induced by HMGB1 (100 ng/ml) in SIRT1 gene silenced fibroblasts, which contrasted to the effects of cilostazol in the negative control cells. Results are the means ±SEM of 4 experiments. $^{**}P<0.01$, $^{***}P<0.001$ vs. no treatment or vehicle (Veh); $^{\#\#}P<0.01$, $^{\#\#\#}P<0.001$ vs. HMGB1; $^{\dagger\dagger}P<0.01$ vs. 10 μM cilostazol.

accumulation, and the absence of IKK-2 resulted in defective induction of VEGF, a HIF-1 target [30]. Consistent with these reports, our results showed that HIF-1α mRNA was significantly suppressed by chetomin [20] and by Bay11–7082 (an inhibitor of IκBα phosphorylation [21]). These reported results indicate the involvements of hypoxia-induced transcription and NF-κB in the action of HMGB1. Thus, we examined the suppression of NF-κB p65 activation by cilostazol in HMGB1-stimulated RA SFs. Indeed, we found that the up-regulation phosphorylated IκBα and nuclear translocation of NF-κB p65 by HMGB1 were significantly attenuated by cilostazol and these were paralleled by a decrease in NF-κB p65 DNA binding activity. In view of several reports issued on the topic [22,30], it appears likely that the down-regulations of HIF-1α and VEGF by cilostazol are due to reductions in NF-κB p65 activity.

Recently, Lim et al. [18] demonstrated that SIRT1 binds to, deacetylates and inactivates HIF-1α, and reported that during hypoxia, SIRT1 is downregulated due to diminished NAD^+ levels, which allows the acetylation and activation of HIF-1α. Interestingly, we found SIRT1 protein expression was significantly decreased in a time (3–24 hr)-dependent manner after exposure to the HMGB1. The stabilization of HIF-1α protein is important in hypoxia, and hypoxia in turn increases extracellular HMGB-1 levels [9]. In the present study, we found that SIRT1 protein up-regulation by cilostazol coincided with enhanced SIRT1 deacetylase activity in SFs, as was reflected by reduced acetylation of the H4 Ac-k16, which support the notion that increased deacetylation of HIF-1α by cilostazol is responsible for the reduced induction of VEGF. Importantly, in the synovial fibroblasts transfected with SIRT1 SiRNA, cilostazol failed to reduce the expression of NF-κB p65 and acetyl-p65, as contrasted to the negative control cells (transfected with scrambled siRNA duplex). These findings strongly suggest that inhibition of NF-κB p65 acetylation by deacetylase activity of SIRT1 is involved in the action mechanism of cilostazol.

As was expected, in the tibiotarsal joint tissues of CIA mice, SIRT1 expression was markedly diminished and in contrast HIF-1α and VEGF were highly up-regulated in concert with CD31. Furthermore, these angiogenic factors were substantially diminished by cilostazol (30 mg/kg/day) and in contrast SIRT1 immunofluorescence was markedly increased. In line with these observations, pronounced vWF staining and increased numbers of vessels, observed in the inflammatory synovial pannus area of CIA

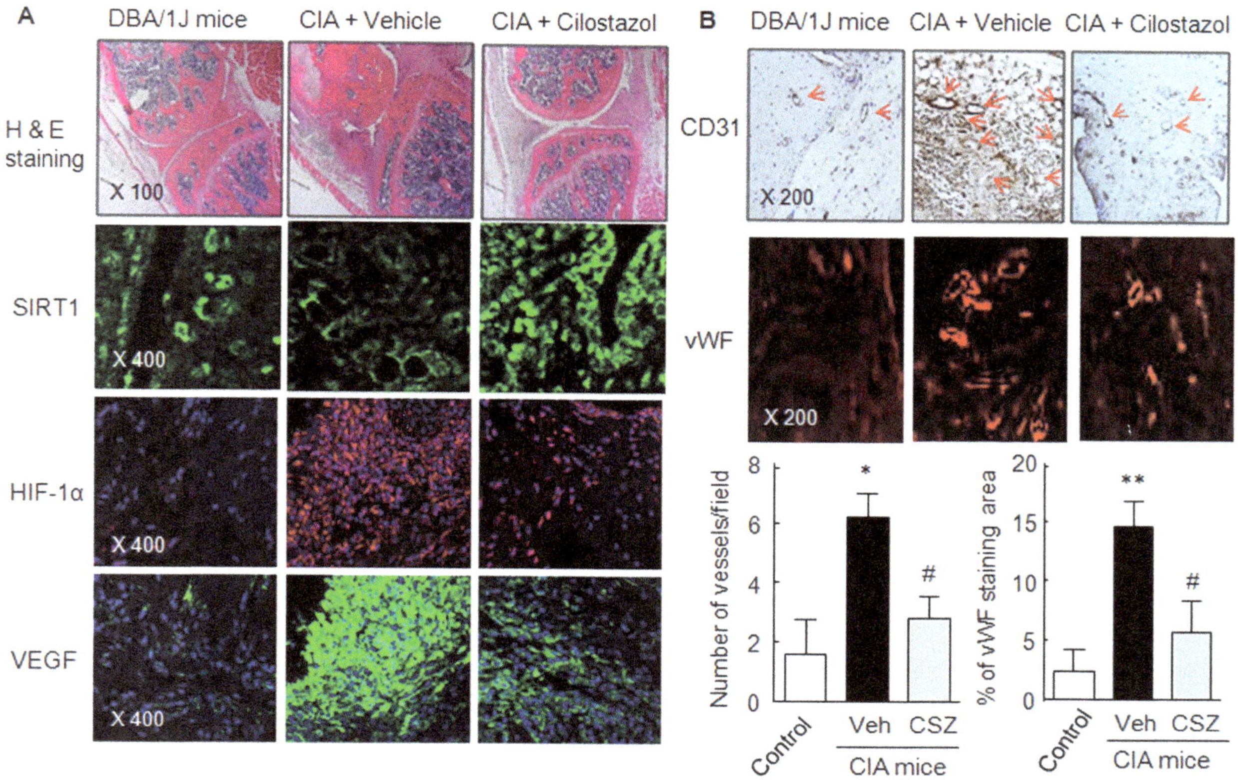

Figure 6. Immunohistochemistry (H & E and CD31) and immunofluorescence (SIRT1, HIF-1α and VEGF) assay. (A) Photographs showing SIRT1(+)-, HIF-1α (+)- and VEGF (+)-spots in joint sections of vehicle control and cilostazol (CSZ)-treated CIA mice. (B) Tibiotarsal joint tissue sections were stained with anti-CD31 antibody, and rabbit anti-human vWF (a marker of endothelial cells). Numbers of blood vessels/field and percentages of vWF stained area were analyzed in joint sections of CIA mice. Results are the means ±SEM of 4 experiments. $^*P<0.05$, $^{**}P<0.01$ vs. control; $^{\#}P<0.05$ vs. vehicle (Veh)-treated CIA mice. The pictures shown are representative of 4 experiments that produced similar results.

mouse, were significantly diminished by cilostazol, which reflects its anti-angiogenic effect.

Summarizing, this study shows cilostazol activates SIRT1, and thus, elicits dual effects in RA SFs, that is, (1) it inhibits NF-κB-mediated transcription, which suggests the suppressions of HIF-1α and VEGF, and (2) it increases HIF-1α deacetylation by enhancing SIRT1 activity, which further blocks VEGF expression and leads to the inhibition of synovial angiogenesis.

Materials and Methods

Animals

All the animals procedures were confirmed in accordance with the Guide for the Care and Use of Laboratory Animals published by the US National Institutes of Health (NIH Publication No. 85-23, revised 1996), and experimental protocols were approved by the Pusan National University Institutional Animal Care and Use Committee. Male DBA/1J mice (aged 8–12 weeks) were purchased from Japan SLC, Inc. (Shizuoka, Japan). All animals were housed in a temperature and humidity controlled animal facility under a 12-h light-dark cycle.

Collagen-induced arthritis (CIA)

CIA was induced in DBA-1 mice as previously described by Park et al. [17]. Briefly, 100 μg of bovine type II collagen (Chondrex, Redmond, WA) dissolved in 0.1 M acetic acid was emulsified with an equal volume of Freund's complete adjuvant (Sigma, St Louis, MO) and administered intradermally at the base of the tails of DBA/1J mice. On day 18 after the first injection, a booster emulsion prepared with type II collagen and Freund's incomplete adjuvant (Sigma) was intradermally administered near the primary injection site. Using the same protocol, adjuvant-treated littermates received phosphate-buffered saline (PBS) in place of type II collagen and served as controls. Cilostazol (30 mg/kg/day) was administered from the day after the booster injection. Thirty-five days after implantation, mice were sacrificed by cervical dislocation.

Cell preparations

Synovial fibroblasts. Synovial fluid samples were obtained from the knees of RA patients, who fulfilled the 1987 revised criteria of the American College of Rheumatology (formerly, the American Rheumatism Association), at the time of therapeutic arthrocentesis. All patients who attended a rheumatology clinic provided informed consent, and the ethics committee of Dong-A University Hospital (Busan, Korea) approved the study protocol. Synovial cells were obtained as described by Neidhart et al. [31]. Briefly, synovial fluid samples were centrifuged at 450×g for 30 min, and pellets were resuspended in Dulbecco's modified Eagle's medium (DMEM) containing 10% fetal bovine serum (FBS), and incubated for 24 hr at 37°C. Non-adherent cells were removed by washing, and medium was changed daily for 3 days. Remaining adherent round monocytes and spindle-shaped fibroblast-like cells were cultured for 2 additional weeks in a flask. The

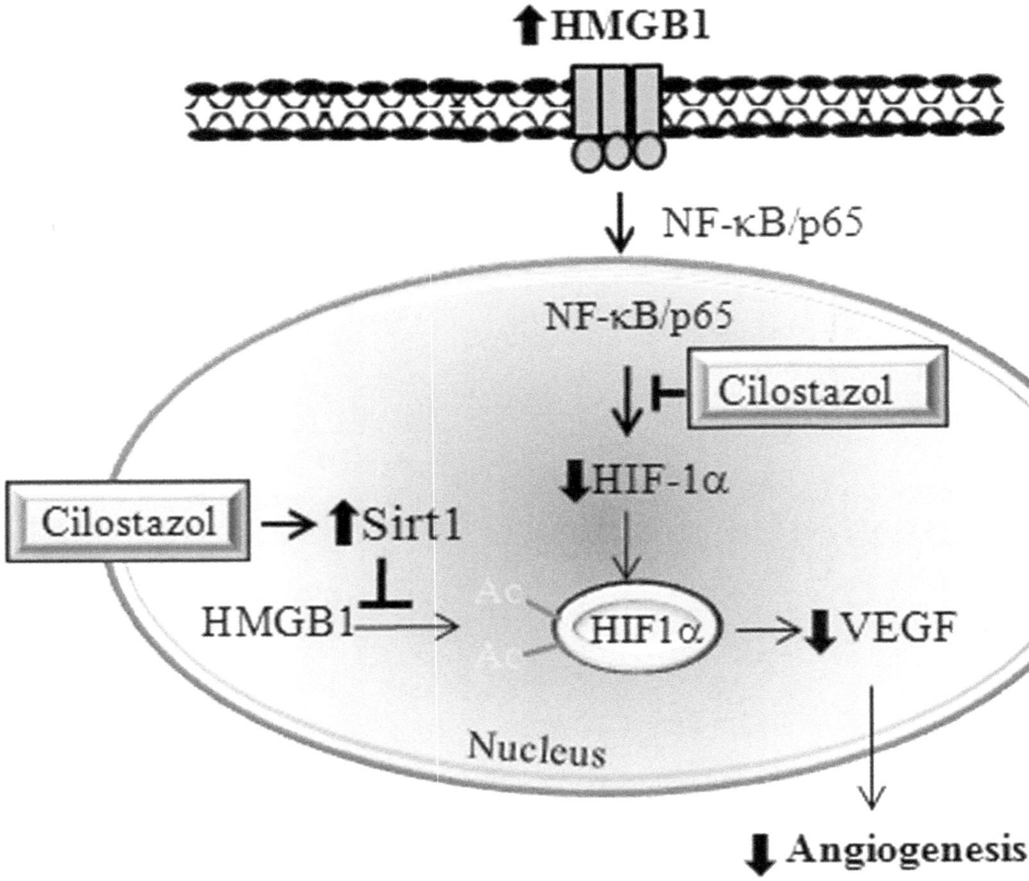

Figure 7. Hypothetical model. Scheme illustrating the dual effects of cilostazol, namely, (1) its inhibition of HMGB1-activated NF-κB nuclear translocation and subsequent HIF-1α expression, and (2) its inactivation of HIF-1α by increasing SIRT1 deacetylase activity in RA SFs. These effects lead to the down-regulation of VEGF and to the inhibition of synovial angiogenesis.

adherent round monocytes that attached to the flask were resistant to trypsinization. In contrast, the spindle-shaped fibroblast-like synovial cells were easily collected by trypsinization. These cells were removed and placed in a new culture flask, and used for experiments at passages 4 to 6.

Endothelial cells. Human microvascular endothelial cells (HMVECs) (Lonza, Waterville, Inc, California) were cultured in endothelial cell basal media-2 (EGM-2) (Bullet kit medium; Clonetics, BioWhittaker, San Diego, CA). HMVECs were grown to confluence at 37°C in 5% CO2 and used for experiments before passage 6.

Reverse transcription–polymerase chain reaction (PCR)

Total RNA was extracted from synovial fibroblast-like cells using TRIzol reagent (Invitrogen, San Diego, CA). The PCR primers used were as follows: for HIF-1α, 5′-AAATCTCC-GTCCCTCAACCT-3′ (sense), 5′-GAAAACTTGGCAACCT-TGGA-3′ (antisense), and VEGF, 5′-ATCTGCATGGTGATG-TTGGA-3′ (sense), 5′-AAGGAGGAGGGCAGAATCAT-3′ (antisense). PCR was conducted using cycles consisting of 95 °C for 1 minute followed by hybridization at 56 °C for 1 minute and an elongation step at 72 °C for 1 minute. Relative mRNA expressions were normalized versus GAPDH mRNA, the levels of which were not altered by treatments. The mRNA expressions of cells treated with vehicle alone were set arbitrarily at 1.

Western blot analysis

Protein (30 μg) samples were loaded onto 10% SDS-polyacrylamide electrophoresis gels and transferred to nitrocellulose membranes (Amersham Biosciences, Inc., Piscataway, NJ). Blocked membranes were then incubated with antibodies for HIF-1α (Cell Signaling Technology, Danvers), NF-κB p65, IκB-α (Santa Cruz Biotechnology, Inc. Santa Cruz), and acetylated histone 4 lysine 16 residue (H4-k16Ac) antibody (Santa Cruz Biotechnology). Immunoreactive bands were visualized using the chemiluminescent reagent in the Supersignal West Dura Extended Duration Substrate Kit (Pierce Chemical, Rockford, IL). Band signals were quantified using a GS-710 calibrated imaging densitometer (Bio-Rad, Hercules, CA). Results are expressed as relative densities.

Tissue preparation and conventional histological analysis

Whole knee joints from mice were dissected and fixed for 1 day in 4% paraformaldehyde, decalcified in 10% EDTA, dehydrated, and embedded in paraffin blocks. Blocks (6-μm thick) were cut and stained with hematoxylin and eosin (H&E) for the assessment of synovial inflammation and bone erosion.

Immunocytochemistry and Immunofluorescence assays

For immunocytochemistry, synovial tissues were fixed with 4% paraformaldehyde, permeabilized with 0.2% Triton X-100, incubated with anti-CD31 antibody for 1 hr, and then with FITC- and Cy3-conjugated secondary antibodies for 30 min. Fluorescent images were obtained using a confocal microscope (OLYMPUS FV-1000, Tokyo, Japan).

In immunofluorescence experiments, preparations were incubated for 1 hr at room temperature with anti-VEGF (Santa Cruz Biotechnology, Inc), anti-HIF-1α (Cell signaling Technology), antibodies against SIRT1 (Covance, Emeryville, CA) and anti-von Willebrand factor (vWF) antibodies. After washing, sections were incubated with a secondary antibody solution for 30 min at room temperature, and mounted using Vectashield mounting medium (Vector Laboratories, Inc.). Fluorescence was detected using a fluorescence microscope (Axiovert 200, Carl Zeiss, Oberkochem, Germany).

Enzyme-linked immunosorbent assay

The levels of IL-6, and MCP-1 in culture supernatants were measured using an ELISA kits (Assay Design Inc., Ann Arbor, MI), according to the manufacturer's instructions.

NF-κB transcription factor assay

To measure levels of NF-κB transcription factor in nuclear extracts, cell lysates were extracted using a nuclear extraction kit (Chemicon International, Temecula, CA). NF-κB p65 DNA binding activities were measured using a colorimetric NF-κB p65 transcription factor assay kit (Rockland Immunochemicals, Gilbertsville, PA), according to the manufacturer's instructions.

Tube formation assay

For obtaining the conditioned medium (CM), RA SF were plated in DMEM containing 1% FBS. The next day, cells were treated with vehicle or HMGB1 (100 ng/ml) for 48 hr. Culture media (CM) were collected and stored at −20°C until required. To perform the tube formation assay, Matrigel Matrix (BD Biosciences, Sanjose, CA) was polymerized for 30 min at 37°C in 48 well plates. HMVECs were then removed from culture by trypsinization and suspended in basal medium (EBM containing 1% FBS). They were then plated onto Matrigel layers, and placed in HMGB1-containing medium or CM (diluted 1:5 in assay medium) at 37°C, and 7~9 hr later cultures were photographed (×100).

Drugs

Cilostazol (OPC-13013) [6-[4-(1-cyclohexyl-1H-tetrazol-5-yl)-butoxy]-3,4-dihydro-2-(1H)-quinolinone] was donated by Otsuka Pharmaceutical Co. Ltd. (Tokushima, Japan), and was dissolved in dimethyl sulfoxide to produce a 10 mM stock solution. Recombinant Human HMGB1 was obtained from R&D Systems (Minneapolis, MN), and chetomin from Enzo Life Sciences (Plymouth Meeting, PA; purity >98% by HPLC analysis). BAY11-7082 [(*E*)3-[(4-methylphenyl)-sulfonyl]-2-propenenitrile], KT5720, resveratrol, and glycyrrhizin (a glycoconjugated triterpene produced by Glycyrrhiza glabra (licorice) from Sigma (St. Louis, MO). YC-1 [3-(5′-hydroxymethyl-2′-furyl)-1-benzylindazole] was from Cayman Chemical (Ann Arbor, MI] and dissolved in 1% DMSO. CD31 polyclonal antibody (1:2,000 dilution; Abcam, Cambridge, UK) and monoclonal anti-vWF antibodies (1:300 dilution; Dako, Glostrup, Denmark) were used to evaluate blood vessel numbers.

Statistical analysis

Results are expressed as means ±SEM. The significances of results were analyzed by one-way analysis of variance (ANOVA) followed by Tukey's multiple comparison test. The Student's *t*-test was used to determine the significances of differences between treated and untreated groups. Statistical significance was accepted for P values <0.05.

Acknowledgments

We are most grateful to Dr. Dai Hyon Yu (Otsuka Pharmaceutical Co., Ltd., Otsuka International Asia Arab Division, Rep of Korea) for his kind donation of cilostazol.

Author Contributions

Conceived and designed the experiments: HYK SYP CDK. Performed the experiments: HYK SYP CDK SWL HRL. Analyzed the data: WSL BYR KWH. Contributed reagents/materials/analysis tools: WSL BYR KWH. Contributed to the writing of the manuscript: KWH.

References

1. Distler JH, Wenger RH, Gassmann M, Kurowska M, Hirth A, et al. (2004) Physiologic responses to hypoxia and implications for hypoxia-inducible factors in the pathogenesis of rheumatoid arthritis. Arthritis Rheum 50: 10–23.
2. Muz B, Khan MN, Kiriakidis S, Paleolog EM (2009) Hypoxia. The role of hypoxia and HIF-dependent signalling events in rheumatoid arthritis. Arthritis Res Ther 11: 201–209.
3. Semenza GL (2007) Vasculogenesis, angiogenesis, and arteriogenesis: mechanisms of blood vessel formation and remodeling. J Cell Biochem 102: 840–847.
4. Thornton RD, Lane P, Borghaei RC, Pease EA, Caro J, et al. (2000) Interleukin 1 induces hypoxia-inducible factor 1 in human gingival and synovial fibroblasts. Biochem J 350: 307–312.
5. Westra J, Brouwer E, Bos R, Posthumus MD, Doornbos-van der Meer B, et al. (2007) Regulation of cytokine-induced HIF-1alpha expression in rheumatoid synovial fibroblasts. Ann N Y Acad Sci 1108: 340–348.
6. Andersson U, Erlandsson-Harris H (2004) HMGB1 is a potent trigger of arthritis. J Intern Med 255: 344–350.
7. Scaffidi P, Misteli T, Bianchi ME (2002) Release of chromatin protein HMGB1 by necrotic cells triggers inflammation. Nature 418: 191–195.
8. Wang H, Bloom O, Zhang M, Vishnubhakat JM, Ombrellino M, et al. (1999) HMG-1 as a late mediator of endotoxin lethality in mice. Science 285: 248–251.
9. Taniguchi N, Kawahara K, Yone K, Hashiguchi T, Yamakuchi M, et al. (2003) High mobility group box chromosomal protein 1 plays a role in the pathogenesis of rheumatoid arthritis as a novel cytokine. Arthritis Rheum 48: 971–981.
10. Hamada T, Torikai M, Kuwazuru A, Tanaka M, Horai N, et al. (2008) Extracellular high mobility group box chromosomal protein 1 is a coupling factor for hypoxia and inflammation in arthritis. Arthritis Rheum 58: 2675–2685.
11. van Beijnum JR, Buurman WA, Griffioen AW (2008) Convergence and amplification of toll-like receptor (TLR) and receptor for advanced glycation end products (RAGE) signaling pathways via high mobility group B1 (HMGB1). Angiogenesis 11: 91–99.
12. Forsythe JA, Jiang BH, Iyer NV, Agani F, Leung SW, et al. (1996) Activation of vascular endothelial growth factor gene transcription by HIF-1. Mol Cell Biol 16: 4604–4613.
13. Carmeliet P, Dor Y, Herbert JM, Fukumura D, Brusselmans K, et al. (1998) Role of HIF-1alpha in hypoxia-mediated apoptosis, cell proliferation and tumour angiogenesis. Nature 394: 485–490.
14. Shin HK, Kim YK, Kim KY, Lee JH, Hong KW (2004) Remnant lipoprotein particles induce apoptosis in endothelial cells by NAD(P)H oxidase-mediated production of superoxide and cytokines via lectin-like oxidized low-density lipoprotein receptor-1 activation: prevention by cilostazol. Circulation 109: 1022–1028.
15. Park SY, Lee JH, Kim YK, Kim CD, Rhim BY, et al. (2005) Cilostazol prevents remnant lipoprotein particle-induced monocyte adhesion to endothelial cells by suppression of adhesion molecules and monocyte chemoattractant protein-1 expression via lectin-like receptor for oxidized low-density lipoprotein receptor activation. J Pharmacol Exp Ther 312: 1241–1248.
16. Park SY, Lee JH, Kim CD, Lee WS, Park WS, et al. (2006) Cilostazol suppresses superoxide production and expression of adhesion molecules in human endothelial cells via mediation of cAMP-dependent protein kinase-mediated maxi-K channel activation. J Pharmacol Exp Ther 317: 1238–1245.
17. Park SY, Lee SW, Shin HK, Chung WT, Lee WS, et al. Cilostazol enhances apoptosis of synovial cells from rheumatoid arthritis patients with inhibition of cytokine formation via Nrf2-linked heme oxygenase 1 induction. Arthritis Rheum 62: 732–741.

18. Lim JH, Lee YM, Chun YS, Chen J, Kim JE, et al. (2010) Sirtuin 1 modulates cellular responses to hypoxia by deacetylating hypoxia-inducible factor 1alpha. Mol Cell 38: 864–878.
19. Chun YS, Yeo EJ, Choi E, Teng CM, Bae JM, et al. (2001) Inhibitory effect of YC-1 on the hypoxic induction of erythropoietin and vascular endothelial growth factor in Hep3B cells. Biochem Pharmacol 61: 947–954.
20. Kung AL, Zabludoff SD, France DS, Freedman SJ, Tanner EA, et al. (2004) Small molecule blockade of transcriptional coactivation of the hypoxia-inducible factor pathway. Cancer Cell 6: 33–43.
21. Pierce JW, Schoenleber R, Jesmok G, Best J, Moore SA, et al. (1997) Novel inhibitors of cytokine-induced IκBα phosphorylation and endothelial cell adhesion molecule expression show anti-inflammatory effects in vivo. J Biol Chem 272: 21096–21103.
22. van Uden P, Kenneth NS, Rocha S (2008) Regulation of hypoxia-inducible factor-1α by NF-κB. Biochem J 412: 477–484.
23. Mollica L, De Marchis F, Spitaleri A, Dallacosta C, Pennacchini D, et al. (2007) Glycyrrhizin binds to high-mobility group box 1 protein and inhibits its cytokine activities. Chem Biol 14: 431–441.
24. Kokkola R, Li J, Sundberg E, Aveberger AC, Palmblad K, et al. (2003) Successful treatment of collagen-induced arthritis in mice and rats by targeting extracellular high mobility group box chromosomal protein 1 activity. Arthritis Rheum 48: 2052–2058.
25. Del Rey MJ, Izquierdo E, Usategui A, Gonzalo E, Blanco FJ, et al. (2010) The transcriptional response of normal and rheumatoid arthritis synovial fibroblasts to hypoxia. Arthritis Rheum 62: 3584–3594.
26. Wang GL, Jiang BH, Rue EA, Semenza GL (1995) Hypoxia-inducible factor 1 is a basic-helix-loop-helix-PAS heterodimer regulated by cellular O_2 tension. Proc Natl Acad Sci USA 92: 5510–5514.
27. Torii S, Okamura N, Suzuki Y, Ishizawa T, Yasumoto K, et al. (2009) Cyclic AMP represses the hypoxic induction of hypoxia-inducible factors in PC12 cells. J Biochem 146: 839–844.
28. Koch AE, Harlow LA, Haines GK, Amento EP, Unemori EN, et al. (1994) Vascular endothelial growth factor. A cytokine modulating endothelial function in rheumatoid arthritis. J Immunol 152: 4149–4156.
29. Paleolog EM, Young S, Stark AC, McCloskey RV, Feldmann M, et al. (1998) Modulation of angiogenic vascular endothelial growth factor by tumor necrosis factor alpha and interleukin-1 in rheumatoid arthritis. Arthritis Rheum 41: 1258–1265.
30. Rius J, Guma M, Schachtrup C, Akassoglou K, Zinkernagel AS, et al. (2008) NF-kappaB links innate immunity to the hypoxic response through transcriptional regulation of HIF-1alpha. Nature 453: 807–811.
31. Neidhart M, Seemayer CA, Hummel KM, Michel BA, Gay RE, et al. (2003) Functional characterization of adherent synovial fluid cells in rheumatoid arthritis: destructive potential in vitro and in vivo. Arthritis Rheum 48: 1873–1880.

iNitro-Tyr: Prediction of Nitrotyrosine Sites in Proteins with General Pseudo Amino Acid Composition

Yan Xu[1]*, Xin Wen[1], Li-Shu Wen[2], Ling-Yun Wu[3], Nai-Yang Deng[4], Kuo-Chen Chou[5,6]

1 Department of Information and Computer Science, University of Science and Technology Beijing, Beijing, China, **2** College of Sciences, Liaoning Shiyou University, FuShun, China, **3** Institute of Applied Mathematics, Academy of Mathematics and Systems Science, Chinese Academy of Sciences, Beijing, China, **4** College of Science, China Agricultural University, Beijing, China, **5** Center of Excellence in Genomic Medicine Research (CEGMR), King Abdulaziz University, Jeddah, Saudi Arabia, **6** Gordon Life Science Institute, Boston, Massachusetts, United States of America

Abstract

Nitrotyrosine is one of the post-translational modifications (PTMs) in proteins that occurs when their tyrosine residue is nitrated. Compared with healthy people, a remarkably increased level of nitrotyrosine is detected in those suffering from rheumatoid arthritis, septic shock, and coeliac disease. Given an uncharacterized protein sequence that contains many tyrosine residues, which one of them can be nitrated and which one cannot? This is a challenging problem, not only directly related to in-depth understanding the PTM's mechanism but also to the nitrotyrosine-based drug development. Particularly, with the avalanche of protein sequences generated in the postgenomic age, it is highly desired to develop a high throughput tool in this regard. Here, a new predictor called "iNitro-Tyr" was developed by incorporating the position-specific dipeptide propensity into the general pseudo amino acid composition for discriminating the nitrotyrosine sites from non-nitrotyrosine sites in proteins. It was demonstrated via the rigorous jackknife tests that the new predictor not only can yield higher success rate but also is much more stable and less noisy. A web-server for iNitro-Tyr is accessible to the public at http://app.aporc.org/iNitro-Tyr/. For the convenience of most experimental scientists, we have further provided a protocol of step-by-step guide, by which users can easily get their desired results without the need to follow the complicated mathematics that were presented in this paper just for the integrity of its development process. It has not escaped our notice that the approach presented here can be also used to deal with the other PTM sites in proteins.

Editor: Reiner Albert Veitia, Institut Jacques Monod, France

Funding: This work is supported by the National Natural Science Foundation of China (No. 11301024, No. 11371365, No. 11101029, No. 31201002, No. 11071013). The funders had no role in study design, data collection and analysis, decision to publish, or preparation of the manuscript.

Competing Interests: The authors have declared that no competing interests exist.

* Email: xuyan@ustb.edu.cn

Introduction

As one of the post-translational modifications (PTMs) of proteins, nitrotyrosine is a product of tyrosine nitration mediated by reactive nitrogen species such as peroxynitrite anion and nitrogen dioxide (**Fig. 1**). Compared with the fluids from healthy people, a remarkably increased level of nitrotyrosine is detected in those suffering from rheumatoid arthritis, septic shock, and coeliac disease. Accordingly, knowledge of nitrotyrosine sites in proteins is very useful for both basic research and drug development. Although conventional experimental methods did provide useful insight into the biological roles of tyrosine nitration [1–3], it is time-consuming and expensive to determine the nitrotyrosine sites based on the experimental approach alone. Particularly, identification of endogenous 3-NTyr modifications remains largely elusive (see, e.g., [4–7]). With the avalanche of protein sequences generated in the postgenomic age, it is highly desired to develop computational methods for identifying the nitrotyrosine sites in proteins. The present study was initiated in an attempt to propose a new method for identifying the nitrotyrosine sites in proteins in hope that it can play a complementary role with the existing methods in this area.

As summarized in [8] and demonstrated in a series of recent publications [9–21], to establish a really useful statistical predictor for a biological system, we need to consider the following procedures: (i) construct or select a valid benchmark dataset to train and test the predictor; (ii) formulate the biological samples with an effective mathematical expression that can truly capture their essence and intrinsic correlation with the target to be predicted; (iii) introduce or develop a powerful algorithm (or engine) to operate the prediction; (iv) properly perform cross-validation tests to objectively evaluate the anticipated accuracy; (v) establish a user-friendly web-server that is accessible to the public. Below, let us describe how to deal with these steps one by one.

Materials and Methods

1. Benchmark Dataset

To develop a statistical predictor, it is fundamentally important to establish a reliable and stringent benchmark dataset to train and test the predictor. If the benchmark dataset contains some errors, the predictor trained by it must be unreliable and the accuracy tested by it would be completely meaningless.

For facilitating description later, let us adopt the Chou's peptide formulation here that was used for studying HIV protease cleavage sites [22,23], specificity of GalNAc-transferase [24], and signal peptide cleavage sites [25]. According to Chou's scheme, a potential nitrotyrosine peptide, i.e., a peptide with Tyr (namely Y) located at its center (**Fig. 2**), can be expressed as

$$\mathbf{P}_\xi(\mathbb{Y}) = \mathrm{R}_{-\xi}\mathrm{R}_{-(\xi-1)}\cdots\mathrm{R}_{-2}\mathrm{R}_{-1}\mathbb{Y}\mathrm{R}_{+1}\mathrm{R}_{+2}\cdots\mathrm{R}_{+(\xi-1)}\mathrm{R}_{+\xi} \quad (1)$$

where the subscript ξ is an integer, $\mathrm{R}_{-\xi}$ represents the ξ−th upstream amino acid residue from the center, R_ξ the ξ−th downstream amino acid residue, and so forth. A $(2\xi+1)$−tuple peptide $\mathbf{P}_\xi(\mathbb{Y})$ can be further classified into the following categories:

$$\mathbf{P}_\xi(\mathbb{Y}) \in \begin{cases} \mathbf{P}_\xi^+(\mathbb{Y}), & \text{if its center is a nitrotyrosine site} \\ \mathbf{P}_\xi^-(\mathbb{Y}), & \text{otherwise} \end{cases} \quad (2)$$

where $\mathbf{P}_\xi^+(\mathbb{Y})$ represents a true nitrotyrosine peptide, $\mathbf{P}_\xi^-(\mathbb{Y})$ a false nitrotyrosine peptide, and $\in$ represents "a member of" in the set theory.

As pointed out by a comprehensive review [26], there is no need to separate a benchmark dataset into a training dataset and a testing dataset for examining the performance of a prediction method if it is tested by the jackknife test or subsampling (K-fold) cross-validation test. Thus, the benchmark dataset for the current study can be formulated as

$$\mathbb{S}_\xi = \mathbb{S}_\xi^+ \bigcup \mathbb{S}_\xi^- \quad (3)$$

where $\mathbb{S}_\xi^+$ only contains the samples of $\mathbf{P}_\xi^+(\mathbb{Y})$, i.e., the nitrotyrosine peptides; $\mathbb{S}_\xi^-$ only contains the samples of $\mathbf{P}_\xi^-(\mathbb{Y})$, i.e., the non-nitrotyrosine peptide (cf. **Eq. 2**); and $\bigcup$ represents the symbol for "union" in the set theory.

Since the length of the peptide $\mathbf{P}_\xi(\mathbb{Y})$ is $2\xi+1$(**Eq. 1**), the benchmark dataset with different values of ξ will contain peptides of different numbers of amino acid residues, as formulated by

$$\mathbb{S}_\xi \text{ contains the peptides of } \begin{cases} 13 \text{ residues}, & \text{when } \xi = 6 \\ 15 \text{ residues}, & \text{when } \xi = 7 \\ 17 \text{ residues}, & \text{when } \xi = 8 \\ 19 \text{ residues}, & \text{when } \xi = 9 \\ 21 \text{ residues}, & \text{when } \xi = 10 \\ \vdots & \vdots \end{cases} \quad (4)$$

The detailed procedures to construct $\mathbb{S}_\xi$ are as follows. (i) Its elements were derived based on the same 546 source proteins used in [27] that contain 1,044 nitrotyrosine sites (see columns 1 and 2 of Supporting Information S1). (ii) Slide a flexible window of $2\xi+1$ amino acids (**Fig. 3**) along each of the 546 protein sequences taken from the Uni-Prot database (version 2014_01). (iii) Collect only those peptide segments with Y (tyrosine) at the center. (iv) If the upstream or downstream in a protein was less than ξ, the lacking residue was filled with a dummy residue "X" [28]. (v) Those peptide samples thus obtained were put into the positive subset $\mathbb{S}_\xi^+$ if their centers have been experimentally confirmed as the nitrotyrosine sites; otherwise, into the negative subset $\mathbb{S}_\xi^-$.

By following the aforementioned procedures, five such benchmark datasets ($\mathbb{S}_{\xi=6}, \mathbb{S}_{\xi=7}, \mathbb{S}_{\xi=8}, \mathbb{S}_{\xi=9}$, and $\mathbb{S}_{\xi=10}$) had been constructed. Each of these datasets contained 1,044 nitrotyrosine peptides and 7,669 non-nitrotyrosine peptides. Note that the sample numbers thus obtained have some minor difference with those in [27]. This is because some proteins originally used in [27] have been removed or replaced in the updated version of the Uni-Prot database.

However, it was observed via preliminary trials that when $\xi=9$, i.e., the peptide samples concerned were formed by 19 residues, the corresponding results were most promising (see **Fig. 4** and **Fig. 5**). Accordingly, we choose $\mathbb{S}_{\xi=9}$ as the benchmark dataset for further investigation. Thus, **Eq. 3** can be reduced to

$$\mathbb{S} = \mathbb{S}^+ \bigcup \mathbb{S}^- \quad (5)$$

where $\mathbb{S} = \mathbb{S}_9$, $\mathbb{S}^+ = \mathbb{S}_9^+$ containing 1,044 nitrotyrosine peptide samples, and $\mathbb{S}^- = \mathbb{S}_9^-$ containing 7,669 non-nitrotyrosine peptide samples. The detailed 19-tuple peptide sequences and their positions in proteins are given in Supporting Information S1.

2. Feature Vector and Pseudo Amino Acid Composition

One of the most important but also most difficult problems in computational biology today is how to effectively formulate a biological sequence with a discrete model or a vector, yet still keep considerable sequence order information. This is because all the existing operation engines, such as correlation angle approach [29], covariance discriminant [30], neural network [31], support vector machine (SVM) [32], random forest [33], conditional random field [28], K-nearest neighbor (KNN) [34], OET-KNN [35], Fuzzy K-nearest neighbor [36], ML-KNN algorithm [37],

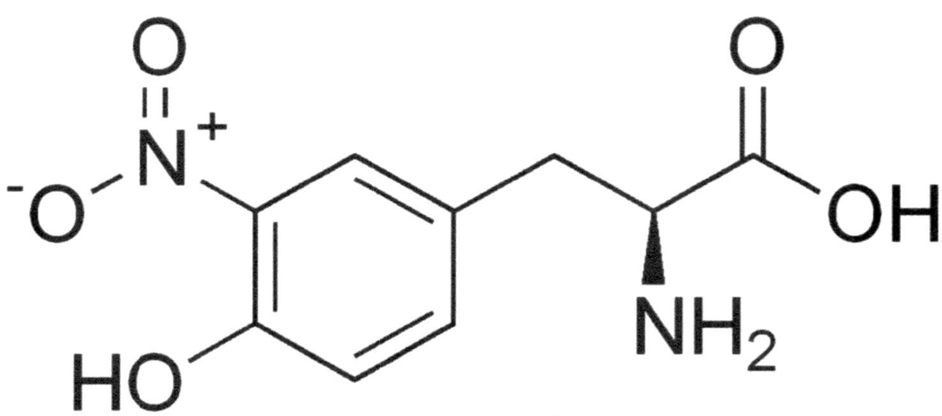

Figure 1. A schematic drawing to show protein nitrotyrosine.

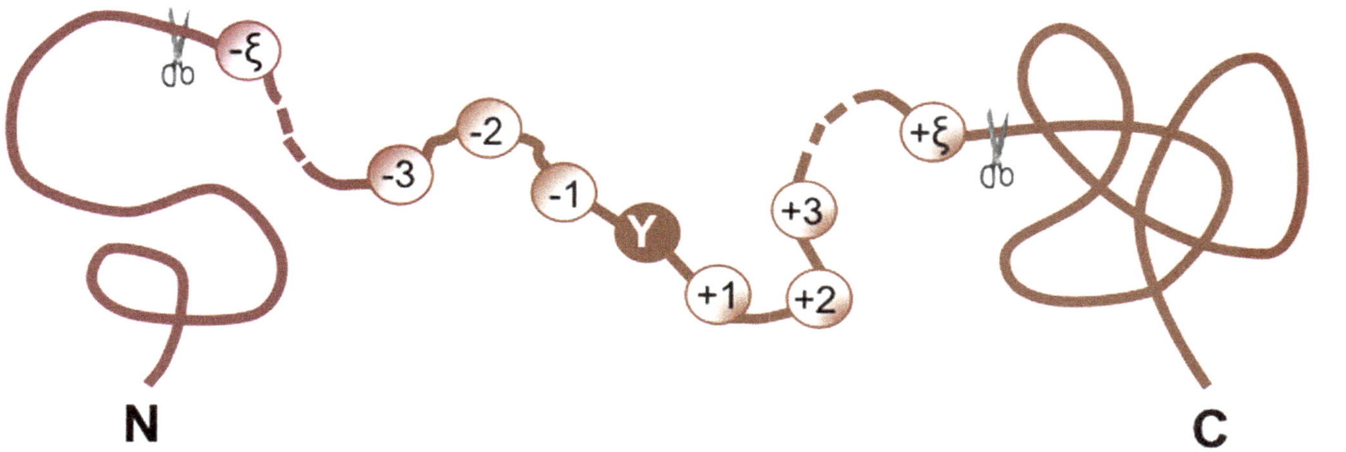

Figure 2. An illustration to show Chou's scheme for a peptide of $(2\xi+1)$ residues with tyrosine (Y) at the center. Adapted from Chou [55,76] with permission.

and SLLE algorithm [30], can only handle vector but not sequence samples. However, a vector defined in a discrete model may totally miss the sequence-order information. To deal with such a dilemma, the approach of pseudo amino acid composition [38] or Chou's PseAAC [39] was proposed. Ever since it was introduced in 2001 [38], the concept of PseAAC has been rapidly penetrated into almost all the areas of computational proteomics, such as in identifying bacterial virulent proteins [40], predicting anticancer peptides [41], predicting protein subcellular location [42], predicting membrane protein types [43], analyzing genetic sequence [44], predicting GABA(A) receptor proteins [45], identifying antibacterial peptides [46], predicting anticancer peptides [41], identifying allergenic proteins [47], predicting metalloproteinase family [48], identifying GPCRs and their types [49], identifying protein quaternary structural attributes [50], among many others (see a long list of references cited in a 2014 article [51]). Recently, the concept of PseAAC was further extended to represent the feature vectors of DNA and nucleotides [9], as well as other biological samples (see, e.g., [52]). Because it has been widely and increasingly used, recently three types of powerful open access soft-ware, called 'PseAAC-Builder' [53], 'propy' [54], and 'PseAAC-General' [51], were established: the former two are for generating various modes of Chou's special PseAAC; while the 3rd one for those of Chou's general PseAAC.

According to a comprehensive review [8], PseAAC can be generally formulated as

$$\mathbf{P}=[\psi_1 \quad \psi_2 \quad \cdots \quad \psi_u \quad \cdots \quad \psi_\Omega]^{\mathbf{T}} \tag{6}$$

where $\mathbf{T}$ is the transpose operator, while Ω an integer to reflect the vector's dimension. The value of Ω as well as the components $\psi_u(u=1,2,\cdots,\Omega)$ in **Eq. 6** will depend on how to extract the desired information from a protein/peptide sequence. Below, let us describe how to extract the useful information from the benchmark datasets to define the peptide samples via **Eq. 6**.

For convenience in formulation, let rewrite **Eq. 1** as follows

$$\mathbf{P}_\xi=\mathrm{R}_1\mathrm{R}_2\cdots\mathrm{R}_\xi\mathrm{R}_{\xi+1}\cdots\mathrm{R}_{2\xi}\mathrm{R}_{2\xi+1} \tag{7}$$

where $\mathrm{R}_{\xi+1}$, the residue at the center of the peptide, is tyrosine (Y), and all the other residues $\mathrm{R}_i(i\neq\xi+1)$ can be any of the 20 native amino acids or the dummy code X as defined above. Hereafter, let us use the numerical codes 1, 2, 3, ..., 20 to represent the 20 native amino acids according to the alphabetic order of their single letter codes, and use 21 to represent the dummy amino acid X. Accordingly, the number of possible different dipeptides will be $21\times21=441$, and the number of dipeptide subsite positions on the sequence of **Eq. 7** will be $(2\xi+1-1)=2\xi$.

Now, let us introduce a positive and a negative PSDP (position-specific dipeptide propensity) matrix, as given below

$$\mathbb{Z}^+(\xi)=\begin{bmatrix} z_{1,1}^+ & z_{1,2}^+ & \cdots & z_{1,2\xi}^+ \\ z_{2,1}^+ & z_{2,2}^+ & \cdots & z_{2,2\xi}^+ \\ \vdots & \vdots & \ddots & \vdots \\ z_{441,1}^+ & z_{441,2}^+ & \cdots & z_{441,2\xi}^+ \end{bmatrix} \tag{8a}$$

$$\mathbb{Z}^-(\xi)=\begin{bmatrix} z_{1,1}^- & z_{1,2}^- & \cdots & z_{1,2\xi}^- \\ z_{2,1}^- & z_{2,2}^- & \cdots & z_{2,2\xi}^- \\ \vdots & \vdots & \ddots & \vdots \\ z_{441,1}^- & z_{441,2}^- & \cdots & z_{441,2\xi}^- \end{bmatrix} \tag{8b}$$

where the element

$$\begin{cases} z_{i,j}^+=F^+(\mathrm{D}_i|j) \\ z_{i,j}^-=F^-(\mathrm{D}_i|j) \end{cases} \quad (i=1,2,\cdots,441;j=1,2,\cdots,2\xi) \tag{9}$$

and

$$\mathrm{D}_1=\mathrm{AA},\mathrm{D}_2=\mathrm{AC},\mathrm{D}_3=\mathrm{AD},\cdots,\mathrm{D}_{440}=\mathrm{XY},\mathrm{D}_{441}=\mathrm{XX} \tag{10}$$

In **Eq. 9**, $F^+(\mathrm{D}_i|j)$ is the occurrence frequency of the $i-$th dipeptide $(i=1,2,\cdots,441)$ at the $j-$th subsite on the sequence of **Eq. 7** (or the $j-$th column in the positive subset dataset $\mathbb{S}^+$) that can be easily derived using the method described in [55] from the sequences in the Supporting Information S1; while $F^-(D_i|j)$ is the corresponding occurrence frequency but derived from the negative subset dataset $\mathbb{S}^-$. Thus, for the peptide sequence of **Eq. 7**, its attribute to the positive set $\mathbb{S}^+$ or negative set $\mathbb{S}^-$ can be formulated by a 2ξ-D (dimension) vector $\mathbf{P}^+$ or $\mathbf{P}^-$, as defined by [23]

$$\mathbf{P}_\xi^+ = [\psi_1^+ \quad \psi_2^+ \quad \cdots \quad \psi_u^+ \quad \cdots \quad \psi_{2\xi}^+]^{\mathrm{T}} \tag{11a}$$

$$\mathbf{P}_\xi^- = [\psi_1^- \quad \psi_2^- \quad \cdots \quad \psi_u^- \quad \cdots \quad \psi_{2\xi}^-]^{\mathrm{T}} \tag{11b}$$

where

$$\psi_u^+ = \begin{cases} z_{1,u}^+ & \text{when } \mathrm{R}_u\mathrm{R}_{u+1} = \mathrm{AA} \\ z_{2,u}^+ & \text{when } \mathrm{R}_u\mathrm{R}_{u+1} = \mathrm{AC} \\ \vdots & \vdots \\ z_{21,u}^+ & \text{when } \mathrm{R}_u\mathrm{R}_{u+1} = \mathrm{AX} \\ z_{22,u}^+ & \text{when } \mathrm{R}_u\mathrm{R}_{u+1} = \mathrm{CA} \\ \vdots & \vdots \\ z_{441,u}^+ & \text{when } \mathrm{R}_u\mathrm{R}_{u+1} = \mathrm{XX} \end{cases} \quad [u = 1,2,\cdots,2\xi = \Omega] \tag{12a}$$

$$\psi_u^- = \begin{cases} z_{1,u}^- & \text{when } \mathrm{R}_u\mathrm{R}_{u+1} = \mathrm{AA} \\ z_{2,u}^- & \text{when } \mathrm{R}_u\mathrm{R}_{u+1} = \mathrm{AC} \\ \vdots & \vdots \\ z_{21,u}^- & \text{when } \mathrm{R}_u\mathrm{R}_{u+1} = \mathrm{AX} \\ z_{22,u}^- & \text{when } \mathrm{R}_u\mathrm{R}_{u+1} = \mathrm{CA} \\ \vdots & \vdots \\ z_{441,u}^- & \text{when } \mathrm{R}_u\mathrm{R}_{u+1} = \mathrm{XX} \end{cases} \quad [u = 1,2,\cdots,2\xi = \Omega] \tag{12b}$$

where R_u and R_{u+1} represent the residues in the u−th and $(u+1)$−th positions of the peptide concerned.

3. Discriminant Function Approach

Now in the 2ξ-D space, let us define an ideal nitrotyrosine peptide $\mathbb{I}^+$ [22] and an ideal non-nitrotyrosine peptide $\mathbb{I}^-$ as expressed by

$$\mathbb{I}_\xi^+ = \begin{bmatrix} \lambda_1^+ \\ \lambda_2^+ \\ \vdots \\ \lambda_u^+ \\ \vdots \\ \lambda_{2\xi}^+ \end{bmatrix} \quad \mathbb{I}_\xi^- = \begin{bmatrix} \lambda_1^- \\ \lambda_2^- \\ \vdots \\ \lambda_u^- \\ \vdots \\ \lambda_{2\xi}^- \end{bmatrix} \tag{13}$$

where $\lambda_i^+ (i=1,2,\cdots,2\xi)$ is the upper limit of the corresponding matrix element in **Eq. 12a**, and $\lambda_i^- (i=1,2,\cdots,2\xi)$ is the upper limit of the corresponding matrix element in **Eq. 12b**. Theoretically speaking, each of these hypothetical upper limits in **Eq. 13** should be 1 [23]. Thus, the similarity score of $\mathbf{P}_\xi^+$ with $\mathbb{I}^+$ and that of $\mathbf{P}_\xi^-$ with $\mathbb{I}^-$ can be defined as

$$\begin{cases} \mathbf{P}_\xi^+ \cdot \mathbb{I}_\xi^+ = \sum_{u=1}^{2\xi} \psi_u^+ \\ \mathbf{P}_\xi^- \cdot \mathbb{I}_\xi^- = \sum_{u=1}^{2\xi} \psi_u^- \end{cases} \tag{14}$$

Similar to the treatment in [23], let us define a discriminant function Δ given by

$$\Delta_\xi = \left(\mathbf{P}_\xi^+ \cdot \mathbb{I}_\xi^+ - \mathbf{P}_\xi^- \cdot \mathbb{I}_\xi^-\right) - \Re = \sum_{u=1}^{2\xi} \left(\psi_u^+ - \psi_u^-\right) - \Re \tag{15}$$

where $\Re$ is the adjust parameter used to optimize the overall success rate when the positive and negative benchmark datasets are highly imbalanced in size. Now the peptide $\mathbf{P}_\xi$ of **Eq. 7** can be identified according to the following rule

$$\begin{cases} \mathbf{P}_\xi \text{ belongs to nitrotyrosine peptide,} & \text{if } \Delta_\xi > 0 \\ \mathbf{P}_\xi \text{ belongs to non-nitrotyrosine peptide,} & \text{if } \Delta_\xi \le 0 \end{cases} \tag{16}$$

The predictor obtained via the above procedures is called **iNitro-Tyr**. How to properly and objectively evaluate the anticipated accuracy of a new predictor and how to make it easily accessible and user-friendly are the two key issues that will have important impacts on its application value [56]. Below, let us address these problems.

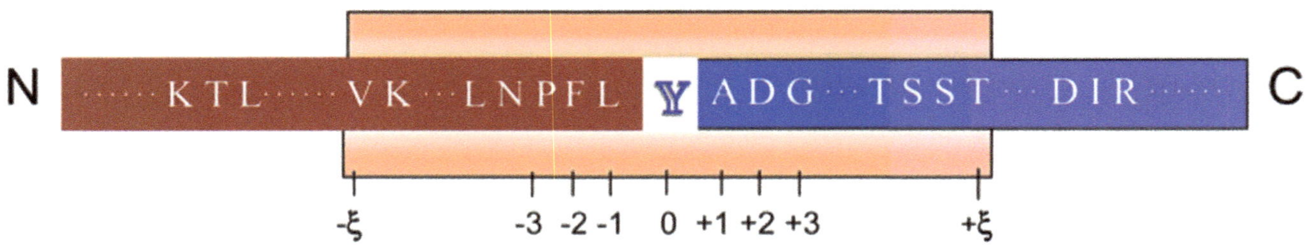

Figure 3. Illustration to show the peptide segment highlighted by sliding the scaled window $[-\xi, +\xi]$ along a protein sequence. During the sliding process, the scales on the window are aligned with different amino acids so as to define different peptide segments. When, and only when, the scale 0 is aligned with Y (tyrosine), is the $(2\xi+1)$−tuble peptide segment seen within the window regarded as a potential nitrotyrosine peptide. Adapted from Chou [55,77] with permission.

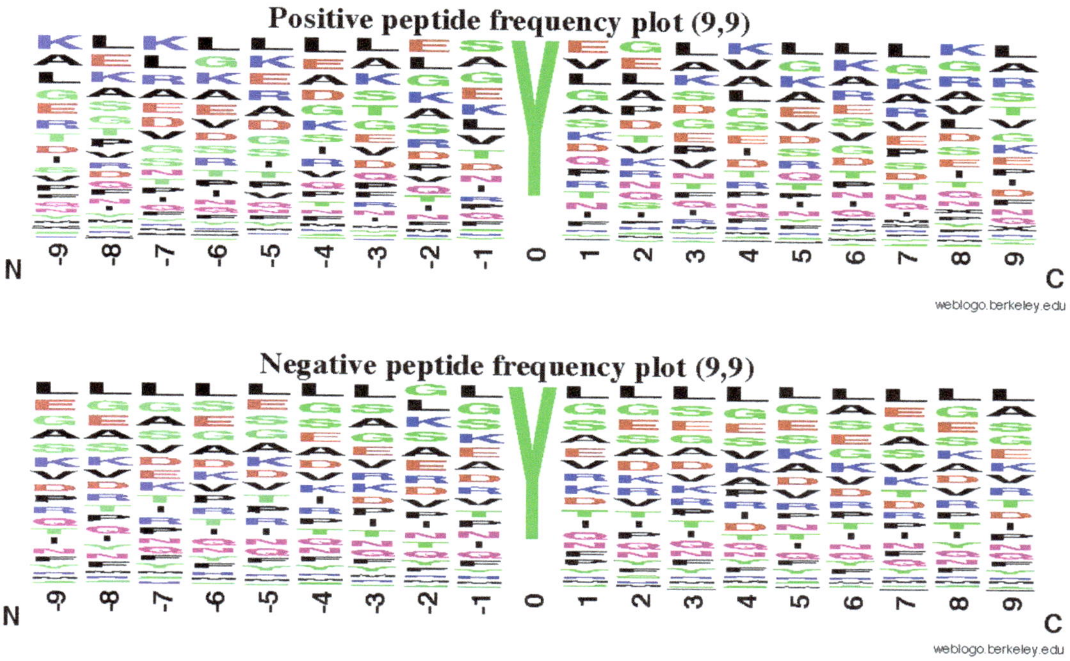

Figure 4. A sequence logo plot to show the difference between the positive and negative peptides. The window's size is 19 when $\xi = 9$. See Eq. 1 and the legend of Fig. 3 for further explanation.

Results and Discussion

1. Metrics for Scoring Prediction Quality

In literature the following four metrics are often used to score the quality of a predictor at four different angles

$$\begin{cases} \mathrm{Sn} = \dfrac{\mathrm{TP}}{\mathrm{TP}+\mathrm{FN}} \\ \mathrm{Sp} = \dfrac{\mathrm{TN}}{\mathrm{TN}+\mathrm{FP}} \\ \mathrm{Acc} = \dfrac{\mathrm{TP}+\mathrm{TN}}{\mathrm{TP}+\mathrm{TN}+\mathrm{FP}+\mathrm{FN}} \\ \mathrm{MCC} = \dfrac{(\mathrm{TP}\times\mathrm{TN})-(\mathrm{FP}\times\mathrm{FN})}{\sqrt{(\mathrm{TP}+\mathrm{FP})(\mathrm{TP}+\mathrm{FN})(\mathrm{TN}+\mathrm{FP})(\mathrm{TN}+\mathrm{FN})}} \end{cases} \tag{17}$$

where TP represents the number of the true positive; TN, the number of the true negative; FP, the number of the false positive; FN, the number of the false negative; Sn, the sensitivity; Sp, the specificity; Acc, the accuracy; MCC, the Mathew's correlation coefficient. To most biologists, unfortunately, the four metrics as formulated in **Eq. 17** are not quite intuitive and easy-to-understand, particularly the equation for MCC. Here let us adopt the formulation proposed recently in [9,11,28] based on the symbols introduced by Chou [25,55] in predicting signal peptides. According to the formulation, the same four metrics can be expressed as

$$\begin{cases} \mathrm{Sn} = 1 - \dfrac{N_-^+}{N^+}, & 0 \le \mathrm{Sn} \le 1 \\ \mathrm{Sp} = 1 - \dfrac{N_+^-}{N^-}, & 0 \le \mathrm{Sp} \le 1 \\ \mathrm{Acc} = 1 - \dfrac{N_-^+ + N_+^-}{N^+ + N^-}, & 0 \le \mathrm{Acc} \le 1 \\ \mathrm{MCC} = \dfrac{1 - \left(\dfrac{N_-^+}{N^+} + \dfrac{N_+^-}{N^-}\right)}{\sqrt{\left(1 + \dfrac{N_+^- - N_-^+}{N^+}\right)\left(1 + \dfrac{N_-^+ - N_+^-}{N^-}\right)}}, & -1 \le \mathrm{MCC} \le 1 \end{cases} \tag{18}$$

where N^+ is the total number of the nitrotyrosine peptides investigated while N_-^+ the number of the nitrotyrosine peptides incorrectly predicted as the non-nitrotyrosine peptides; N^- the total number of the non-nitrotyrosine peptides investigated while N_+^- the number of the non-nitrotyrosine peptides incorrectly predicted as the nitrotyrosine peptides [57].

Now, it is crystal clear from **Eq. 18** that when $N_-^+ = 0$ meaning none of the nitrotyrosine peptides was incorrectly predicted to be a non-nitrotyrosine peptide, we have the sensitivity $\mathrm{Sn} = 1$. When $N_-^+ = N^+$ meaning that all the nitrotyrosine peptides were incorrectly predicted as the non-nitrotyrosine peptides, we have the sensitivity $\mathrm{Sn} = 0$. Likewise, when $N_+^- = 0$ meaning none of the non-nitrotyrosine peptides was incorrectly predicted to be the nitrotyrosine peptide, we have the specificity $\mathrm{Sp} = 1$; whereas $N_+^- = N^-$ meaning all the non-nitrotyrosine peptides were incorrectly predicted as the nitrotyrosine peptides, we have the specificity $\mathrm{Sp} = 0$. When $N_-^+ = N_+^- = 0$ meaning that none of nitrotyrosine peptides in the positive dataset $\mathbb{S}^+$ and none of the non- nitrotyrosine peptides in the negative dataset $\mathbb{S}^-$ was incorrectly predicted, we have the overall accuracy $\mathrm{Acc} = 1$ and $\mathrm{MCC} = 1$; when $N_-^+ = N^+$ and $N_+^- = N^-$ meaning that all the nitrotyrosine peptides in the positive dataset $\mathbb{S}^+$ and all the non- nitrotyrosine peptides in the negative dataset $\mathbb{S}^-$ were incorrectly predicted, we have the overall accuracy $\mathrm{Acc} = 0$ and $\mathrm{MCC} = -1$; whereas when $N_-^+ = N^+/2$ and $N_+^- = N^-/2$ we have $\mathrm{Acc} = 0.5$ and $\mathrm{MCC} = 0$ meaning no better than random prediction. As we can see from the above discussion based on **Eq. 18**, the meanings of sensitivity, specificity, overall accuracy, and Mathew's correlation coefficient have become much more intuitive and easier-to-understand.

It is instructive to point out, however, the set of metrics in **Eqs. 17–18** is valid only for the single-label systems. For the multi-label systems, such as those for the subcellular localization of multiplex proteins (see, e.g., [58–62]) where a protein may have two or more

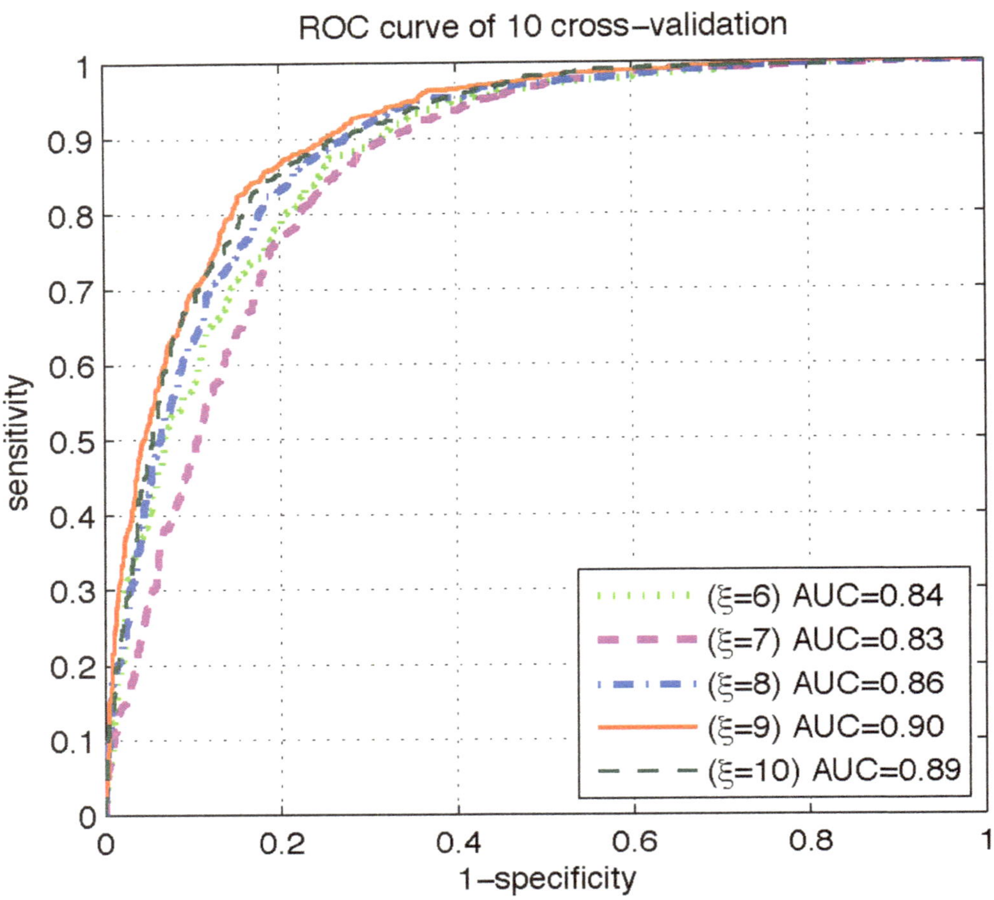

Figure 5. A plot to show the different ROC curves obtained by the 10-fold cross-validation under different ξ values. As we can see, when $\xi = 9$, the corresponding AUC (i.e., the area under its curve) is the largest, meaning the most promising compared with the other values of ξ.

locations, and those for the functional types of antimicrobial peptides (see, e.g., [63] where a peptide may possess two or more functional types, a completely different set of metrics is needed as elaborated in [37].

2. Jackknife Cross-Validation

With a set of clear and valid metrics as defined in **Eq. 18** to measure the quality of a predictor, the next thing we need to consider is how to objectively derive the values of these metrics for a predictor.

In statistical prediction, the following three cross-validation methods are often used to calculate the metrics of **Eq. 18** for evaluating the quality of a predictor: independent dataset test, subsampling test, and jackknife test [64]. However, of the three test methods, the jackknife test is deemed the least arbitrary that can always yield an unique result for a given benchmark dataset [65]. The reasons are as follows. (i) For the independent dataset test, although all the samples used to test the predictor are outside the training dataset used to train it so as to exclude the "memory" effect or bias, the way of how to select the independent samples to test the predictor could be quite arbitrary unless the number of independent samples is sufficiently large. This kind of arbitrariness might result in completely different conclusions. For instance, a predictor achieving a higher success rate than the other predictor for a given independent testing dataset might fail to keep so when tested by another independent testing dataset [64]. (ii) For the subsampling test, the concrete procedure usually used in literatures is the 5-fold, 7-fold or 10-fold cross-validation. The problem with this kind of subsampling test is that the number of possible selections in dividing a benchmark dataset is an astronomical figure even for a very simple dataset, as demonstrated by Eqs.28–30 in [8]. Therefore, in any actual subsampling cross-validation tests, only an extremely small fraction of the possible selections are taken into account. Since different selections will always lead to different results even for a same benchmark dataset and a same predictor, the subsampling test cannot avoid the arbitrariness either. A test method unable to yield an unique outcome cannot be deemed as a good one. (iii) In the jackknife test, all the samples in the benchmark dataset will be singled out one-by-one and tested by the predictor trained by the remaining samples. During the process of jackknifing, both the training dataset and testing dataset are actually open, and each sample will be in turn moved between the two. The jackknife test can exclude the "memory" effect. Also, the arbitrariness problem as mentioned above for the independent dataset test and subsampling test can be avoided because the outcome obtained by the jackknife cross-validation is always unique for a given benchmark dataset. Accordingly, the jackknife test has been increasingly used and widely recognized by investigators to examine the quality of various predictors (see, e.g., [33,41,43,45–47,66–72]).

Table 1. Comparison of the new iNitro-Tyr predictor with the existing predictors in identifying the nitrotyrosine sites; the rates listed below were derived by the jackknife cross-validation on the 546 source proteins used in [27].

Predictor	Threshold	Acc (%)	MCC	Sn (%)	Sp (%)
GPS-YNO2[a]	High	82.57	0.1884	28.89	90.02
	Medium	79.60	0.2171	40.53	85.02
	Low	76.51	0.2335	50.09	90.18
iNitro-Tyr[b]		84.52	0.4905	81.76	85.89

[a]As reported in [27], where $\xi=7$, i.e., the length of the potential nitrotyrosine peptides considered is $(2\xi+1)=15$.
[b]See Eqs. 15–16, where $\Re=0.70$ and $\xi=9$, i.e., the length of the potential nitrotyrosine peptides considered is $(2\xi+1)=19$.

Accordingly, in this study we also used the jackknife cross-validation method to calculate the metrics in **Eq. 18** although it would take more computational time.

3. Comparison with Other Methods

The jackknife test results by iNitro-Tyr on the benchmark dataset $\mathbb{S}=\mathbb{S}^{+}\bigcup\mathbb{S}^{-}$ (cf. Supporting Information S1) for the four metrics defined in **Eq. 18** are listed in **Table 1**, where for facilitating comparison, the corresponding results by GPS-YNO2 [27] with different thresholds are also given.

From the table, we can see the following facts. (i) The overall accuracy by the current iNitro-Tyr predictor is Acc = 84.52%, which is higher than the overall accuracy by GPS-YNO2 regardless what threshold is used for the latter. (ii) The Mathew's correlation coefficient obtained by iNitro-Tyr is MCC = 0.4905, which is significantly higher than that by GPS-YNO2, indicating that the new predictor is more stable and less noisy. (iii) The sensitivity and specificity obtained by iNitro-Tyr are Sn = 81.76% and Sp = 85.89%, which are much more evenly distributed than those by the GPS-YNO2 predictor.

It is instructive to point out that, as shown by **Eqs. 12a** and **b**, the amino acid pairwise coupling effects [11] has been incorporated via the general form of PseAAC [8] to formulate the peptide samples. If, however, we just used the single amino acid specific position occurrence frequency to formulate the peptide samples, the corresponding prediction quality would drop down to Acc = 44.88% and MCC = 0.1656, clearly indicating that consideration of the amino acid pairwise coupling effects could significantly enhance the prediction quality, fully consistent with the reports by previous investigators [73,74], where it was observed that the prediction of protein secondary structural contents had been remarkably improved by taking into account the amino acid pairwise coupling effects.

Accordingly, compared with the best of existing predictors for identifying the nitrotyrosine sites in proteins, the new **iNitro-Tyr** predictor not only can yield higher or comparable accuracy, but is also much more stable and less noisy. It is anticipated that **iNitro-Tyr** may become a useful high throughput tool in this area, or at the very least play a complementary role to the existing predictors.

4. Web-Server and User Guide

For the convenience of most experimental scientists, we have established a web-server for the **iNitro-Tyr** predictor, with which users can easily get their desired results according to the steps below without the need to understand the mathematical equations in the method section.

Step 1. Open the web server at http://app.aporc.org/iNitro-Tyr/and you will see the top page of the predictor on your computer screen, as shown in **Fig. 6**. Click on the Read Me button to see a brief introduction about **iNitro-Tyr** predictor and the caveat when using it.

Step 2. Either type or copy/paste the sequences of query proteins into the input box shown at the center of **Fig. 6**. All the input sequences should be in the FASTA format. A sequence in FASTA format consists of a single initial line beginning with the symbol ">" in the first column, followed by lines of sequence data in which amino acids are represented using single-letter codes. Except for the mandatory symbol ">", all the other characters in the single initial line are optional and only used for the purpose of identification and description. The sequence ends if another line starting with the symbol ">" appears; this indicates the start of another sequence. Example sequences in FASTA format can be seen by clicking on the Example button right above the open box. Note that if your input protein sequences should be formed by the 20 native amino acid codes (ACDEFGHIKLMNPQRSTVWY).

Step 3. Click on the Submit button to see the predicted results. For example, if you use the two query protein sequences in the Example window as the input, after clicking the Submit button, you will see the following on your screen. (i) The 1st protein (P05181) contains 18 Y residues; of which only those located at the sequence position 71, 318, 349, 381, and 423 are of nitrotyrosine site, while all the others are of non-nitrotyrosine site. (ii) The 2nd protein (P03023) contains 8 Y residues; of which only those located at the sequence positions 7, 12, 17, and 47 belong to the nitrotyrosine site, while all the others belong to non-nitrotyrosine site. All these results are fully consistent with experimental observations except for one Y residue at the position 349 in the 1st protein (P05181) that is actually non-nitrotyrosine site but was overpredicted as nitrotyrosine site.

Step 4. As shown on the lower panel of **Fig. 6**, you may also submit your query proteins in an input file (with FASTA format) via the "Browse" button. To see the sample of input file, click on the Example button right under the input box.

Step 5. Click on the Data button to download the benchmark dataset used to train and test the iNitro-Tyr predictor.

Conclusions

As one of the important posttranslational modifications (PTMs), nitrotyrosine is a product occurring in proteins when their tyrosine (Tyr or Y) residue is nitrated. Since a remarkably increasing level of nitrotyrosine is detected for those patients who have suffered from rheumatoid arthritis, septic shock, and coeliac disease, knowledge of nitrotyrosine is very useful for developing drugs against these diseases.

A new predictor was developed for identifying the nitrotyrosine sites in proteins based on a set of 19-tuple peptides generated as follows. Sliding a window of 19 amino acids along each of the 546 protein sequences taken from a protein database, collected were

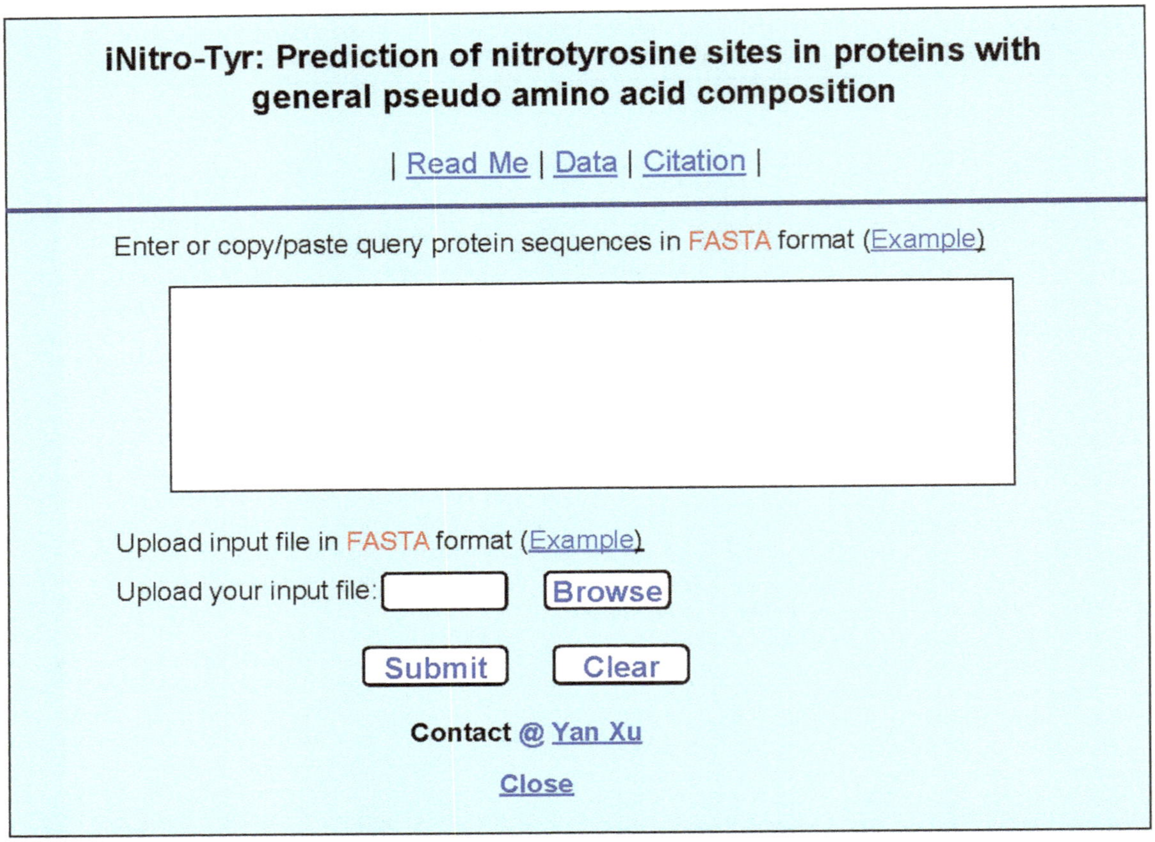

Figure 6. A semi-screenshot to show the top page of the iNitro-Tyr srver. Its website address is at http://app.aporc.org/iNitro-Tyr/.

only those peptide segments with Y (tyrosine) at the center, i.e., the potential nitrotyrosine-site-containing peptides. The benchmark dataset thus obtained contains 1,044 experiment-confirmed nitrotyrosine peptides and 7,669 non-nitrotyrosine peptides.

The new predictor is called iNitro-Tyr, in which each of the potential nitrotyrosine-site-containing peptides was formulated with a 18-D vector formed by incorporating the position-specific dipeptide propensity (PSDP) into the general form [8] of pseudo amino acid composition [38,75] or Chou's PseAAC [39,51,54].

It has been observed by the rigorous cross validations that the iNitro-Tyr not only yields higher success rates but also is more stable and less noisy as reflected by a set of four metrics generally used to measure the quality of a predictor from different angles.

For the convenience of most experimental scientists, the web-server of iNitro-Tyr has been established at http://app.aporc.org/iNitro-Tyr/. Furthermore, to maximize their convenience, a step-by-step guide has been provided, by which users can easily get their desired results without the need to follow the complicated mathematics that were presented in this paper just for the integrity of the predictor.

It has not escaped our notice that the current approach can also be used to develop various effective methods for identifying the sites of other PTM sites in proteins.

Supporting Information

Supporting Information S1 The benchmark dataset used in this study contains 8,713 peptides formed by 19 amino acid residues with Y (tyrosine) at the center. Of these peptides, 1,044 are of nitrotyrosine and 7,669 of non-nitrotyrosine. Listed are also the codes of the source proteins from which these 19-tuple peptide sequences are derived as well as their corresponding sites in proteins. See the main text for further explanation.

Acknowledgments

The authors wish to thank the three anonymous reviewers, whose constructive comments are very helpful for strengthening the presentation of this paper.

Author Contributions

Conceived and designed the experiments: YX. Performed the experiments: YX LSW. Analyzed the data: KCC XW. Contributed reagents/materials/analysis tools: YX XW LSW. Wrote the paper: YX NYD KCC. Collected the data: XW LSW. Revised the manuscript: LYW NYD KCC.

References

1. Casoni F, Basso M, Massignan T, Gianazza E, Cheroni C, et al. (2005) Protein nitration in a mouse model of familial amyotrophic lateral sclerosis: possible multifunctional role in the pathogenesis. J Biol Chem 280: 16295–16304.
2. Ghesquiere B, Colaert N, Helsens K, Dejager L, Vanhaute C, et al. (2009) In vitro and in vivo protein-bound tyrosine nitration characterized by diagonal chromatography. Mol Cell Proteomics 8: 2642–2652.

3. Zhan X, Du Y, Crabb JS, Gu X, Kern TS, et al. (2008) Targets of tyrosine nitration in diabetic rat retina. Mol Cell Proteomics 7: 864–874.
4. Jarmula A, Rode W (2013) Computational study of the effects of protein tyrosine nitrations on the catalytic activity of human thymidylate synthase. J Comput Aided Mol Des 27: 45–66.
5. Abello N, Kerstjens HA, Postma DS, Bischoff R (2009) Protein tyrosine nitration: selectivity, physicochemical and biological consequences, denitration, and proteomics methods for the identification of tyrosine-nitrated proteins. J Proteome Res 8: 3222–3238.
6. Feeney MB, Schoneich C (2013) Proteomic Approaches to Analyze Protein Tyrosine Nitration. Antioxid Redox Signal.
7. Dekker F, Abello N, Wisastra R, Bischoff R (2012) Enrichment and detection of tyrosine-nitrated proteins. Curr Protoc Protein Sci Chapter 14: Unit 14 13.
8. Chou KC (2011) Some remarks on protein attribute prediction and pseudo amino acid composition (50th Anniversary Year Review). Journal of Theoretical Biology 273: 236–247.
9. Chen W, Feng PM, Lin H (2013) iRSpot-PseDNC: identify recombination spots with pseudo dinucleotide composition Nucleic Acids Research 41: e69.
10. Min JL, Xiao X (2013) iEzy-Drug: A web server for identifying the interaction between enzymes and drugs in cellular networking. BioMed Research International 2013: 701317.
11. Xu Y, Shao XJ, Wu LY, Deng NY (2013) iSNO-AAPair: incorporating amino acid pairwise coupling into PseAAC for predicting cysteine S-nitrosylation sites in proteins. PeerJ 1: e171.
12. Xiao X, Min JL, Wang P (2013) iCDI-PseFpt: Identify the channel-drug interaction in cellular networking with PseAAC and molecular fingerprints. Journal of Theoretical Biology 337C: 71–79.
13. Fan YN, Xiao X, Min JL (2014) iNR-Drug: Predicting the interaction of drugs with nuclear receptors in cellular networking. Intenational Journal of Molecular Sciences 15: 4915–4937.
14. Guo SH, Deng EZ, Xu LQ, Ding H, Lin H, et al. (2014) iNuc-PseKNC: a sequence-based predictor for predicting nucleosome positioning in genomes with pseudo k-tuple nucleotide composition. Bioinformatics 30: 1522–1529.
15. Liu B, Zhang D, Xu R, Xu J, Wang X, et al. (2014) Combining evolutionary information extracted from frequency profiles with sequence-based kernels for protein remote homology detection. Bioinformatics 30: 472–479.
16. Qiu WR, Xiao X (2014) iRSpot-TNCPseAAC: Identify recombination spots with trinucleotide composition and pseudo amino acid components. Int J Mol Sci 15: 1746–1766.
17. Xu Y, Wen X, Shao XJ, Deng NY (2014) iHyd-PseAAC: Predicting hydroxyproline and hydroxylysine in proteins by incorporating dipeptide position-specific propensity into pseudo amino acid composition. International Journal of Molecular Sciences 15: 7594–7610.
18. Ding H, Deng EZ, Yuan LF, Liu L, Lin H, et al. (2014) iCTX-Type: A sequence-based predictor for identifying the types of conotoxins in targeting ion channels. BioMed Research International 2014: 286419.
19. Qiu WR, Xiao X, Lin WZ (2014) iMethyl-PseAAC: Identification of protein methylation sites via a pseudo amino acid composition approach. BioMed Research International 2014: ID 947416.
20. Chen W, Feng PM, Lin H (2014) iSS-PseDNC: identifying splicing sites using pseudo dinucleotide composition. Biomed Research International 2014: 623149.
21. Chen W, Feng PM, Deng EZ, Lin H (2014) iTIS-PseTNC: a sequence-based predictor for identifying translation initiation site in human genes using pseudo trinucleotide composition. Analytical Biochemistry 10.1016/j.ab.2014.1006.1022.
22. Chou KC (1993) A vectorized sequence-coupling model for predicting HIV protease cleavage sites in proteins. Journal of Biological Chemistry 268: 16938–16948.
23. Chou KC (1996) Review: Prediction of human immunodeficiency virus protease cleavage sites in proteins. Analytical Biochemistry 233: 1–14.
24. Chou KC (1995) A sequence-coupled vector-projection model for predicting the specificity of GalNAc-transferase. Protein Science 4: 1365–1383.
25. Chou KC (2001) Prediction of signal peptides using scaled window. Peptides 22: 1973–1979.
26. Chou KC, Shen HB (2007) Review: Recent progresses in protein subcellular location prediction. Analytical Biochemistry 370: 1–16.
27. Liu Z, Cao J, Ma Q, Gao X, Ren J, et al. (2011) GPS-YNO2: computational prediction of tyrosine nitration sites in proteins. Mol Biosyst 7: 1197–1204.
28. Xu Y, Ding J, Wu LY (2013) iSNO-PseAAC: Predict cysteine S-nitrosylation sites in proteins by incorporating position specific amino acid propensity into pseudo amino acid composition PLoS ONE 8: e55844.
29. Chou JJ (1993) A formulation for correlating properties of peptides and its application to predicting human immunodeficiency virus protease-cleavable sites in proteins. Biopolymers 33: 1405–1414.
30. Wang M, Yang J, Xu ZJ (2005) SLLE for predicting membrane protein types. Journal of Theoretical Biology 232: 7–15.
31. Feng KY, Cai YD (2005) Boosting classifier for predicting protein domain structural class. Biochemical & Biophysical Research Communications 334: 213–217.
32. Feng PM, Chen W, Lin H (2013) iHSP-PseRAAAC: Identifying the heat shock protein families using pseudo reduced amino acid alphabet composition. Analytical Biochemistry 442: 118–125.
33. Kandaswamy KK, Martinetz T, Moller S, Suganthan PN, et al. (2011) AFP-Pred: A random forest approach for predicting antifreeze proteins from sequence-derived properties. Journal of Theoretical Biology 270: 56–62.
34. Chou KC, Shen HB (2006) Predicting eukaryotic protein subcellular location by fusing optimized evidence-theoretic K-nearest neighbor classifiers. Journal of Proteome Research 5: 1888–1897.
35. Shen HB (2009) A top-down approach to enhance the power of predicting human protein subcellular localization: Hum-mPLoc 2.0. Analytical Biochemistry 394: 269–274.
36. Xiao X, Min JL, Wang P (2013) iGPCR-Drug: A web server for predicting interaction between GPCRs and drugs in cellular networking. PLoS ONE 8: e72234.
37. Chou KC (2013) Some Remarks on Predicting Multi-Label Attributes in Molecular Biosystems. Molecular Biosystems 9: 1092–1100.
38. Chou KC (2001) Prediction of protein cellular attributes using pseudo amino acid composition. PROTEINS: Structure, Function, and Genetics (Erratum: ibid, 2001, Vol44, 60) 43: 246–255.
39. Lin SX, Lapointe J (2013) Theoretical and experimental biology in one. J Biomedical Science and Engineering (JBiSE) 6: 435–442.
40. Nanni L, Lumini A, Gupta D, Garg A (2012) Identifying Bacterial Virulent Proteins by Fusing a Set of Classifiers Based on Variants of Chou's Pseudo Amino Acid Composition and on Evolutionary Information. IEEE/ACM Trans Comput Biol Bioinform 9: 467–475.
41. Hajisharifi Z, Piryaiee M, Mohammad Beigi M, Behbahani M, Mohabatkar H (2014) Predicting anticancer peptides with Chou's pseudo amino acid composition and investigating their mutagenicity via Ames test. Journal of Theoretical Biology 341: 34–40.
42. Mei S (2012) Predicting plant protein subcellular multi-localization by Chou's PseAAC formulation based multi-label homolog knowledge transfer learning. Journal of Theoretical Biology 310: 80–87.
43. Chen YK, Li KB (2013) Predicting membrane protein types by incorporating protein topology, domains, signal peptides, and physicochemical properties into the general form of Chou's pseudo amino acid composition. Journal of Theoretical Biology 318: 1–12.
44. Georgiou DN, Karakasidis TE, Megaritis AC (2013) A short survey on genetic sequences, Chou's pseudo amino acid composition and its combination with fuzzy set theory. The Open Bioinformatics Journal 7: 41–48.
45. Mohabatkar H, Mohammad Beigi M, Esmaeili A (2011) Prediction of GABA(A) receptor proteins using the concept of Chou's pseudo-amino acid composition and support vector machine. Journal of Theoretical Biology 281: 18–23.
46. Khosravian M, Faramarzi FK, Beigi MM, Behbahani M, Mohabatkar H (2013) Predicting Antibacterial Peptides by the Concept of Chou's Pseudo-amino Acid Composition and Machine Learning Methods. Protein & Peptide Letters 20: 180–186.
47. Mohabatkar H, Beigi MM, Abdolahi K, Mohsenzadeh S (2013) Prediction of Allergenic Proteins by Means of the Concept of Chou's Pseudo Amino Acid Composition and a Machine Learning Approach. Medicinal Chemistry 9: 133–137.
48. Mohammad Beigi M, Behjati M, Mohabatkar H (2011) Prediction of metalloproteinase family based on the concept of Chou's pseudo amino acid composition using a machine learning approach. Journal of Structural and Functional Genomics 12: 191–197.
49. Zia Ur R, Khan A (2012) Identifying GPCRs and their Types with Chou's Pseudo Amino Acid Composition: An Approach from Multi-scale Energy Representation and Position Specific Scoring Matrix. Protein & Peptide Letters 19: 890–903.
50. Sun XY, Shi SP, Qiu JD, Suo SB, Huang SY, et al. (2012) Identifying protein quaternary structural attributes by incorporating physicochemical properties into the general form of Chou's PseAAC via discrete wavelet transform. Molecular BioSystems 8: 3178–3184.
51. Du P, Gu S, Jiao Y (2014) PseAAC-General: Fast building various modes of general form of Chou's pseudo-amino acid composition for large-scale protein datasets. International Journal of Molecular Sciences 15: 3495–3506.
52. Jiang Y, Huang T, Chen L, Gao YF, Cai Y, et al. (2013) Signal propagation in protein interaction network during colorectal cancer progression. Biomed Res Int 2013: 287019.
53. Du P, Wang X, Xu C, Gao Y (2012) PseAAC-Builder: A cross-platform stand-alone program for generating various special Chou's pseudo-amino acid compositions. Analytical Biochemistry 425: 117–119.
54. Cao DS, Xu QS, Liang YZ (2013) propy: a tool to generate various modes of Chou's PseAAC. Bioinformatics 29: 960–962.
55. Chou KC (2001) Using subsite coupling to predict signal peptides. Protein Engineering 14: 75–79.
56. Chou KC, Shen HB (2009) Review: recent advances in developing web-servers for predicting protein attributes. Natural Science 2: 63–92.
57. Chou KC (2001) Prediction of protein signal sequences and their cleavage sites. PROTEINS: Structure, Function, and Genetics 42: 136–139.
58. Chou KC, Wu ZC, Xiao X (2012) iLoc-Hum: Using accumulation-label scale to predict subcellular locations of human proteins with both single and multiple sites. Molecular Biosystems 8: 629–641.
59. Xiao X, Wu ZC (2011) iLoc-Virus: A multi-label learning classifier for identifying the subcellular localization of virus proteins with both single and multiple sites. Journal of Theoretical Biology 284: 42–51.
60. Wu ZC, Xiao X (2011) iLoc-Plant: a multi-label classifier for predicting the subcellular localization of plant proteins with both single and multiple sites. Molecular BioSystems 7: 3287–3297.

61. Lin WZ, Fang JA, Xiao X (2013) iLoc-Animal: A multi-label learning classifier for predicting subcellular localization of animal proteins Molecular BioSystems 9: 634–644.
62. Chou KC, Wu ZC, Xiao X (2011) iLoc-Euk: A Multi-Label Classifier for Predicting the Subcellular Localization of Singleplex and Multiplex Eukaryotic Proteins. PLoS One 6: e18258.
63. Xiao X, Wang P, Lin WZ, Jia JH (2013) iAMP-2L: A two-level multi-label classifier for identifying antimicrobial peptides and their functional types. Analytical Biochemistry 436: 168–177.
64. Chou KC, Zhang CT (1995) Review: Prediction of protein structural classes. Critical Reviews in Biochemistry and Molecular Biology 30: 275–349.
65. Chou KC, Shen HB (2008) Cell-PLoc: A package of Web servers for predicting subcellular localization of proteins in various organisms. Nature Protocols 3: 153–162.
66. Shen HB, Yang J, Liu XJ (2005) Using supervised fuzzy clustering to predict protein structural classes. Biochem Biophys Res Commun 334: 577–581.
67. Mei S (2012) Multi-kernel transfer learning based on Chou's PseAAC formulation for protein submitochondria localization. Journal of Theoretical Biology 293: 121–130.
68. Chen W, Lin H, Feng PM, Ding C, Zuo YC, et al. (2012) iNuc-PhysChem: A Sequence-Based Predictor for Identifying Nucleosomes via Physicochemical Properties. PLoS ONE 7: e47843.
69. Sahu SS, Panda G (2010) A novel feature representation method based on Chou's pseudo amino acid composition for protein structural class prediction. Computational Biology and Chemistry 34: 320–327.
70. Huang C, Yuan JQ (2013) Predicting protein subchloroplast locations with both single and multiple sites via three different modes of Chou's pseudo amino acid compositions. Journal of Theoretical Biology 335: 205–212.
71. Kong L, Zhang L, Lv J (2014) Accurate prediction of protein structural classes by incorporating predicted secondary structure information into the general form of Chou's pseudo amino acid composition. J Theor Biol 344: 12–18.
72. Jia C, Lin X, Wang Z (2014) Prediction of Protein S-Nitrosylation Sites Based on Adapted Normal Distribution Bi-Profile Bayes and Chou's Pseudo Amino Acid Composition. Int J Mol Sci 15: 10410–10423.
73. Liu W (1999) Protein secondary structural content prediction. Protein Engineering 12: 1041–1050.
74. Chou KC (1999) Using pair-coupled amino acid composition to predict protein secondary structure content. Journal of Protein Chemistry 18: 473–480.
75. Chou KC (2005) Using amphiphilic pseudo amino acid composition to predict enzyme subfamily classes. Bioinformatics 21: 10–19.
76. Chou KC (2002) Review: Prediction of protein signal sequences. Current Protein and Peptide Science 3: 615–622.
77. Chou KC, Shen HB (2007) Signal-CF: a subsite-coupled and window-fusing approach for predicting signal peptides. Biochem Biophys Res Comm 357: 633–640.

Comparative Persistence of the TNF Antagonists in Rheumatoid Arthritis – A Population-Based Cohort Study

Anat Fisher[1,2]*, Ken Bassett[1,2,3], James M. Wright[1,2,4], M. Alan Brookhart[5], Hugh Freeman[4], Colin R. Dormuth[1,2]

1 Therapeutics Initiative, University of British Columbia, Vancouver, Canada, **2** Department of Anesthesiology, Pharmacology & Therapeutics, University of British Columbia, Vancouver, Canada, **3** Department of Family Practice, University of British Columbia, Vancouver, Canada, **4** Department of Medicine, University of British Columbia, Vancouver, Canada, **5** Department of Epidemiology, Gillings School of Global Public Health, University of North Carolina, Chapel Hill, North Carolina, United States of America

Abstract

Objective: To compare persistence with tumor necrosis factor alpha (TNF) antagonists among rheumatoid arthritis patients in British Columbia. Treatment persistence has been suggested as a proxy for real-world therapeutic benefit and harm of treatments for chronic non-curable diseases, including rheumatoid arthritis. We hypothesized that the different pharmacological characteristics of infliximab, adalimumab and etanercept cause statistically and clinically significant differences in persistence.

Methods: We conducted a population-based cohort study using administrative health data from the Canadian province of British Columbia. The study cohort included rheumatoid arthritis patients who initiated the first course of a TNF antagonist between 2001 and 2008. Persistence was measured as the time between first dispensing to discontinuation. Drug discontinuation was defined as a drug-free interval of 180 days or switching to another TNF antagonist, anakinra, rituximab or abatacept. Persistence was estimated and compared using survival analysis.

Results: The study cohort included 2,923 patients, 63% treated with etanercept. Median persistence in years (95% confidence interval) with infliximab was 3.7 (2.9–4.9), with adalimumab 3.3 (2.6–4.1) and with etanercept 3.8 (3.3–4.3). Similar risk of discontinuation was observed for the three drugs: the hazard ratio (95% confidence interval) was 0.98 (0.85–1.13) comparing infliximab with etanercept, 0.95 (0.78–1.15) comparing infliximab with adalimumab and 1.04 (0.88–1.22) comparing adalimumab with etanercept.

Conclusions: Similar persistence was observed with infliximab, adalimumab and etanercept in rheumatoid arthritis patients during the first 9 years of use. If treatment persistence is a good proxy for the therapeutic benefit and harm of these drugs, then this finding suggests that the three drugs share an overall similar benefit-harm profile in rheumatoid arthritis patients.

Editor: Paul Proost, University of Leuven, Rega Institute, Belgium

Funding: The study was supported by the University of British Columbia Graduate Fellowship and a grant to the University of British Columbia from the British Columbia Ministry of Health. The funders had no role in study design, data collection and analysis, decision to publish, or preparation of the manuscript.

Competing Interests: The authors have declared that no competing interests exist.

* Email: anat.fisher@ti.ubc.ca

Introduction

The tumor necrosis factor alpha (TNF) antagonists are a relatively new class of drugs used to treat multiple inflammatory diseases, including rheumatoid arthritis (RA). These drugs bind and inactivate TNF, a cytokine that primarily acts as a proinflammation mediator and is thought to be important in the pathogenesis of RA [1].

Treatment with a TNF antagonist is not a cure [2] but rather reduces the symptoms of inflammation, possibly inducing remission and preventing long-term complications.

Randomized clinical trials (RCTs) are limited in their ability to provide evidence on the relative benefit and harm of TNF antagonists in real-world setting for several reasons. First, there are no head-to-head RCTs comparing two (or more) individual TNF antagonists. Multiple indirect comparisons have reported inconsistent estimates of relative efficacy and safety [3–9]. Second, the duration of RCTs is considerably shorter than the lifetime of the disease. Since RA is characterized by a variation in disease activity and deterioration over time, effects observed in a short-term trial may not be significant in the long-term and a drug which had no short-term effects may prevent complications or progression of the disease over the long-term [10,11]. Last, RA patients who participate in RCTs designed to assess therapeutic benefit and harm of TNF antagonists are not representative of actual RA populations treated with TNF antagonists in routine clinical settings [12–15]. Furthermore, patients eligible to participate in RCTs had an improved response compared to ineligible patients

[12–14], and therefore an overestimation of therapeutic benefit is likely.

Real-life drug persistence was suggested as a simple indirect approach for assessing long-term therapeutic benefit and harm [10]. This suggestion is based on the assumption that when using a drug that reduces symptoms and prevents complications (but does not cure the disease), patients persist with the treatment as long as they experience or perceive a benefit and they do not experience (or perceive) an unacceptable amount of harm. This theoretical perspective on persistence seems to hold for TNF antagonist drugs – the main reasons for discontinuing or switching these drugs in RA were decreased benefit (36–67% of the discontinuations) or perceived harm (30–58%) [16–21].

Estimates of comparative persistence with TNF antagonists in RA patients remain controversial and estimates could not be pooled due to differences in measures of persistence (e.g. median, mean, percentage of persistent patients after 1-year) [22,23]. Hence, high quality research is warrant to provide evidence on comparative persistence of these drugs.

Each TNF antagonist has different pharmacological properties [24–26] and therefore substantive differences in therapeutic benefit and harm are expected. Since most discontinuations of these drugs are due to decreased benefit or increased harm, we hypothesized that differences in therapeutic effects would lead to differences in persistence between the TNF anatgonists in RA patients. The main objective of the current study was to compare persistence with infliximab, adalimumab and etanercept in RA in the Canadian province of British Columbia.

Patients and Methods

Patients were identified using four British Columbia Ministry of Health administrative databases: PharmaNet (pharmacy dispensing data), Medical Service Plan (MSP) registration information (demographic data), MSP payment information (fee-for-service payments to physicians and alternative providers), and the Discharge Abstract Database (hospital separations). The databases were linked using a unique anonymized identifier. Follow-up data were available until December 31, 2009. The study protocol was approved by the Clinical Research Ethics Board of the University of British Columbia. Patient records and physician information were anonymized and de-identified prior to analysis.

The study cohort was identified based on (1) exposure to infliximab, adalimumab or etanercept and (2) diagnosis of RA. Exposure to TNF antagonist was defined as at least one recorded dispensing claim of infliximab, adalimumab or etanercept between March 2001 and December 31, 2008. The index date was the date of the first dispensing event. We defined a pre-study period of three years preceding the index date during which patients were required to have continuous provincial MSP coverage. A gap shorter than 30 days was not considered to be an interruption in MSP coverage. The pre-study period ensured a standard run-in period of at least three years without TNF antagonist exposure and a standard period during which diagnosis of RA was required.

RA patients were selected into the study cohort if they had two outpatient visits in physician clinics with a diagnosis code of RA (ICD-9 714.XX) at least 60 days apart, or at least one hospitalization with a recorded discharge diagnosis of RA in the pre-study period. This method was similar, though not identical, to criteria previously used in British Columbia data [27]. Patients entering the cohort were assigned to mutually exclusive exposure categories based on the first TNF antagonist they received (i.e., infliximab, adalimumab or etanercept). None of the patients was dispensed two or more different TNF antagonists at the index date. Patients were excluded if they were previously treated with anakinra, rituximab or abatacept, or if either sex or date of birth was not available. In addition, patients were excluded if they had a concurrent diagnosis of Crohn's disease (based on at least one outpatient or inpatient diagnosis code in the pre-study period) or if they were younger than 18 years at the index date (to remove patients with juvenile RA).

During the study period, clinical guidelines and the provincial drug coverage policy considered the drugs comparable [28,29]; nevertheless, the choice of a specific TNF antagonist could be associated with factors that influence drug persistence, such as age or disease severity. Demographic and clinical status variables were included in the multivariate regression model to minimize the effect of such possible confounders. Patient demographic variables included sex, age and a proxy variable for socio-economic status (the annual deductible for prescription cost, which was based on family annual income [30]). We used four mutually exclusive age categories: 18–30, 30–70 (reference), 70–80 and >80 years old, based on a preliminary analysis that demonstrated homogeneous persistence within each age category. Clinical status variables included the number of inpatient and outpatient encounters in the year prior to index, the duration of disease (defined as time from the first recording of diagnostic code of RA in the data to the index) and the presence and severity of comorbidities. We used Quan's algorithm for administrative databases [31] to determine the Charlson comorbidity score [32] during the year preceding the index, but excluding rheumatic diseases. The regression model also contained three variables for other antirheumatic (synthetic) drugs. Two binary variables were: (1) concomitant methotrexate in the 200 days prior to index, where the dispensing period of 200 days reflected average plus two standard deviations of between-dispensing intervals of methotrexate in the study cohort; and (2) dispensing of any nonsteroidal anti-inflammatory drug (NSAID) in the year preceding the index. The third drug variable was the number of previous antirheumatic drugs in the pre-study period. Dispensing records for nine drugs were sought: methotrexate, hydroxychloroquine, sulfasalazine, azathioprine, cyclosporine, minocycline, penicillamine, sodium aurothiomalate, prednisone and intra-articular triamcinolone/methylprednisolone acetate. We included a categorical variable for the calendar year of the index date, which allowed adjustment for possible secular trends in clinical practice [33,34] and late availability of adalimumab (3 years after infliximab and etanercept).

Finally, we included a series of 12 binary variables for high-volume prescribers who initiated more than 70 courses in the study cohort. This series allowed adjustment for differences (an increase or a decrease) in the risk of discontinuing any TNF antagonist in patients treated by a particular physician. We used the prescriber recorded on the first dispensing claim for TNF antagonist as a proxy of the care-providing physician. The prescribers were determined using an anonymized identifier.

Our outcome was persistence (continuous variable), measured in years from index until drug discontinuation. Drug discontinuation was defined as either switching to another 'biologic' antirheumatic drug (TNF antagonists including certolizumab and golimumab, anakinra, rituximab and abatacept) or elapsing of a drug-free interval of 180 days. A drug-free interval was defined as a period without additional dispensing of the same pharmaceutical component after the days-supply of the latest dispensing claim was exhausted. Adding-on a synthetic antirheumatic drug was not considered discontinuation. We selected a long drug free interval that was previously used in similar studies [35] to ensure that we capture events of discontinuation and not only temporary decrease in adherence (patients who had short gaps in treatment and then

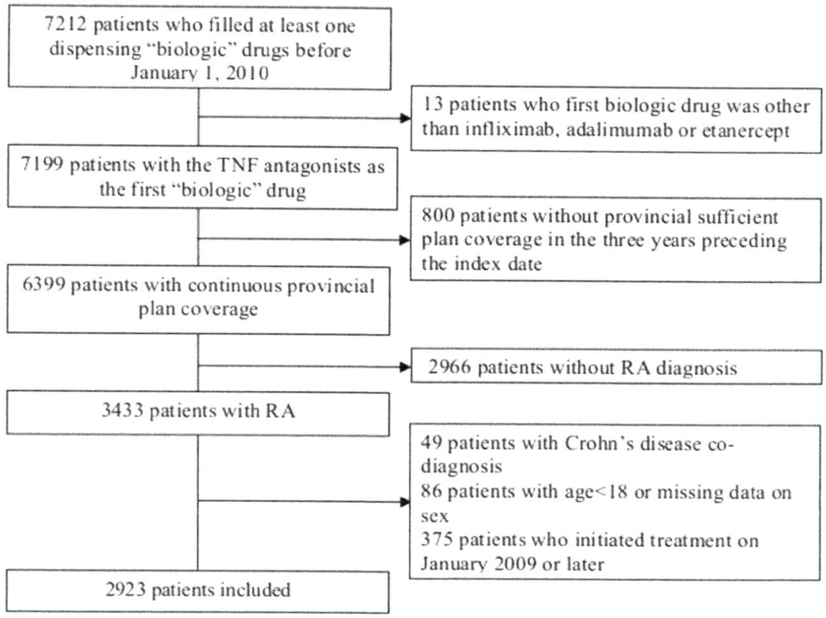

"Biologic" drugs = infliximab, adalimumab, etanercept, anakinra, rituximab, abatacept, certolizumab and golimumab; RA – rheumatoid arthritis, TNF – tumour necrosis factor alpha

Figure 1. Patients' Flow.

resume the same drug). Discontinuation date was set to the end of days-supply of the latest dispensing event or the date of the first dispensing claim of a different 'biologic' antirheumatic drug, whichever was earliest. Patients were considered censored if they were continuously treated with the first TNF antagonist on December 31, 2009 (end of follow-up period) or during an interruption of more than six days in the provincial MSP coverage. The most common causes of prolonged or infinite interruptions were emigration from the province and death.

Original data on the number of days-supply recorded in PharmaNet were unreliable and frequently did not match the quantity dispensed. Therefore we also calculated days-supply based on dispensed quantity, which, if required, was imputed using the recorded total cost. We considered the prescription cost to be the most accurate and reliable quantity field; given the high cost of these medications, the number of vials or milligrams dispensed could be easily defined. We used the longest duration of days-supply, recorded or calculated, to determine both the length of a drug-free interval and the date of drug discontinuation.

Statistical Methods

Baseline characteristics were presented and compared across the three drug groups. We assumed normality of continuous variables and the significance of differences between groups was assessed with one-way analysis of variance (ANOVA) F-test for continuous variables and the Pearson's Chi-square test for categorical variables. The crude and adjusted hazard ratios for drug discontinuation were estimated using Cox proportional hazards regression. Three pairwise comparisons were presented: infliximab versus adalimumab, infliximab versus etanercept and adalimumab versus etanercept. Drug-sex and drug-age interactions were examined but were included in the final models only if the overall significance was <0.1. We also presented the adjusted hazard ratios for all variables included in the model. We tested linearity of continuous variables and categorized non-linear variables. We also tested model assumptions including the proportional hazards and absence of interactions and found them to be valid. All calculations were performed using the SAS software package Version 9.1 (SAS Institute Inc., Cary, NC).

Results

The study cohort included 2,923 RA patients who initiated TNF antagonists by December 31, 2008 and met all selection criteria (Figure 1). The cohort was predominantly women (72%) and patients treated with etanercept (63%) (Table 1). Ages ranged from 18–92 years (median 56). Patients treated with infliximab had the highest prevalence of concomitant methotrexate therapy and patients with etanercept the lowest. This reflects differences in the indications mentioned in the product monographs; while infliximab is indicated for use in combination with methotrexate [36], the monograph of etanercept mentioned that it "can be initiated in combination with methotrexate … or used alone" [37]. Similarly, while the provincial special authority policy requires that infliximab is used in combination with methotrexate (or other drug), such requirement does not exist for treatment with etanercept or adalimumab [29].

The three TNF antagonist drugs had similar persistence (median roughly 3.5 years, Figure 2). In the multivariable analysis, the estimated adjusted hazards were comparable for the three TNF antagonists (Table 2). Drug-sex and drug-age interactions were insignificant and were not included in the final model.

The following patients' subgroups had a decreased discontinuation hazard (improved persistence): males, age 30–70, patients without admission to hospital in the year preceding treatment initiation, patients on concomitant MTX or NSAIDs treatment

Table 1. Baseline Characteristics of Patients.

Factor	Infliximab (n = 620, 21%)	Adalimumab (N = 474, 16%)	Etanercept (n = 1829, 63%)
Females, n (%)	438 (71)	344 (73)	1322 (72)
Age	56 (18–87)	58 (22–91)	56 (18–92)
Low deductible ($1–500), n (%)	34 (5)	56 (12)	162 (9)
Medium deductible ($501–2250) n (%)	96 (15)	118 (25)	356 (19)
High deductible (>$2250) n (%)	40 (6)	46 (10)	169 (9)
No deductible n (%)	49 (8)	83 (18)	213 (12)
Number of outpatient visits	33 (3–158)	31 (2–112)	32 (3–136)
Number of admissions	0 (0–6)	0 (0–5)	0 (0–8)
Number of comorbidity	0 (0–6)	0 (0–8)	0 (0–7)
RA duration in years	9.1 (0.1–17.9)	7.7 (0.3–17.9)	8.2 (0–17.8)
MTX users n (%)	417 (67)	277 (59)	902 (49)
NSAID users n (%)	332 (54)	224 (47)	983 (54)
Number of previous drugs	4 (0–8)	4 (0–8)	4 (0–9)
Calendar year	2003 (2001–2008)	2007 (2004–2008)	2005 (2001–2008)

Values are median (range) unless otherwise specified. Please refer to text (Patients and methods) for further details on the variables.
%- percent; MTX- methotrexate; NSAID- nonsteroidal anti-inflammatory drug; RA – rheumatoid arthritis; $ Canadian dollars.

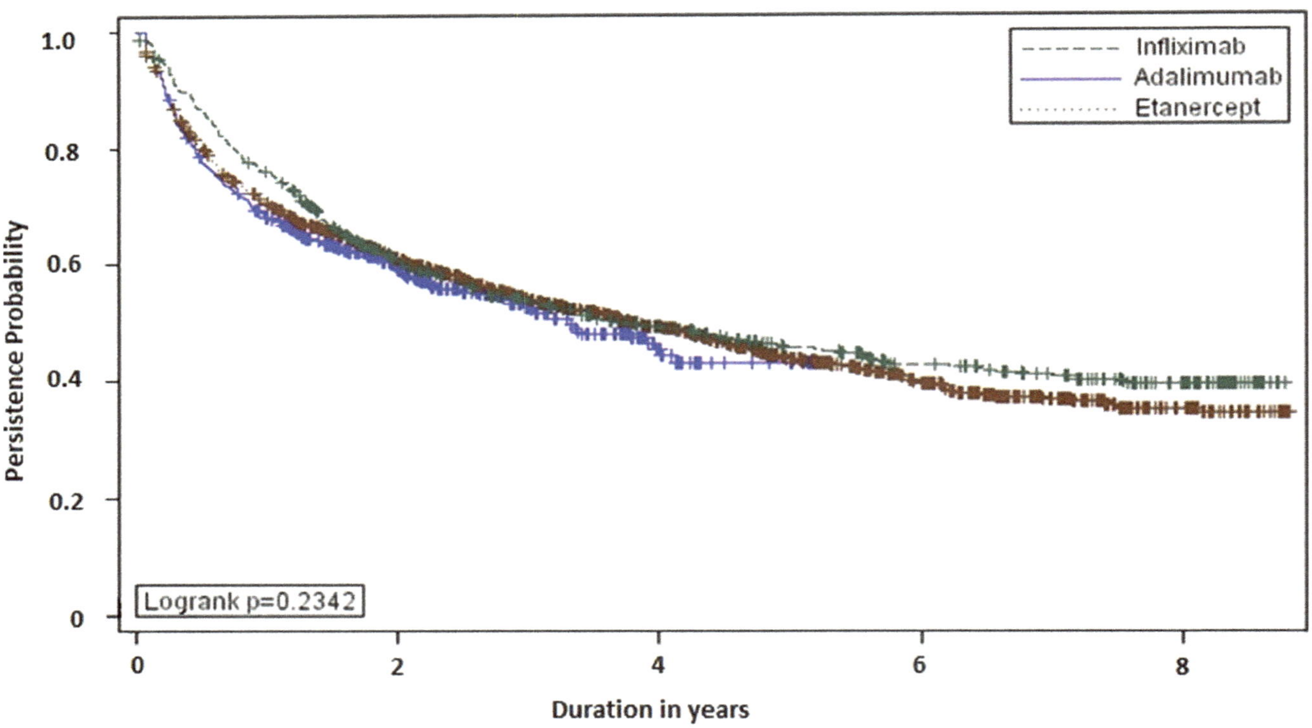

	Number of patients	Events	Censored	Median survival (95% confidence interval)
Infliximab	620	53% (328)	47% (292)	3.68 (2.88-4.95)
Adalimumab	474	46% (219)	54% (255)	3.33 (2.63-4.10)
Etanercept	1829	52% (960)	48% (869)	3.78 (3.31-4.32)

Figure 2. Drug Persistence Curves.

Table 2. Hazard Ratios for Discontinuation of Tumor Necrosis Factor Alpha Antagonists.

Comparison	Crude hazard ratio (95% CI)	Adjusted hazard ratio (95% CI)
Infliximab versus etanercept	0.92 (0.81–1.04)	0.98 (0.85–1.13)
Infliximab versus adalimumab	0.87 (0.73–1.03)	0.95 (0.78–1.15)
Adalimumab versus etanercept	1.06 (0.92–1.23)	1.04 (0.88–1.22)

CI – confidence interval.

and patients previously treated with less than 7 antirheumatic drugs (Table 3).

We demonstrated variation in prescribing practice between the physicians, expressed as differences in the risk for discontinuing any TNF antagonist in patients treated by different physicians (Table 3). Physician-specific risk was estimated through a series of binary variables for each of 12 heavy-volume prescribers who initiated more than 70 courses in the study cohort. Each binary variable represented deviation in 'baseline risk of discontinuing' for patients treated by a particular prescriber. We found that patients treated by two 'heavy-volume' prescribers had an increased risk of discontinuation (hazard ratios significantly higher than 1) and patients treated by another two had a significantly lower risk (hazard ratios significantly lower than 1) (Table 3) compared to patients treated with low to medium-volume prescribers. This physician-specific baseline risk of discontinuation was a significant predictor of persistence (p-value of log likelihood test <0.0001). None of the remaining covariates were associated with persistence.

Discussion

This study found no significant difference in persistence between infliximab, adalimumab and etanercept prescribed for RA patients in British Columbia despite known differences in their pharmacological properties. The theory that treatment persistence can serve as a measurable proxy for real-world therapeutic benefit and harm implies similar long-term benefit and harm of the three drugs in RA patients. In the absence of any safety concerns that are specific to a particular TNF antagonist, it would be reasonable to base the TNF antagonist drug formulary, at least in part, on non-therapeutic factors such as cost, convenience and availability. Even if persistence is not a suitable proxy for harm-benefit in these patients, we showed that differences in convenience of administration - intravenous infusion of infliximab compared with subcutaneous injection of etanercept and adalimumab - were not associated with differences in persistence and therefore should not be considered when selecting a treatment.

Three alternative explanations are suggested for the finding of similar persistence with the three drugs. First, similar persistence could reflect similarities in the benefits and harms of the three drugs despite their different pharmacological properties. This explanation is based on the assumption that not all pharmacological properties strongly influence therapeutic effects, and the differences in these properties between the drugs would therefore not influence the clinical outcome of these drugs.

Second, similar persistence amongst the three TNF antagonists may result from benefit and harm differences in different directions. For example, some properties of infliximab might cause increased benefits compared to etanercept (e.g. apoptosis of

Table 3. Predictors of Discontinuation of Tumor Necrosis Factor Alpha Antagonists.

Factor (reference)	P value (log likelihood test)	Adjusted hazard ratio (95% CI)
Sex (female)	<0.0001	0.76 (0.68–0.86)
Age (30–69 years)	<0.0001	18–29 years 1.53 (1.20–1.96); 70–79 years 1.32 (1.14–1.54); ≥80 years 1.83 (1.39–2.41
Deductible	0.8	
Outpatient visits	0.051	
Admissions (no admission)	0.006	1 admission 1.26 (1.09–1.47); 2 admissions 1.10 (0.86–1.42); >2 admissions 1.51 (1.09–2.10)
Comorbidity	0.23	
RA duration	0.07	
MTX use	<0.0001	0.79 (0.71–0.88)
NSAIDs use	0.03	0.89 (0.80–0.99)
Previous drugs (3–6 RA drugs)	0.03	No drug 1.38 (0.99–1.92); 1–2 drugs 1.04 (0.90–1.20); 7–9 drugs 1.40 (1.09–1.81)
Index year (categories)	0.08	
Prescriber-specific risk (a group of prescribers with <70 courses)	<0.0001	Physician 0.57 (0.42–0.76); physician 0.67 (0.47–0.98); physician 1.38 (1.03–1.84); physician 1.57 (1.26–1.96)

Hazard ratios are presented only for factors that are significant predictors of persistence (p-value of log likelihood test ≤0.05) and for 4 prescribers with hazard ratios that are significantly different than the reference.
CI – confidence interval, MTX – methotrexate; NSAID – nonsteroidal anti-inflammatory drug, RA – rheumatoid arthritis.

activated T cells and circulating monocytes [38] or lack of binding of lymphotoxin alpha. [39,40]). Potentially cancelling the increased benefit is the higher immunogenicity of infliximab which could lead to harm such as an infusion reaction [41] or the wide fluctuations in serum concentration of infliximab [39] which could increase the risk of exceeding the maximum tolerated concentration (leading to harm), or reaching suboptimal concentrations (leading to lack of therapeutic benefit).

Alternatively, persistence may be influenced by factors unrelated to therapeutic benefit or harm and the influence of these factors might be different between the drugs. For example, infliximab requires intravenous administration by health care professionals while both adalimumab and etanercept are self-injectable (subcutaneous administration). Patients treated with infliximab may discontinue treatment due to patient or physician preference for subcutaneous administered drugs [42]. This negative influence on persistence due to intravenous administration may be counter balanced by regular physician follow-up that has been shown to improve adherence and persistence to drug therapy in a variety of diseases [43,44].

Similar persistence with the infliximab, adalimumab and etanercept has previously been demonstrated in some studies [45–48], while differences in persistence was observed in others [18,19,49–55]. Controversial results of previous studies may be due to different population or methodology (e.g. crude versus adjusted estimates). An in-depth systematic exploration of the reasons for the differences between the studies is beyond the scope of current study and requires further research.

The two main strengths of our study are: the characteristics of the data used and accounting for differences in practice between physicians. The universal nature of the Canadian health care system minimized selection bias and thus increased the external validity of our results. Patients were included regardless of age, employment status, socioeconomic status and heath facility use, all factors that could potentially caused biases in previous research that used administrative data, clinical chart review, or registries. Furthermore, the British Columbia Ministry of Health uses a largely systematic and standardized approach to data collection, which ensures the better representativeness of real life treatment patterns and drug-taking behavior. Access to complete information on all dispensed prescription drugs and multiple sources of data (physician encounters, hospital separation and pharmacies) contributed to the usefulness of the data. The data also granted a large sample (N = 2923), which provided ample power, as well as relatively long durations of follow up; roughly nine years.

We accounted for differences in prescribing practice between physicians by adjusting for the baseline risk of discontinuing any TNF antagonist in patients treated by different physicians. Differences in prescribing habits could be caused by differences in knowledge or adherence to different guidelines. Alternatively, patients treated by the same physician may be more similar than patients treated by different physicians in parameters such as geography, socioeconomic status, ethnic background, or age [56], and that could cause differences in the baseline risk of discontinuation. Confirming our finding, Zhang et al 2011 [57] demonstrated differences in physician response to decreased benefit with TNF antagonist therapy.

Several limitations are apparent in in analysis of administrative health data and are caused by absence of clinical information. We were unable to identify reasons for drug discontinuation in our cohort. However, based on previous studies, we assumed that the most common reasons were decreased benefit or increased harm. We also did not have access to possible clinical confounders, and therefore used proxies. This may result in residual confounding that has the potential to bias the results.

Diagnostic accuracy might be compromised or biased because disease diagnoses are coded and recorded in the databases for payment purpose. In addition, differences in accuracy of codes between the care-providers (e.g., different physicians) and variation in coding precision in different diseases are to be expected. To minimize the effect of these sources of inaccuracy, and in the absence of validated algorithm appropriate for our data, we designed a disease algorithm requiring at least two outpatient encounters with RA diagnosis.

We identified errors in recording days-supply in our data, which may be the result of refill policy of the provincial drug-coverage plan, different interpretations of days-supply, or dose titration. To overcome these inaccuracies we used a conservative estimate of days-supply (the longest among several possible approaches to estimation) that might have led to underestimation of the actual length of drug-free intervals, false late ascertainment of drug discontinuation and overestimation of drug persistence. Dispensing data for the three drugs were treated similarly to ensure that the relative hazard ratios were not systematically biased in this regard.

Inaccuracies in recording days-supply also limited our ability to identify patients with dose adjustment. Two analyses of administrative databases [48,55] previously evaluated the frequency of dose escalation in RA patients treated with TNF antagonists showed that dose escalating was more common in patients treated with infliximab. The limited ability to identify dose adjustment in our study may have resulted in overestimation of the days-supply for patients who experienced dose escalation, mainly patients treated with infliximab, and biased estimated comparative persistence of infliximab versus adalimumab or etanercept.

We used a long drug-free interval to ascertain discontinuation rather than direct recording of discontinuation (e.g., medical records or patient reporting). This long drug-free interval algorithm minimized the number of patients considered discontinuers for a temporary interruption. We claim that temporary interruptions should be considered noncompliance, not discontinuation. By using short drug-free intervals, previous studies captured a complex measure of both persistence and compliance and therefore the end point in these studies should not be considered discontinuation. However, by using a long drug-free interval, our analysis was more vulnerable to immortal person-time bias. Patients were required to be alive at the end of drug-free interval to be considered discontinuers; otherwise, their data was censored. Patients who died due to drug effects (harm) were not considered discontinuers but their follow-up time was accounted for. This bias might have affected our comparative estimates if death related to drug effects was significantly more frequent with one of the drug, a condition we did not expected to exist.

The study results indicate that persistence with infliximab, adalimumab and etanercept is similar in RA patients – a finding that does not disapproves the hypothesis that the drugs' benefit and harm could be considered equivalent. Accordingly, clinical and policy decisions for treatment with TNF antagonist could be based on convenience and cost. Even if persistence is not a suitable proxy for harm-benefit profile, our results show that persistence should not be a consideration when selecting a TNF antagonist in RA patients.

Author Contributions

Conceived and designed the experiments: AF KB JMW MAB HF CRD. Performed the experiments: AF. Analyzed the data: AF. Contributed reagents/materials/analysis tools: AF MAB CRD. Contributed to the writing of the manuscript: AF KB JMW MAB HF CRD.

References

1. Brennan FM, Maini RN, Feldmann M (1992) TNF alpha–A pivotal role in rheumatoid arthritis? Br J Rheumatol 31: 293–298.
2. Feldmann M, Maini RN (2001) Anti-TNF alpha therapy of rheumatoid arthritis: What have we learned? Annu Rev Immunol 19: 163–196.
3. Hochberg MC, Tracy JK, Hawkins-Holt M, Flores RH (2003) Comparison of the efficacy of the tumour necrosis factor alpha blocking agents adalimumab, etanercept, and infliximab when added to methotrexate in patients with active rheumatoid arthritis. Ann Rheum Dis 62: ii13–ii16.
4. Gartlehner G, Hansen RA, Jonas BL, Thieda P, Lohr KN (2006) The comparative efficacy and safety of biologics for the treatment of rheumatoid arthritis: A systematic review and metaanalysis. J Rheumatol 33: 2398–2408.
5. Nixon RM, Bansback NJ, Brennan A (2007) Using mixed treatment comparisons and meta-regression to perform indirect comparison to estimate the efficacy of biologic treatments in rheumatoid arthritis. Stat Med 26: 1237–1254.
6. Singh JA, Christensen R, Wells GA, Suarez-Almazor ME, Buchbinder R, et al. (2009) Biologics for rheumatoid arthritis: An overview of Cochrane reviews. Cochrane Database Syst Rev 4: CD007848.
7. Ingham M, Carter C (2010) Meta-analysis and biologics comparing apples to apples: An example using radiographic outcomes in rheumatoid arthritis Arthritis Rheum 62: 76.
8. Wiens A, Venson R, Correr CJ, Otuki MF, Pontarolo R (2010) Meta-analysis of the efficacy and safety of adalimumab, etanercept, and infliximab for the treatment of rheumatoid arthritis. Pharmacotherapy 30: 339–353.
9. Devine EB, Alfonso-Cristancho R, Sullivan SD (2011) Effectiveness of biologic therapies for rheumatoid arthritis: An indirect comparisons approach. Pharmacotherapy 31: 39–51.
10. Wolfe F (1995) The epidemiology of drug treatment failure in rheumatoid arthritis. Baillieres Clin Rheumatol 9: 619–632.
11. Pincus T, Sokka T (2004) Clinical trials in rheumatic diseases: Designs and limitations. Rheum Dis Clin North Am 30: 701–724.
12. Kievit W, Fransen J, Oerlemans AJ, Kuper HH, van der Laar MA, et al. (2007) The efficacy of anti-TNF in rheumatoid arthritis, a comparison between randomised controlled trials and clinical practice. Ann Rheum Dis 66: 1473–1478.
13. Zink A, Strangfeld A, Schneider M, Herzer P, Hierse F, et al. (2006) Effectiveness of tumor necrosis factor inhibitors in rheumatoid arthritis in an observational cohort study: Comparison of patients according to their eligibility for major randomized clinical trials. Arthritis Rheum 54: 3399–3407.
14. Berthelot JM, Benoist-Gerard S, le Goff B, Muller-Chevalet F, Maugars Y (2010) Outcome and safety of TNFalpha antagonist therapy in 475 consecutive outpatients (with rheumatoid arthritis or spondyloarthropathies) treated by a single physician according to their eligibility for clinical trials. Joint Bone Spine 77: 564–569.
15. Sokka T, Pincus T (2003) Eligibility of patients in routine care for major clinical trials of anti-tumor necrosis factor alpha agents in rheumatoid arthritis. Arthritis Rheum 48: 313–318.
16. Hyrich KL, Lunt M, Watson KD, Symmons DPM, Silman AJ (2007) Outcomes after switching from one anti-tumor necrosis factor alpha agent to a second anti-tumor necrosis factor alpha agent in patients with rheumatoid arthritis: Results from a large UK national cohort study. Arthritis Rheum 56: 13–20.
17. Carmona L, Gomez-Reino JJ, on behalf of the BIOBADASER Group (2006) Survival of TNF antagonists in spondylarthritis is better than in rheumatoid arthritis. Data from the Spanish registry BIOBADASER. Arthritis Res Ther 8: R72.
18. Hetland ML, Christensen IJ, Tarp U, Dreyer L, Hansen A, et al. (2010) Direct comparison of treatment responses, remission rates, and drug adherence in patients with rheumatoid arthritis treated with adalimumab, etanercept, or infliximab: Results from eight years of surveillance of clinical practice in the nationwide danish DANBIO registry. Arthritis Rheum 62: 22–32.
19. Fernandez-Nebro A, Irigoyen MV, Urena I, Belmonte-Lopez MA, Coret V, et al. (2007) Effectiveness, predictive response factors, and safety of anti-tumor necrosis factor (TNF) therapies in anti-TNF-naive rheumatoid arthritis. J Rheumatol 34: 2334–2342.
20. Kievit W, Fransen J, Adang EMM, den Broeder AA, Bernelot Moens HJ, et al. (2011) Long-term effectiveness and safety of TNF-blocking agents in daily clinical practice: Results from the Dutch rheumatoid arthritis monitoring register. Rheumatology (Oxford) 50: 196–203.
21. Filippini M, Bazzani C, Favalli EG, Marchesoni A, Atzeni F, et al. (2010) Efficacy and safety of anti-tumour necrosis factor in elderly patients with rheumatoid arthritis: An observational study. Clin Rev Allergy Immunol 38: 90–96.
22. Blum MA, Koo D, Doshi JA (2011) Measurement and rates of persistence with and adherence to biologics for rheumatoid arthritis: A systematic review. Clin Ther 33: 901–913.
23. Koncz T, Pentek M, Brodszky V, Ersek K, Orlewska E, et al. (2010) Adherence to biologic DMARD therapies in rheumatoid arthritis. Expert Opin Biol Ther 10: 1367–1378.
24. Anderson PJ (2005) Tumor necrosis factor inhibitors: Clinical implications of their different immunogenicity profiles. Semin Arthritis Rheum 34: 19–22.
25. Nestorov I (2005) Clinical pharmacokinetics of TNF antagonists: How do they differ? Semin Arthritis Rheum 34: 12–18.
26. Rigby WF (2007) Drug insight: Different mechanisms of action of tumor necrosis factor antagonists-passive-aggressive behavior? Nat Clin Pract Rheumatol 3: 227–233.
27. Lacaille D, Anis AH, Guh DP, Esdaile JM (2005) Gaps in care for rheumatoid arthritis: A population study. Arthritis Rheum 53: 241–248.
28. Furst DE, Keystone EC, Braun J, Breedveld FC, Burmester GR, et al. (2011) Updated consensus statement on biological agents for the treatment of rheumatic diseases, 2010. Ann Rheum Dis 70: i2–i36. 10.1136/ard.2010.146852.
29. British Columbia Ministry of Health (2011) Special authority request; abatacept/ adalimumab/ certolizumab/ etanercept/ golimumab/ infliximab rheumatoid arthritis (initial or switch). British Columbia Ministry of Health website. Available: https://www.health.gov.bc.ca/exforms/pharmacare/5345fil.pdf. Accessed 2012 May 14.
30. British Columbia Ministry of Health (2011) Your level of fair PharmaCare coverage in fair PharmaCare. British Columbia Ministry of Health website. Available: http://www.health.gov.bc.ca/pharmacare/plani/planiindex.html#7. Accessed 2011 Mar 29.
31. Quan H, Sundararajan V, Halfon P, Fong A, Burnand B, et al. (2005) Coding algorithms for defining comorbidities in ICD-9-CM and ICD-10 administrative data. Med Care 43: 1130–1139.
32. Charlson ME, Pompei P, Ales KL, MacKenzie CR (1987) A new method of classifying prognostic comorbidity in longitudinal studies: Development and validation. J Chronic Dis 40: 373–383.
33. Bensen B, Atkins C, Sheriff M, Kelsall J, Khalil H (2011) Profile of patients with rheumatoid arthritis treated with infliximab in Canada-trends toward less DMARD use prior to a biologic, earlier use of infliximab and differences in baseline disease [abstract]. J Rheumatol 38: 1155.
34. Hyrich KL, Watson KD, Lunt M, Symmons DP, on behalf of the British Society for Rheumatology Biologics Register (BSRBR) (2011) Changes in disease characteristics and response rates among patients in the United Kingdom starting anti-tumour necrosis factor therapy for rheumatoid arthritis between 2001 and 2008. Rheumatology (Oxford) 50: 117–123.
35. Ogale S, Hitraya E, Henk HJ (2011) Patterns of biologic agent utilization among patients with rheumatoid arthritis: A retrospective cohort study. BMC Musculoskelet Disord 12: 204.
36. eCPS (online Compendium of Pharmaceuticals and Specialties) (2008) Remicade® (infliximab). 2008. 2009 Jun.
37. eCPS (online Compendium of Pharmaceuticals and Specialties) (2009) Enbrel® (etanercept). 2009. 2009 Jun.
38. Furst DE, Wallis R, Broder M, Beenhouwer DO (2006) Tumor necrosis factor antagonists: Different kinetics and/or mechanisms of action may explain differences in the risk for developing granulomatous infection. Semin Arthritis Rheum 36: 159–167.
39. Tracey D, Klareskog L, Sasso EH, Salfeld JG, Tak PP (2008) Tumor necrosis factor antagonist mechanisms of action: A comprehensive review. Pharmacol Ther 117: 244–279.
40. Ware CF (2005) Network communications: Lymphotoxins, LIGHT, and TNF. Annu Rev Immunol 23: 787–819.
41. Emi Aikawa N, de Carvalho JF, Artur Almeida Silva C, Bonfa E (2010) Immunogenicity of anti-TNF-alpha agents in autoimmune diseases. Clin Rev Allergy Immunol 38: 82–89.
42. Vander Cruyssen B, Van Looy S, Wyns B, Westhovens R, Durez P, et al. (2006) Four-year follow-up of infliximab therapy in rheumatoid arthritis patients with long-standing refractory disease: Attrition and long-term evolution of disease activity. Arthritis Res Ther 8: R112.
43. Amuah JE, Hogan DB, Eliasziw M, Supina A, Beck P, et al. (2010) Persistence with cholinesterase inhibitor therapy in a population-based cohort of patients with alzheimer's disease. Pharmacoepidemiol Drug Saf 19: 670–679.
44. Brookhart MA, Patrick AR, Schneeweiss S, Avorn J, Dormuth C, et al. (2007) Physician follow-up and provider continuity are associated with long-term medication adherence: A study of the dynamics of statin use. Arch Intern Med 167: 847–852. 10.1001/archinte.167.8.847.
45. Finckh A, Simard JF, Gabay C, Guerne PA, SCQM physicians (2006) Evidence for differential acquired drug resistance to anti-tumour necrosis factor agents in rheumatoid arthritis. Ann Rheum Dis 65: 746–752.
46. Flendrie M, Creemers MCW, Welsing PMJ, Den Broeder AA, Van Riel PLCM (2003) Survival during treatment with tumour necrosis factor blocking agents in rheumatoid arthritis. Ann Rheum Dis 62: i30–i33.
47. Pocock JM, Albreshni S, Slack R, Polydoropoulou V, O'Reilly D, et al. (2009) A comparison of drug survival times for infliximab, adalimumab and etanercept [abstract]. Rheumatology (Oxford) 48: 69.
48. Wu E, Chen L, Birnbaum H, Yang E, Cifaldi M (2008) Retrospective claims data analysis of dosage adjustment patterns of TNF antagonists among patients with rheumatoid arthritis. Curr Med Res Opin 24: 2229–2240.
49. Du Pan SM, Dehler S, Ciurea A, Ziswiler HR, Gabay C, et al. (2009) Comparison of drug retention rates and causes of drug discontinuation between anti-tumor necrosis factor agents in rheumatoid arthritis. Arthritis Rheum 61: 560–568.

50. Kristensen LE, Saxne T, Nilsson JA, Geborek P (2006) Impact of concomitant DMARD therapy on adherence to treatment with etanercept and infliximab in rheumatoid arthritis. results from a six-year observational study in southern Sweden. Arthritis Res Ther 8: R174.
51. Marchesoni A, Zaccara E, Gorla R, Bazzani C, Sarzi-Puttini P, et al. (2009) TNF-alpha antagonist survival rate in a cohort of rheumatoid arthritis patients observed under conditions of standard clinical practice. Ann N Y Acad Sci 1173: 837–846.
52. Brocq O, Roux CH, Albert C, Breuil V, Aknouche N, et al. (2007) TNFalpha antagonist continuation rates in 442 patients with inflammatory joint disease. Joint Bone Spine 74: 148–154.
53. Kristensen LE, Saxne T, Geborek P (2006) The LUNDEX, a new index of drug efficacy in clinical practice: Results of a five-year observational study of treatment with infliximab and etanercept among rheumatoid arthritis patients in southern Sweden. Arthritis Rheum 54: 600–606.
54. Ostergaard M, Unkerskov J, Linde L, Krogh NS, Ravn T, et al. (2007) Low remission rates but long drug survival in rheumatoid arthritis patients treated with infliximab or etanercept: Results from the nationwide Danish DANBIO database. Scand J Rheumatol 36: 151–154.
55. Yazici Y, Krasnokutsky S, Barnes JP, Hines PL, Wang J, et al. (2009) Changing patterns of tumor necrosis factor inhibitor use in 9074 patients with rheumatoid arthritis. J Rheumatol 36: 907–913.
56. Donner A, Klar N (2000) Design and analysis of cluster randomization trials in health research. London: Arnold. 178 p.
57. Zhang J, Shan Y, Reed G, Kremer J, Greenberg JD, et al. (2011) Thresholds in disease activity for switching biologics in rheumatoid arthritis patients: Experience from a large US cohort. Arthritis Care Res 63: 1672–1679. 10.1002/acr.20643; 10.1002/acr.20643.

22

Identification of Urinary Peptide Biomarkers Associated with Rheumatoid Arthritis

Angelique Stalmach[1*], Hanna Johnsson[2], Iain B. McInnes[3], Holger Husi[1], Julie Klein[4], Mohammed Dakna[4], William Mullen[1], Harald Mischak[1,4], Duncan Porter[3]

1 University of Glasgow, Institute of Cardiovascular and Medical Sciences, Glasgow, United Kingdom, 2 Western General Infirmary, Edinburgh, United Kingdom, 3 University of Glasgow, Institute of Infection, Immunity and Inflammation, Glasgow, United Kingdom, 4 Mosaiques-Diagnostics GmbH, Hannover, Germany

Abstract

Early diagnosis and treatment of rheumatoid arthritis are associated with improved outcomes but current diagnostic tools such as rheumatoid factor or anti-citrullinated protein antibodies have shown limited sensitivity. In this pilot study we set out to establish a panel of urinary biomarkers associated with rheumatoid arthritis using capillary electrophoresis coupled to mass spectrometry. We compared the urinary proteome of 33 participants of the Scottish Early Rheumatoid Arthritis inception cohort study with 30 healthy controls and identified 292 potential rheumatoid arthritis-specific peptides. Amongst them, 39 were used to create a classifier model using support vector machine algorithms. Specific peptidic fragments were differentially excreted between groups; fragments of protein S100-A9 and gelsolin were less abundant in rheumatoid arthritis while fragments of uromodulin, complement C3 and fibrinogen were all increasingly excreted. The model generated was subsequently tested in an independent test-set of 31 samples. The classifier demonstrated a sensitivity of 88% and a specificity of 93% in diagnosing the condition, with an area under the receiver operating characteristic curve of 0.93 ($p<0.0001$). These preliminary results suggest that urinary biomarkers could be useful in the early diagnosis of rheumatoid arthritis. Further studies are currently being undertaken in larger cohorts of patients with rheumatoid arthritis and other athridities to assess the potential of the urinary peptide based classifier in the early detection of rheumatoid arthritis.

Editor: Paul Proost, University of Leuven, Rega Institute, Belgium

Funding: The Scottish Early Rheumatoid Arthritis (SERA) inception cohort and biobank is funded by the Chief Scientist's Office, Scottish Government and Pfizer; neither funder was involved in this study design, execution, analysis, decision to publish or preparation of the manuscript.

Competing Interests: HM is the founder and co-owner of Mosaiques Diagnostics, who developed the CE-MS technology. This does not alter the authors' adherence to all the PLOS ONE policies on sharing data and materials.

* Email: Angelique.Stalmach@glasgow.ac.uk

These authors contributed equally to this work.

Introduction

Rheumatoid arthritis (RA) is a systemic autoimmune condition that primarily affects the joints and can lead to joint damage, disability and premature mortality. Early diagnosis and treatment of RA are associated with better patient response to treatment [1,2], reduced co-morbidity and lower mortality [3]. In the initial stages of the disease, accurate diagnosis can be challenging. In 2010, the American College of Rheumatology and European League Against Rheumatism (ACR/EULAR) developed a new approach to classifying RA based on scoring criteria [4]. This classification system improves sensitivity for the early detection of the disease compared to the former ACR 1987 classification criteria. However it has been shown to lead to both over- and under-diagnosis [5]. The biomarkers rheumatoid factor (RF) and anti-citrullinated protein antibodies (ACPA) form one of the current classification criteria, but in isolation the markers lack sensitivity [6]. Novel biomarkers which could assist in accurate, early diagnosis would facilitate more effective early intervention whilst limiting exposure to disease modifying therapy in patients otherwise destined to remit spontaneously. Recent studies have sought novel RA biomarkers in peripheral blood and synovial fluid [7–10]. Despite early promises, none of these approaches have yet yielded combinations of biomarkers with better specificity and sensitivity than ACPA used alone.

A novel approach for identification of diagnostic biomarkers in RA uses capillary electrophoresis coupled to mass spectrometry (CE-MS). This method has already enabled the identification of urinary biomarker classifiers for the diagnosis of diseases like chronic kidney disease [11], acute kidney injury [12], stroke [13], and cardiovascular diseases [14]. It allows classification of case versus control groups with good accuracy [15]. The use of urine rather than blood for the identification of biomarkers has several advantages, including non-invasive sample collection, a high stability due to absence of proteolytic agents and a low dynamic range of analyte concentration which facilitates the detection and quantification of peptides [16]. Furthermore, discovery of proteomic biomarkers may be useful in understanding the molecular mechanisms involved in the onset and progression of disease [17]. In this study, we aimed to identify potential biomarkers for the early diagnosis of RA. We hypothesized that RA-specific peptides would be measured in urine samples of patients and produce a unique fingerprint of peptides compared to healthy controls. This was achieved by comparing the urinary peptide profile of patients with RA with that of healthy controls. Our secondary objective was to identify the proteases involved in generating the RA-specific peptide fragments, using an in silico approach.

Materials and Methods

RA population and data collection

Patients are recruited to the Scottish Early RA (SERA) inception cohort if they have newly diagnosed undifferentiated arthritis or rheumatoid arthritis. Detailed demographic and clinical data are recorded; samples of blood, urine and synovial fluid are taken every 6 months, and stored for future analyses.

Patients enrolled in SERA who fulfilled the ACR/EULAR diagnostic criteria for RA at diagnosis were identified, and 25 ACPA positive (>20 units) and 24 ACPA negative (<7 units) patients were selected at random. Clinical information on gender, age, disease duration from onset of symptoms, 28 joint count disease activity score (DAS28) [18], health assessment questionnaire (HAQ), C-reactive protein (CRP), ACPA and RF values were collected. Laboratory tests had been analysed in routine National Health Service (NHS) laboratories across Scotland.

Control population

Controls were volunteers who agreed to participate in nutritional-based interventions, were at least 18 years of age, non-smokers and in general good health. They were enrolled in other on-going proteomic studies and had given written informed consent prior to starting the studies.

Ethics statement

Cases provided enduring and generic written consent for their samples to be used in analyses, and the SERA study was approved by the West of Scotland Research Ethics Committee. Controls gave written informed consent prior to participating in on-going proteomic studies approved by the University of Glasgow Faculty of Medicine Ethics Committee.

Urine collection

For both cases and controls, spot urine samples were collected in sterile containers at the time of the study visit. One millilitre aliquots of unprocessed samples were stored at −80°C prior to being processed as recommended by the European Kidney and Urine Proteomics and Human Kidney and Urine Proteome Project and described previously [16]. Most samples were frozen within 4 hours of collection but samples from remote parts of Scotland were couriered in chilled containers overnight. Once frozen, samples were left to defrost at room temperature, occasionally mixing by gentle inversion, and samples were defrosted only once.

Urinary proteomic analysis

The urine samples were prepared as previously described by removing large proteins (>20 kDa), urea, electrolytes and salts, and by enriching polypeptides [11]. Briefly, 700 µL of urine were defrosted with the addition of 0.1% PMSF saturated in ethanol and diluted with 700 µL of a solution containing 2 M urea, 0.1 M NaCl, 10 mM NH_4OH and 0.02% SDS. The mixture was then filtered through a 20 kDa MW cut-off ultra-centrifugation filter device (Sartorius Stedim UK Ltd, United Kingdom) at 2,600 × *g* for one hour at 4°C. A volume of 1.1 mL of the filtrate was then loaded onto a pre-equilibrated PD-10 desalting column (GE Healthcare, Sweden) and eluted using 0.01% aqueous NH_4OH. The eluate was subsequently freeze-dried and stored at 4°C prior to being resuspended in HPLC-grade water to a final protein concentration of 2 mg/mL for capillary electrophoresis-mass spectrometry analysis.

Table 1. Baseline characteristics of the training and test set populations (case and control)[1].

	RA cohort		Controls	
	Training set (n = 33)	**Test set (n = 16)**	**Training set (n = 30)**	**Test set (n = 15)**
Age (Years)[2]	59 (39; 65)	58 (55; 68)	31 (23; 60)	36 (29; 58)
Female[3]	23 (70%)	13 (76%)	11 (37%)	10 (67%)
Duration of disease (Days)	113 (74; 261)	91 (54; 225)	nd	nd
ACPA positive	16 (48%)	9 (56%)	nd	nd
ACPA (Units)	5.7 (3; 161)	47 (2; 214)	nd	nd
RF[4] positive	11 (73%)	6 (86%)	nd	nd
RF[4] (Units)	15 (11; 30)	20 (18; 55)	nd	nd
DAS28 score	5.5 (4.3; 6.2)	4.5 (3.9; 5.5)	nd	nd
HAQ score	1.1 (0.8; 1.9)	1.1 (0.5; 1.6)	nd	nd
CRP abnormal	19 (63%)	11 (73%)	nd	nd
CRP (mg/l)	20.5 (6. 0; 41.0)	19 (8.3; 38.5)	nd	nd

nd, not determined; ACPA, anti-citrullinated protein antibodies; RF, rheumatoid factor; DAS28, 28 joint count disease activity score; HAQ, health assessment questionnaire score; CRP, C-reactive protein.

[1]Differences between training set and test set within both RA and control groups were not statistically significant (Mann-Whitney for continuous values and Chi Square for categorical values; $p<0.05$) with the exception for the proportion of female in the control group between the training and test sets ($p<0.05$).

[2]Difference in the median age value between groups is statistically significant between RA and control groups of the training set ($p = 0.0023$) and between RA and control groups of the test set ($p = 0.0059$).

[3]Difference in the gender distribution between groups is statistically significant between RA and control groups of the training set ($p<0.01$) but not between RA and control groups of the test set ($p>0.05$) (Chi Square test).

[4]Data missing for 18 patients in the training set and 9 patients in test set, percentage refers to proportion of patients tested.

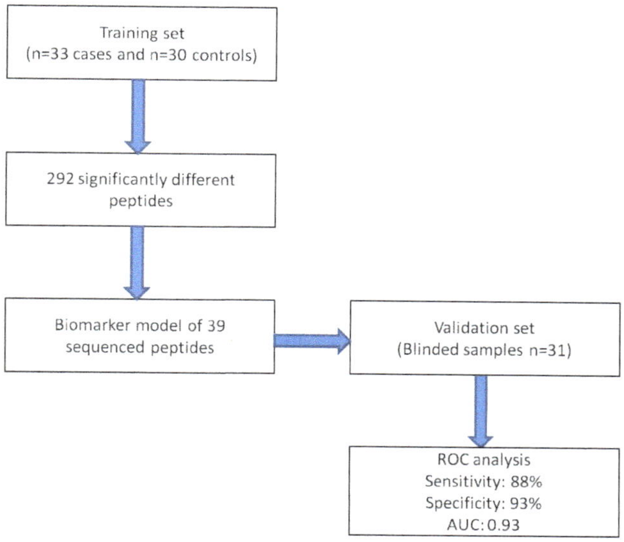

Figure 1. Work flow used for the determination of urinary biomarkers associated with RA.

Capillary Electrophoresis-Mass Spectrometry (CE-MS) analysis and Data processing

CE-MS analysis was performed as previously described using a P/ACE MDQ capillary electrophoresis system (Beckman Coulter, Fullerton, USA) on line coupled to a MicroTOF MS (BrukerDaltonic, Bremen, Germany) [19]. Samples were injected hydrodynamically at 2.0 psi for 99 sec (ca. 250 nL) and separation of peptides was achieved by reverse polarity at 25 kV for the first 30 min, and with increasing pressure (up to 0.5 psi) for another 34 min. The cartridge temperature was maintained at 25°C. Running buffer contained 79:20:1 (v/v) deionised filtered (0.2 μm) water, acetonitrile and formic acid. Sheath liquid consisted of 30% 2-propanol and 0.4% formic acid in deionised filtered (0.2 μm) water. The ESI sprayer (Agilent Technologies, Palo Alto, CA, USA) was grounded, and the ion spray interface potential was set between −4 and −4.5 kV. Spectra were accumulated every 3 seconds over a range of mass-to-charge ratios from 50 to 3000. Details on accuracy, precision, selectivity, sensitivity, reproducibility, and stability of the CE-MS method have been previously described [11,20]. MosaiquesVisu was used to analyse the CE-MS data [21]. Peptides are initially characterised by their molecular mass, CE-migration time, and ion signal intensity (amplitude) value. Internal standard peptides were used for calibration, as previously described [22]. All detected peptides were deposited, matched, and annotated in a MicrosoftSQL database, allowing for further analysis and comparison between case and control groups.

Statistical analysis and classifier development

Of the initial cohort of RA patients (n = 49) and healthy controls (n = 45), 33 cases and 30 controls were selected at random to establish a panel of RA-specific urinary peptides. After testing for normal distribution, continuous data were compared by the Mann-Whitney test, as this test has proven to be of superior statistical power in proteomics datasets [23]. This test is particularly suited for proteomics data as such data suffer from missing values leading to non-normal skewed distributions even after log-transformation. A p-value of <0.05 was considered to be statistically significant, after correction for multiple testing. Only peptides with a frequency of at least 40% in either group were considered for further analysis. In order to control for the false discovery rate at 0.05, the p-values were adjusted by the Benjamini and Hochberg method [24] implemented in the Bioconductor package multtest [25].

Correlative association between significantly excreted peptides and potential confounding factors such as age and gender was assessed in both case and control groups using Spearman's rank coefficient correlation (age) and Mann-Whitney test (gender) followed by p-value adjustment using the Benjamini and Hochberg method as previously described. Due to the small sample size of the study, we further analyzed the correlation of the potential biomarkers with age and gender in a cohort of 500 healthy patients from our database.

Significantly differentially excreted peptides were subsequently identified using MS-MS and used to develop a biomarker model to classify between RA and non-RA patients. The remaining 31 samples (16 cases and 15 controls) were used as an independent validation subset in the support-vector-machine (SVM) based MosaCluster software [14,19]. The sensitivity, specificity and area under the receiver operating characteristic (ROC) curve of the resulting model were calculated using MedCalc version 12.1.3.0 (MedCalc Software bvba, Belgium).

The SVM classifier uses the log transformed intensities of n peptides as coordinates in an n dimensional space. It then builds an n-1 hyper plane that spans this space by performing a quadratic programming optimization of a Lagrangian using the training labels only while allowing for samples to lie on the wrong side of the plane. For such misclassification, the SVM introduces a cost parameter C. Due to the fact that non separable problems in low dimensions may be separable in higher dimensions, the SVM uses the so-called Kernel-trick to transform the samples to a higher dimensional space. Mosacluster uses the standard radial basis functions as kernel. These functions are Gaussians with the parameter gamma controlling for the width. The optimal parameters C and gamma are found via a leave-one-out cross validation error estimation. Implantation of SMV is popular in data mining software, and the Kernel-based Machine Learning Lab (kernlab) package in R in particular is used as a versatile tool for building SVM-based classifiers [26].

Proteases prediction

In order to link urinary fragments to the proteases involved in their generation, a predictive analysis was carried out using Proteasix. This is an open-source tool used to predict the proteases involved in naturally occurring peptide generation in silico, as previously described [27]. Briefly, Proteasix is a cleavage site database that can associate proteases with their corresponding cleavage site sequences based on octopeptides (P4P3P2P1-P1′P2′P3′P4′). Each peptide is described by the respective substrate SWISS-PROT identifier or name, peptide start and peptide end. The search predicts protease association with 0 and up to 3 mismatches in the cleavage site sequence. After entering the peptide list, the tool aligns each peptide sequence with the full-length SWISS-PROT sequence to identify N- and C-term cleavage sites. Each cleavage site is searched in the database to retrieve all predicted protease/cleavage site combinations. This required the generation of a discovery matrix of unique peptide versus protease, and every matrix point is either 0 (no cut), 1 (cut) or 2 (cuts both N-and C-terminus). The matrix was subsequently divided between peptides that were up- or down-regulated based on the absolute fold-change values, and the occurrences were computed by summing the matrix points. Data were assessed using a mathematical approach of frequency analysis. Frequency analysis uses the calculated frequencies of protease association

Table 2. Urinary peptides which were significantly less abundant in patients with RA.

Fold change	Sequence	Identification
0.018	PpGpPGKNGDDGEAGKPG	Collagen alpha-1(I) chain
0.047	SpGERGETGPpGPA	Collagen alpha-1(III) chain
0.074	VADEAQVQKVKELEDLEHLQ	Carboxypeptidase A1
0.117 *	PpGKNGDDGEAGKPGRpGERGppGP	Collagen alpha-1(I) chain
0.138	pGLPGKAGASGFPGTKGEMGmmGPPGPpGP	Collagen alpha-5(IV) chain
0.138	HAHKLRVDPVNF	Hemoglobin subunit alpha
0.151	GEAGKpGEQGVpGDLGApGP	Collagen alpha-1(I) chain
0.151	TGLSmDGGGSPKGDVDP	Sodium/potassium-transporting ATPase subunit gamma
0.176	VVHTNYDEY	Alpha-1-microglobulin
0.183	EAGENQKQPEKNAGPTAR	C-X-C motif chemokine 16
0.270 *	TTLASHSTK	Mucin-1 subunit alpha
0.312	NpGPPGpSGSpGKDGPpGPAG	Collagen alpha-1(III) chain
0.383	EDLDTNADKQLSFEEF	Protein S100-A9
0.399 *	NRGERGSEGSPGHpGQPGPpGPPGApGP	Collagen alpha-1(III) chain
0.421 *	PpGKNGDDGEAGKPGRpGERGppGPQ	Collagen alpha-1(I) chain
0.432 *	EGSpGRDGSpGAKGDRG	Collagen alpha-1(I) chain
0.439	GSpGSpGPDGKTGPpGPAG	Collagen alpha-1(I) chain
0.456	LSSHIANVERVPFDAATLHTSTA	Gelsolin
0.460 *	DQGPVGRTGEVGAVGpPGFAGEKGPSGEAGTAGPpGTpGP	Collagen alpha-2(I) chain
0.460 *	GLpGTGGpPGENGKpGEPGPKG	Collagen alpha-1(III) chain
0.466	SDGLAHLDNLKG	Hemoglobin subunit delta
0.504	DGVPGKDGPRGP	Collagen alpha-1(III) chain
0.512 *	SpGSPGPDGKTGpP	Collagen alpha-1(I) chain
0.514 *	DGPpGRDGQpGHKG	Collagen alpha-2(I) chain
0.540	ApGPAGSRGApGPQGpRGDKGETGERG	Collagen alpha-1(III) chain
0.548	DpGKNGDKG	Collagen alpha-2(I) chain
0.579 *	pPGADGQPGAKGEpGDAGAKGDAGPpGPAGPAGPPGPIG	Collagen alpha-1(I) chain
0.580 *	GEHNPFKGAI	T calcium channel alpha 1G subunit variant 249
0.617	DDGEAGKpGRpG	Collagen alpha-1(I) chain
0.623 *	GKNGDDGEAGKPGRpGERGPpGp	Collagen alpha-1(I) chain
0.632 *	SpGSPGPDGKTGPpGPAG	Collagen alpha-1(I) chain
0.667 *	PpGPPGPpGPPGPPS	Collagen alpha-1(I) chain
0.700 *	pPGADGQpGAKGEPGDAGAKGDAGPpGPAGPAGPpGPIG	Collagen alpha-1(I) chain
0.733 *	pPGEAGKpGEQGVPGDLG	Collagen alpha-1(I) chain

*Peptides not included in the RA classifying biomarker model.

with peptides per protease in either up- or down-regulated groups. The analysis was done using the normal/equal distribution as a reference. Frequency scores were calculated, per protease, using the absolute ratios of the difference over the sum of the frequencies of peptide occurrences that were found up- and down- regulated, multiplied by the difference of occurrences in the up- and down-regulated groups. This mathematical model provides an indication of the distribution of peptide occurrences from the normal distribution, where clustering of peptides around the normal distribution line being interpreted as a lack of specificity in the protease activity.

Results

Descriptive data

Median and interquartile ranges are shown in Table 1 for age, duration of symptoms, ACPA, RF, DAS28, HAQ and CRP values for the training and test sets. The patients all fulfilled the 2010 ACR/EULAR diagnostic criteria for RA [4], and had a median duration of symptoms of 113 days in the training set and 91 days in the test set. Most patients had moderate to severe disease activity in both groups, with a DAS28 of greater than 3.2 [28]. In the training set, 48% were positive for ACPA compared to 56% in the test set. A preliminary analysis investigating the correlation between DAS28, HAQ and CRP revealed a poor correlation between CRP and DAS28, and CRP and HAQ (coefficient of determination between DAS28 and HAQ of 0.310 with p-

Table 3. Urinary peptides which were found in significantly higher concentration in patients with RA.

Fold change	Sequence	Identification
1.398 *	DGQpGAKGEpGDAGAKGDAGPpGP	Collagen alpha-1(I) chain
1.452 *	EpGSpGENGApGQmGPR	Collagen alpha-1(I) chain
1.522	NSGEpGApGSKGDTGAKGEpGpVG	Collagen alpha-1(I) chain
1.613 *	SGHPGSPGSPGYQGPpGEPGQAGPSGPpGP	Collagen alpha-1(III) chain
1.705	ApGGKGDAGApGERGPpG	Collagen alpha-1(III) chain
1.732 *	NGEpGGKGERGApGEKGEGGPpG	Collagen alpha-1(III) chain
1.749 *	PAPAPPPEPERPKEVE	Myosin light chain 3
1.816	AGERGHPGAPGpSGSpGLPGVPGSMGDMVNYDEIK	Collagen alpha-1(XVI) chain
1.857 *	KGDRGETGpAGPPGApGAPGAPGPVGP	Collagen alpha-1(I) chain
1.960	NGApGEAGRDGNpGNDGPpG	Collagen alpha-2(I) chain
1.984	PpGDEGEmAIISQKGTpGEpGP	Collagen alpha-4(IV) chain
2.074 *	ADGQpGAKGEpGDAGAKGDAGppGP	Collagen alpha-1(I) chain
2.142	SGSVIDQSRVLNLGPITRK	Uromodulin
2.421	QGKTGpPGPPGVVGpQGPTGETGPMGERGHpGPpGP	Collagen alpha-1(V) chain
2.426	NGEpGGKGERGApGEKGEGGppG	Collagen alpha-1(III) chain
2.434 *	GPpGEAGKpGEQGVP	Collagen alpha-1(I) chain
2.607 *	GPpGKNGDDGEAGKPG	Collagen alpha-1(I) chain
2.942	TPEEKSAVTALWGKVNVDEV	Hemoglobin subunit beta
3.084	IDQSRVLNLGPITRK	Uromodulin
3.242 *	ADGQpGAKGEpGDAGAKGDAGPpGPAGP	Collagen alpha-1(I) chain
3.681 *	SGEpGApGSKGDTGAKGEpGP	Collagen alpha-1(I) chain
3.699	GEVGpAGSpGSNGApGQRGEPGPQGHAGAQGPPGpPG	Collagen alpha-1(III) chain
3.910 *	GppGPpGPAGKEG	Collagen alpha-1(I) chain
3.928	VIDQSRVLNLGPIT	Uromodulin
4.016	SGSVIDQSRVL	Uromodulin
4.080	NSGEpGApGSKGDTG	Collagen alpha-1(I) chain
4.547 *	GPpGPTGPGGDKGDTGPpGP	Collagen alpha-1(III) chain
5.569 *	LSMDGGGSPKGDVDP	Sodium/potassium-transporting ATPase subunit gamma
7.564 *	GDpGPpGPpGPpG	Collagen alpha-1(XV) chain
8.523	pGPQGPLGKPGAPGEPGPQG	Collagen alpha-1(VIII) chain
8.928	FGASAGTGDLSDNHDIISMK	Vesicular integral-membrane protein VIP36
11.494	EGVQKEDIPPADLSDQVPDTESETRILLQGTPVA	Complement C3
15.096	RPGApGPAGARGNDGATGAAGPPGPTGpAGpP	Collagen alpha-1(I) chain
16.970	DEAGSEADHEGTHSTKRGHAKS	Fibrinogen alpha chain
23.336	FDSDPITVTVPVEV	Clusterin
27.407	NPPKPMPNPNPNHPSSSGS	CD99 antigen

*Peptides not included in the RA classifying biomarker model.

value = 0.001; coefficient of determination between CRP and DAS28 of 0.053 with p-value = 0.124; coefficient of determination between CRP and HAQ of 0.126 with p-value = 0.015).

Urinary biomarkers associated with RA

The work flow used for establishing urinary biomarkers associated with RA is shown in Figure 1. In order to establish potential urinary biomarkers associated with RA, urines samples from 33 RA patients and 30 healthy volunteers were run using CE-MS and analysed for their peptidomic profile.

A total of 292 peptides were significantly differentially regulated in the RA patients compared to controls, after adjustment for multiple testing using the Benjamini-Hochberg procedure for false discovery rate. Of the 292 potential biomarkers, 70 peptides were identified by MS/MS sequencing.

Of these, 34 were found in lower (Table 2) and 36 in higher concentrations (Table 3) in RA patients. Peptide fragments found in significantly lower abundance were identified as protein S100-A9, gelsolin, alpha-1-microglobulin, C-X-C motif chemokine 16, mucin-1 subunit alpha, carboxypeptidase A1 and T calcium channel alpha 1G subunit variant 249. Peptide fragments with higher abundance in RA urine were myosin light chain 3, uromodulin, vesicular integral-membrane protein VIP36, complement 3, fibrinogen alpha chain, clusterin and CD99 antigen. There were also proteins from which peptide fragments were found in both higher and lower concentrations in patients with RA

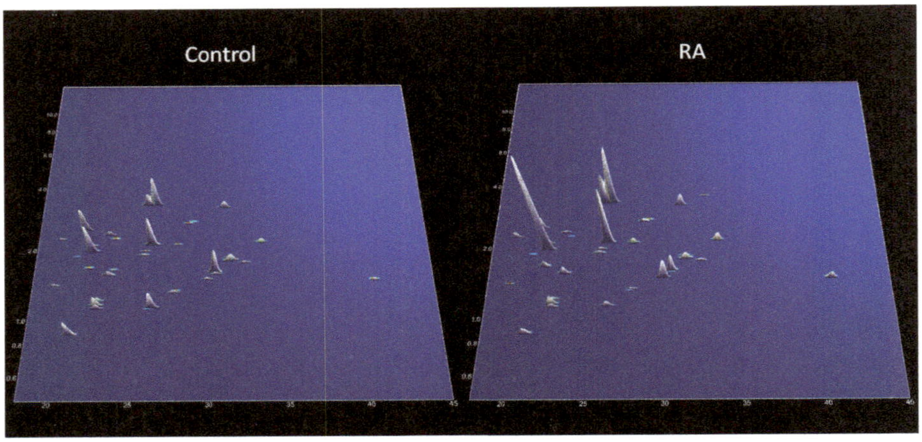

Figure 2. Urinary polypeptide signatures in cases and controls from the validation set based on 39 significantly different sequenced peptides. Normalized molecular weight (500–15000 Da) in logarithmic scale is plotted against normalized migration time (18–45 minutes). The mean signal intensity of the polypeptide peak is given in 3-dimensional depiction (n = 15 controls and 16 cases).

and these were fragments of collagen 1A1 and 1A3, sodium/potassium transporting-ATPase subunit gamma and haemoglobin subunits.

Model of RA-specific classifier biomarkers

As the RA population and the controls showed systematic differences in age and gender, their confounding aspect was checked by correlating each of the 70 biomarkers with age and gender in a cohort of 500 healthy patients from our database. This resulted in 31 biomarkers showing a correlation with age, gender or both (see Table S1). These biomarkers were therefore excluded from the RA classifier biomarker model. The biomarker model was established using the remaining 39 sequenced peptides that were significantly different between controls and cases. Accuracy of the model in the training set was 100% when tested employing complete take-one-out crossvalidation.

When tested on the blinded test set of 31 samples (16 cases and 15 controls), the proteomic signal was significantly different between groups, and the polypeptidic profiles obtained are shown in Figure 2. Accuracy of the model in the independent test set was

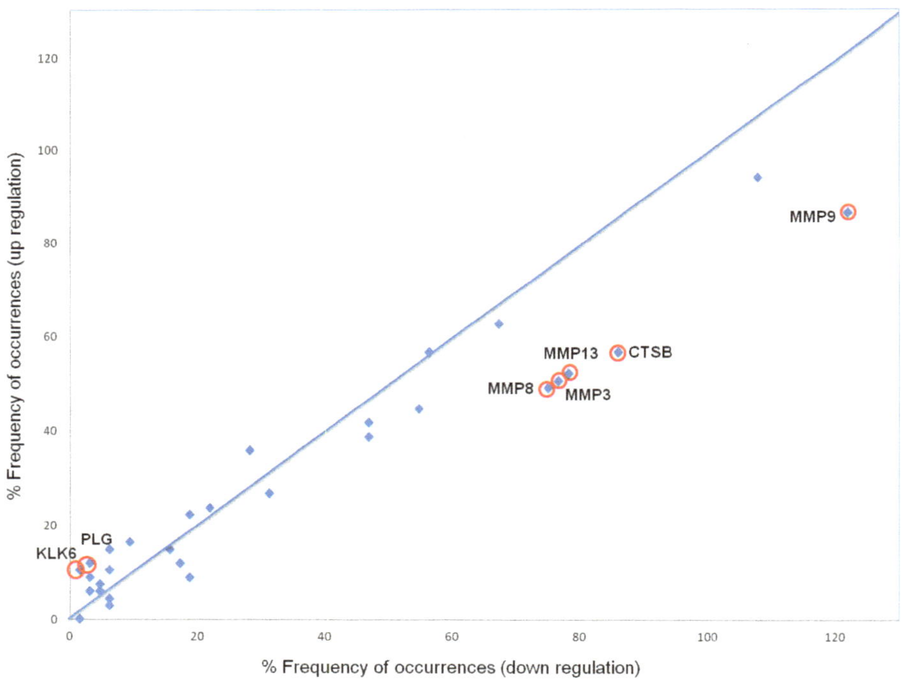

Figure 3. Graphical representation of the frequency distribution of proteases with modified activity associated with RA. Percentage frequency of peptide occurrences in the down-regulation group is plotted on the x-axis, whereas the percentage frequency of occurrences in the up-regulated group is plotted on the y-axis. Circled data points represent the proteases which activity is the most affected in RA compared to that of healthy controls (see Table 4).

Table 4. Predictive analysis of changes in protease activity associated with peptides differentially regulated in RA [1].

Protease	occ(up) [N(up) = 67]	occ(down) [N(down) = 64]	% frequency (up)	% frequency (down)	% frequency difference ratio	Frequency scores
Kallikrein 6	**7**	**1**	**10.5**	**1.6**	**74.0**	**443.9**
Plasminogen	**8**	**2**	**11.9**	**3.1**	**58.5**	**351.1**
Cathepsin B	**38**	**55**	**56.7**	**85.9**	**20.5**	**−348.2**
MMP9	**58**	**78**	**86.6**	**121.9**	**16.9**	**−338.8**
MMP8	**33**	**48**	**49.3**	**75.0**	**20.7**	**−310.8**
MMP13	**34**	**49**	**50.8**	**76.6**	**20.3**	**−304.2**
MMP3	**35**	**50**	**52.2**	**78.1**	**19.9**	**−297.9**
Prolyl endopeptidase	10	4	14.9	6.3	41.0	245.8
ADAMTS4	6	12	9.0	18.8	35.4	−212.1
Kallikrein 4	6	2	9.0	3.1	48.3	193.1
Granzyme A	11	6	16.4	9.4	27.3	136.5
KLK3	0	1	0.0	1.6	100.0	−100.0
MMP20	7	4	10.5	6.3	25.1	75.4
Cathepsin L1	24	18	35.8	28.1	12.0	72.2
Thimet oligopeptidase	2	4	3.0	6.3	35.4	−70.7
MMP25	4	2	6.0	3.1	31.3	62.6
Thrombin	4	2	6.0	3.1	31.3	62.6
Signal peptidase complex catalytic subunit	8	11	11.9	17.2	18.0	−54.0
MMP14	30	35	44.8	54.7	10.0	−49.8
Kallikrein 2	5	3	7.5	4.7	22.8	45.7
MMP12	63	69	94.0	107.8	6.8	−41.0
MMP1	26	30	38.8	46.9	9.4	−37.7
Cathepsin S	15	12	22.4	18.8	8.8	26.5
Triptidyl-peptidase 1	3	4	4.5	6.3	16.5	−16.5
ADAMTS5	18	20	26.9	31.3	7.5	−15.1
Kallikrein 5	4	3	6.0	4.7	12.0	12.0
MMP2	28	30	41.8	46.9	5.7	−11.5
Cathepsin K	16	14	23.9	21.9	4.4	8.8
MMP7	42	43	62.7	67.2	3.5	−3.5
Meprin A	38	36	56.7	56.3	0.4	0.8
Calpain 2	10	10	14.9	15.6	2.3	0.0
Neprilysin	10	10	14.9	15.6	2.3	0.0

[1]Frequency distribution analysis based on all peptides (n = 131).
Mathematical calculations are based on the following parameter and calculations:
occ(up) = Sum of all occurrences for each individual protease in the up-regulated peptides,
occ(down) = Sum of all occurrences for each individual protease in the down-regulated peptides,
N(up) = Total number of peptides being up-regulated,
N(down) = Total number of peptides being down-regulated,
% frequency(up) = (occ(up)/N(up)) * 100.
% frequency(down) = (occ(down)/N(down)) * 100.
% frequency difference ratio = | ((freq%(up) − freq%(down))/(freq%(up)+freq%(down)) * 100 |.
Frequency scores = %freq * (occ(up)-occ(down)).

91%, and an area under the curve (AUC) of 0.93 on ROC analysis. Median value of the 39 biomarker classifier model was 0.955 (−2.563; 2.394) with sensitivity of 88% and specificity of 93% for identification of RA ($p<0.0001$). Median values (range) of the classifier model obtained for the case and control groups were 1.542 (0.175; 2.394) and −0.087 (−2.563; 1.809) respectively.

Prediction of changes in protease activity based on RA-associated urinary biomarkers

Predicted changes in protease activity, based on the association between a protease and its corresponding cleavage site sequence in the octapeptide form, was carried out on peptides which were significantly differentially regulated on the entire cohort of cases (n = 49) and controls (n = 45). Proteasix search and subsequent analysis resulted in the identification of 131 peptides associated with 32 proteases, resulting in 1271 protease-peptide pairs. The frequency distribution analysis presented here (computed as frequency scores) provides a mathematical modelling of the data taking into account the frequency of peptide occurrences per protease weighed by the difference of occurrences. This analysis, as opposed to a statistical approach based on chi-squared frequency distribution or test of independency, takes into account not only the frequency of distribution but also the difference of occurrences, therefore discarding proteases resulting in a similar number of peptides found equally up- and down- regulated. As plotted in Figure 3, proteases found the furthest away from the normal distribution line (demonstrating an increased specificity in cleavage activity) and with a greater difference in the number of occurrences between the up- and down- regulated groups (as indicated by the higher frequency score in Table 4, with negative scores emphasising a down-regulation) are potential candidates involved in the pathophysiology of RA. Amongst the 32 proteases associated with urinary fragments of RA-related peptides, the potential predicted activities of kallikrein 6 (KLK6) and plasminogen (PLG) were up-regulated, whereas the associated activities of matrix metalloproteinase 3 (MMP3), MMP8, MMP9 and MMP13 and cathepsin B were down-regulated in cases compared to controls (Table 4).

Discussion

Based on the comparison of 33 newly diagnosed patients with RA and 30 healthy controls, we were able to identify 292 potential urinary biomarkers associated with the diagnosis of RA. Of these, 70 were sequenced and identified by MS/MS, and 39 used to develop a biomarker model for RA after adjusting for age and gender. This is the first study to show that a urinary biomarker model has potential to assist with the early diagnosis of RA, with good sensitivity and specificity (88% and 93% respectively). Although repeat analysis with better matched controls is required to evaluate if the model is truly specific for RA, these initial results compare favourably to ACPA [6]. Furthermore, a panel of biomarkers like this usually performs better as a diagnostic tool than single or few biomarkers alone [29].

Urinary peptides and protein fragments are the end products of upstream proteolytic processes so the differential urinary excretion of peptides between controls and RA patients may indicate their role in the pathophysiology of the disease. Some of the protein fragments identified originated from proteins known to be up/down regulated in RA, including collagens [30,31], gelsolin [32], and fibrinogen alpha [7,33]. To identify which proteases might be responsible for the urinary biomarkers identified, we performed a Proteasix prediction analysis. This suggested an increased activity of KLK-6 and PLG and a reduced activity of cathepsin B, MMP3, MMP8, MMP9 and MMP13.

The kallikrein-kinin system with activation plasma (KLKB1) as well as tissue kallikrein (KLK1) has been implicated in inflammation, and raised levels of both have been found in plasma and synovial fluid of patients with RA [34–38]. Less is known about the role of KLK6 in the pathogenesis of RA, but KLK6 has been found in synovial fluid in patients with psoriatic arthritis [39], and KLK6 promotes survival of murine lymphocytes with actions on proteinase-activated receptor 1 [40].

PLG has been implicated in early RA and although the mechanism remains to be fully established, it may cleave components of the complement system and activate protease-activated receptors and MMPs [41]. Both MMPs and cathepsin B contribute to joint destruction in RA [42,43] and elevated levels of serum MMP1 and MMP3 correlate well with the progression of erosive disease in early disease [44]. It is therefore unexpected that the protease prediction analysis consistently suggested down-regulation of MMPs and cathepsin B in our RA cohort. Future studies are required to evaluate and explain these findings which may reflect technical elements of our approach or allude to as yet unexplained renal biology in RA patients.

Further validation is also needed to confirm the diagnostic value of urinary biomarkers in early RA. In particular, comparison should be made between the urinary proteome of patients with RA and aged and gender matched patients with other chronic inflammatory conditions and arthritidies. This will establish if the peptides and peptidases identified are specific to RA or reflect chronic inflammation and joint degradation in general. It would also be informative to take into account disease characteristics such as the 2010 classification score and the presence of erosions. This was not possible in the current study due to the small sample size, which also has implications for the power of the study as a whole. It will therefore be necessary to use a bigger and better characterised cohort when validating our findings. This will allow for estimations of sensitivity and specificity of our biomarker profile for diagnostic purposes and will also allow more powerful correlations between individual peptides and disease markers and characteristics. The current study is based on a cross-sectional design but a longitudinal design would be required to monitor disease progression, to investigate if the urinary proteome at baseline is predictive of outcome. A longitudinal design would also allow monitoring changes in the urinary proteome over time in the same patients with correlation to clinical assessments and response to treatment. In cardiovascular disease, for example, it has been shown that the urinary biomarker pattern becomes healthier in patients who had received treatment [14].

Supporting Information

Table S1 31 biomarkers showed a correlation with age, gender or both.

Author Contributions

Conceived and designed the experiments: DP HM IM. Performed the experiments: AS. Analyzed the data: AS HH HJ MD. Contributed reagents/materials/analysis tools: JK WM. Wrote the paper: AS DP HJ. Obtained SERA samples: HJ.

References

1. Anderson JJ, Wells G, Verhoeven AC, Felson DT (2000) Factors predicting response to treatment in rheumatoid arthritis: the importance of disease duration. Arthritis Rheum 43: 22–29.
2. O'Dell JR (2002) Treating rheumatoid arthritis early: a window of opportunity? Arthritis Rheum 46: 283–285.
3. Symmons DP, Jones MA, Scott DL, Prior P (1998) Longterm mortality outcome in patients with rheumatoid arthritis: early presenters continue to do well. The Journal of Rheumatology 25: 1072–1077.
4. Aletaha D, Neogi T, Silman AJ, Funovits J, Felson DT et al. (2010) 2010 Rheumatoid arthritis classification criteria: an American College of Rheumatology/European League Against Rheumatism collaborative initiative. Annals of the Rheumatic Diseases 69: 1580–1588.
5. Cader MZ, Filer A, Hazlehurst J, de Pablo P, Buckley CD et al. (2011) Performance of the 2010 ACR/EULAR criteria for rheumatoid arthritis: comparison with 1987 ACR criteria in a very early synovitis cohort. Ann Rheum Dis 70: 949–955.
6. Whiting PF, Smidt N, Sterne JA, Harbord R, Burton A et al. (2010) Systematic review: accuracy of anti-citrullinated Peptide antibodies for diagnosing rheumatoid arthritis. Ann Intern Med 152: W155–W166.

7. Chandra PE, Sokolove J, Hipp BG, Lindstrom TM, Elder JT et al. (2011) Novel multiplex technology for diagnostic characterization of rheumatoid arthritis. Arthritis Res Ther 13: R102.
8. De Franceschi L, Bosello S, Scambi C, Biasi D, De Santis M et al. (2011) Proteome analysis of biological fluids from autoimmune-rheumatological disorders. Proteomics Clin Appl 5: 78–89.
9. Kriegsmann M, Seeley EH, Schwarting A, Kriegsmann J, Otto M et al. (2012) MALDI MS imaging as a powerful tool for investigating synovial tissue. Scand J Rheumatol 41: 305–309.
10. Wild N, Karl J, Grunert VP, Schmitt RI, Garczarek U et al. (2008) Diagnosis of rheumatoid arthritis: multivariate analysis of biomarkers. Biomarkers 13: 88–105.
11. Good DM, Zurbig P, Argiles A, Bauer HW, Behrens G et al. (2010) Naturally occurring human urinary peptides for use in diagnosis of chronic kidney disease. Mol Cell Proteomics 9: 2424–2437.
12. Metzger J, Kirsch T, Schiffer E, Ulger P, Mentes E et al. (2010) Urinary excretion of twenty peptides forms an early and accurate diagnostic pattern of acute kidney injury. Kidney Int 78: 1252–1262.
13. Dawson J, Walters M, Delles C, Mischak H, Mullen W (2012) Urinary proteomics to support diagnosis of stroke. PLoS One 7: e35879.
14. Delles C, Schiffer E, von Zur Muhlen C, Peter K, Rossing P et al. (2010) Urinary proteomic diagnosis of coronary artery disease: identification and clinical validation in 623 individuals. J Hypertens 28: 2316–2322.
15. Mischak H, Schanstra JP (2011) CE-MS in biomarker discovery, validation, and clinical application. Proteomics – Clinical Applications 5: 9–23.
16. Mischak H, Kolch W, Aivaliotis M, Bouyssié D, Court M et al. (2010) Comprehensive human urine standards for comparability and standardization in clinical proteome analysis. Proteomics – Clinical Applications 4: 464–478.
17. Mischak H, Rossing P (2010) Proteomic biomarkers in diabetic nephropathy-reality or future promise? Nephrology Dialysis Transplantation 25: 2843–2845.
18. Prevoo ML, van 't Hof MA, Kuper HH, van Leeuwen MA, van de Putte LB et al. (1995) Modified disease activity scores that include twenty-eight-joint counts. Development and validation in a prospective longitudinal study of patients with rheumatoid arthritis. Arthritis Rheum 38: 44–48.
19. Carty DM, Siwy J, Brennand JE, Zurbig P, Mullen W et al. (2011) Urinary proteomics for prediction of preeclampsia. Hypertension 57: 561–569.
20. Mischak H, Vlahou A, Ioannidis JP (2013) Technical aspects and inter-laboratory variability in native peptide profiling: the CE-MS experience. Clin Biochem 46: 432–443.
21. Wittke S, Fliser D, Haubitz M, Bartel S, Krebs R et al. (2003) Determination of peptides and proteins in human urine with capillary electrophoresis-mass spectrometry, a suitable tool for the establishment of new diagnostic markers. Journal of Chromatography A 1013: 173–181.
22. Jantos-Siwy J, Schiffer E, Brand K, Schumann G, Rossing K et al. (2009) Quantitative urinary proteome analysis for biomarker evaluation in chronic kidney disease. J Proteome Res 8: 268–281.
23. Dakna M, Harris K, Kalousis A, Carpentier S, Kolch W et al. (2010) Addressing the challenge of defining valid proteomic biomarkers and classifiers. BMC Bioinformatics 11.
24. Benjamini Y, Hochberg Y (1995) Controlling the false discovery rate: a practical and powerful approach to multiple testing. Journal of the Royal Statistical Society Series B (Methodological) 57: 289–300.
25. Gentleman R, Carey V, Bates D, Bolstad B, Dettling M et al. (2004) Bioconductor: open software development for computational biology and bioinformatics. Genome Biology 5: R80. 10.1186/gb-2004-5-10-r80.
26. Karatzoglou A, Smola A, Hornik K, Zeileis A (2004) kernlab – An S4 Package for Kernel Methods in R. Journal of Statistical Software 11: 1–20.
27. Klein J, Eales J, Zürbig P, Vlahou A, Mischak H et al. (2013) Proteasix: A tool for automated and large-scale prediction of proteases involved in naturally occurring peptide generation. Proteomics 13: 1077–1082.
28. Fransen J, van Riel PLCM (2005) The Disease Activity Score and the EULAR response criteria. Clin Exp Rheumatol 23: S93–S99.
29. Schiffer E, Bick C, Grizelj B, Pietzker S, SchÂfer W (2012) Urinary proteome analysis for prostate cancer diagnosis: Cost-effective application in routine clinical practice in Germany. International Journal of Urology 19: 118–125.
30. Mullan RH, Matthews C, Bresnihan B, FitzGerald O, King L et al. (2007) Early changes in serum type ii collagen biomarkers predict radiographic progression at one year in inflammatory arthritis patients after biologic therapy. Arthritis & Rheumatism 56: 2919–2928.
31. Verstappen SMM, Poole AR, Ionescu M, King LE, Abrahamowicz M et al. (2006) Radiographic joint damage in rheumatoid arthritis is associated with differences in cartilage turnover and can be predicted by serum biomarkers: an evaluation from 1 to 4 years after diagnosis. Arthritis Research & Therapy 8: R31. 10.1186/ar1882.
32. Osborn T, Verdrengh M, Stossel T, Tarkowski A, Bokarewa M (2008) Decreased levels of the gelsolin plasma isoform in patients with rheumatoid arthritis. Arthritis Research & Therapy 10: R117. 10.1186/ar2520.
33. Zhao X, Okeke N, Sharpe O, Batliwalla F, Lee A et al. (2008) Circulating immune complexes contain citrullinated fibrinogen in rheumatoid arthritis. Arthritis Research & Therapy 10: R94. 10.1186/ar2478.
34. Isordia-Salas I, Pixley RA, Sainz IM, Martinez-Murillo C, Colman RW (2004) The role of plasma high molecular weight kininogen in experimental intestinal and systemic inflammation. Archives of Medical Research 35: 369–377.
35. Rahman MM, Bhoola KD, Elson CJ, Lemon M, Dieppe PA (1995) Identification and functional importance of plasma kallikrein in the synovial fluids of patients with rheumatoid, psoriatic, and osteoarthritis. Annals of the Rheumatic Diseases 54: 345–350.
36. Williams RJ, Henderson LM, Naidoo Y, Cassim B, Elson CJ et al. (1997) Immunocytochemical analysis of tissue kallikrein and the kinin moiety in rheumatoid synovial fluid neutrophils. Rheumatology 36: 420–425.
37. Cassim B, Shaw OM, Mazur M, Misso NL, Naran A et al. (2009) Kallikreins, kininogens and kinin receptors on circulating and synovial fluid neutrophils: role in kinin generation in rheumatoid arthritis. Rheumatology 48: 490–496.
38. Rahman MM, Lemon MJC, Elson CJ, Dieppe PA, Bhoola KD (1994) Proinflammatory role of tissue kallikrein in modulating pain in inflamed joints. British Journal of Rheumatology 34: 88–90.
39. Eissa A, Cretu D, Soosaipillai A, Thavaneswaran A, Pellett F et al. (2013) Serum kallikrein-8 correlates with skin activity, but not psoriatic arthritis, in patients with psoriatic disease. Clin Chem Lab Med 51: 317–325.
40. Scarisbrick IA, Epstein B, Cloud BA, Yoon H, Wu J et al. (2011) Functional role of kallikrein 6 in regulating immune cell survival. PLoS One 6: e18376. doi:10.1371/journal.pone.0018376.
41. Judex MO, Mueller BM (2005) Plasminogen activation/plasmin in rheumatoid arthritis: matrix degradation and more. Am J Pathol 166: 645–647.
42. Vincenti M, Brinckerhoff C (2002) Transcriptional regulation of collagenase (MMP-1, MMP-13) genes in arthritis: integration of complex signaling pathways for the recruitment of gene-specific transcription factors. Arthritis Res 4: 157–164. 10.1186/ar401.
43. Trabandt A, Gay RE, Fassbender HG, Gay S (1991) Cathepsin B in synovial cells at the site of joint destruction in rheumatoid arthritis. Arthritis Rheum 34: 1444–1451.
44. Green MJ, Gough AKS, Devlin J, Smith J, Astin P et al. (2003) Serum MMP-3 and MMP-1 and progression of joint damage in early rheumatoid arthritis. Rheumatology 42: 83–88.

23

Effect of Combination Therapy on Joint Destruction in Rheumatoid Arthritis: A Network Meta-Analysis of Randomized Controlled Trials

Niels Graudal[1]*, Thorbjørn Hubeck-Graudal[2], Simon Tarp[3], Robin Christensen[3,4], Gesche Jürgens[5]

1 Department of Rheumatology IR4242, Copenhagen University Hospital, Rigshospitalet, Denmark, **2** Department of Radiology, Copenhagen University Hospital, Gentofte, Denmark, **3** Musculoskeletal Statistics Unit, the Parker Institute, Department of Rheumatology, Copenhagen University Hospital, Frederiksberg, Denmark, **4** Institute of Sports Science and Clinical Biomechanics, University of Southern Denmark, Odense, Denmark, **5** Department of Clinical Pharmacology, Copenhagen University Hospital, Bispebjerg, Denmark

Abstract

Background: Despite significant cost differences, the comparative effect of combination treatments of disease modifying anti-rheumatic drugs (DMARDs) with and without biologic agents has rarely been examined. Thus we performed a network meta-analysis on the effect of combination therapies on progression of radiographic joint erosions in patients with rheumatoid arthritis (RA).

Methods and Findings: The following combination drug therapies compared versus single DMARD were investigated: Double DMARD: 2 DMARDs (methotrexate, sulfasalazine, leflunomide, injectable gold, cyclosporine, chloroquine, azathioprin, penicillamin) or 1 DMARD plus low dose glucocorticoid (LDGC); triple DMARD: 3 DMARDs or 2 DMARDs plus LDGC; biologic combination: 1 DMARD plus biologic agent (tumor necrosis factor α inhibitor (TNFi) or abatacept or tocilizumab or CD20 inhibitor (CD20i)). Randomized controlled trials were identified in a search of electronic archives of biomedical literature and included in a star-shaped network meta-analysis and reported according to the Preferred Reporting Items for Systematic Reviews and Meta-Analyses (PRISMA) statement protocol. Effects are reported as standardized mean differences (SMD). The effects of data from 39 trials published in the period 1989–2012 were as follows: Double DMARD: −0.32 SMD (CI: −0.42, −0.22); triple DMARD: −0.46 SMD (CI: −0.60, −0.31); 1 DMARD plus TNFi: −0.30 SMD (CI: −0.36, −0.25); 1 DMARD plus abatacept: −0.20 SMD (CI: −0.33, −0.07); 1 DMARD plus tocilizumab: −0.34 SMD (CI: −0.48, −0.20); 1 DMARD plus CD20i: −0.32 SMD (CI: −0.40, −0.24). The indirect comparisons showed similar effects between combination treatments apart from triple DMARD being significantly better than abatacept plus methotrexate (−0.26 SMD (CI: −0.45, −0.07)) and TNFi plus methotrexate (−0.16 SMD (CI: −0.31, −0.01)).

Conclusion: Combination treatment of a biologic agent with 1 DMARD is not superior to 2–3 DMARDs including or excluding LDGC in preventing structural joint damage. Future randomized studies of biologic agents should be compared versus a combination of DMARDs.

Editor: Adrian V. Hernandez, Universidad Peruana de Ciencias Aplicadas (UPC), Peru

Funding: This study was supported by The A.P. Møller Foundation for the Advancement of Medical Science. The Musculoskeletal Statistics Unit, the Parker Institute are supported by grants from the The Oak Foundation, Frederiksberg Hospital, and The Danish Medicines Agency. The A.P.M. Foundation, The Oak Foundation, and The Danish Medicines Agency are non-profit funding sources and had no role in the design and conduct of the study or in the collection, analysis, and interpretation of the data or in the preparation, review, and approval of the manuscript.

Competing Interests: Niels Graudal, Thorbjørn Hubeck-Graudal, Simon Tarp, and Gesche Jürgens had no financial or other conflicts of interest to disclose. On behalf of Robin Christensen, the Parker Institute received consultancies from Axellus, Abbott, BMS, Roche, MSD, Pfizer, norpharma, mundipharma, IPSEN, Cambridge Weight Plan (UK) in the previous 3 years; RC is one of the statistical editors in Cochrane Musculoskeletal Group (CMSG) and is a consultant for Danish Guideline Panels (unrelated to industry) making recommendations on how and when to apply expensive biological therapies in rheumatology, gastroenterology, and dermatology and is a member of the GRADE Working Group. This does not alter the authors' adherence to PLOS ONE policies on sharing data and materials.

* Email: graudal@dadlnet.dk

Introduction

In a meta-analysis of 70 randomized controlled trials (RCTs) of rheumatoid arthritis (RA) patients investigating the effect of drug treatment on radiographic joint destruction (erosions), disease modifying anti rheumatic drugs (DMARDs), low-dose glucocorticoids (LDGC), biologic agents, and combinations of these significantly reduced radiographic progression with a relative effect of 48–84% compared with placebo treatment [1]. Although several biologic agents have been investigated as single therapy, biologic treatment is usually given in combination with a DMARD (typically methotrexate) in order to minimize the risk of developing neutralizing antibodies and to improve efficacy. A biologic agent plus methotrexate is superior to single methotrexate and superior to a single biologic agent [1]. Furthermore a combination of DMARDs is superior to a single DMARD [1]. Due to the lack of combination DMARD arms in the studies of biological drugs

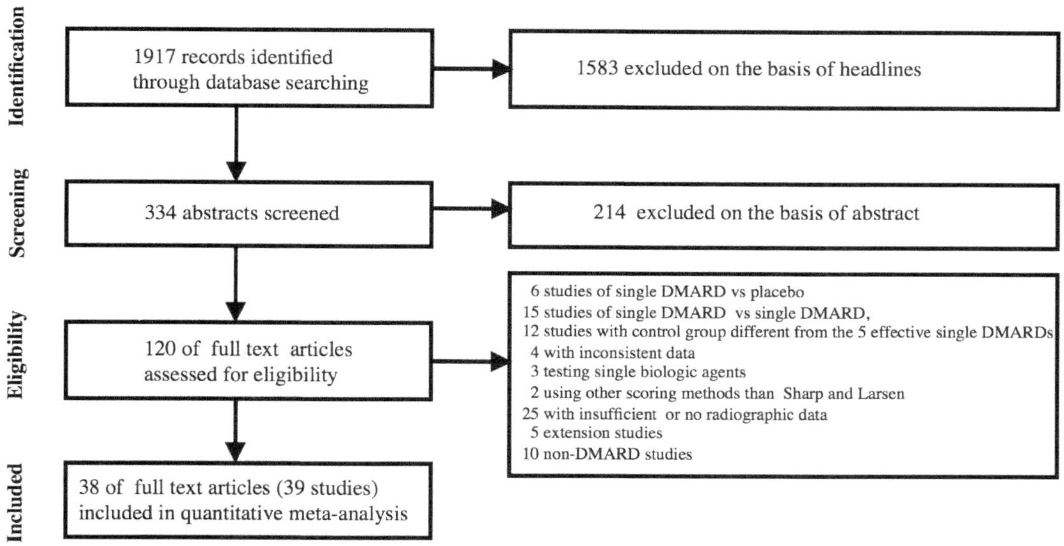

Figure 1. Flow diagram of literature search.

[1,2], the comparative effect of combination treatments with and without biologic agents is unclear.

Hitherto only one randomized trial has directly compared the combination of a biologic agent plus methotrexate with a combination of DMARDs [3]. This study and its follow-up study [4] showed no difference between these two treatment principles. Very recently, additionally three studies have confirmed these observations [5–7]. Due to the shortage of direct comparisons, network (or mixed treatment comparison (MTC)) meta-analyses [8] have been performed to indirectly compare the effects of different biologic agents [9–10]. In contrast, the combination of conventional DMARDs versus biologic agents plus DMARDs have not been analysed in network meta-analyses, although such comparisons seem more interesting due to the cost differences between treatments with and without biologic agents. As our previous study [1] indicated that combination drug treatment was effective irrespective of the drugs involved in the combination, we intended to test the hypothesis that in patients with RA combination treatments of at least two DMARDs, or at least one DMARD plus LDGC or one DMARD plus a biologic agent do not differ significantly in their ability to reduce radiographic joint destruction (erosions) when compared with a single DMARD. Consequently we performed a network meta-analysis of the available direct and indirect evidence from RCTs comparing combination treatment versus single DMARD treatment.

Methods

The analysis is reported according to the Preferred Reporting Items for Systematic reviews and Meta-Analyses (PRISMA) [11] and supplied with an analysis of consistency between indirect and direct evidence [12]. The first version of a protocol for the present study was performed on October 12, 2010 and was based on our previous meta-analysis [1].

Definition of network

Unlike a traditional meta-analysis, which summarizes the results of trials that have evaluated the same treatment/placebo combination (direct comparison), a network meta-analysis consist of a network of treatment effects for all possible pairwise comparisons from RCTs, whether or not they have been compared head to head (i.e. include both direct and indirect comparisons). The fundamental principle of the network is that the indirectly compared treatment effects have a common comparator on which they are anchored. In a simple network there is only one common comparator, whereas more complex networks may have several comparators, which are connected in the network.

The disadvantage of complex networks with many anchor treatments is that at least some of the many different treatment principles usually will be unbalanced and thus contribute to heterogeneity, which may complicate the interpretation of the outcome of the analysis. Furthermore, many of the treatments in a complex network often originates from a single study and thus do not benefit from the statistical power, which is the advantage of a conventional meta-analysis. Thus a complex network meta-analysis may result in numerous pairwise comparisons with low power and a high degree of undefined heterogeneity. Consequently, although the universality of the complex models is appealing, it is important to design a network with caution to avoid creating statistical results of limited clinical value.

For instance the total number of treatment principles in our first analysis [1] was 34. If all these principles should be compared in one network meta-analysis the result would be 561 comparisons, many of which would be clinically uninteresting and most of which would have low power. Inclusion of different doses of the same treatment would increase the problem.

In order to minimize the number of low power comparisons and the amount of heterogeneity we intended to create a simple network focussing on the interesting question and eliminating repetition of established evidence on the ability of drugs to reduce inflammation and joint destruction in RA.

First it is established in several conventional meta-analyses of direct comparisons that a single DMARD is better than placebo. Furthermore direct comparisons have shown that DMARDs generally have similar effects. Finally it has been established in direct comparisons that 2–3 DMARDs are better than one DMARD. In addition treatment principles, which are not fully investigated, should be avoided in the network. For instance the 10 known DMARDs can be combined in 45 different double

Table 1. Study Characteristics and Risk of Bias Factors.

Reference no.	Sequence generation	Concealed allocation	Study blinding	Outcome blinding	Radiographic sequence	Incomplete outcome	Sponsor	Test drug	Treatment group	N_ (radiograph)	Duration RA, years	Scoring system	Initial radiographic score	Radiographic score, Max	Duration of study, months	PARPR	Mean Dose GC mg	Strategy change allowed	DMARD inadequate response
[3]	A	A	C	A	A	C	C	Mt	Single	115	0,5	Sharp	2,0	280	12	1,4	0,03	Yes	No
[3]	A	A	C	A	A	C	C	MtSu	Double	110	0,5	Sharp	2,0	280	12	1,4	0,04	Yes	No
[3]	A	A	C	A	A	C	C	MtSuGc	Triple	125	0,5	Sharp	2,0	280	12	1,4	0,01	Yes	No
[3]	A	A	C	A	A	C	C	InMt	TNFiMt	119	0,5	Sharp	2,0	280	12	1,4	0,02	Yes	No
[17]	B	B	A	A	C	C	C	Mt	Single	49	1,5	Sharp	3,8	280	12	0,9	0,00	No	No
[17]	B	B	A	A	C	C	C	Su	Single	46	0,9	Sharp	2,8	280	12	1,1	0,00	No	No
[17]	B	B	A	A	C	C	C	MtSu	Double	49	0,9	Sharp	4,3	280	12	1,7	0,00	No	No
[18]	B	B	C	A	C	C	A	Mt	Single	30	0,9	Sharp	1,2	280	12	0,5	2,10	Yes	No
[18]	B	B	C	A	C	C	A	MtCs	Double	28	0,9	Sharp	1,1	280	12	0,4	2,10	Yes	No
[19]	B	B	C	A	B	C	B	Cs	Single	30	1,3	Larsen	14,5	200	12	5,6	2,20	No	No
[19]	B	B	C	A	B	C	B	CsMt	Double	30	1,3	Larsen	13,5	200	12	5,2	3,25	No	No
[19]	B	B	C	A	B	C	B	CsCl	Double	29	1,5	Larsen	13,7	200	12	4,6	2,15	No	No
[20]	B	B	A	A	A	C	C	Au	Single	32	2,0	Larsen	30,5	240	12	6,4	0,00	No	No
[20]	B	B	A	A	A	C	C	AuCl	Double	27	2,0	Larsen	31,2	240	12	6,5	0,00	No	No
[21]	A	A	A	A	C	C	A	Su	Single	66	1,0	Sharp	6,0	448	12	1,3	0,09	No	No
[21]	A	A	A	A	C	C	A	SuGc	Double	64	1,0	Sharp	8,0	448	12	1,8	0,09	No	No
[22]	B	B	A	B	B	C	A	Mt	Single	30	16,0	Larsen	37,0	240	12	1,0	0,09	Yes	No
[22]	B	B	A	B	B	C	A	MtGc	Double	32	13,0	Larsen	47,0	240	12	1,5	0,06	Yes	No
[23]	A	B	C	A	A	C	A	Mt	Single	39	8,5	Larsen	31,5	160	12	2,3	0,04	Yes	No
[23]	A	B	C	A	A	C	A	MtGc	Double	43	2,8	Larsen	28,5	160	12	6,4	0,05	Yes	No
[24]	B	A	A	A	A	C	A	Su	Single	49	1,3	Larsen	6,2	140	12	3,4	0,00	No	No
[24]	B	A	A	A	A	C	A	SuGc	Double	54	1,3	Larsen	2,7	140	12	1,5	0,00	No	No
[25]	A	B	C	A	C	C	A	Mt	Single	115	0,5	Sharp	1,9	280	12	1,4	0,62	Yes	No
[25]	A	B	C	A	C	C	A	MtGc	Double	99	0,5	Sharp	1,9	280	12	1,4	0,28	Yes	No
[26]	B	B	A	B	B	A	A	Au	Single	20	2,5	Sharp	17,0	280	10	2,4	0,04	Yes	No
[26]	B	B	A	B	B	A	A	AuGc	Double	20	1,8	Sharp	11,0	280	10	2,2	0,01	Yes	No
[27]	A	B	A	A	C	C	C	Mt	Single	72	0,8	Sharp	4,7	280	12	2,1	0,00	No	No
[27]	A	B	A	A	C	C	C	MtGc	Double	70	0,8	Sharp	6,0	280	12	2,7	0,00	No	No
[28]	A	A	A	A	B	A	A	Mt	Single	117	0,2	Larsen	7,0	240	24	14,6	0,82	Yes	No
[28]	A	A	A	A	B	A	A	MtCs	Double	119	0,3	Larsen	8,0	240	24	11,1	0,82	Yes	No
[28]	A	A	A	A	B	A	A	MtGc	Double	115	0,4	Larsen	5,0	240	24	5,2	0,82	Yes	No
[28]	A	A	A	A	B	A	A	MtCsGc	Triple	116	0,3	Larsen	5,0	240	24	6,9	0,82	Yes	No

Table 1. Cont.

Reference no.	Sequence generation	Concealed allocation	Study blinding	Outcome blinding	Radiographic sequence	Incomplete outcome	Sponsor	Test drug	Treatment group	N_ (radiograph)	Duration RA, years	Scoring system	Initial radiographic score	Radiographic score, Max	Duration of study, months	PARPR	Mean Dose GC mg	Strategy change allowed	DMARD inadequate response
[29]	B	B	C	A	B	C	B	Mt	Single	57	2,3	Larsen	32,8	200	24	7,1	1,50	Yes	No
[29]	B	B	C	A	B	C	B	MtSu	Double	56	2,5	Larsen	33,6	200	24	6,7	1,50	Yes	No
[29]	B	B	C	A	B	C	B	MtSuCl	Triple	58	2,2	Larsen	33,4	200	24	7,6	1,50	Yes	No
[30]	A	A	C	A	C	C	A	Su	Single	47	1,7	Sharp	32,0	280	18	6,7	1,15	Yes	No
[30]	A	A	C	A	C	C	A	MtSuCl	Triple	52	1,6	Sharp	28,0	280	18	6,3	4,08	Yes	No
[31]	A	A	C	A	B	A	A	Mt	Single	98	0,7	Larsen	2,0	240	24	1,2	3,59	No	No
[31]	A	A	C	A	B	A	A	MtSuCl	Triple	97	0,6	Larsen	2,0	240	24	1,4	5,14	No	No
[32]	A	A	A	A	C	C	B	Su	Single	65	0,3	Sharp	5,0	280	13	6,0	0,27	No	No
[32]	A	A	A	A	C	C	B	SuMtGc	Triple	70	0,3	Sharp	2,0	280	13	2,4	0,27	No	No
[33]	B	A	A	A	A	C	C	Mt	Single	212	6,8	Sharp	11,5	280	12	0,6	3,20	No	No
[33]	B	A	A	A	A	C	C	EtMt	TNFiMt	218	6,8	Sharp	9,5	280	12	0,5	3,10	No	No
[34]	A	A	A	A	A	C	C	Mt	Single	230	0,8	Sharp	5,0	448	12	1,4	2,50	No	No
[34]	A	A	A	A	A	C	C	EtMt	TNFiMt	246	0,7	Sharp	5,0	448	12	1,6	2,45	No	No
[35]	B	B	B	A	A	C	C	Mt	Single	64	11,0	Sharp	82,0	280	12	2,7	3,20	No	Yes
[35]	B	B	B	A	A	C	C	InMt	TNFiMt	71	10,0	Sharp	79,0	280	12	2,8	3,15	No	Yes
[36]	A	A	A	A	A	C	C	Mt	Single	226	0,9	Sharp	8,3	280	12	3,3	1,90	Yes	No
[36]	A	A	A	A	A	C	C	InMt	TNFiMt	306	0,8	Sharp	8,8	280	12	3,9	1,85	Yes	No
[37]	B	B	A	A	A	A	C	Mt	Single	251	0,8	Sharp	13,6	230	12	7,4	2,27	No	No
[37]	B	B	A	A	A	A	C	AdMt	TNFiMt	267	0,7	Sharp	11,0	230	12	6,8	2,40	No	No
[38]	B	B	A	A	A	C	C	Mt	Single	172	10,9	Sharp	37,2	230	12	1,5	2,71	Yes	Yes
[38]	B	B	A	A	A	C	C	AdMt	TNFiMt	183	11,0	Sharp	41,4	230	12	1,6	2,46	Yes	Yes
[39]	B	B	A	A	A	A	C	Mt	Single	199	6,2	Sharp	20,0	440	12	0,7	1,70	No	Yes
[39]	B	B	A	A	A	A	C	CzMt	TNFiMt	393	6,1	Sharp	20,0	440	12	0,7	1,70	No	Yes
[40]	B	B	A	A	A	A	C	Mt	Single	127	5,6	Sharp	23,1	280	6	1,5	2,85	No	Yes
[40]	B	B	A	A	A	A	C	CzMt	TNFiMt	246	6,1	Sharp	19,0	280	6	1,1	2,75	No	Yes
[41]	A	A	B	A	A	A	C	Mt	Single	195	8,9	Sharp	21,8	145	12	1,7	3,45	Yes	Yes
[41]	A	A	B	A	A	A	C	AbMt	ABAMt	391	8,5	Sharp	21,7	145	12	1,8	3,60	Yes	Yes
[42]	B	B	A	A	B	C	C	Mt	Single	223	0,5	Sharp	4,8	145	12	6,6	4,56	Yes	No
[42]	B	B	A	A	B	C	C	AbMt	ABAMt	218	0,5	Sharp	5,4	145	12	7,4	3,63	Yes	No
[43]	B	B	C	A	A	C	C	Mt	Single	184	11,6	Sharp	46,2	145	12	2,7	3,05	No	Yes
[43]	B	B	C	A	A	C	C	RtMt	CD20iMt	273	12,0	Sharp	46,2	145	12	2,7	3,25	No	Yes
[44]	A	A	A	A	B	C	A	Mt	Single	15	0,7	Sharp	24	448	22	7,7	1.6	Yes	No

Table 1. Cont.

Reference no.	Sequence generation	Concealed allocation	Study blinding	Outcome blinding	Radiographic sequence	Incomplete outcome	Sponsor	Test drug	Treatment group	N_ (radiograph)	Duration RA, years	Scoring system	Initial radiographic score	Radiographic score, Max	Duration of study, months	PARPR	Mean Dose GC mg	Strategy change allowed	DMARD inadequate response
[44]	A	A	A	A	B	C	A	MtBu	Double	15	0,8	Sharp	14	448	22	3,9	0.8	Yes	No
[45]	A	A	A	A	A	A	C	Mt	Single	232	0,90	Sharp	3,70	145	12	2,8	2,40	No	No
[45]	A	A	A	A	A	A	C	RtMt	CD20iMt	244	0,90	Sharp	3,50	145	12	2,7	2,20	No	No
[46a]	B	A	A	B	B	A	C	Mt	Single	160	2,9	Sharp	19,7	448	12	1,5	3,40	Yes	No
[46a]	B	A	A	B	B	A	C	GoMt	TNFiMt	159	3,5	Sharp	18,7	448	12	1,2	3,50	Yes	No
[46b]	B	A	A	B	B	A	C	Mt	Single	133	6,5	Sharp	36,7	448	12	1,3	4,80	Yes	Yes
[46b]	B	A	A	B	B	A	C	GoMt	TNFiMt	89	4,5	Sharp	29,7	448	12	1,5	5,60	Yes	Yes
[47]	B	B	A	B	B	B	C	Mt	Single	393	9	Sharp	28,8	145	12	2,2	3,45	Yes	Yes
[47]	B	B	A	B	B	B	C	TzMt	TZMt	398	9,3	Sharp	29,1	145	12	2,2	3,10	Yes	Yes
[48]	A	A	A	A	C	C	A	Mt	Single	110	0,6	Sharp	0	280	24	0,0	0	Yes	No
[48]	A	A	A	A	C	C	A	MtGc	Double	112	0,6	Sharp	0	280	24	0,0	0	Yes	No
[49]	B	B	A	A	A	B	C	Mt	Single	84	8,7	Sharp	30,8	280	6	1,3	NA	Yes	Yes
[49]	B	B	A	A	A	B	C	GoMt	TNFiMt	81	8,8	Sharp	32,1	280	6	1,3	NA	Yes	Yes
[50]	B	A	A	A	B	C	C	Mt	Single	285	7,2	Sharp	NA	448	11	NA	3,54	No	Yes
[50]	B	A	A	A	B	C	C	OcMt	CD20iMt	324	7,6	Sharp	NA	448	11	NA	3,83	No	Yes
[51]	B	B	A	A	C	C	C	Mt	Single	282	11,8	Sharp	NA	448	11	NA	4,07	No	Yes
[51]	B	B	A	A	A	C	C	OcMt	CD20iMt	277	12,3	Sharp	NA	448	11	NA	3,81	No	Yes
[52]	B	A	A	A	B	C	C	Mt	Single	196	1,23	Sharp	13,3	448	12	2,4	2	No	No
[52]	B	A	A	A	B	C	C	OcMt	CD20iMt	194	1,2	Sharp	12,4	448	12	2,3	2,11	No	No
[53]	B	A	A	A	B	A	C	Mt	Single	514	4,5	Sharp	5,1	280	6	0,4	2,3	No	No
[53]	B	A	A	A	B	A	C	AdMt	TNFiMt	508	4	Sharp	5,4	280	6	0,5	2,05	No	No

*Percentage of Annual Radiographic Progression Rate

Ref. no., comparison	Std. Mean Difference Fixed, 95% CI
03 2 DMARDs vs DMARD	-0.15 [-0.52, 0.21]
03 In+Mt vs Mt	-0.63 [-1.00, -0.26]
03 2 DMARDs+Gc vs DMARD	-0.60 [-0.97, -0.24]
17 Mt+Su vs Mt/Su	-0.12 [-0.51, 0.28]
18 Mt+Cs vs Mt	-0.71 [-1.25, -0.18]
19 Mt+Cs vs Cs	-0.82 [-1.46, -0.17]
19 Cl+Cs vs Cs	-0.12 [-0.74, 0.50]
20 Au,ij+Cl vs Au,ij	-0.16 [-0.68, 0.35]
28 Mt+Cs vs Mt	-0.29 [-0.65, 0.07]
28 Mt+Gc vs Mt	-0.32 [-0.69, 0.04]
28 Mt+Cs+Gc vs Mt	-0.62 [-0.98, -0.25]
29 2 DMARDs vs DMARD	-0.18 [-0.64, 0.27]
29 3 DMARDs vs DMARD	-0.22 [-0.66, 0.23]
30 3 DMARDs vs DMARD	-0.56 [-0.96, -0.16]
31 Mt+Su+Cl vs Su	-0.46 [-0.75, -0.18]
32 Su+Mt+Gc vs Su	-0.25 [-0.59, 0.09]
21 Gc+Su vs Su	0.13 [-0.21, 0.48]
22 Gc+DMARD vs DMARD	-0.51 [-1.02, -0.01]
23 Gc+DMARD vs DMARD	-0.25 [-0.69, 0.18]
24 Gc+DMARD vs DMARD	-0.31 [-0.70, 0.07]
25 Gc+DMARD vs DMARD	-0.51 [-0.78, -0.24]
26 Gc+Au,ij vs Au,ij	-0.25 [-0.87, 0.37]
27 Gc+DMARD vs DMARD	-3.71 [-4.25, -3.16]
33 Et+Mt vs Mt	-0.34 [-0.53, -0.15]
34 Et+Mt vs Mt	-0.38 [-0.56, -0.20]
35 In+Mt vs Mt	-0.65 [-0.99, -0.30]
36 In+Mt vs Mt	-0.43 [-0.60, -0.25]
37 Ad+Mt vs Mt	-0.23 [-0.40, -0.06]
38 Ad+Mt vs Mt	-0.44 [-0.65, -0.23]
39 Cz+Mt vs Mt	-0.31 [-0.48, -0.14]
40 Cz+Mt vs Mt	-0.28 [-0.49, -0.06]
41 Ab+Mt vs Mt	-0.19 [-0.37, -0.02]
42 Ab+Mt vs Mt	-0.20 [-0.39, -0.02]
43 Rt+Mt vs Mt	-0.24 [-0.43, -0.05]
44 Mt+Bu vs Mt	-0.63 [-1.36, 0.11]
45 Rt+Mt vs Mt	-0.32 [-0.50, -0.13]
46 Go+Mt vs Mt	-0.04 [-0.30, 0.23]
46 Go+Mt vs Mt	-0.13 [-0.35, 0.09]
47 Tz+Mt vs Mt	-0.34 [-0.48, -0.20]
48 Mt+Gc vs Mt	-0.52 [-0.79, -0.25]
49 Go+Mt vs Mt	-0.39 [-0.69, -0.08]
50 Oc+Mt vs Mt	-0.42 [-0.58, -0.26]
51 Oc+Mt vs Mt	-0.27 [-0.43, -0.10]
52 Oc+Mt vs Mt	-0.33 [-0.53, -0.13]
53 Ad+Mt vs Mt	-0.21 [-0.33, -0.09]
Total (95% CI)	**-0.31 [-0.35, -0.28]**

Heterogeneity: Chi² = 53.69, df = 43 (P = 0.13); I² = 20%
Test for overall effect: Z = 16.81 (P < 0.00001)

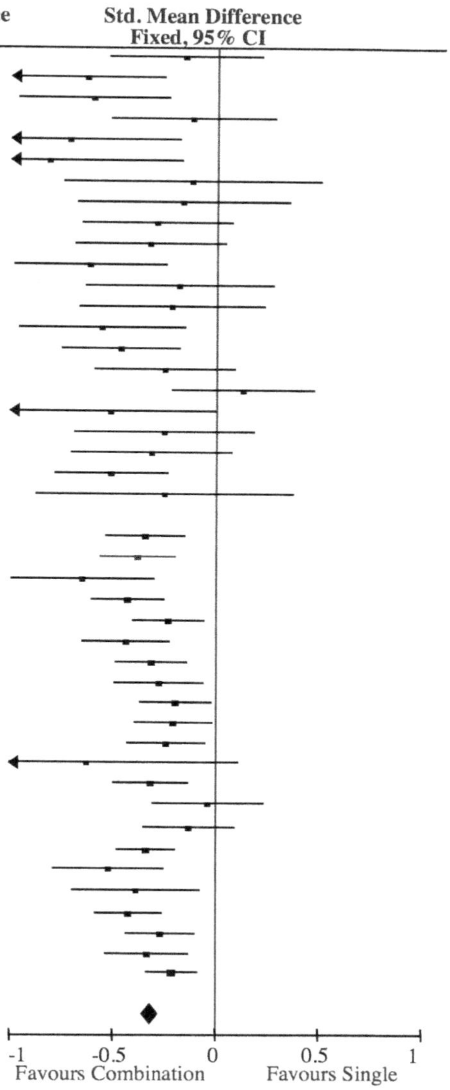

Figure 2. Combination treatment versus single DMARD. The effect on all studies is −0.33 SMD (CI: −0.36, −0.29). Test for overall effect: Z = 17.66 (P<0.00001). Heterogeneity: Chi^2 = 201.54, df = 44 (P<0.00001); I^2 = 78%. One study [27] contributed to heterogeneity due an extreme effect (−3.71 SMD). The elimination of this study resulted in a little more conservative estimate (−0.31 SMD (CI: −0.35, −0.28), Z = 16.81), but eliminated the significant heterogeneity (I^2 = 20, p = 0.13). Consequently, reference [27] was excluded from all comparisons. N, combination: 6725; N, single: 5446.

combinations. However only 6 of these combinations have been tested, and therefore it is not possible to determine the most effective of the 45 combinations. Furthermore 4 of the combinations have only been tested in one study. Therefore statistical conclusions based on indirect comparisons of these combinations would be weak. In contrast, a comparison of a group of combination DMARD studies with other treatments would be powerful. The different biologic drugs combined with methotrexate have all been investigated in large studies, and therefore these combinations could all be included in powerful comparisons. Elimination of non-standard doses of biologics, which in direct comparisons have been shown to be inferior, would contribute to the reduction of heterogeneity.

The issue of interest does not only depend on the effect of the treatment, but also on the cost of the treatment. For instance a large difference between cheap DMARDs is interesting, whereas a small difference is not. Similarly a large difference between expensive biologics may be interesting, whereas a small difference is not. In contrast, it would be very interesting if there was only a small or no difference in effect between DMARDs and biologics.

We already know from previous conventional meta-analyses and network meta-analyses that the mutual effects of DMARDs and the mutual effects of biologics are similar, and that biologics as single treatment are better than single DMARD treatment. Furthermore we know the optimal standard dose of the biologics. Considering the 100 fold difference in cost, the remaining interesting question is whether a combination of a standard dose of a biologic plus methotrexate is better than a combination of cheap DMARDs. Consequently it was the intention to create a network to answer that question. Existing evidence was used to simplify the network in order to decrease heterogeneity and increase the power of the comparisons:

1) Placebo controlled single DMARD studies are eliminated, because the effects of single DMARDs are established
2) Single DMARD controlled single DMARD studies are eliminated, because the similar effects of single DMARDs are established
3) The combination DMARD studies are combined in one group and the comparison of different DMARD combinations are eliminated due to lack of investigations and power
4) To ensure the comparability with other network meta-analyses, the different biologic combinations are not combined but compared separately.
5) Only standard doses of biologics are investigated
6) IL1i treatment (anakinra) was excluded as IL1i has been shown to be inferior to other biologics in several network meta-analyses.

Eligibility criteria

Types of studies. Full-length studies published in peer-reviewed journals that were performed according to a RCT design and that scored joint radiographs as the primary or secondary outcome at 2 separate time points with a time interval of at least 3 months were included, irrespective of sample size and publication year.

Types of participants. Patients with RA diagnosed according to the 1958 or the 1987 criteria of the American College of Rheumatology (ACR; formerly, the American Rheumatism Association) were included. In studies performed before 1959, the stated study definitions of RA were accepted.

Type of outcome. The outcome was the difference between follow-up radiographic erosion score and baseline radiographic erosion score.

Types of intervention. As our previous meta-analysis [1] showed no statistically significant difference in radiographic progression between methotrexate (Mt), sulfasalazine (Su), cyclosporine (Cs), leflunomide (Lf) and injectable gold (Au, ij), we included combination DMARD studies, which had one of these effective DMARDs in the single DMARD arm, but excluded those that included the less effective DMARDs (chloroquine (Cl), D-penicillamine (Dp) and Dp analogue bucillamin (Bu), azathioprine (Az), cyclophosphamide (Cph) and peroral gold (Au, po)) in the single DMARD arm. Furthermore, we showed that LDGC, defined as maximally 7.5 mg prednisone or prednisolone per day, had an effect similar to the effective DMARDs [1], and therefore LDGC was included as a DMARD equivalent. Any DMARD was allowed in the combination arm. Finally, we included combination treatments of methotrexate plus TNF inhibitors (etanercept (Et), infliximab (In), adalimumab (Ad), certolizumab (Cz), and golimumab (Go)), methotrexate plus abatacept (Ab), methotrexate plus tocilizumab (Tz), and methotrexate plus CD20 inhibitors (rituximab (Rt), ocrelizumab (Oc)).

Information sources

Trials were identified by searching the electronic databases (PubMed, the Cochrane database, and ClinicalTrials.gov) and by scanning the lists of references from the identified randomized trials.

Search methods for identification of studies

The search was based on the following combination of search terms:

"rheumatoid arthritis and randomized and methotrexate OR rheumatoid arthritis and randomized and sulfasalazine OR rheumatoid arthritis and randomized and leflunomide OR rheumatoid arthritis and randomized and gold OR rheumatoid arthritis and randomized and cyclosporine OR rheumatoid arthritis and randomized and infliximab OR rheumatoid arthritis and randomized and etanercept OR rheumatoid arthritis and randomized and adalimumab OR rheumatoid arthritis and randomized and certolizumab OR rheumatoid arthritis and randomized and golimumab OR rheumatoid arthritis and randomized and tocilizumab OR rheumatoid arthritis and randomized and abatacept OR rheumatoid arthritis and randomized and rituximab OR rheumatoid arthritis and randomized and ocrelizumab OR rheumatoid arthritis and randomized and ofatumumab OR rheumatoid arthritis and randomized and glucocorticoid OR rheumatoid arthritis and randomised and methotrexate OR rheumatoid arthritis and randomised and sulfasalazine OR rheumatoid arthritis and randomised and leflunomide OR rheumatoid arthritis and randomised and gold OR rheumatoid arthritis and randomised and cyclosporine OR rheumatoid arthritis and randomised and infliximab OR rheumatoid arthritis and randomised and etanercept OR rheumatoid arthritis and randomised and adalimumab OR rheumatoid arthritis and randomised and certolizumab OR rheumatoid arthritis and randomised and golimumab OR rheumatoid arthritis and randomised and tocilizumab OR rheumatoid arthritis and randomised and abatacept OR rheumatoid arthritis and randomised and rituximab OR rheumatoid arthritis and randomised and ocrelizumab OR rheumatoid arthritis and randomised and ofatumumab OR rheumatoid arthritis and randomised and glucocorticoid."

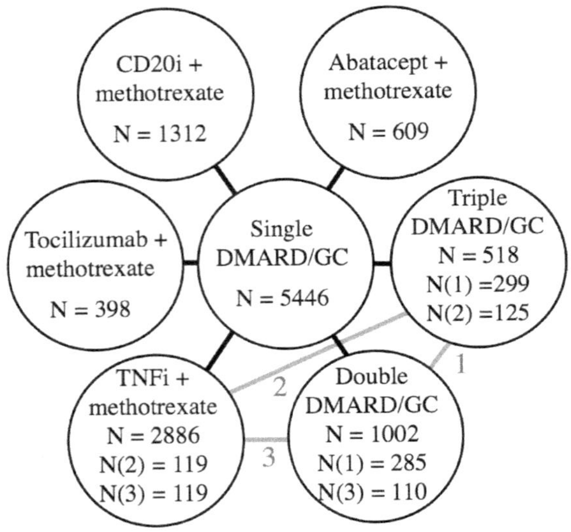

Figure 3. Star shaped network showing the 6 different combination treatments anchored on single treatment as the common comparator. The loops (grey lines) with corresponding numbers (1, 2, 3) show the subgroups, which were directly compared in addition to being indirectly compared. N indicates the number of patients in the groups.

Data collection

Selection of trials. Titles were screened, abstracts read, and possible papers retrieved. Trials fulfilling eligibility criteria were included in the systematic review.

Data extraction. Eligibility assessment, data collection and risk of bias assessment were performed independently by two

Ref. no., comparison	Weight	Std. Mean Difference Fixed, 95% CI
03 2 DMARDs vs DMARD	7.2%	-0.15 [-0.52, 0.21]
17 Mt+Su vs Mt/Su	6.2%	-0.12 [-0.51, 0.28]
18 Mt+Cs vs Mt	3.5%	-0.71 [-1.25, -0.18]
19 Mt+Cs vs Cs	2.4%	-0.82 [-1.46, -0.17]
19 Cl+Cs vs Cs	2.5%	-0.12 [-0.74, 0.50]
20 Au,ij+Cl vs Au,ij	3.7%	-0.16 [-0.68, 0.35]
28 Mt+Cs vs Mt	7.4%	-0.29 [-0.65, 0.07]
28 Mt+Gc vs Mt	7.4%	-0.32 [-0.69, 0.04]
29 2 DMARDS vs DMARD	4.7%	-0.18 [-0.64, 0.27]
21 Gc+Su vs Su	8.3%	0.13 [-0.21, 0.48]
22 Gc+DMARD vs DMARD	3.8%	-0.51 [-1.02, -0.01]
23 Gc+DMARD vs DMARD	5.2%	-0.25 [-0.69, 0.18]
24 Gc+DMARD vs DMARD	6.5%	-0.31 [-0.70, 0.07]
25 Gc+DMARD vs DMARD	13.2%	-0.51 [-0.78, -0.24]
26 Gc+Au,ij vs Au,ij	2.5%	-0.25 [-0.87, 0.37]
27 Gc+DMARD vs DMARD	0.0%	-3.71 [-4.25, -3.16]
44 Mt+Bu vs Mt	1.8%	-0.63 [-1.36, 0.11]
48 Mt+Gc vs Mt	13.7%	-0.52 [-0.79, -0.25]
Total (95% CI) (Excl. 27)	**100.0%**	**-0.32 [-0.42, -0.22]**

Heterogeneity: $Chi^2 = 19.23$, $df = 16$ ($P = 0.26$); $I^2 = 17\%$
Test for overall effect: $Z = 6.40$ ($P < 0.00001$)

Total (95% CI) (Incl. 27)	**100.0%**	**-0.43 [-0.53, -0.33]**

Heterogeneity: $Chi^2 = 161.42$, $df = 17$ ($P < 0.00001$); $I^2 = 89\%$
Test for overall effect: $Z = 8.67$ ($P < 0.00001$)

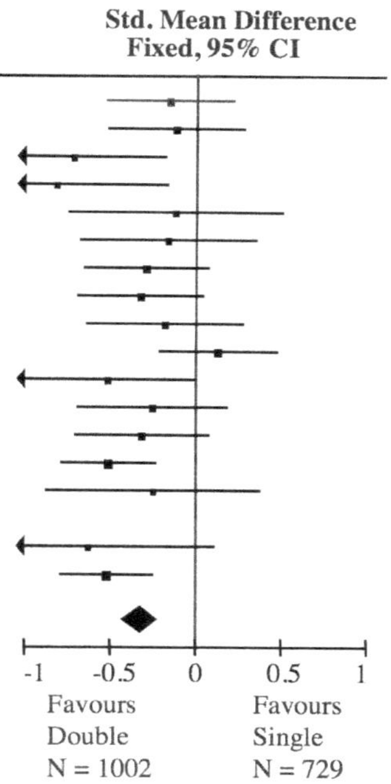

Figure 4. Double DMARD versus single DMARD: The effect of the Double DMARD treatment was highly significant (Z = 6.40). All 18 Double studies showed heterogeneity ($I^2 = 89\%$). The exclusion of one reference [27], which had an extreme effect (−3.71 SMD), eliminated the significant heterogeneity ($I^2 = 17\%$).

authors and disagreement resolved by consensus. All data were entered into standardized extraction forms.

Data items. Mean radiographic scores and standard deviations (SD) were assessed based on the change scores from baseline to follow-up for each treatment arm. In addition the following variables were recorded: Study identification, year of publication, scoring system, initial radiographic score, maximum radiographic score of scoring system, number of patients in each treatment arm, duration of RA at baseline, duration of study, DMARD inadequate response (i.e. whether included patients previously had had an inadequate response to a least one DMARD), strategy change (i.e. whether a change of treatment strategy was allowed during the course of the study) and mean daily glucocorticoid use in all treatment arms. We used the baseline radiographic score, the maximum radiographic score of scoring system and the duration of RA to calculate the percentage annual radiographic progression rate (PARPR) [1] in the period before baseline as a marker of disease activity at baseline.

Risk of bias in individual studies

Six different risk-of-bias domains defined by Cochrane [13] were assessed on the outcome level: sequence generation, allocation concealment, study blinding, outcome assessor blinding, incomplete outcome data and selective outcome reporting. In

Ref. no., comparison	Weight	Std. Mean Difference Fixed, 95% CI
03 2 DMARDs+GC vs DMARD	15.9%	-0.60 [-0.97, -0.24]
28 Mt+Cs+Gc vs Mt	15.6%	-0.62 [-0.98, -0.25]
29 3 DMARDS vs DMARD	10.6%	-0.22 [-0.66, 0.23]
30 3 DMARDs vs DMARD	13.1%	-0.56 [-0.96, -0.16]
31 3 DMARDs vs Su	26.2%	-0.46 [-0.75, -0.18]
32 Su+Mt+Gc vs Su	18.5%	-0.25 [-0.59, 0.09]
Total (95% CI)	**100.0%**	**-0.46 [-0.60, -0.31]**

Heterogeneity: $Chi^2 = 4.08$, $df = 5$ ($P = 0.54$); $I^2 = 0\%$
Test for overall effect: $Z = 6.13$ ($P < 0.00001$)

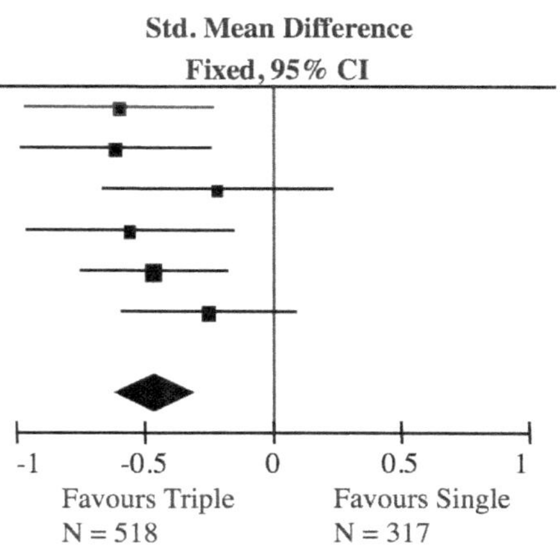

Figure 5. Triple DMARD versus single DMARD: The effect of the Triple DMARD treatment was highly significant (Z = 6.13). The 6 Triple studies showed no heterogeneity ($I^2 = 0$).

Ref. No., comparison	Weight	Std. Mean Difference Fixed, 95% CI
03 In+Mt vs Mt	2.2%	-0.63 [-1.00, -0.26]
33 Et+Mt vs Mt	8.4%	-0.34 [-0.53, -0.15]
34 Et+Mt vs Mt	9.2%	-0.38 [-0.56, -0.20]
35 In+Mt vs Mt	2.5%	-0.65 [-0.99, -0.30]
36 In+Mt vs Mt	10.0%	-0.43 [-0.60, -0.25]
37 Ad+Mt vs Mt	10.2%	-0.23 [-0.40, -0.06]
38 Ad+Mt vs Mt	6.8%	-0.44 [-0.65, -0.23]
39 Cz+Mt vs Mt	10.3%	-0.31 [-0.48, -0.14]
40 Cz+Mt vs Mt	6.6%	-0.28 [-0.49, -0.06]
46 Go+Mt vs Mt	6.3%	-0.13 [-0.35, 0.09]
46 Go+Mt vs Mt	4.2%	-0.04 [-0.30, 0.23]
49 Go+Mt vs Mt	3.2%	-0.39 [-0.69, -0.08]
53 Ad+Mt vs Mt	20.1%	-0.21 [-0.33, -0.09]
Total (95% CI)	**100.0%**	**-0.30 [-0.36, -0.25]**

Heterogeneity: $Chi^2 = 20.67$, df = 12 (P = 0.06); $I^2 = 42\%$

Test for overall effect: Z = 10.84 (P < 0.00001)

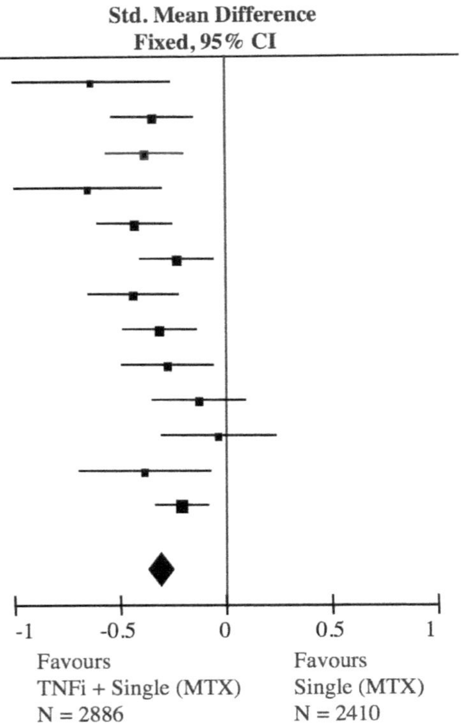

Figure 6. TNF inhibitor combined with methotrexate versus single DMARD (methotrexate): The effect of TNF inhibitor was highly significant (Z = 10.84). The 13 TNF inhibitor studies showed no significant heterogeneity ($I^2 = 42\%$, p = 0.06). The borderline heterogeneity was due to two golimumab studies (GoBefore, GoForward) [46]. The exclusion of these, did, however, not change the overall result (−0.33 SMD (CI: −0.39, −0.27)).

addition we included radiographic sequence blinding and company sponsoring as risk of bias domains.

Measures of treatment effect

For each randomized combination drug group and single DMARD group the difference between follow-up radiographic erosion score and baseline radiographic erosion score and the corresponding SDs were recorded. The difference between the mean effect in the combination drug group and the single DMARD group was the treatment effect.

Data analysis

Unit of analysis issues. If radiographic scoring was performed more than once during follow-up, the scoring with the most complete data was recorded. In trials with multi dose arms, only the defined standard dose arm was included. If the treatment arms of multi-armed trials consisted of different combination treatments (direct comparisons), these treatment arms were included in the network meta-analysis and additionally analyzed separately for the purposes of a consistency analysis of indirect comparisons versus direct comparisons. In this case the shared control group was split into a number of subgroups corresponding to the number of treatment arms to avoid multiple count of the control group.

Missing data. In articles where the median, but not the mean, was given, the median value was used in the calculations. If SD was not given, it could often be calculated from a 95% confidence interval, a standard error or a p-value [13]. An

Ref. No., comparison	Weight	Std. Mean Difference Fixed, 95% CI
41 Ab+Mt vs Mt	54.2%	-0.19 [-0.37, -0.02]
42 Ab+Mt vs Mt	45.8%	-0.20 [-0.39, -0.02]
Total (95% CI)	**100.0%**	**-0.20 [-0.33, -0.07]**

Heterogeneity: $Chi^2 = 0.01$, df = 1 (P = 0.94); $I^2 = 0\%$

Test for overall effect: Z = 3.08 (P = 0.002)

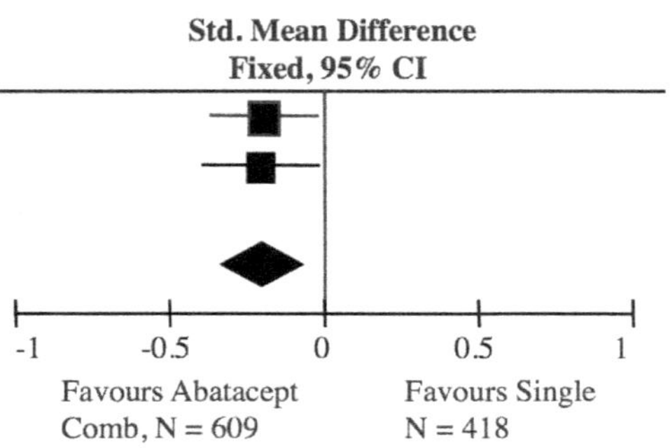

Figure 7. Abatacept combined with methotrexate versus single DMARD (methotrexate): The effect of abatacept was significant (Z = 3.08). The 2 abatacept studies showed no heterogeneity ($I^2 = 0$).

Ref. No., comparison	Weight	Std. Mean Difference Fixed, 95% CI
43 Rt+Mt vs Mt	17.9%	-0.24 [-0.43, -0.05]
45 Rt+Mt vs Mt	19.3%	-0.32 [-0.50, -0.13]
50 Oc+Mt vs Mt	24.3%	-0.42 [-0.58, -0.26]
51 Oc+Mt vs Mt	22.7%	-0.27 [-0.43, -0.10]
52 Oc+Mt vs Mt	15.8%	-0.33 [-0.53, -0.13]
Total (95% CI)	**100.0%**	**-0.32 [-0.40, -0.24]**

Heterogeneity: Chi² = 2.64, df = 4 (P = 0.62); I² = 0%
Test for overall effect: Z = 7.87 (P < 0.00001)

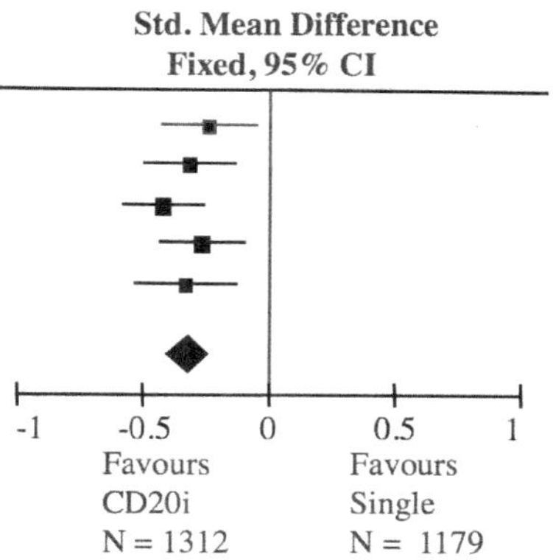

Figure 8. CD20 inhibitor treatment combined with single DMARD versus single DMARD: The effect of CD20 inhibitor treatment was highly significant (Z = 7.87). The 5 CD20 inhibitor studies showed no heterogeneity ($I^2 = 0$).

interquartile range (2 quartiles) was made equivalent to 1.35 x SD [13] and a full range was converted to an SD according to a conversion factor defined by Walther and Yao [14].

Heterogeneity. Heterogeneity between studies was tested statistically for all studies and each intervention by a χ^2 (chi square) test, and quantified by means of the I^2 statistic, which describes the percentage of the variability in effect estimates that is due to heterogeneity rather than sampling error: I^2, 0%–30%, unimportant heterogeneity; I^2, 30%–60%, moderate heterogeneity; I^2, > 60%, substantial heterogeneity [13]. Both fixed and random effect models were used, but the existence of statistically significant heterogeneity would determine whether a fixed effect model (non-significant heterogeneity test) or a random effect model (significant heterogeneity test) would be used in the primary or secondary analysis [13]. Potential heterogeneity would be explored by means of subgroup analyses of extracted data.

Outcome data synthesis. A network meta-analysis consist of a network of treatment effects for all possible pairwise comparisons from RCTs, whether or not they have been compared head to head (i.e. include both direct and indirect comparisons) [7,8]. We used a stepwise approach [15,16], first performing multiple pairwise meta-analyses of the direct comparisons of each of the combination treatments versus single DMARD followed by an indirect comparison of the pooled results of each of these meta-analyses. As the outcome measure (radiographic progression) was estimated at different time points (6–24 months) and as the maximum score of the different scoring systems (Sharp, Larsen) differed, we standardized the outcome measure by dividing the outcome with the SD, thus converting the outcome unit to the unitless standardized mean difference (SMD) [13]. Consequently, we interpreted our analyses of the pairwise meta-analyses on the basis of the SMD, whereas the indirect comparisons were performed as weighted mean differences of the SMDs calculated in the pairwise meta-analyses.

Consistency analysis. Consistency analyses of the effects obtained in the trials directly comparing combination treatments versus the effects obtained by means of the exclusively indirect comparisons were performed to explore possible differences between the direct and the indirect comparisons [12].

Risk of bias across studies. Each of the above eight assessed risk of bias domains were evaluated in 3 groups: A: Low risk; B: Unclear risk; C: High risk [13]. In addition publication bias was evaluated visually by means of a funnel plot in which the effect of each trial was plotted by the inverse of its standard error [13].

Additional analyses. The outcome effect (radiographic progression) of combination DMARD treatments including LDGC was compared versus combination DMARD treatments not including LDGC.

Measures of bias domains and of other possible confounders were compared between the combination treatment groups with the purpose of performing sensitivity analyses for those, which differed. The outcome effect was compared between the grading (A, B, C) of the relevant bias domains and between the upper and lower 50% percentiles of possible confounders of continuous variables (PARPR (as a marker of disease activity at baseline), disease duration, differences in the mean use of glucocorticoids) and between groups of possible confounders of category variables (DMARD inadequate response and strategy change).

Data synthesis method. The combined effect measures of the direct comparisons of the individual combination treatments,

Ref. No., comparison	Weight	Std. Mean Difference Fixed, 95% CI
47 Tz+Mt vs Mt	100.0%	-0.34 [-0.48, -0.20]
Total (95% CI)	**100.0%**	**-0.34 [-0.48, -0.20]**

Heterogeneity: Not applicable
Test for overall effect: Z = 4.70 (P < 0.00001)

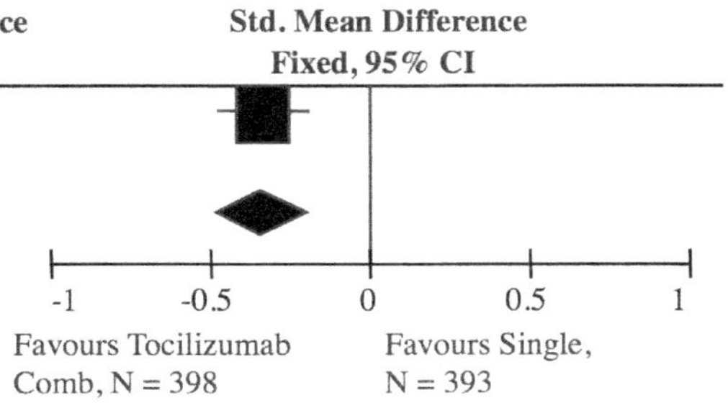

Figure 9. Tocilizumab combined with methotrexate versus single DMARD (methotrexate): The effect of tocilizumab is significant (Z = 4.70).

Combination 1 vs Combination 2	Combination 1 SMD1	SD	Total	Combination 2 SMD2	SD	Total	WMD 95% CI
Double vs Triple	-0.32	2.12	1731	-0.46	2.06	835	0.14 [-0.03, 0.31]
Double vs TNFi	-0.32	2.12	1731	-0.3	2.04	5296	-0.02 [-0.13, 0.09]
Double vs Abatacept	-0.32	2.12	1731	-0.2	2.11	1027	-0.12 [-0.28, 0.04]
Double vs Tocilizumab	-0.32	2.12	1731	-0.34	2.01	797	0.02 [-0.15, 0.19]
Double vs CD20i	-0.32	2.12	1731	-0.32	2.04	2491	0.00 [-0.13, 0.13]
Triple vs TNFi	-0.46	2.06	835	-0.3	2.04	5296	-0.16 [-0.31, -0.01]
Triple vs Abatacept	-0.46	2.06	835	-0.2	2.11	1027	-0.26 [-0.45, -0.07]
Triple vs Tocilizumab	-0.46	2.06	835	-0.34	2.01	797	-0.12 [-0.32, 0.08]
Triple vs CD20i	-0.46	2.06	835	-0.32	2.04	2491	-0.14 [-0.30, 0.02]
TNFi vs Abatacept	-0.3	2.04	5296	-0.2	2.11	1027	-0.10 [-0.24, 0.04]
TNFi vs Tocilizumab	-0.3	2.04	5296	-0.34	2.01	797	0.04 [-0.11, 0.19]
TNFi vs CD20i	-0.3	2.04	5296	-0.32	2.04	2491	0.02 [-0.08, 0.12]
Abatacept vs Tocilizumab	-0.2	2.11	1027	-0.34	2.01	797	0.14 [-0.05, 0.33]
Abatacept vs CD20i	-0.2	2.11	1027	-0.32	2.04	2491	0.12 [-0.03, 0.27]
Tocilizumab vs CD20i	-0.34	2.01	797	-0.32	2.04	2491	-0.02 [-0.18, 0.14]

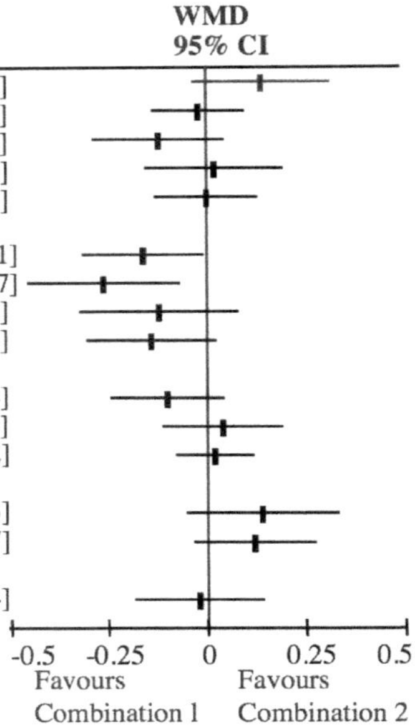

Figure 10. Indirect comparisons of different combination treatments. There is a trend towards triple treatment being superior to abatacept and TNFi. All other differences between the combination treatments are non-significant. Abbreviations: SMD: Standardized mean difference. WMD: Weighted mean difference (SMD1-SMD2).

the indirect comparisons of the combined effect measures of the individual combination treatments, the consistency analyses and the additional analyses were compared by means of the inverse variance method in Review Manager (RevMan) (Computer program), version 5.1. Copenhagen: The Nordic Cochrane Centre, the Cochrane Collaboration, 2008 [13].

Results

Trial selection

The search was repeated during the review period, by two authors by turns. The final search was performed July 5, 2012. A flow diagram of the literature search is shown in Figure 1.

The PubMed search revealed 1917 references. A search of ClinicalTrials.gov using the key-words "rheumatoid arthritis" and "radiographic progression" revealed 3 published studies with radiographic data, which also were identified during our primary search, 1 published study with no radiographic data and 2 finished but not published studies out of a total of 21 ongoing studies.

This search was supplied with a search in Cochrane Central Register of Controlled Trials using the terms "rheumatoid arthritis and radiographic progression" or "rheumatoid arthritis and joint destruction" resulting in 65 hits, none of which supplied the list of included studies.

After eliminating references which were considered irrelevant according to the headlines, 334 abstracts were read. On the basis of the abstracts 120 articles were retrieved in full length. From these a total of 38 references were identified (Figure 1). Until December 31 2009 the present search identified all 28 combination studies [3,17–43] identified in our previous search [1] plus one additional study published in 2005 [44]. In addition the present search revealed three new references [45–47] (4 investigations) published in 2011 and 6 studies published in 2012 [48–53]. In total 38 "combination treatment" references (39 trials, 45 treatment groups) were included.

Characteristics of included studies

All were parallel studies. Individual study characteristics and risk of bias domains are shown in Table 1. A forest plot of the individual study results is shown in Figure 2. Heterogeneity seemed to be unimportant ($I^2 = 20\%$, $p = 0.13$).

Description of network

On the basis of the included treatment arms and doses, we defined 6 combination treatments versus single DMARD:

1) Two DMARDs/LDGC (Double);
2) Three DMARDs/LDGC (Triple);
3) Standard dose of TNFi (Infliximab: 3 mg/kg/8 weeks; etanercept: 50 mg/1 week; adalimumab: 40 mg/2 weeks; certolizumab: 200 mg/2 weeks; golimumab: 50 mg/4 weeks);
4) Standard dose of CD20 inhibitor treatment (rituximab 2 g/6 months; ocrelizumab 1 g/6 months);
5) Abatacept 10 mg/kg/4 weeks;
6) Tocilizumab 8 mg/kg/4 weeks.

The star shaped network is shown in Figure 3. As one study included a direct comparison between TNFi, double and triple [3] and additionally two studies included direct comparisons between double and triple [28,29], the star includes loops to indicate the direct comparisons between TNFi, double and triple.

Synthesis of results

Only one study [27] contributed to heterogeneity in the analyses of all 45 treatment groups ($I^2 = 78\%$) (Figure 2) and in the analysis of double DMARD vs. single DMARD ($I^2 = 89\%$) (Figure 4). All other heterogeneity analyses were non-significant (I^2 varying in the range 0–42%, Figures 5–9). Consequently we eliminated this study [27] from the statistical analyses (reducing I^2 to 17–20%) and used a fixed effect model in the primary analyses and a random effect model in the secondary analyses. The results of the conventional meta-analyses of the 6 combination treatments are

Table 2. Observed Frequencies of bias factors for treatment groups.

	Double	Triple	TNFi	ABA	CD20i	TZ	χ^2	p
Sequence generation								
A	9	5	3	1	1	0		
B	9	1	10	1	4	1		
C	0	0	0	0	0	0	8.3	0.14
Allocation concealment								
A	7	5	7	1	3	0		
B	11	5	6	1	2	1		
C	0	0	0	0	0	0	4.8	0.44
Study blinding								
A	11	2	11	1	4	1		
B	0	0	1	1	0	0		
C	7	4	1	0	1	0	19.7	0.03
Outcome blinding								
A	16	11	6	2	5	0		
B	2	2	1	0	0	1		
C	0	0	0	0	0	0	9.7	0.09
Radiographic sequence								
A	4	1	10	1	3	0		
B	8	3	3	1	2	1		
C	6	2	0	0	0	0	16.3	0.09
Incomplete outcome data								
A	3	2	6	1	1	0		
B	0	0	1	0	0	1		
C	15	4	6	1	4	0	27.7	0.002
Selective outcome reporting								
A	18	6	13	2	5	1		
B	0	0	0	0	0	0		
C	0	0	0	0	0	0	-	-
Sponsorship								
A	11	3	0	0	0	0		
B	3	2	0	0	0	0		
C	4	1	13	2	5	1	30.1	0.001

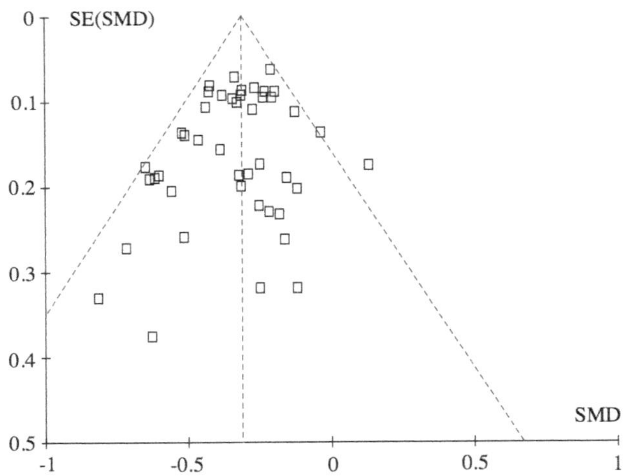

Figure 11. Funnel plot of all combination studies ([27] eliminated). The left lower corner is empty compared with the right lower corner. This asymmetry may indicate that small studies with no effect was not published (publication bias). However, this asymmetry is quantitatively small, and probably does not affect the overall result. Exclusion of the three lower right studies [18,19,44] to eliminate the asymmetry did not change the overall result shown in Figure 2: −0.31 SMD (CI: −0.35, −0.27), test for overall effect: Z = 16.49 (P<0.00001). Heterogeneity: $Chi^2 = 48.41$, df = 40 (P = 0.17); $I^2 = 17\%$. Abbreviations: SMD: Standardized mean difference.

shown in Figures 4–9. The borderline heterogeneity in the TNFi analysis ($I^2 = 42\%$) (Figure 6) was due to two golimumab studies [46]. Elimination of these studies reduced heterogeneity ($I^2 = 27\%$) but did not change the overall result (SMD: −0.33 (CI: −0.39, −0.27)).

Because all interventions are connected in the network (i.e. each pair has a path from one to the other) indirect comparisons can be performed for each of the combination treatments in the star versus each other. Figure 10 shows the results of the indirect comparisons of the 6 combination treatments. The effects varied between −0.46 SMD (triple) and −0.20 SMD (abatacept). Statistically, triple treatment with DMARDs was a little better than abatacept plus methotrexate (−0.26 SMD (CI: −0.45, −0.07)) and TNFi plus methotrexate (−0.16 SMD (CI: −0.31, −0.01)), but no other significant differences between the different combination treatments were identified (Figure 10).

Risk of bias across studies

The cumulated grade (A, B, C) frequencies are shown in Table 2. Six of the eight bias domains are predominantly graded as being of low (A) or unclear (B) risk, whereas two domains (incomplete outcome reporting and study sponsoring) are predominantly classified as being of high risk. Concerning the 6 Cochrane bias domains, 28 of 39 trials contained at least one high risk (C) grade.

A funnel plot indicates a minor degree of publication bias (Figure 11).

Consistency analysis

Three trials [3,28,29] of the 39 trials contributed with treatment arms to three combination treatment groups (TNFi, Double and Triple). Pairwise consistency analyses of the SMD effects obtained in the trials directly comparing combination treatments versus the SMD effects obtained by means of the exclusively indirect comparisons were performed to explore possible differences between the direct and the indirect comparisons.

Triple versus Double: Direct comparison (n = 584) versus indirect comparison (n = 1616): Weighted mean difference = 0.20 SMD (CI: −0.08, 0.48).

Double versus TNFi plus methotrexate:

1) Direct comparison (BeSt study [3], 1. year data) (n = 229) versus indirect comparison (n = 6722): Weighted mean difference = 0.55 SMD (CI: 0.28, 0.82).
2) Supplementary analysis including the second year data from the BeSt study [4]: Direct comparison (n = 236) versus indirect

Combination 1 vs Combination 2	Combination 1 SMD1	SD	Total	Combination 2 SMD2	SD	Total	WMD 95% CI
1) 2 DM vs DM+GC	-0.29	2.06	724	-0.35	2.10	1007	0.06 [-0.14, 0.26]
2) 3 DM vs 2 DM+GC	-0.44	1.99	381	-0.48	2.17	454	0.04 [-0.24, 0.32]
3) CD20i: DN vs DIA	-0.32	2.10	866	-0.32	2.06	1625	0.00 [-0.17, 0.17]
4) TNFi: DN vs DIA	-0.30	1.95	3456	-0.33	2.08	1842	0.03 [-0.09, 0.15]
5) D+T: NonSp vs Sp	-0.37	1.98	1253	-0.33	1.64	321	-0.04 [-0.25, 0.17]
6) D: DB vs Open	-0.32	2.19	1088	-0.32	2.20	643	0.00 [-0.21, 0.21]
7) D: CO vs IO	-0.3	2.29	352	-0.33	2.08	1379	0.03 [-0.23, 0.29]
8) T: CO vs IO	-0.52	2.19	350	-0.41	2.13	485	-0.11 [-0.41, 0.19]
9) TNFi: CO vs IO	-0.22	1.97	3046	-0.42	2.18	2250	0.20 [0.09, 0.31]
10) TNFi: Dur:<1.3y vs >1.3y	-0.36	2.09	1683	-0.28	1.84	3613	-0.08 [-0.20, 0.04]
11) TNFi: GC <2.1mg vs >2.1mg	-0.3	1.90	2828	-0.31	1.96	2303	0.01 [-0.10, 0.12]
12) D: PARPR, L vs H	-0.34	2.17	1035	-0.3	2.22	696	-0.04 [-0.25, 0.17]
13) T: PARPR L vs H	-0.52	2.12	359	-0.41	2.11	476	-0.11 [-0.40, 0.18]
14) TNFi: PARPR L vs H	-0.29	1.76	4111	-0.36	1.98	1185	0.07 [-0.06, 0.20]

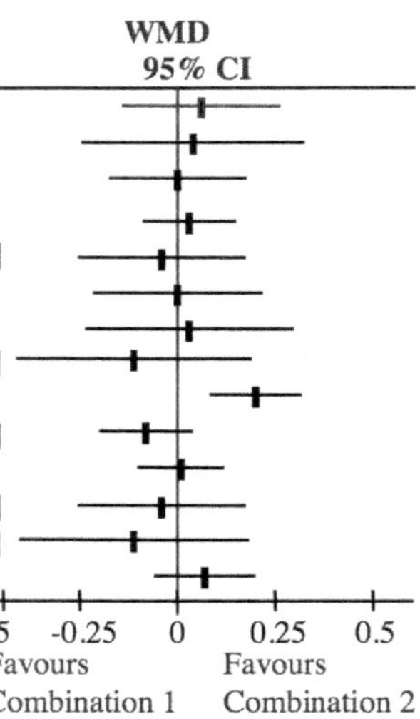

Figure 12. Analyses of bias factors and confounders, which differed significantly across treatment groups. Only 1 bias factor (TNFi studies: Complete outcome versus incomplete outcome, line 9) had a significant influence on the outcome. Abbreviations: SMD: Standardized mean difference. WMD: Weighted mean difference (SMD1-SMD2); DM: DMARD; GC: Glucocorticoid; DN: DMARD naive; DIA: DMARD inadequate responder; D: double; T: Triple; Sp: Sponsoring; DB: double-blind; CO: Complete outcome; IO: Incomplete outcome; Dur: Disease duration at baseline; PARPR: Percentage of annual radiographic progression rate; L: low; H: High.

comparison (n = 6722): Weighted mean difference = 0.05 SMD (CI: −0.32, 0.42).

Triple versus TNFi plus methotrexate: Direct comparison (n = 244) versus indirect comparison (n = 5810): Weighted mean difference = 0.23 SMD (CI: −0.07, 0.53).

Table 3. Other possible confounders across treatment groups.

	Double	Triple	TNFi	ABA	CD20i	TZ	p
N	18	6	13	2	5	1	
Duration (years) of RA at baseline							
Mean	2.1	0.9	5.0	4.6	6.7	9.2	
SD	3.4	0.8	3.6	4.7	5.1	0.2	0.0001
Percentage of annual radiographic progression rate at baseline							
Mean	3.5	5.2	1.9	4.4	2.6	2.2	
SD	3.3	3.9	1.7	3.1	0.2	0.04	0.03
Glucocorticoid use during study							
Mean	0.6	1.6	2.6	3.8	3.0	3.3	
SD	0.9	1.7	1.2	0.5	0.8	0.2	0.0001
Strategy change during study							
No	7	2	7	0	5	0	
Yes	11	4	6	2	0	1	0.09

Additional analyses

Using a random effect model instead of a fixed effect model eliminated the small significant difference between triple DMARD and TNFi (weighted mean difference: −0.14 SMD (CI: −0.30; 0.02)), but all other indirect comparisons as shown in Figure 10 were unchanged.

There was no difference between DMARD combination studies using LDGC as a DMARD equivalent and those using only DMARDs (Figure 12, lines 1–2). There was no difference between biologic studies performed in DMARD naïve (DN) patients and DMARD inadequate responders (DIA) (Figure 12, lines 3–4).

Table 3 shows other possible confounders across treatment groups. Sensitivity analyses were performed for the bias domains (Table 2) and possible confounding variables (Table 3), which differed across studies and the results are shown in Figure 12. The results of these analyses showed that these factors did not influence the results significantly (Figure 12, lines 5–14) with the exception TNFi studies with incomplete outcome reporting (high risk of bias), which had a significantly higher effect than those with complete outcome reporting (low risk of bias) (Figure 12, line 9).

Discussion

In contrast to our previous meta-analysis [1], which was a compilation of conventional meta-analyses, the present network meta-analysis indirectly compared the different treatment principles arranged in a network anchored on single DMARD therapy. The analysis is the first network meta-analysis to use the essential outcome (joint destruction) and to show that different biologic treatments combined with methotrexate may not be superior to treatments with 2–3 DMARDs or 1–2 DMARDs + LDGC (Figure 10). Furthermore the different biologic treatments did not differ from each other. The latter finding confirms the reliability of the analysis, as it is in agreement with previous network meta-analyses using ACR50 as an outcome [9–10,54–59], which indicate that TNF inhibitors, tocilizumab and rituximab have similar effects, abatacept is borderline inferior and IL1i is clinically and statistically inferior. Most of these used a Bayesian framework, but one used a statistical method based on Bucher's design, similar to ours [57]. The outcome of this analysis corresponded to the outcome of the others and ours. A limitation is that the outcomes of the present and previous network meta-analyses are based on indirect data. Therefore doubt can be raised that the treatment arms compared may not be as comparable as randomized treatment arms from one population. This doubt can never be completely eliminated and therefore some reservation concerning the outcomes should be acknowledged. Consequently, the present analysis cannot be considered to be definite evidence that two or more DMARDs prevent structural joint damage to the same degree as a biologic agent combined with methotrexate. The reverse conclusion is also not definite. Therefore confirmation of the present results in direct comparison studies and meta-analyses would be desirable. Recently, a few such studies did confirm that the effect of triple DMARD therapy was comparable with the effect of TNFi plus methotrexate [5–7]. These studies, which were published after the date of our final literature search, did not fulfill our inclusion criteria, as they did not use a single DMARD therapy treatment arm. Similar direct comparisons of the other biologic drugs (tocilizumab, abatacept and rituximab) with combination DMARD treatment have not been performed.

Our approach to reduce heterogeneity was successful, as there was no heterogeneity after exclusion of a single study, neither when the studies were analyzed in one group (Figure 2) nor when the treatments were analyzed separately (Figures 4–9). Most within study bias sources (Table 1) were equally distributed across the defined treatment groups (Table 2) and only one of the Cochrane defined bias domains (incomplete outcome data) was dominated by the high risk of bias grade C (26 of 39). Sensitivity analyses of the bias sources, which were unequally distributed in the combination treatment groups (Tables 2 and 3), did not change the results (Figure 12) with the exception TNFi studies with incomplete outcome data (Figure 12, line 9). This bias could inflate the effect of TNFi, but not change the main finding of the study. In general the results were robust. The amount of evidence in the network was significant (Figure 3), the heterogeneity analysis of the study effects was insignificant indicating similar results from study to study (Figure 2) and direct and indirect comparisons were consistent when comparing treatment balanced data. The main reason for the low degree of heterogeneity was probably that all comparisons were anchored on a similar comparator (single DMARD) and that the baseline differences between included populations were moderate. Finally, publication bias (Figure 11), or other possible confounders such as different disease duration , different disease activity at baseline (PARPR), different use of glucocorticoid or treatment strategy change during the treatment period (Table 3) could not explain the similar outcome effects (Figure 12).

A recent study indicated that patients included in newer studies have a lower baseline disease activity than in older studies [60]. This could in theory explain why the effect of the biologics did not exceed the effect of the DMARDs. This theory is in part confirmed by the fact that there was a difference in baseline disease activity between TNFi studies (PARPR = 1.9%) and triple DMARD studies (PARPR = 5.2%). However, the sensitivity analyses of studies with high baseline activity versus low baseline activity showed no differences (Figure 12, lines 12–14). Furthermore, the baseline activity of the double DMARD studies did not differ from the baseline activity of the other biologic studies (Table 3). Consequently the different time periods of the different studies could probably not explain the similar effects.

The chosen outcome (joint destruction) is the essential outcome of RA [61–62]. Furthermore, the ACR response criteria used in the meta-analyses of biologic studies [9–10,54–59] are not available in older DMARD studies. We accepted two different scoring methods as our previous analysis showed concordant results for both methods [1]. This outcome and other outcome measures of RA are mutually dependent. Although joint inflammation and joint destruction are not always linked, several studies have shown that on the average there is a very high association between integrated measures of inflammatory variables (i.e. ESR, CRP, swollen joint count) and the radiographic score, as shown and reviewed previously [63–64]. Therefore, the radiographic score is a cumulative measure that not only shows the existing status of the patient, but also reflects the preceding disease course [63–64]. The assumption that the radiographic progression sufficiently reflects the outcome of RA is further verified by the fact that network-meta-analyses comparing biologic drugs using ACR response criteria as outcome measure also do not find differences between the different biologic drugs except that the IL1 inhibitor has an inferior effect [9–10,54–59].

All approved treatment principles were investigated. The grouping of DMARDs and LDGC was based on the findings of our previous analyses, which showed that these drugs had similar effects [1]. The present study confirms that the effect of LDGC corresponds to the effect of a DMARD (Figure 12, line 1–2). Our assumption of equality between methotrexate, sulfasalazine and leflunomide has recently been verified in an independent review [65], which, however, did not investigate cyclosporine and gold.

In general, our results agree with those of an independent research group [66], which in an analysis of pairwise meta-analyses indicated that DMARD and TNFi/methotrexate combinations had equal efficacy on ACR response, withdrawals for inefficacy, disability and erosive progression.

Because of the high prices of biologics, their cost-effectiveness is a matter of debate [67]. This may be a reason why different official treatment recommendations are not completely concordant.

Our results are not consistent with the European League against Rheumatism (EULAR) recommendations [68], which suggest that in DMARD naive patients, irrespective of the addition of glucocorticoids, DMARD mono therapy rather than combination therapy of DMARDs may be applied followed by switching to another single DMARD or addition of a biologic agent. In contrast to the EULAR guidelines, the American College of Rheumatology (ACR) guidelines does recommend combination DMARD treatment [69]. However, ACR also recommends biologic treatment to subgroups of patients with poor prognostic factors, who have either received single DMARD therapy or never received DMARDs.

A recent analysis concluded that the continued use of placebo arms instead of active arms in the controlled trials of new biologic agents exposed patients in the control arms to possible deterioration [2]. In an accompanying editorial [70], the previous use of placebo was in part defended, but it was also acknowledged that new designs were necessary to reduce the risk of patients in the control arms. In our opinion there is now evidence that combination treatment with at least two DMARDs, one of which could be LDGC, may prevent structural joint damage to the same degree as a biologic agent combined with methotrexate. Therefore future study designers should not seek superiority of the new drug compared with placebo, but should design studies with sufficient power to demonstrate equality with a combination of conventional DMARDs. Biologic agents should, as originally intended, be reserved for patients that are insufficiently treated with a combination of at least two conventional DMARDs.

Supporting Information

Checklist S1 PRISMA Checklist.

Author Contributions

Conceived and designed the experiments: NG. Performed the experiments: NG THG ST RC GJ. Analyzed the data: NG THG RC. Contributed reagents/materials/analysis tools: NG THG ST RC GJ. Wrote the paper: NG.

References

1. Graudal N, Jürgens G (2010) Similar effects of disease-modifying antirheumatic drugs, glucocorticoids and biologics on radiographic progression in rheumatoid arthritis: meta-analysis of 70 randomized placebo or drug controlled studies including 112 comparisons. Arthritis Rheum 62: 2852–2863.

2. Estellat C, Ravaud P (2012) Lack of head-to-head trials and fair control arms: randomized controlled trials of biologic treatment for rheumatoid arthritis. Arch Intern Med 172: 237–44.
3. Goekoop-Ruiterman YP, de Vries-Bouwstra JK, Allaart CF, van Zeben D, Kerstens PJ, et al. (2005) Clinical and radiographic outcomes of four different treatment strategies in patients with early rheumatoid arthritis (the BeSt study): a randomized, controlled trial. Arthritis Rheum 52: 3381–90.
4. Goekoop-Ruiterman YP, de Vries-Bouwstra JK, Allaart CF, van Zeben D, Kerstens PJ, et al. (2007) Comparison of treatment strategies in early rheumatoid arthritis: a randomized trial. Ann Intern Med 146: 406–15.
5. Van Vollenhoven RF, Geborek P, Forslind K, Albertsson K, Ernestam S, et al. (2012) Conventional combination treatment versus biological treatment in methotrexate-refractory early rheumatoid arthritis: 2 year follow-up of the randomised, non-blinded, parallel-group Swefot trial. Lancet 379: 1712–20.
6. Moreland LW, O'Dell JR, Paulus HE, Curtis JR, Bathon JM, et al. (2012) A randomized comparative effectiveness study of oral triple therapy versus etanercept plus methotrexate in early aggressive rheumatoid arthritis: the treatment of early aggressive rheumatoid arthritis trial. Arthritis Rheum 64: 2824–35.
7. O'Dell JR, Mikuls TR, Taylor TH, Ahluwalia V, Brophy M, et al. (2013) Therapies for active rheumatoid arthritis after methotrexate failure. N Engl J Med 369: 307–18.
8. Caldwell DM, Ades AE, Higgins JP (2005) Simultaneous comparison of multiple treatments: combining direct and indirect evidence. BMJ 331: 897–900.
9. Nixon RM, Bansback N, Brennan A (2007) Using mixed treatment comparisons and meta-regression to perform indirect comparisons to estimate the efficacy of biologic treatments in rheumatoid arthritis. Stat Med 26: 1237–54.
10. Singh JA, Christensen R, Wells GA, Suarez-Almazor ME, Buchbinder R, et al. (2009) A network meta-analysis of randomized controlled trials of biologics for rheumatoid arthritis: a Cochrane overview. CMAJ 181: 787–96.
11. Liberati A, Altman DG, Tetzlaff J, Mulrow C, Gøtzsche PC, et al. (2009) The PRISMA statement for reporting systematic reviews and meta-analyses of studies that evaluate healthcare interventions: explanation and elaboration. BMJ 339: b2700.
12. Song F, Loke YK, Walsh T, Glenny AM, Eastwood AJ, et al. (2009) Methodological problems in the use of indirect comparisons for evaluating healthcare interventions: survey of published systematic reviews. BMJ 338: b1147
13. The Nordic Cochrane Centre, Higgins JP, Green S, editors (2009) Cochrane handbook for systematic reviews of interventions version 5.0.1, section 7.7.3. The Cochrane Collaboration. Available: www.cochrane-handbook.org.
14. Walter SD, Yao X (2009) Effect sizes can be calculated for studies reporting ranges for outcome variables in systematic reviews. J Clin Epidemiol 60: 849–52.
15. Jansen JP, Fleurence R, Devine B, Itzler R, Barrett A, et al. (2011) Interpreting indirect treatment comparisons and network meta-analysis for health-care decision making: report of the ISPOR Task Force on Indirect Treatment Comparisons Good Research Practices: part 1. Value Health; 14: 417–28.
16. Bucher HC, Guyatt GH, Griffith LE, Walter SD (1997) The results of direct and indirect treatment comparisons in meta-analysis of randomized controlled trials. J Clin Epidemiol 50: 683–91.
17. Dougados M, Combe B, Cantagrel A, Goupille P, Olive P, et al. (1999) Combination therapy in early rheumatoid arthritis: a randomised, controlled, double blind 52 week clinical trial of sulphasalazine and methotrexate compared with the single components. Ann Rheum Dis 58: 220–225.
18. Marchesoni A, Battafarano N, Arreghini M, Panni B, Gallazzi M, et al. (2003) Radiographic progression in early rheumatoid arthritis: a 12-month randomized controlled study comparing the combination of cyclosporin and methotrexate with methotrexate alone. Rheumatology 42: 1545–49.
19. Sarzi-Puttini P, D'Ingianna E, Fumagalli M, Scarpellini M, Fiorini T, et al. (2005) An open, randomized comparison study of cyclosporine A, cyclosporine A + methotrexate and cyclosporine A + hydroxychloroquine in the treatment of early severe rheumatoid arthritis. Rheumatol Int 25: 15–22.
20. Scott DL, Dawes PT, Tunn E, Fowler PD, Shadforth MF, et al. (1989) Combination therapy with gold and hydroxychloroquine in rheumatoid arthritis: a prospective, randomized, placebo-controlled study. Br J Rheumatol 28: 128–33.
21. Capell HA, Madhok R, Hunter JA, Porter D, Morrison E, et al. (2004) Lack of radiological and clinical benefit over two years of low dose prednisolone for rheumatoid arthritis: results of a randomised controlled trial. Ann Rheum Dis 63: 797–803.
22. Choy EH, Kingsley GH, Khoshaba B, Pipitone N, Scott DL (2005) Intramuscular Methylprednisolone Study. A two year randomised controlled trial of intramuscular depot steroids in patients with established rheumatoid arthritis who have shown an incomplete response to disease modifying antirheumatic drugs. Ann Rheum Dis 64: 1288–93
23. Hansen M, Podenphant J, Florescu A, Stoltenberg M, Borch A, et al. (1999) A randomised trial of differentiated prednisolone treatment in active rheumatoid arthritis. Clinical benefits and skeletal side effects. Ann Rheum Dis 58: 713–18.
24. Kirwan JR, The Arthritis and Rheumatism Council Low-Dose Glucocorticoid Study (1995) The effect of glucocorticoids on joint destruction in rheumatoid arthritis. N Engl J Med 333: 142–46.
25. Svensson B, Boonen A, Albertsson K, van der Heijde D, Keller C, et al. (2005) Low-dose prednisolone in addition to the initial disease-modifying antirheumatic drug in patients with early active rheumatoid arthritis reduces joint destruction and increases the remission rate: a two-year randomized trial. Arthritis Rheum 52: 3360–3370.
26. Van Gestel AM, Laan RF, Haagsma CJ, Van de Putte LB, van Riel PL (1995) Oral steroids as bridge therapy in rheumatoid arthritis patients starting with parenteral gold. A randomized double-blind placebo-controlled trial. Br J Rheumatol 34: 347–51.
27. Wassenberg S, Rau R, Steinfeld P, Zeidler H (2005) Very low-dose prednisolone in early rheumatoid arthritis retards radiographic progression over two years: a multicenter, double-blind, placebo-controlled trial. Arthritis Rheum 52: 3371–80.
28. Choy EH, Smith CN, Farewell V, Walker D, Hassell A, et al. (2008) Factorial randomised controlled trial of glucocorticoids and combination disease modifying drugs in early rheumatoid arthritis. Ann Rheum Dis 67: 656–63.
29. Calgüneri M, Pay S, Caliskaner Z, Apras S, Kiraz S, et al. (1999) Combination therapy versus monotherapy for the treatment of patients with rheumatoid arthritis. Clin Exp Rheumatol 17: 699–704.
30. Grigor C, Capell H, Stirling A, McMahon AD, Lock P, et al. (2004) Effect of a treatment strategy of tight control for rheumatoid arthritis (the TICORA study): a single-blind randomised controlled trial. Lancet 364: 263–69.
31. Möttönen T, Hannonen P, Leirisalo-Repo M, Nissilä M, Kautiainen H, et al. (1999) Comparison of combination therapy with single-drug therapy in early rheumatoid arthritis: a randomised trial. FIN-RACo trial group. Lancet 353: 1568–73.
32. Boers M, Verhoeven AC, Markusse HM, van de Laar MA, Westhovens R, et al. (1997) Randomised comparison of combined step-down prednisolone, methotrexate and sulphasalazine with sulphasalazine alone in early rheumatoid arthritis. Lancet 350: 309–18.
33. Klareskog L, van der Heijde D, de Jager JP, Gough A, Kalden J, et al. (2004) Therapeutic effect of the combination of etanercept and methotrexate compared with each treatment alone in patients with rheumatoid arthritis: double-blind randomised controlled trial. Lancet. 363: 675–81.
34. Emery P, Breedveld FC, Hall S, Durez P, Chang DJ, et al. (2008) Comparison of methotrexate monotherapy with a combination of methotrexate and etanercept in active, early, moderate to severe rheumatoid arthritis (COMET): a randomised, double-blind, parallel treatment trial. Lancet 372: 375–82.
35. Lipsky PE, van der Heijde DM, St Clair EW, Furst DE, Breedveld FC, et al. (2000) Infliximab and methotrexate in the treatment of rheumatoid arthritis. Anti-Tumor Necrosis Factor Trial in Rheumatoid Arthritis with Concomitant Therapy Study Group. N Engl J Med 343: 1594–602.
36. St Clair EW, van der Heijde DM, Smolen JS, Maini RN, Bathon JM, et al. (2004) Combination of infliximab and methotrexate therapy for early rheumatoid arthritis: a randomized, controlled trial. Arthritis Rheum 50: 3432–43.
37. Breedveld FC, Weisman MH, Kavanaugh AF, Cohen SB, Pavelka K, et al. (2006) The PREMIER study: A multicenter, randomized, double-blind clinical trial of combination therapy with adalimumab plus methotrexate versus methotrexate alone or adalimumab alone in patients with early, aggressive rheumatoid arthritis who had not had previous methotrexate treatment. Arthritis Rheum 54: 26–37.
38. Keystone EC, Kavanaugh AF, Sharp JT, Tannenbaum H, Hua Y, et al. (2004) Radiographic, clinical, and functional outcomes of treatment with adalimumab (a human anti-tumor necrosis factor monoclonal antibody) in patients with active rheumatoid arthritis receiving concomitant methotrexate therapy: a randomized, placebo-controlled, 52-week trial. Arthritis Rheum 50: 1400–1411.
39. Keystone E, van der Heijde D, Mason D, Landewé R, Vollenhoven RV, et al. (2008) Certolizumab pegol plus methotrexate is significantly more effective than placebo plus methotrexate in active rheumatoid arthritis: findings of a fifty-two-week phase III, multicenter, randomized, double-blind, placebo-controlled, parallel-group study. Arthritis Rheum 58: 3319–29.
40. Smolen JS, Landewé RB, Mease PJ, Brzezicki J, Mason D, et al. (2009) Efficacy and Safety of Certolizumab Pegol plus Methotrexate in Active Rheumatoid Arthritis: The RAPID 2 Study. Ann Rheum Dis 68: 797–804.
41. Kremer JM, Genant HK, Moreland LW, Russell AS, Emery P, et al. (2006) Effects of abatacept in patients with methotrexate-resistant active rheumatoid arthritis: a randomized trial. Ann Intern Med 144: 865–76.
42. Westhovens R, Robles M, Ximenes AC, Nayiager S, Wollenhaupt J, et al. (2009) Clinical efficacy and safety of abatacept in methotrexate-naive patients with early rheumatoid arthritis and poor prognostic factors. Ann Rheum Dis 68: 1870–7.
43. Keystone EC, Emery P, Peterfy CG, Tak PP, Cohen S, et al. (2009) Rituximab inhibits structural joint damage in rheumatoid arthritis patients with an inadequate response to tumour necrosis factor inhibitor therapies. Ann Rheum Dis 68: 216–221.
44. Ichikawa Y, Saito T, Yamanaka H, Akizuki M, Kondo H, et al. (2005) Therapeutic effects of the combination of methotrexate and bucillamine in early rheumatoid arthritis: a multicenter, double-blind, randomized controlled study. Mod Rheumatol 15: 323–8.
45. Tak PP, Rigby WF, Rubbert-Roth A, Peterfy CG, van Vollenhoven RF, et al. (2011) Inhibition of joint damage and improved clinical outcomes with rituximab plus methotrexate in early active rheumatoid arthritis: the IMAGE trial. Ann Rheum Dis 70: 39–46.
46. Emery P, Fleischmann R, van der Heijde D, Keystone EC, Genovese MC, et al. (2011) The Effects of Golimumab on Radiographic Progression in Rheumatoid Arthritis: Results of randomized controlled studies on Golimimab before

methotrexate therapy and golimumab after methotrexate therapy. Arthritis Rheum 63: 1200–1210.

47. Kremer JM, Blanco R, Brzosko M, Burgos-Vargas R, Halland AM, et al. (2011) Tocilizumab Inhibits Structural Joint Damage in Rheumatoid Arthritis Patients with an Inadequate Response to Methotrexate: results from the double-blind treatment phase of a randomized placebo-controlled trial of tocilizumab safety and prevention of structural joint damage at one year. Arthritis Rheum 63: 609–621.
48. Bakker MF, Jacobs JW, Welsing PM, Verstappen SM, Tekstra J, et al. (2012) Low-dose prednisone inclusion in a methotrexate-based, tight control strategy for early rheumatoid arthritis: a randomized trial. Ann Intern Med 156: 329–39.
49. Tanaka Y, Harigai M, Takeuchi T, Yamanaka H, Ishiguro N, et al. (2012) Golimumab in combination with methotrexate in Japanese patients with active rheumatoid arthritis: results of the GO-FORTH study. Ann Rheum Dis 71: 817–24.
50. Rigby W, Tony HP, Oelke K, Combe B, Laster A, et al. (2012) Safety and efficacy of ocrelizumab in patients with rheumatoid arthritis and an inadequate response to methotrexate: results of a forty-eight-week randomized, double-blind, placebo-controlled, parallel-group phase III trial. Arthritis Rheum 64: 350–9.
51. Tak PP, Mease PJ, Genovese MC, Kremer J, Haraoui B, et al. (2012) Safety and efficacy of ocrelizumab in patients with rheumatoid arthritis and an inadequate response to at least one tumor necrosis factor inhibitor: results of a forty-eight-week randomized, double-blind, placebo-controlled, parallel-group phase III trial. Arthritis Rheum 64: 360–70.
52. Stohl W, Gomez-Reino J, Olech E, Dudler J, Fleischmann RM, et al. (2012) Safety and efficacy of ocrelizumab in combination with methotrexate in MTX-naive subjects with rheumatoid arthritis: the phase III FILM trial. Ann Rheum Dis 71: 1289–96.
53. Kavanaugh A, Fleischmann RM, Emery P, Kupper H, Redden L, et al. (2013) Clinical, functional and radiographic consequences of achieving stable low disease activity and remission with adalimumab plus methotrexate or methotrexate alone in early rheumatoid arthritis: 26-week results from the randomised, controlled OPTIMA study. Ann Rheum Dis 72: 64–71.
54. Bergman GJ, Hochberg MC, Boers M, Wintfeld N, Kielhorn A, et al. (2010) Indirect comparison of tocilizumab and other biologic agents in patients with rheumatoid arthritis and inadequate response to disease-modifying antirheumatic drugs. Semin Arthritis Rheum 39: 425–41.
55. Devine EB, Alfonso-Cristancho R, Sullivan SD (2011). Effectiveness of biologic therapies for rheumatoid arthritis: an indirect comparisons approach. Pharmacotherapy 31: 39–51.
56. Launois R, Avouac B, Berenbaum F, Blin O, Bru I, et al. (2011) Comparison of certolizumab pegol with other anticytokine agents for treatment of rheumatoid arthritis: a multiple-treatment Bayesian metaanalysis. J Rheumatol 38: 835–45.
57. Salliot C, Finckh A, Katchamart W, Lu Y, Sun Y, et al. (2011) Indirect comparisons of the efficacy of biological antirheumatic agents in rheumatoid arthritis in patients with an inadequate response to conventional diseasemodifying antirheumatic drugs or to an anti-tumour necrosis factor agent: a meta-analysis. Ann Rheum Dis 70: 266–71.
58. Schmitz S, Adams R, Walsh CD, Barry M, Fitzgerald O (2012) A mixed treatment comparison of the efficacy of anti-TNF agents in rheumatoid arthritis for methotrexate non-responders demonstrates differences between treatments: a Bayesian approach. Ann Rheum Dis 71: 225–30.
59. Turkstra E, Ng SK, Scuffham PA (2011) A mixed treatment comparison of the short term efficacy of biologic disease modifying anti-rheumatic drugs in established rheumatoid arthritis. Curr Med Res Opin 27: 1885–97.
60. Rahman MU, Buchanan J, Doyle MK, Hsia EC, Gathany T, et al. (2011) Changes in patient characteristics in anti-tumour necrosis factor clinical trials for rheumatoid arthritis: results of an analysis of the literature over the past 16 years. Ann Rheum Dis 70: 1631–40.
61. Brower AC (1990) Use of the radiograph to measure the course of rheumatoid arthritis. The gold standard versus fool's gold. Arthritis Rheum 33: 316–24.
62. Graudal NA, Jurik AG, de Carvalho A, Graudal HK (1998) Radiographic progression in rheumatoid arthritis: a long-term prospective study of 109 patients. Arthritis Rheum 41: 1470–80.
63. Graudal N, Tarp U, Jurik AG, Galloe AM, Garred P, et al. (2000) Inflammatory patterns in rheumatoid arthritis estimated by the number of swollen and tender joints, the erythrocyte sedimentationrate, and hemoglobin: long-term course and association to radiographic progression. J Rheumatol 27: 47–57.
64. Graudal N (2004) The natural history and prognosis of rheumatoid arthritis: association of radiographic outcome with process variables, joint motion and immune proteins. Scand J Rheumatol 33 (Suppl 118): 1–37.
65. Donahue KE, Jonas DE, Hansen RA, Roubey R, Jonas B, et al. (2012) Drug Therapy for Rheumatoid Arthritis in Adults: An Update [Internet]. Agency for Healthcare Research and Quality (US). Report No.: 12-EHC025-EF. AHRQ Comparative Effectiveness Reviews.
66. Ma MH, Kingsley GH, Scott DL (2010) A systematic comparison of combination DMARD therapy and tumour necrosis inhibitor therapy with methotrexate in patients with early rheumatoid arthritis. Rheumatology (Oxford). 49: 91–8.
67. Scott DL (2012) Biologic based therapy for the treatment of rheumatoid arthritis. CPT 91: 30–43.
68. Smolen JS, Landewé R, Breedveld FC, Dougados M, Emery P, et al. (2010) EULAR recommendations for the management of rheumatoid arthritis with synthetic and biological disease-modifying antirheumatic drugs. Ann Rheum Dis 69: 964–75.
69. Singh JA, Furst DE, Bharat A, Curtis JR, Kavanaugh AF, et al. (2012) 2012 Update of the 2008 American College of Rheumatology Recommendations for the Use of Disease-Modifying Antirheumatic Drugs and Biologic Agents in the Treatment of Rheumatoid Arthritis. Arthritis Care Res 64: 625–639.
70. Pearson SD (2012) Placebo-controlled trials, ethics, and the goals of comparative effectiveness research: comment on "lack of head-to-head trials and fair control arms". Arch Intern Med 172: 244–5.

Permissions

All chapters in this book were first published in PLOS ONE, by The Public Library of Science; hereby published with permission under the Creative Commons Attribution License or equivalent. Every chapter published in this book has been scrutinized by our experts. Their significance has been extensively debated. The topics covered herein carry significant findings which will fuel the growth of the discipline. They may even be implemented as practical applications or may be referred to as a beginning point for another development.

The contributors of this book come from diverse backgrounds, making this book a truly international effort. This book will bring forth new frontiers with its revolutionizing research information and detailed analysis of the nascent developments around the world.

We would like to thank all the contributing authors for lending their expertise to make the book truly unique. They have played a crucial role in the development of this book. Without their invaluable contributions this book wouldn't have been possible. They have made vital efforts to compile up to date information on the varied aspects of this subject to make this book a valuable addition to the collection of many professionals and students.

This book was conceptualized with the vision of imparting up-to-date information and advanced data in this field. To ensure the same, a matchless editorial board was set up. Every individual on the board went through rigorous rounds of assessment to prove their worth. After which they invested a large part of their time researching and compiling the most relevant data for our readers.

The editorial board has been involved in producing this book since its inception. They have spent rigorous hours researching and exploring the diverse topics which have resulted in the successful publishing of this book. They have passed on their knowledge of decades through this book. To expedite this challenging task, the publisher supported the team at every step. A small team of assistant editors was also appointed to further simplify the editing procedure and attain best results for the readers.

Apart from the editorial board, the designing team has also invested a significant amount of their time in understanding the subject and creating the most relevant covers. They scrutinized every image to scout for the most suitable representation of the subject and create an appropriate cover for the book.

The publishing team has been an ardent support to the editorial, designing and production team. Their endless efforts to recruit the best for this project, has resulted in the accomplishment of this book. They are a veteran in the field of academics and their pool of knowledge is as vast as their experience in printing. Their expertise and guidance has proved useful at every step. Their uncompromising quality standards have made this book an exceptional effort. Their encouragement from time to time has been an inspiration for everyone.

The publisher and the editorial board hope that this book will prove to be a valuable piece of knowledge for researchers, students, practitioners and scholars across the globe.

List of Contributors

Katsunori Ikari, Koichiro Yano, Eisuke Inoue, Atsuo Taniguchi, Hisashi Yamanaka and Shigeki Momohara
Institute of Rheumatology, Tokyo Women's Medical University, Shinjuku, Tokyo, Japan

Taku Suzuki
Institute of Rheumatology, Tokyo Women's Medical University, Shinjuku, Tokyo, Japan
Department of Orthopaedic Surgery, Keio University School of Medicine, Shinjuku, Tokyo, Japan

Yoshiaki Toyama
Department of Orthopaedic Surgery, Keio University School of Medicine, Shinjuku, Tokyo, Japan

Louise Berg
Rheumatology Unit, Department of Medicine, Karolinska Institutet, Stockholm, Sweden

Agneta J. Laurent
Rheumatology Unit, Department of Medicine, Karolinska Institutet, Stockholm, Sweden
Neurogenetics Unit, Department of Molecular Medicine and Surgery, Karolinska Institutet, Stockholm, Sweden

Niels Bindslev
Department of Biomedical Sciences, Faculty of Health and Medical Sciences, University of Copenhagen, Copenhagen, Denmark

Björn Johansson
Neurogenetics Unit, Department of Molecular Medicine and Surgery, Karolinska Institutet, Stockholm, Sweden

Shirley R. Utiyama, Renato M. Nisihara and Iara J. T. Messias-Reason
Department of Medical Pathology, Federal University of Paraná, Curitiba, Brazil

Isabela Goeldner
Department of Medical Pathology, Federal University of Paraná, Curitiba, Brazil
Institute of Tropical Medicine, University of Tübingen, Tübingen, Germany

Hoang van Tong
Institute of Tropical Medicine, University of Tübingen, Tübingen, Germany

Thirumalaisamy P. Velavan
Institute of Tropical Medicine, University of Tübingen, Tübingen, Germany
Fondation Congolaise pour la Recherche Medicale, Brazzaville, Republic of Congo

Thelma L. Skare
Rheumatology Unit, Evangelical Hospital, Curitiba, Brazil

Yanxia Fu, Hailing Zhou, Shuangyan Wang and Qun Wei
Department of Biochemistry and Molecular Biology, Beijing Normal University, Gene Engineering and Biotechnology Beijing Key Laboratory, Beijing, P. R. of China

Erich Dolejsi and Florian Frommlet
Center for Medical Statistics, Informatics, and Intelligent Systems/Section of Medical Statistics, Medical University Vienna, Vienna, Austria

Bernhard Bodenstorfer
cogiti e.U., Karlstift, Austria

Sreejoyee Ghosh, Lalit Kumar Singh, Ashish Sarkar, Yogendra Singh and Sagarika Biswas
Department of Genomics & Molecular Medicine, CSIR-Institute of Genomics and Integrative Biology, Delhi, India

Saurabh Sharma
Department of Genomics & Molecular Medicine, CSIR-Institute of Genomics and Integrative Biology, Delhi, India
Department of Environmental Studies, Delhi University, Delhi, India

Radhey Shyam Sharma
Department of Environmental Studies, Delhi University, Delhi, India

Darshan Singh Bhakuni and Onkar Prasad Garg
Department of Clinical Immunology and Rheumatology, Army Hospital (Research and Referral), New Delhi, India

Rajesh Malhotra
Department of Orthopaedic, All India Institute of Medical Sciences, New Delhi, India

Taposh Kumar Das
Department of Anatomy, All India Institute of Medical Sciences, New Delhi, India

Jana Burkhardt and Grit Wolfram
Translational Centre for Regenerative Medicine (TRM), Universität Leipzig, Leipzig, Germany

Frank Emmrich
Translational Centre for Regenerative Medicine (TRM), Universität Leipzig, Leipzig, Germany
University Leipzig, Institute for Clinical Immunology and Tranfusion Medicine (IKIT), Universität Leipzig, Leipzig, Germany
Fraunhofer Institute for Celltherapy and Immunology (IZI), Leipzig, Germany

Mechthild Blume and Anke Steiner
University Leipzig, Institute for Clinical Immunology and Tranfusion Medicine (IKIT), Universität Leipzig, Leipzig, Germany

Elisabeth Petit-Teixeira and Céline Pierlot
Genhotel-EA 3886, Université d'Evry-Val d'Essonne, Evry, France

Vitor Hugo Teixeira
Centre for Respiratory Research, University College London, London, United Kingdom

Elfi Quente
Fraunhofer Institute for Celltherapy and Immunology (IZI), Leipzig, Germany

Holger Kirsten
Fraunhofer Institute for Celltherapy and Immunology (IZI), Leipzig, Germany
LIFE – Leipzig Research Center for Civilization Diseases, Universität Leipzig, Leipzig, Germany
Institute for Medical Informatics, Statistics and Epidemiology (IMISE), Universität Leipzig, Leipzig, Germany

Markus Scholz
LIFE – Leipzig Research Center for Civilization Diseases, Universität Leipzig, Leipzig, Germany

Peter Ahnert
LIFE – Leipzig Research Center for Civilization Diseases, Universität Leipzig, Leipzig, Germany
Institute for Medical Informatics, Statistics and Epidemiology (IMISE), Universität Leipzig, Leipzig, Germany

Paola Migliorini and Stefano Bombardieri
Pisa University, Pisa, Italy

Alejandro Balsa
La Paz Hospital, Madrid, Spain

René Westhovens
Rheumatology KU Leuven, Leuven, Belgium

Pilar Barrera
Nijmegen University, Nijmegen, the Netherlands

Timothy R. D. J. Radstake
University Medical Center Utrecht, Utrecht, the Netherlands

Helena Alves
Porto San Joao Hospital, Porto, Portugal

Thomas Bardin
Fédération de Rhumatologie, Lariboisière Hospital, Paris, France

Bernard Prum
Laboratoire Statistique & Génome, Université d'Evry-Val d'Essonne, Evry, France

François Cornelis
GenHotel-Auvergne, Université d'Auvergne, Clermont-Ferrand, France
Institute for Medical Informatics, Statistics and Epidemiology (IMISE), Universität Leipzig, Leipzig, Germany

Taras Lyubchenko
Division of Rheumatology, University of Colorado School of Medicine, Aurora, Colorado, United States of America

Gary O. Zerbe
Department of Biostatistics and Informatics, University of Colorado School of Public Health, Aurora, Colorado, United States of America

Balázs Szalay
Department of Laboratory Medicine, Faculty of Medicine, Semmelweis University, Budapest, Hungary

Áron Cseh and Gergő Mészáros
First Department of Pediatrics, Faculty of Medicine, Semmelweis University, Budapest, Hungary

László Ková cs and Attila Balog
Department of Rheumatology, Faculty of Medicine, Albert Szent-Györgyi Health Center, University of Szeged, Szeged, Hungary

Barna Vásá rhelyi
Department of Laboratory Medicine, Faculty of Medicine, Semmelweis University, Budapest, Hungary
MTASE, Pediatrics and Nephrology Research Group, Budapest, Hungary

Burcu Ayoglu, Jochen M. Schwenk and Peter Nilsson
Affinity Proteomics, SciLifeLab, School of Biotechnology, KTH Royal Institute of Technology, Stockholm, Sweden

Eszter Szarka, Krisztina Huber, Anita Orosz and Gabriella Sármay
Department of Immunology, Eötvös Loránd University, Budapest, Hungary

Fruzsina Babos and Anna Magyar
3 MTA-ELTE Research Group of Peptide Chemistry, Budapest, Hungary

Ferenc Hudecz
MTA-ELTE Research Group of Peptide Chemistry, Budapest, Hungary
Department of Organic Chemistry, Eötvös Loránd University, Budapest, Hungary

Bernadette Rojkovich and Tamás Gáti
Department of Rheumatology, Polyclinic of the Hospitaller Brothers of St. John of God, Budapest, Hungary

György Nagy
Department of Rheumatology, Polyclinic of the Hospitaller Brothers of St. John of God, Budapest, Hungary
Department of Genetics, Cell and Immunobiology, Semmelweis University, Medical School, Budapest, Hungary

József Prechl
MTA-ELTE Immunology Research Group, Budapest, Hungary
Diagnosticum Ltd., Budapest, Hungary

Krisztián Papp
Affinity Proteomics, SciLifeLab, School of Biotechnology, KTH Royal Institute of Technology, Stockholm, Sweden
MTA-ELTE Immunology Research Group, Budapest, Hungary

Christie Fitch-Rogalsky, Whitney Steber, Terri Lupton, Liam Martin, Susan G. Barr, Dianne P. Mosher, James Wick and Marvin J. Fritzler
Faculty of Medicine, University of Calgary, Calgary, Alberta, Canada

Michael Mahler
INOVA Diagnostics Inc., San Diego, California, United States of America

Imad Abugessaisa, Giorgos Tsipras and Jesper Tegnér
Unit of Computational Medicine, Department of Medicine, Center for Molecular Medicine, Karolinska Institutet, Stockholm, Sweden

Saedis Saevarsdottir, Charlotta Sandin, Vivianne Malmström and Lars Klareskog
Rheumatology Unit, Department of Medicine, Center for Molecular Medicine, Karolinska Institutet, Stockholm, Sweden

Staffan Lindblad
Medical Management Center, Department of Learning, Informatics, Management and Ethics, Karolinska Institutet, Stockholm, Sweden

Pernilla Nikamo4, Mona Ståhle
Dermatology and Venereology Unit, Department of Medicine, Karolinska Institutet, Karolinska University Hospital, Stockholm, Sweden

Georges Haour and Sandy Lucier
URC Eco Île-de-France (AP-HP), Hôtel Dieu, Paris, France

Karine Chevreul
URC Eco Île-de-France (AP-HP), Hôtel Dieu, Paris, France
Inserm, ECEVE, U1123, Paris, France
Univ Paris Diderot, Sorbonne Paris Cité, ECEVE, UMRS 1123, Paris, France

Isabelle Durand-Zaleski
URC Eco Île-de-France (AP-HP), Hôtel Dieu, Paris, France
Inserm, ECEVE, U1123, Paris, France
Univ Paris Diderot, Sorbonne Paris Cité, ECEVE, UMRS 1123, Paris, France
Department of Public Health, Henri Mondor-Albert Chenevilier Hospitals (AP-HP), Créteil, France

Stephanie Harvard
URC Eco Île-de-France (AP-HP), Hôtel Dieu, Paris, France
Pierre and Marie Curie University (UPMC) - Paris 6, UPMC GRC 08, Institut Pierre Louis d'Epidémiologie et Santé Publique, Paris, France

Marie-Laure Laroche
Pharmacology and Toxicology Unit, Centre of Pharmacovigilance-Pharmacoepidemiology CHU, Limoges, France
Limoges University, EA 6310 HAVAE, Faculty of Medicine, Limoges, France

Xavier Mariette
Paris XI University, Department of Rheumatology, Bicêtre University Hospital (AP-HP), Le Kremlin Bicêtre, France

Alain Saraux
Brest University, Department of Rheumatology, La Cavale Blanche Hospital, Brest, France

Francis Guillemin
Lorraine University, EA 4360 APEMAC; INSERM CIC-EC CIE6, Nancy, France

Bruno Fautrel
Pierre and Marie Curie University (UPMC) - Paris 6, UPMC GRC 08, Institut Pierre Louis d'Epidémiologie et Santé Publique, Paris, France
AP-HP, Department of Rheumatology, La Pitié Salpêtrière University Hospital, Paris, France

Yutaro Nakamura, Noriyuki Enomoto, Dai Hashimoto, Tomoyuki Fujisawa, Naoki Inui, Takafumi Suda and Kingo Chida
Second Division, Department of Internal Medicine, Hamamatsu University School of Medicine, Hamamatsu, Japan

Masato Kono
Second Division, Department of Internal Medicine, Hamamatsu University School of Medicine, Hamamatsu, Japan
Department of Laboratory Medicine, Hamamatsu University School of Medicine, Hamamatsu, Japan

Masato Maekawa
Department of Laboratory Medicine, Hamamatsu University School of Medicine, Hamamatsu, Japan

Thomas V. Colby
Department of Laboratory Medicine and Pathology, Mayo Clinic, Scottsdale, Arizona, United Sates of America

Ondřej Sglunda, Hana Hulejová, Marké ta Kuklová, Lenka Pleštilová and Mária Filková
Institute of Rheumatology, Prague, Czech Republic

Heřman Mann, Karel Pavelka, Jiří Vencovský and Ladislav Šenolt
Institute of Rheumatology, Prague, Czech Republic
Department of Rheumatology, First Faculty of Medicine, Charles University in Prague, Prague, Czech Republic

Ondřej Pecha
Technology Centre ASCR, Prague, Czech Republic

Ping-Wei Zhao, Wei-Guang Jiang, Li Wang, Yu-Xing Shan and Yan-Fang Jiang
Key Laboratory of Zoonosis Research, Ministry of Education, The First Hospital, Jilin University, Changchun, China

Zhen-Yu Jiang
Department of Rheumatism, The First Hospital, Jilin University, Changchun, China

Katsunori Ikari, Takefumi Furuya, Atsuo Taniguchi, Hisashi Yamanaka and Shigeki Momohara
Institute of Rheumatology, Tokyo Women's Medical University, Tokyo, Japan

Shinji Yoshida
Institute of Rheumatology, Tokyo Women's Medical University, Tokyo, Japan
Department of Orthopaedic Surgery, Keio University School of Medicine, Tokyo, Japan

Yoshiaki Toyama
Department of Orthopaedic Surgery, Keio University School of Medicine, Tokyo, Japan

Ivy Y. Choi
Division of Clinical Immunology and Rheumatology, Academic Medical Center/University of Amsterdam, Amsterdam, the Netherlands

Danielle M. Gerlag
Division of Clinical Immunology and Rheumatology, Academic Medical Center/University of Amsterdam, Amsterdam, the Netherlands
GlaxoSmithKline Research & Development, Cambridge, United Kingdom

Paul P. Tak
Division of Clinical Immunology and Rheumatology, Academic Medical Center/University of Amsterdam, Amsterdam, the Netherlands
University of Cambridge, Cambridge, United Kingdom
GlaxoSmithKline Research & Development, Stevenage, United Kingdom

Dirk Holzinger
Department of Paediatric Rheumatology and Immunology, University Children's Hospital Muenster, Muenster, Germany
Institute of Immunology, University Hospital Muenster, Muenster, Germany

Johannes Roth
Institute of Immunology, University Hospital Muenster, Muenster, Germany

Hye Young Kim, So Youn Park, Hye Rin Lee and Ki Whan Hong
Medical Research Center for Ischemic Tissue Regeneration, Pusan National University, Yangsan, Gyeongnam, Republic of Korea

Chi Dae Kim and Won Suk Lee
Medical Research Center for Ischemic Tissue Regeneration, Pusan National University, Yangsan, Gyeongnam, Republic of Korea
Department of Pharmacology, School of Medicine, Pusan National University, Yangsan, Gyeongnam, Republic of Korea

Byung Yong Rhim
Department of Pharmacology, School of Medicine, Pusan National University, Yangsan, Gyeongnam, Republic of Korea

Sung Won Lee
Department of Internal Medicine, College of Medicine, Dong-A University, Busan, Republic of Korea

Yan Xu and Xin Wen
Department of Information and Computer Science, University of Science and Technology Beijing, Beijing, China

Li-Shu Wen
College of Sciences, Liaoning Shiyou University, FuShun, China

Ling-Yun Wu
Institute of Applied Mathematics, Academy of Mathematics and Systems Science, Chinese Academy of Sciences, Beijing, China

Nai-Yang Deng
College of Science, China Agricultural University, Beijing, China

Kuo-Chen Chou
Center of Excellence in Genomic Medicine Research (CEGMR), King Abdulaziz University, Jeddah, Saudi Arabia
Gordon Life Science Institute, Boston, Massachusetts, United States of America

Anat Fisher and Colin R. Dormuth
Therapeutics Initiative, University of British Columbia, Vancouver, Canada
Department of Anesthesiology, Pharmacology & Therapeutics, University of British Columbia, Vancouver, Canada

Ken Bassett
Therapeutics Initiative, University of British Columbia, Vancouver, Canada
Department of Anesthesiology, Pharmacology & Therapeutics, University of British Columbia, Vancouver, Canada
Department of Family Practice, University of British Columbia, Vancouver, Canada

James M. Wright
Therapeutics Initiative, University of British Columbia, Vancouver, Canada
Department of Anesthesiology, Pharmacology & Therapeutics, University of British Columbia, Vancouver, Canada
Department of Medicine, University of British Columbia, Vancouver, Canada

Hugh Freeman
Department of Medicine, University of British Columbia, Vancouver, Canada

M. Alan Brookhart
Department of Epidemiology, Gillings School of Global Public Health, University of North Carolina, Chapel Hill, North Carolina, United States of America

Angelique Stalmach, Holger Husi and William Mullen
University of Glasgow, Institute of Cardiovascular and Medical Sciences, Glasgow, United Kingdom

Hanna Johnsson
Western General Infirmary, Edinburgh, United Kingdom

Duncan Porter and Iain B. McInnes
University of Glasgow, Institute of Infection, Immunity and Inflammation, Glasgow, United Kingdom

Julie Klein and Mohammed Dakna
Mosaiques-Diagnostics GmbH, Hannover, Germany

Harald Mischak
University of Glasgow, Institute of Cardiovascular and Medical Sciences, Glasgow, United Kingdom
Mosaiques-Diagnostics GmbH, Hannover, Germany

Niels Graudal
Department of Rheumatology IR4242, Copenhagen University Hospital, Rigshospitalet, Denmark

Thorbjørn Hubeck-Graudal
Department of Radiology, Copenhagen University Hospital, Gentofte, Denmark

Simon Tarp
Musculoskeletal Statistics Unit, the Parker Institute, Department of Rheumatology, Copenhagen University Hospital, Frederiksberg, Denmark

Robin Christensen
Musculoskeletal Statistics Unit, the Parker Institute, Department of Rheumatology, Copenhagen University Hospital, Frederiksberg, Denmark
Institute of Sports Science and Clinical Biomechanics, University of Southern Denmark, Odense, Denmark

Gesche Jürgens
Department of Clinical Pharmacology, Copenhagen University Hospital, Bispebjerg, Denmark

Index

A

Allelic Expression, 68-69, 71, 73-74

Anti-nuclear Antibody, 105, 143-144

Anti-rheumatic Drugs, 2-3, 57, 131, 155, 210, 226

Anti-tnf Therapy, 85, 90

Antibody Isotypes, 92-93, 95, 97

Articular Cartilage, 36, 155

Autoantibody, 1, 8, 56, 67, 96, 99, 102-103, 105-106, 108-112, 117, 123

Autoimmune Disease, 2, 29, 32, 34, 41-42, 56, 62, 65, 68, 76, 85, 101, 107-108, 112, 131, 144

Autoreactive B Cell, 78, 83

B

B Cell Immune, 78, 82

Bcr Signaling, 78-83

Bcr Signaling Proteins, 78-79, 81-82

Bone Erosion, 34, 41-42, 180

C

C3 Deposition, 92-93, 95-97, 101-102

Capillary Electrophoresis, 201-203, 209

Cardiovascular Diseases, 9, 75, 154, 201

Cartilage Destruction, 9, 56, 67

Cellular Adhesion, 68-69, 74

Cellular Adhesion Processes, 68-69, 74

Central Triage, 105-107, 109

Chronic Synovitis, 2, 5

Cilostazol, 172-181

Citrullinated Fibrinogen, 92, 102, 209

Collagen Vascular Disease, 140, 142, 144-146, 148-149

Collagen-induced Arthritis, 34, 36, 38, 42, 161, 172, 179, 182

D

Deacetylase Activity, 172-173, 175, 177-178, 180

Disease Activity, 2, 5, 7, 23, 57, 69, 75, 79, 84, 86-87, 94, 115, 120-122, 125, 132-134, 137-139, 150-156, 159-161, 163, 167-171, 193, 200, 202, 209, 217, 219, 224, 226

Dmard Treatment, 134, 155, 157-158, 160-161, 215, 217, 224

E

Endothelial Cells, 68-69, 75, 172-173, 179-181

Erythrocyte, 57, 67, 87, 132, 156, 168-169, 226

Ethanol, 9-20, 202

Extractable Nuclear Antigen, 105

F

Fetal Bovine Serum, 60, 179

Fibromyalgia, 106-109

G

Gene Expression, 69, 71-72, 75, 77, 155

Glucocorticsteroid, 85

Glycyrol Attenuates, 36, 38, 41

H

High-resolution Computed Tomography, 141-142, 145, 148

Hip Fracture, 162-163, 165-166

Hmvecs, 172-174, 176, 180-181

I

Idiopathic Pulmonary Fibrosis, 140, 142, 144-148

Immune Cells, 41, 56, 68, 150-152

Immune Reactions, 22

Immunoelectron Microscopy, 64

Infectious Diseases, 22, 29, 93, 104

Interstitial Pneumonia, 140, 142-149

Isopentenyl, 9

Isopentenyl Pyrophosphate, 9

J

Joint Deformation, 56

Joint Destruction, 1-2, 4-7, 32, 34, 66, 70, 93, 155, 161-162, 208-211, 223-225

Joint Inflammation, 41, 155

M

Mannose-biding Lectin, 22, 29

Methothrexate, 85

Microscopic Polyangiitis, 140-141, 143

Mixed Connective Tissue Disease, 105, 107

Molecular Masses, 58

N
Nitric Oxide, 85-86, 88-91

Non-dmard, 131, 133-135

Non-genetic Factors, 1-3, 7, 163

O
Osteoarthritis, 33, 56-57, 62, 67, 106-109, 209

P
Peripheral Blood, 9-10, 23, 71, 78, 83, 85-86, 90, 120-121, 159, 167-168, 170, 201

Peripheral Immune Tolerance, 78-79, 81, 83

Phosphorylation Levels, 78-81

Plasma Proteins, 56, 58-61

R
Reactive Oxygen Species, 85, 89, 91

S
Serum Dilution, 94-97, 101, 109

Serum Lipids, 150-151

Serum Visfatin, 150-152, 154

Single Nucleotide Polymorphisms, 2, 23, 68-69, 162-163

Surgical Lung Biopsy, 141-143

Synovial Fibroblast, 76, 150, 180

Synovial Fluid, 9-10, 15, 17, 20, 33, 57-58, 61, 64-68, 117, 119-120, 161, 172, 177, 179, 182, 201, 208-209

Synovial Hyperplasia, 34, 36-37, 155

Systemic Lupus Erythematosus, 7, 29, 33, 56-57, 62, 83, 91, 105, 107, 111-112, 141, 149, 159, 161

T
Therapeutic Intervention, 2, 42, 91

Thyroid Hormone, 57, 66

Transcription Factor, 40-41, 68, 72, 74-76, 177, 181

Transthyretin, 56, 60, 66-67

Tumour Necrosis Factor, 29, 154, 161, 170, 199, 225-226